Realities of
Canadian Nursing
Professional, Practice, and Power Issues

EDITION 2

Realities of Canadian Nursing

Professional, Practice, and Power Issues

Marjorie McIntyre, RN, PhD
Associate Professor
University of Victoria
Victoria, BC

Elizabeth Thomlinson, RN, PhD

Carol McDonald, RN, PhD
Assistant Professor
University of Victoria
Victoria, BC

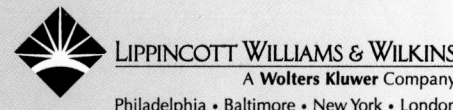
LIPPINCOTT WILLIAMS & WILKINS
A **Wolters Kluwer** Company
Philadelphia • Baltimore • New York • London
Buenos Aires • Hong Kong • Sydney • Tokyo

Acquisitions Editor: Quincy McDonald
Managing Editor: Dana Irwin
Editorial Assistant: Marivette Torres
Production Editor: Audrey Lickwar
Senior Production Manager: Helen Ewan
Senior Managing Editor/Production: Erika Kors
Creative Director: Doug Smock
Design Coordinator: Brett MacNaughton
Cover Designer: Melissa Walter
Interior Designer: B. J. Crim
Manufacturing Coordinator: Karin Duffield
Indexer: Angie Wiley
Compositor: TechBooks
Printer: RR Donnelley/Crawfordsville

2nd Edition

9 8 7 6 5 4 3

Library of Congress Cataloging-in-Publication Data

Realities of Canadian nursing : professional, practice, and power issues / [edited by] Marjorie McIntyre, Elizabeth (Betty) Thomlinson, Carol McDonald.—2nd ed.
     p. ; cm.
  ISBN 13: 978-0-7817-6132-1
  ISBN 10: 0-7817-6132-8
  1. Nursing—Canada. 2. Nurses—Canada. I. McIntyre, Marjorie, RN, PhD. II. Thomlinson, Elizabeth. III. McDonald, Carol. [DNLM: 1. Nursing—Canada. 2. Nurses—Canada. WY 16
R288 2006]
RT6.A1R435 2006
610.73'0971—dc22

                                                                    2005008134

Care has been taken to confirm the accuracy of the information presented and to describe generally accepted practices. However, the authors, editors, and publisher are not responsible for errors or omissions or for any consequences from application of the information in this book and make no warranty, express or implied, with respect to the content of the publication.

The authors, editors, and publisher have exerted every effort to ensure that drug selection and dosage set forth in this text are in accordance with the current recommendations and practice at the time of publication. However, in view of ongoing research, changes in government regulations, and the constant flow of information relating to drug therapy and drug reactions, the reader is urged to check the package insert for each drug for any change in indications and dosage and for added warnings and precautions. This is particularly important when the recommended agent is a new or infrequently employed drug.

Some drugs and medical devices presented in this publication have Food and Drug Administration (FDA) clearance for limited use in restricted research settings. It is the responsibility of the health care provider to ascertain the FDA status of each drug or device planned for use in his or her clinical practice.

LWW.com

Elizabeth (Betty) Thomlinson, RN, PhD
(1942–2004)

Remembering Betty . . . our friend, colleague, and coauthor

For making a difference in nursing education, in practice, in research,

and in the world

Acknowledging her gift for championing nursing issues, for honoring diversity,

and for mentoring students and colleagues

We miss you, Betty . . . never more than as we revisited and revised

this new edition.

Authors Carol McDonald (left) and Marjorie McIntyre (right)

Marjorie McIntyre, RN, PhD, attended the Royal Alexander School of Nursing in Edmonton and practised in both acute care and community settings. She earned a BN at the University of Victoria, an MN at the University of British Columbia, and a PhD at the University of Colorado in Denver. As an associate professor, she currently teaches at the University of Victoria, where her interests include critical feminist philosophy, hermeneutics, and issues in nursing and health care.

Carol McDonald, RN, PhD, is currently an assistant professor at the University of Victoria School of Nursing. Following a 20-year practice career in the areas of mental health and group psychotherapy, Carol earned a PhD in nursing from the University of Calgary. Among her passions are women's health issues, including lesbian health, and feminist hermeneutics.

Geertje Boschma, RN, PhD
Assistant Professor
School of Nursing
University of British Columbia
Vancouver, BC
■ Chapter 7

Isobel Boyle, RN, MN
Clinical Director
Children's Program
Grand River Hospital
Kitchner, ON
■ Chapter 20

Anne Bruce, RN, PhD
Assistant Professor
School of Nursing
University of Victoria
Victoria, BC
■ Chapter 25

Laurel Brunke, RN, MSN
Executive Director
Registered Nurses Association of
   British Columbia
Vancouver, BC
■ Chapter 9

Barbara Brush, RNC, PhD, FAAN
Associate Professor
School of Nursing
University of Michigan
Ann Arbor, MI
■ Chapter 7

W. Dean Care, BN, MEd, EdD
Associate Professor
Faculty of Nursing
University of Manitoba
Winnipeg, MB
■ Chapter 14

Christine Ceci, PhD
Postdoctoral Fellow
University of Victoria
Victoria, BC
■ Chapter 23

Wanda Chernomas, RN, PhD
Associate Professor and Associate Dean
Undergraduate Programs, Academic Affairs
Faculty of Nursing
University of Manitoba
Winnipeg, MB
■ Chapter 14

Heather Clark, RN, PhD
Principal
Health and Nursing Policy
Research and Evaluation Consulting
Vancouver, BC
■ Chapter 5

Elizabeth Cragg, RN, EdD
Professor
School of Nursing
University of Ottawa
Ottawa, ON
■ Chapter 11

Diana Davidson Dick, RN, MEd
Dean, Nursing Division
Saskatchewan Institute of Applied
   Science and Technology
Saskatoon, SK
■ Chapter 11

David Gregory, RN, PhD
Professor
Faculty of Nursing
University of Manitoba
Winnipeg, MB
■ Chapter 14

Laurie Hardingham, RN, MA
Clinical Ethicist
St. Joseph's Health Care London
London, ON
■ Chapter 18

Fjola Hart-Wasekeesikaw, RN, MN
Doctoral Student
Faculty of Nursing
University of Calgary
Calgary, AB
■ Chapter 24

Sioban Nelson, RN, PhD
Professor and Head of School
School of Nursing
University of Melbourne
Melbourne, Australia
■ Chapter 13

Dorothy Pringle, RN, PhD
Professor
Faculty of Nursing
University of Toronto
Toronto, ON
■ Chapter 15

Mary Ellen Purkis, RN, PhD
Dean, Faculty of Human and Social
   Development
University of Victoria
Victoria, BC
■ Chapter 13

Sandra Reilly, RN, EdD
Associate Professor
Faculty of Nursing
University of Calgary
Calgary, AB
■ Chapter 4

Ginette Lemire Rodger, RN, PhD
Vice President, Professional Practice
   and Chief Nursing Executive
The Ottawa Hospital
Ottawa, ON
■ Chapter 8

Judith Shamian, RN, PhD
President and Chief Executive Officer
Victorian Order of Nurses Canada
Ottawa, ON
■ Chapter 6

Judith Skelton-Green, RN, PhD
President
TRANSITIONS: HOD Consultants, Inc.
Penetanguishene, ON
■ Chapter 6

Janet Storch, RN, PhD
Professor
School of Nursing
University of Victoria
Victoria, BC
■ Chapter 3

Meryn Stuart, PhD, RN
Associate Professor
School of Nursing
University of Ottawa
Ottawa, Ontario
■ Chapter 7

Deborah Tamlyn, RN, PhD
President, Canadian Nurses Association
■ Chapter 4

Sally Thorne, RN, PhD
Professor and Director
School of Nursing
University of British Columbia
Vancouver, BC
■ Chapter 12

Hanneke van Maanen, DrNSc
Professor
Faculty of Health and Human Services
Department of Nursing Science
University of Breman
Breman, Germany
■ Chapter 10

Michael Villeneuve, RN, MSc
Senior Nurse Consultant
Canadian Nurses Association
Ottawa, ON
■ *Chapter 6*

Christina Whittaker, RN, MN
Nurse Educator
Child Health Program
Winnipeg Regional Health Authority
Winnipeg, MB
■ *Chapter 14*

Sandra Bassendowski, EdD, RN
Assistant Professor
University of Saskatchewan
Saskatoon, SK

Dana S. Edge, RN, BSN, MSN, PhD
Associate Professor
University of Calgary
Calgary, AB

Sonya Grypma, BN, MN, PhD(c)
Doctoral Candidate
University of Alberta
Edmonton, AB

Pauline O'Reilly, MSN
Program Head
Specialty Nursing Degree
British Columbia Institute of Technology
Burnaby, BC

n 2000, when we were first approached by Margaret Zuccarini, who, at the time, was a senior acquisitions editor for Lippincott Williams & Wilkins, we could never have imagined the enthusiastic response that the text would receive from students, teaching faculty, and practicing nurses. Nor could we have foreseen that in 2005 we would be preparing to release the second edition of the text. Needless to say, we are thrilled at the success of the first edition and in particular at its apparent resonance with nurses across the country. As we put the final touches on the second edition, complete with both new and revised chapters, we find ourselves curious about how our latest creative endeavor will be received in the nursing community.

But first, we must thank those of you who embraced the ideas in the first edition with such generosity. Next, and perhaps even more importantly, we want to express our gratitude to those of you who forwarded your critiques and suggestions, which have assisted us in producing this new edition. As in the first edition, we wish to acknowledge the amazing support and technical expertise of the Lippincott Williams & Wilkins team, and in particular the work of Dana Irwin and Audrey Lickwar. In addition to the team in Philadelphia, we want to give recognition to the dedicated work of the Canadian book representatives, with special thanks to Corey Wolfe.

One of the biggest challenges in writing an issues textbook is the nature of issues as emerging and evolving. While many of the issues that we address in health care have been with us over time, others can be seen as uniquely located in the realities of our current situation. At the outset of this second edition, we approached the contributors of previous chapters with an invitation to revise or update their work. In addition, we had imagined some revisions to the text arising from changes in political and practice realities as well as from feedback received from reviewers. Specifically, in Chapter 2 of the second edition, we plunge ourselves and our readers into one of today's—and perhaps one of Canadian nursing history's—most controversial and politically laden issues: the nurse practitioner movement. This chapter brings into question the realities that infiltrate every nursing issue—power, professionalization, regulation, and education. While we have made every effort to provide a comprehensive and current presentation of this issue—with the assistance of some excellent, in-depth reviews and critiques—we are acutely aware of its emergent nature. As such, we look forward to continuing this conversation and to providing new iterations of the topic in future editions!

Equally controversial but in a different realm is another new chapter, Chapter 25, "Opening the Conversation: Dilemmas and Possibilities of Spirituality and Spiritual Care." In this contribution, Anne Bruce leads us into a reflection that opens spaces for understanding the many possibilities of spiritual practices. Anne deliberately pulls away from the tendency to define spirituality and spiritual care once and for all and instead takes us on a journey where we encounter human suffering, philosophical assumptions, faith traditions, and, perhaps most importantly, ourselves. The opportunity to write this chapter with Anne expanded our thinking about spirituality, and, again, we anticipate continued discussions on this topic with students, with reviewers, and in future writing.

Other changes that are evident in this edition include the repositioning of Deborah Tamlyn and Sandra Reilly's leadership chapter into the first part of the textbook, and Chapters 15 and 16 were recast as a single chapter to reflect the inseparability of the nature of nurses' work from the settings in which this work takes place. Also in this edition, rather than a chapter focusing on the topic of the nursing shortage, this important content has been integrated in various chapters throughout the book. Finally, we have revisited Chapter 1, "Nursing Issues: A Call to Political Action," and included a new chapter, Chapter 26, "Professional, Practice, and Power Issues: Thinking Back, Looking Ahead," with a renewed vision for political action, social justice, and historical understandings.

Books are written for many reasons, and the first edition of *Realities of Canadian Nursing: Professional, Practice, and Power Issues* was no exception. At first glance, it might seem that the decision to edit a book on nursing issues was simple. On one level, we convinced ourselves that a new and different book for teaching nursing issues was needed. On another level, we were looking for a book that would do more than provide the material needed to understand issues; we wanted to prepare and inspire students to participate in political action alongside the generations of nurses who have already taken the lead. We imagined a book that would engage readers in such a way that they would be prepared to work with others in addressing the long-standing barriers to many of the issues that confront nurses and the people who seek nurses' services. We further speculated that, in addressing these issues, nurses who understood the barriers to resolving these issues were in the best position to make significant contributions to their resolutions. We wanted to dispel the many myths that question the need for nurses to be political and the notion that others will act on our behalf. This book is unapologetically feminist, shows respect for our history, and is deeply invested in our future.

We hope that the second edition of *Realities of Canadian Nursing: Professional, Practice, and Power Issues* will not only influence students to engage with nursing issues in new ways but that its chapters will stimulate new writing among Canadian scholars on nursing issues. An additional goal of this book is to disrupt the notion that changes to nursing and health care will happen without informed political action on the part of nurses: We hope to instill in more nurses the obligation to use their regulatory power, collectively and individually, to influence decision making in professional associations, collective bargaining units, government, and workplaces.

The intention of *Realities of Canadian Nursing: Professional, Practice, and Power Issues* has been, from its inception, to provide readers with a critical analysis of the tensions and contradictions that exist between nurses' legislated authority to self-regulate and the changing nature and realities of nurses' work. The changing conditions of nurses' workplaces, the changing settings and contexts of nurses' work, and the realities of contemporary society that challenge, on a daily basis, nurses' practice are all covered, as is the centrality of nurses' work and its contribution to the health of Canadians. Additionally, reference to earlier publications on professional regulation, health care systems, leadership, education, research, ethics, and legal issues is also included. Drawing on feminist and other forms of critical analysis, our contributors offer strategic points of resistance to dominant discourses by attributing significance to that too often considered insignificant—the underlying experiences and unheard concerns of nurses. Thoughtful exploration of these issues calls us all, nurses and non-nurses, to reflect on the ways in which we disrupt and maintain complicity in dominant discourses and on how we can deliberately use our knowledge to break through barriers and act strategically to resolve issues.

The audience for this second edition is nursing students taking issues courses offered at the third and fourth years of undergraduate programs. The text is meant to serve as a resource for related courses and as a reference text for practicing nurses and graduate students. Our ambition is to engage students in relevant issues in health, health care, and the nursing profession and to prepare students to identify, articulate, critically analyze, and generate possible solutions to relevant issues for nursing. *Realities of Canadian Nursing: Professional, Practice, and Power Issues* presents a comprehensive exploration of nursing issues with subtopics related to the Canadian health care system, professional associations, nursing ethics, and societal issues on current practice. Our approach to this material is intended to both restate what is already known in the field of nursing issues and to expand on this knowledge through the reconceptualization of issues for the purpose of generating new understandings for resolution, for which we also employed a pragmatic approach to developing and evaluating strategies.

A few additional comments about this edition. We have endeavored to provide consistent use of Canadian English throughout the text and have drawn on the *Gage Canadian Dictionary* as the authority in spelling. Also, since the first edition of this text, the Canadian Association of University Schools of Nursing (CAUSN) has become the Canadian Association of Schools of Nursing (CASN). Our intention is to have the writings in this edition reflect this June 2002 change to CASN.

On a closing note, we would like to acknowledge the change in authorship for the second edition. When conversations first began about this new edition, Betty was already aware of her failing health. Marjorie and Betty invited Carol McDonald, contributor coordinator for the first edition, to join them as third author. While we lost Betty a short time later, her contributions remain very present, both in the works that she has authored and through the continued influence of her ideas in our writings.

Contents

PART 2 Regulatory Power 115

PART 3   **Nursing Knowledge: How We Come to Know What We Know**   **187**

PART 4 Workplace Realities 283

PART 5   **Societal Issues: Challenges for Nursing Practice   349**

NURSES, NURSING, and the HEALTH CARE SYSTEM

Critical Questions

As a way of engaging with the ideas in this chapter, consider the following:

1. What comes to mind when you think of political action?
2. Do you think of yourself as a social activist?
3. Would you consider nursing practice a political act?

CHAPTER

1

Marjorie McIntyre
Elizabeth Thomlinson
Carol McDonald

Nursing Issues: A Call to Political Action

Nurses in Saskatchewan took very public steps to communicate their response to nursing cutbacks and other work environment issues that "invalidate their concerns, their practices, and disallow their understandings." They marched and left their shoes as a calling card, inviting officials and others to "run a mile in [a nurse's] shoes." (Photography by Larry Lemoal, Saskatchewan Union of Nurses. Used with permission from *Canadian Nurse*.)

After completing this chapter, you will be able to:

1. Understand the importance of political action for nurses.
2. Distinguish between problem solving and a process of issue articulation and resolution.
3. Use a framework for the articulation and analysis of an issue.
4. Begin to understand the complexity of issues arising in health care and nursing practice.
5. Describe strategies for addressing barriers and moving issues toward resolution.

Nurses across Canada are grappling with what seems at times to be irresolvable issues embedded in health care delivery, nursing practice, and education. Nurses struggle to solve recurring problems within a context of inadequate resources and insufficient support. In this text, we raise the questions of how we might understand these problems differently. How might we move beyond a short-term problem-solving approach, where problems are viewed in isolation, to facilitate an understanding of issues as complex and interrelated, with a breadth and scope not accounted for in a problem-solving approach? How might we benefit from a new approach to issue articulation and issue resolution? The premise of this chapter and, in fact, of this entire book is that reconceptualizing short-term, seemingly unresolvable problems as issues situated in political, material, and social contexts opens us to the realities and possibilities previously obscured. It is important for nurses to question the ways in which issues are conceptualized because how a nursing situation is understood by nurses and other decision makers will have implications for how it is likely to be addressed. The many issues affecting nurses, the profession, and the health care system can be understood and articulated as political issues in that they ultimately involve influencing others for the purpose of quality patient care.

Thoughtful exploration of these political questions calls us all, nurses and non-nurses, to reflect on that which constrains—and enables—the ways we can communicate and think about nursing. When nurses find themselves unable to nurse as they had envisioned, as they believe they can or should, or when their interpretations of what is occurring in health care are excluded from policy discussions, a sense of being incorrect, in some essential sense, in their understanding of themselves and their work, comes into play. A profound dissonance emerges between what one believes one is called on to be and do and what the world, and one's relationship to it, allows. This distress deepens when it remains unheard, when what is of concern to nurses remains stubbornly invisible to others (Ceci & McIntyre, 2001). The ability to articulate and act on issues is one of the means of preparing nurses for political action. Box 1.1 presents a health care issue identified by nurses.

This chapter introduces nursing issues and provides an overview of issue articulation and its significance to nursing. Specifically, it provides a framework to explore, articulate, analyze, and generate possibilities for increased understanding and, when feasible, for resolution of nursing issues. Examples of barriers to issue resolution and specific strategies to generate possibilities for resolution are also discussed.

■ SIGNIFICANCE FOR NURSES

What is the significance of understanding problems in health care as complex and multilayered issues? Issues are best served by an approach that questions and interrogates the taken-for-granted view of the particular subject. Rather than a move to solve problems, an in-depth analysis of issues includes an exploration of barriers that makes visible the complexity of the issue. This moves us past the notion that any one strategy could move an issue to resolution. To articulate an issue fully means to consider the political, historical, social, and economic realities on and through which issues are constructed.

The nursing shortage is an excellent example of how we might distinguish between issue analysis/resolution and problem solving. If we think of the shortage as a problem of not enough nurses—a problem of numbers—the shortage could be solved by producing more nurses. If we think of the shortage as reflecting

Health Care Issue: Political Action Results in Screening Program

Four community nurses working with homeless people suspected there was an increase in tuberculosis (TB) based on several cases of active TB and an increase in positive skin tests among their patients. However, when they approached the public health department, they were informed that the statistics did not indicate an increase. Although the nurses asked that TB screening be conducted in homeless shelters and drop-in centers, the health department refused.

The nurses believed that TB was increasing and, therefore, decided to press the health department to initiate a screening program. They proceeded with the following steps:

■ Calling a meeting with other health care workers, shelter and drop-in staff, and homeless people
■ Forming an action group
■ Educating group members about TB
■ Researching the experiences of other cities
■ Making representations to health departments
■ Offering to assist with screenings

These efforts resulted in a major screening program that demonstrated the increased numbers of people with TB. The group then expanded its focus to include other issues.

From Canadian Nurses Association. (2000) *CNA Today, 10*(2), 11. Used with permission.

nurses' dissatisfaction with their work, we might move to improve nurses' salaries and other contractual issues. However, regardless of what might be accomplished by addressing these individual problems in the short term, studies have shown that it is not one but many problems, and the interrelationship between them, that contribute to the shortage (Baumann et al., 2001). The recurrence of the nursing shortage over time suggests that it would be more beneficially analyzed and addressed as a complex issue including many overlapping and interconnected problems.

Analyzing the nursing shortage as an issue raises many questions. How might we account for the cycle of surplus and shortages historically? What constitutes a shortage of nurses? Who is the authority on what counts as a shortage? How do the prevailing attitudes in society about what it means to be a nurse contribute to the shortage? What of the status of nurses' work and nursing knowledge in the recruitment and retention of nurses? Is it possible that nursing shortages are created? Who might benefit from such a shortage? Who suffers? What are the economic implications of a shortage for nurses for the health care system and for the health of Canadians? Moving the shortage past the idea of individual problems to be solved to the depth and scope of an issue illuminates the potential barriers for resolution. Barriers to resolving the nursing shortage include the incongruity between the complex nature of nursing practice and the lesser status attributed to nurses' work and nursing knowledge, the reality that many decisions made about nurses' work are not made by nurses, and the use of nurses as temporary workers prepared to fill a gap in services. Strategies that emerge from such an analysis would necessarily include the multiple stakeholders involved and consideration of these barriers so that solutions are long-term.

■ SIGNIFICANCE FOR THE PROFESSION

The significance of clear articulation of issues for the profession goes beyond the individual nurse to include the organization of nurses and their ideas into a larger collective. To be effective in supporting political action within the profession, nurses need to speak in unison on issues and organize themselves to act provincially/territorially, nationally, and internationally. In 1977, Mussallem (1977, p. 156) claimed what is still true today: In the context of state-provided health care, the link between health care and political action is inseparable. The *raison d'etre* of nursing is health care. The quality of health care depends to a large extent on the nature of the nursing component determined by four elements:

- Standards of education and preparation for those entering the profession
- Quality of care provided by the practitioner—a quality closely associated with education and preparation
- Number of nurses available—a determination considered in modern times largely by the social and economic status the profession offers its members
- Milieu in which care is offered

If nurses are concerned about health care, they must accept responsibility for safeguarding these four dynamic elements of nursing practice. This can be achieved only by the participation of nurses in political action.

In addition, the Canadian Nurses Association (CNA) *Code of Ethics* mandates that nurses represent nursing interests and perspectives before legislature, employers, other disciplines, and the media (Banks, 1988, p. 31; CNA, 1997). Particular issues around which professional organizations have pledged their support include the following:

- Acting as advocates for patients
- Speaking out on issues that directly affect the health status of Canadians
- Lobbying for positive changes in health policy
- Improving the image of nursing

■ UNDERSTANDING ISSUES HISTORICALLY

An in-depth analysis of issues brings us the opportunity to reopen our nursing and health care history. This reopening is more than a return to the history that has been dominantly recorded; rather, it can be seen as an occasion to excavate the historical understandings that have been silenced, diminished, or erased. This approach to history reminds us that each telling of history is necessarily situated in the standpoint or the assumptions of the one who recounts the story. Each telling of our past is, in some sense, a partial and incomplete interpretation. In this way, history is understood as multiple histories; each account presents a reality, although only a limited depiction of our recorded past. McPherson (1996), a nurse historian, points out that events from nursing history are understood quite differently depending on who has been responsible for the documentation or analysis of the event. For example, in her discussion of the subordination of nurses, McPherson highlights the difference in viewing historical events through a lens of class analysis, gender analysis, or academic/professional analysis. The view of a particular history through these multiple lenses for analysis yields different historical realities, each of which contributes to a full understanding of the issue.

■ NURSING PRACTICE AS POLITICAL ACTION

The need for problem-solving and decision-making abilities has been ingrained in the discipline of nursing since its inception. Although one cannot argue that many problems are amenable to deductive thinking/ problem solving, it is also apparent that nurses face increasingly complex issues in a continually expanding array of practice settings. And so, although nursing practice and education have historically privileged a deductive approach to decision making, the changing world in which practice occurs and the advancing education level of nurses underscore the need for more inductive, interpretive approaches. In recent years, there has been an increased focus on nurses' advocacy. Legislative changes in the scope of practice and in the code of ethics have contributed to the politicization of nursing practice. Where once many nurses were identified as nonpolitical, today, political awareness, political action, and social justice are increasingly—and necessarily—embedded in nursing education and nursing practice. The advancement of nursing education underpins the movement of nurses into leadership positions in the health care system and in education. Concurrent with their increasing social consciousness, nurse leaders experience an awareness of the limitations of approaching complex social-political issues with short-term approaches to change.

In the face of a health care system in which there are seemingly continual therapeutic and technological advances, it is easy to think of health care and indeed of nursing practice as progressively advancing. However, the reality for many Canadians is diminished access to nursing and health care services. Perhaps more than ever before, nurses are in a position to bring attention to the health care needs of underserved populations. Increasing numbers of nurses are employed in the community, in home care work, and in agencies and institutions providing care to elderly individuals (CNA, 2004). In these work environments, nurses face issues of health and health care that are mediated by the social and material realities of the lives of the people to whom they provide care. Community and home care nursing magnifies our awareness of the realities of poverty, lack of education, inadequate housing, and isolation, and the influence of these on the health of Canadians. Although we can expect that many people would have intellectual awareness of these impoverished circumstances within our society, nurses, through their privileged access to underserved populations in the provision of care, live alongside this knowledge in practice. Nurses are then caught in the tension of knowing what is needed and knowing that these resources are not forthcoming. This disparity is what incites the political will to challenge existing structures and processes that limit access to health and health care for underserved Canadians.

■ FRAMING AND ANALYZING AN ISSUE

To begin examining and acting on an issue, one identifies the topic of interest and from this selects a particular issue and articulates, or expresses, it clearly. An issue can be expressed as a dilemma, conundrum, question or series of questions, or simple statement. Once the issue is articulated clearly, the analysis may proceed as outlined in the following section. Some issues call for a particular framework or approach to analysis, but most issues benefit from more than one approach. However, it is unlikely that all approaches to analysis would be undertaken with every issue. Some categories of analysis or frameworks, discussed later and constructed as guidelines, are intended to generate rather than limit possibilities for discussion, and you may generate other questions as you work. The purpose of asking these questions is to increase understanding of all aspects of the issue and to move the discussion toward resolution. In Chapter 2, the framework for analysis presented here is explicitly used to articulate and analyze the issues arising from the nurse practitioner movement. Box 1.2 summarizes the steps used in articulating and analyzing an issue.

BOX 1.2	Articulation and Analysis of an Issue

1. Identify the topic of interest.
2. Select a particular issue and articulate it clearly. Define your own beliefs and assumptions about the issue.
3. Proceed with the analysis by addressing appropriate frameworks.
4. Identify barriers to resolution.
5. Explore strategies for resolution.

Before beginning an analysis, you need to make explicit your own beliefs and assumptions about the issue. An assumption is an idea that is held to be true without any support or substantiation, and all of us operate from day to day under assumptions.

Nature of the Issue

The following are some questions to ask when analyzing what you assume to be a nursing issue:

- What makes this issue a nursing issue?
- In what ways are nurses involved in the issue?
- Who are the other participants and what is their involvement in the issue?
- Who first became concerned with the subject?
- Who began to raise the subject as an issue and why?

Historical Analysis of the Issue

- When did the issue originate?
- What are the conditions that led to the development of the issue?
- How have these conditions changed over time?
- What has contributed to the stance taken by participants in the issue?
- What have been the barriers to resolution?
- What strategies for resolution have already been tried?

Ethical and Legal Analysis of the Issue

- What are the laws that influence this issue?
- What professional codes or legislative acts mandate participants' responses to this issue?
- What professional, organizational, and governmental (municipal, provincial/territorial, and national) documents inform, constrain, or influence the issue? Possibilities include the CNA *Code of Ethics* (1997), provincial/territorial standards of practice, the British North America Act, the Health Professions Act, and the Canada Health Act.

Social and Cultural Analysis of the Issue

Every issue develops in a societal context that shapes the issue and influences the possibilities for resolution.

- What contexts shape this particular issue?
- What are the prevailing attitudes in society about this issue?
- What values and priorities of the dominant culture influence this issue? In what ways, if any, do these values and priorities privilege the dominant culture over other members of society?

Political Analysis of the Issue

- Who benefits from the issue staying the same?
- Who benefits from the issue being resolved?
- What is the relationship between knowledge and power in this situation?
- How do ageist, sexist, racist, and ablest ideologies influence our understanding of this issue?

Critical Feminist Analysis of the Issue

■ Are there errors or myths about women's abilities or realities contained in this issue?
■ Is this issue influenced by the power inequities or the hierarchical or patriarchal structures of institutions over nurses or patients?
■ In this situation, is expert power given authority over personal power and the right to be the subject of one's own life?

Economic Analysis of the Issue

■ In what ways are the forces of supply and demand at work in this issue?

■ BARRIERS TO RESOLUTION

One of the most important strategies for moving an issue toward resolution is identifying barriers that may impede the resolution process. Once the barriers are identified, there may be an increased opportunity for resolution through mediation, collaboration, or negotiation. The following are some potential barriers to resolution of nursing issues:

■ Limited accessibility to resources, such as human and financial resources, knowledge, or expertise, may obstruct resolution.
■ Issues are not clearly understood or are understood in a limited way. For example, a barrier to resolving the nursing shortage is conceptualizing the issue as only a problem of numbers of nurses entering the profession.
■ Irresolvable differences or competing interests between participants may block the resolution of issues.
■ Circumstances in which some participants benefit from the issue remaining unresolved limit the opportunity for resolution.
■ Power inequities between parties invested in the issue can contribute to resistance to resolution.
■ Participants in the issue may experience unconscious resistance to change.
■ Key stakeholders in the issue may lack tolerance for multiple viewpoints.
■ Stakeholders may ascribe to differing underlying assumptions or beliefs that influence the way the issue is understood and the way resolution is undertaken.
■ Alienation from coworkers, hostility from bureaucratic and administrative officials, and fear of job loss may isolate nurses from the supports needed for resolution.
■ Lack of time, energy, role models, and mentors seriously undermines possibilities for effective resolution.

■ DEVISING STRATEGIES FOR RESOLUTION

After an issue relevant to the profession of nursing or health care is articulated and analyzed, multiple strategies can be implemented to address and resolve the issue. Essential to the success of any effort is the communication of a well-developed plan of action. Strategies for resolution include, but are not limited to, the following:

■ Formation of lobby groups
■ Preparation of resolutions for presentation to agencies, associations, and organizations
■ Establishment of a letter-writing campaign
■ Involvement of the news media through letters to the editor and articles that solicit public support

The use of any of these strategies depends on the following:

- People affected by the issue
- Interest that is generated
- Time available
- Human and financial resources available

To generate the maximum amount of support, it is important to enlist the assistance of as many people as possible who are affected by the issue. A greater response and resolution can be anticipated if the affected parties are unified in their efforts to address the specific issue. The following sections include specific, detailed examples of strategies that have been employed by individuals from multiple segments of the population in their efforts to create change and to address issues of relevance to them.

Lobbying Strategies

Although lobby groups are usually associated with persuading elected officials to vote a certain way on an issue or to carry an issue forward for debate, change within an organization can be promoted by lobbying key individuals. Regardless of whether the issue is of national or international importance, or whether the issue affects nurses and health care on a particular unit or agency, the same techniques are available and applicable.

Lobbying may occur through direct contact with people who are in positions to address the issue and through indirect methods by which others influence the officials (Hood, 1998). Table 1.1 provides a comparison of direct and indirect strategies.

Nurses must keep several key points in mind when initiating a lobby and planning meetings with key officials, including the following:

- Become informed about the issue by reading newspapers, documents, and reports; watching television and listening to the radio; and knowing the professional associations' positions.
- Use simple statistics and avoid percentages. The clearer the statistics, the more attention they will generate. Then apply the numbers in human terms, and illustrate the statistics with personal stories.
- Be sure to articulate clearly why the issue is an issue and identify its importance.
- Know what other people are saying about the issue.
- Keep in mind that the more people supporting the issue, the more effective the lobby.
- If you are lobbying government officials or bodies, remember to include members of the opposition parties.
- Follow meetings with written submissions that are accurate and succinct.

TABLE 1.1   Comparing Direct and Indirect Lobbying Strategies

Direct Strategies	Indirect Strategies
Engaging in letter, phone call, and e-mail campaigns to elected officials or others in power	Writing reports, articles, and books
Meeting with key people professionally	Enlisting the support of key people
Taking opportunities to meet key people socially	Using the media through news announcements on the radio and on television, in newspaper and magazine columns, and in advertisements
Submitting resolutions to professional organizations and unions	

Letters to Officials

One popular and well-used lobbying strategy is writing letters. Prepare the letter so it outlines a selected issue and the possibilities for resolution. Send the letter to a public official such as the dean of your school or faculty, the unit manager in your facility or organization, a city councilor, members of the legislative assembly (MLA) of your provincial government, or members of parliament (MP) of the government of Canada. Consider sending a copy of the letter to other stakeholders and interested parties, and keep a copy of letters for your own files. See Box 1.3 for an example of a lobbying letter, and see the Appendix for additional samples of written documents.

BOX 1.3   **Lobbying and Letter Writing: An Example**

Whether you are writing to your MP or to the minister of health or finance, adapt these letters to fit your own situation. Personalized letters have more impact. The sample letter presented here is to the minister of health.

The Honorable _____, P.C., M.P. Minister of Health

House of Commons Ottawa, Ontario K1A OA6

Dear Minister,

At the CNA Biennial Convention in Ottawa in June, you noted that "since Jeanne Mance set foot in this land, nurses have been caring for this country, and now, more than ever, it is time for Canada to show how much it cares for nurses." I thank you for these words and am writing you today to encourage you to demonstrate your willingness to invest in the nursing profession.

    Canadians are worried about the state of the health care system and associate the declining quality of care with the decreasing availability of nurses. (*Note: Add a personal example from your own area as appropriate.*) As you are aware, Canada faces a severe shortage of nurses with the knowledge and skills to meet the future health needs of Canadians. Care is becoming increasingly complex and technologically advanced. As you work to create an integrated continuum of care, Canadians will require highly qualified nurses to plan and deliver that care.

    As the federal government examines its fiscal priorities and resources for the coming year, the nurses of Canada urge you to take a leadership role in making sustainable investments in the health care system, including:

- Increasing federal transfer payments
- Expanding the continuum of care to include accessible home and community care
- Making a modest investment of $200 million over 5 years to support nursing recruitment, retention, research, and the dissemination and uptake of evidence to provide the best patient care

The nurses of Canada are looking to the federal government to demonstrate the strength of your commitment to ensure that all Canadians continue to enjoy ready access to the best health care system in the world.

Sincerely,

[Your name & address]

From Canadian Nurses Association. (1998). *The quiet crisis in health care*. Lobby Kit. Ottawa: Author. Used with permission.

Letters to the Editor

To be published, letters to the editor should comment on a public issue, and they usually are a response to a particular article or editorial published in the newspapers. An example may be a letter that responds to an editorial discussing the next federal budget, which is expected to be a "health budget." Keeping the letter short and punchy will enhance its chances of being published. Remember to sign the letter and add a daytime telephone number in case the editor wants verification or more information from you. Information on where to send letters is usually found in the letters section of the newspaper.

News Releases

A news release is much like a letter but does not have a salutation. Information should include relevant facts—the who, what, when, where, why, and how of the issue that you want to highlight. The release should also include the name and telephone number of a person whom the media can contact for further comments or to arrange for an interview. The following example of a news release may be adapted to fit various needs:

In (name of region), *registered nurses will be meeting with politicians and holding events, such as news conferences, to build support for the nursing investment. A meeting with* (name of politician) *will be held* (insert date) *at* (insert place). *A photo opportunity and brief statement by the nursing group will follow at* (time and place). *The event is scheduled in response to a public meeting held* (insert when and where), *when nurses joined their voices with the growing number of Canadian nurses calling for a federal investment in health care. Canadian nurses are warning the government that Canadians will soon be deprived of care if action is not taken to avert a massive nursing shortage.*

"Nurses make up 75% of health professionals. Without registered nurses at the bedside, who will care for Canadians?" asked (insert name). *"You can't open beds in hospitals or deliver quality home care if there are no nurses."*

Earlier, in Ottawa, in meetings with members of parliament and government officials, the Canadian Nurses Association (CNA) called on the federal government to support recruitment and retention of registered nurses, nursing research, and the dissemination and uptake of evidence. The CNA estimates the federal government investment should be $40 million a year over the next 5 years. "Our support of this is essential. We know firsthand the impact of the nursing shortage on patient care," said (insert name).

Resolutions

Prepare a written resolution for presentation at a professional organization's annual general meeting, such as one for a provincial association, a college of nursing, or the CNA. To be most effective, resolutions should be submitted in writing before the meeting date, so be sure to check deadlines, as resolutions received after the deadline may not be able to be considered by the resolutions committee. Although resolutions can usually be presented from the floor of the meeting, this means that time for consideration and discussion may be limited. You will be most effective if you allow participants time to formulate their own responses and opinions on the topic.

A resolution is an original main motion written with great formality. A resolution generally has two parts: a preamble (optional) and the resolution.

The preamble states the reasons for making the resolution and is the equivalent to debating the question before it is on the floor. Each paragraph begins with the word *whereas*—underscored or in italics and followed by a comma—and each paragraph closes with a semicolon. Additionally, the word after *whereas* begins with a capital letter (e.g., *Whereas,* The). There is no limit to the number of times you use *whereas*.

A resolution is introduced with the word *resolved*, and, as with *whereas*, the word is underscored or put in italics and followed by a comma. Additionally, the word after *resolved* begins with a capital letter (e.g., *Resolved,* That). You may have more than one "resolved" sentence.

All proposed resolutions must include supporting documentation, including the financial implications relevant to the proposal. Also, it is helpful if the proposed resolution includes an implementation date.

BOX 1.4   What to Ask About Resolutions

1. Does each *Whereas* support the resolution?
2. Does the resolution conflict with the act under which the association is legislated?
3. Have you indicated who will carry out the action (e.g., a taskforce of members, a staff person)?
4. Have you projected the cost of the resolution (e.g., will the resolution for a lobby be limited to one letter from the association to a minister, or will the campaign be expanded to a major letter-writing campaign involving all members [10,000 × 0.48 = 4,800], for mail plus paper, envelopes, staff time, and phone for a total of 6,000)?
5. Have you included supporting documentation for the resolution, if appropriate?
6. Have you indicated a deadline for completion?
7. If the action requires reporting back, have you identified to whom and when?
8. Have you considered the intended effect of your resolution, political implications, and so forth?

An example follows:

Whereas, *The biennial meeting will be held in Vancouver; and*
Whereas, *There will be business, education sessions, and special awards; therefore*
Resolved, *That all the members of the Canadian Nurses Association be encouraged to attend the 2000 Biennial Meeting from June 19 to 23, 2000.*

Each resolution must be moved and seconded.

Questions regarding the preparation of a resolution can usually be answered by contacting the association office to which you will be submitting the resolution. Box 1.4 summarizes the resolution process. See the Appendix for an example of a complete resolution.

Additional Resources and Political Action

Nurses can obtain information to assist with political action from their national and provincial nursing associations. The use of electronic media has made resources available to nurses across the country; most associations can be accessed through the Internet.

Other sources of information include nursing unions. The Web sites and e-mail addresses for several nursing unions can be found in Chapter 17.

■ SUMMARY

This chapter addresses the significance of nurses understanding the inherently political nature of nursing and being able to articulate clearly the relevant issues in nursing, in health care, and in advocating for the health of Canadians. Articulation of an issue involves selecting the particular issue from a topic of interest. The nature of the issue is articulated by asking questions, such as Who are the participants in the issue? What makes this a nursing issue? and Who first raised this as an issue and why?

Beliefs and assumptions inform an understanding of the issue, and the importance of articulating these assumptions is the first step of issue analysis. A framework for the analysis of issues includes raising questions of historical, ethical-legal, social-cultural, political, critical feminist, and economic natures. The purpose of asking these questions is to increase understanding of all aspects of the issue and to move the discussion toward resolution. The categories of analysis are, however, not intended to be exclusive; pertinent questions may arise during the analysis process.

Identifying barriers to the resolution of an issue is an important step in moving the issue toward resolution. Potential barriers to resolution include inaccessibility of resources, irresolvable differences or competing interests between participants, and differing underlying assumptions on the part of key stakeholders.

Essential to the success of any effort in issue resolution is the communication of a well-developed plan of action. Strategies for resolution include, but are not limited to, formation of lobby groups; establishment of letter-writing campaigns; submission of letters to the editor; distribution of news releases to print, radio, and television; and preparation of resolutions for presentation to agencies, associations, and organizations.

Online Resources

Add to your knowledge of this issue:

Canadian Journal of Nursing Research   www.cjnr.nursing.mcgill.ca/archive/30/
30_4_Baumgart.html

Canadian Nursing Association   can-aiic.ca/cna/documents/pdf/publications/
Nursing_Political_Act_May_2000_e.pdf

Canadian Student Nurses' Association   www.cnsa.ca

REFLECTIONS on the Chapter . . .

1. From your practice experience, identify examples of nursing as political action.

2. There is evidence to suggest that nurses take a variety of stances in relation to using their knowledge and influence to address relevant issues in their practice. How might you account for these differences?

3. Identify at least one issue in your practice experience. Using the questions highlighted in the chapter, begin to explore the nature of this issue and possibilities for why it has remained an issue. Identify your own assumptions and beliefs that influence your interpretation of this issue.

4. What are the barriers to this issue being resolved?

5. Review the strategies for issue resolution offered at the end of the chapter, and discuss the advantages and limitations of each for the issue you have selected.

References

Banks, P. (1988). Lobbying: A legitimate, critical nursing intervention. *RNABC News, 12*(5), 31–32.

Baumann, A., O'Brien-Pallas, L., Armstrong-Strassen, B., et al. (2001). *Commitment and care: The benefit of healthy work places for nurses, their patients and the system. A policy synthesis. Canadian Health Research Foundation.* Ottawa: Government of Canada.

Canadian Nurses Association. (1997). *Code of ethics.* Ottawa: Author.

_____. (1998). *The quiet crisis in health care. Lobby kit.* Ottawa: Author.

_____. (2000). CNA Today. *Canadian Nurse, 10*(2), 11.

_____. (2004). Highlights of the 2003 nursing statistics. Ottawa: Author.

Ceci, C., & McIntyre, M. (2001). A "quiet" crisis in health care: Developing our capacity to hear. *Nursing Philosophy, 2*(2), 122–130.

Hood, L. (1998). The professional nurse's role in public policy. In S. Leddy (Ed.), *Conceptual bases of professional nursing* (4th ed., pp. 275–298). Philadelphia: Lippincott Williams & Wilkins.

Manitoba Association of Registered Nurses. (1997). *Directions for a pharmaceutical policy in Canada.* Report prepared for the National Forum on Health. Winnipeg: Author.

McPherson, K. (1996). *Bedside matters: The transformation of Canadian nursing 1900–1990.* Oxford University Press: Don Mills.

Mussallem, H. (1977). Nurses and political action. In B. LaSor & R. Elliott (Eds.), *Issues in Canadian nursing.* Ontario: Prentice Hall.

Critical Questions

As a way of engaging with the ideas in this chapter, consider the following:

1. What do you already know about nurse practitioner practice and education in Canada?

2. On the surface, what appeals to you about pursuing a career as a nurse practitioner?

3. What do you imagine would be the benefits of graduate education for nurse practitioners?

CHAPTER

2

Marjorie McIntyre
Carol McDonald

The Nurse Practitioner Movement: Recurring Issues

The outgoing president ▶
of the Canadian Nurses
Association talks with
nurse practitioner
students attending the
Summer Institute at the
University of Victoria
School of Nursing.

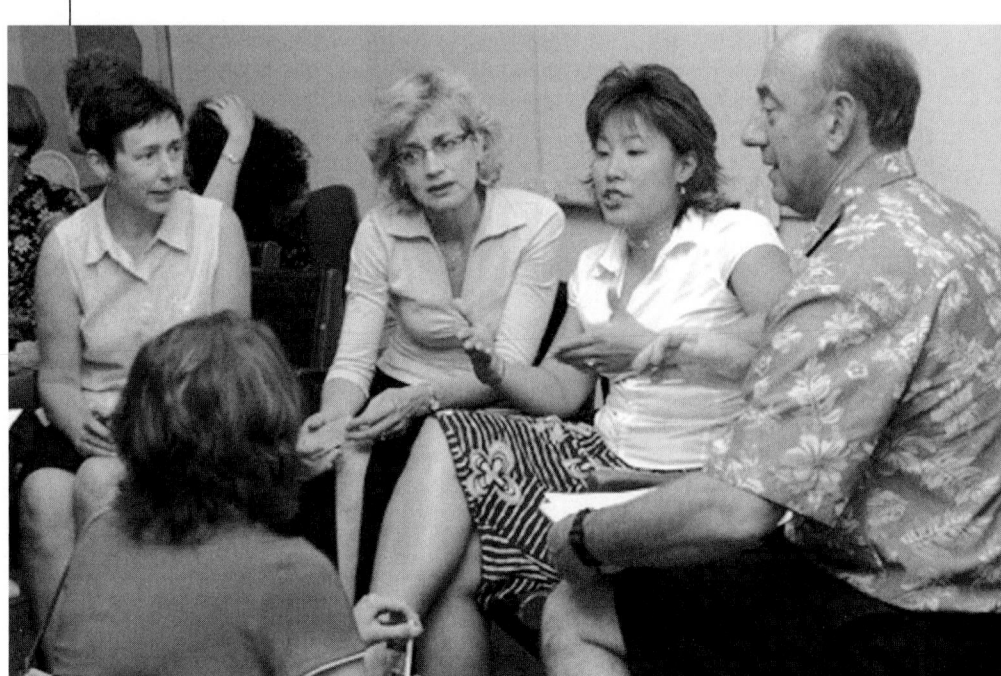

After completing this chapter, you will be able to:

1. Identify relevant issues in relation to the nurse practitioner movement.
2. Articulate selected ways of understanding the issue.
3. Understand different interpretations of the recurring issues in the nurse practitioner movement.
4. Identify past and current barriers to the resolution of issues affecting the movement.
5. Identify strategies that might facilitate resolution of issues surrounding the nurse practitioner movement.

All across Canada in the offices of ministries of education and health, at curriculum meetings in schools/faculties of nursing, on boards of national and provincial professional nursing associations/colleges, plans are under way to implement educational programs and to standardize and regulate the work of nurse practitioners. Although it is not entirely clear what or who initiated this movement or what directs and sustains it, what is clear is that plans, big plans, are under way. One could speculate that a movement of such a grand scale would have only been undertaken after careful consideration of the current strengths, limitations, and resources of our current health care system. A closer look, however, suggests that no such consideration has occurred and that the current situation is based on the belief that nurse practitioners variously conceptualized can do many things—not the least of which is to address Canada's current shortage of primary care physicians.

SITUATING THE TOPIC: THE NATURE OF THE ISSUE

This chapter opens by making explicit those assumptions that for us, as authors and professional nurses, make this a topic worthy of study. Our first assumption is that the current interest in nurse practitioners is a response primarily to a political rather than a health agenda. Historically, the evolution of nurse practitioner practice in Canada has been sporadic and inconsistent—often created to address short-term problems. Second, despite the numerous studies exploring the benefits of nurse practitioners in primary or acute care settings in Canada, the United States, and the United Kingdom over the past several decades, the evidence supporting these benefits is inconclusive (Horrocks et al., 2002; Martin-Misener et al., 2004; Sidani et al., 2000; Spitzer et al., 1974; Spitzer, 1984). Third, there is wide variability in the requirements to practice as a nurse practitioner across provinces/territories and practice settings. Educational programs preparing nurse practitioners often reflect institutional (university/college) rather than health care priorities. Fourth, the history of nurse practitioner practice and employment in Canada has been irregular and uncertain (Chambers & West, 1978; LeFort & Kergin, 1978; Spitzer, 1984). The lack of definitive information about nurse practitioner employment (where they will work) and scope of practice (activities nurses are educated and authorized to perform) is the major concern for employers and practitioners alike. Last, we assume that the conceptualization of nurse practitioner practice as roles and competencies rather than as nursing knowledge developed within the discipline for professional nursing practice will make their integration into that practice problematic (Baer, 2003; Fagin, 2003).

ARTICULATING THE TOPIC AS AN ISSUE

The conundrum for nurses—educators, regulators, and potential employers of nurse practitioners—is that our complicity in this movement communicates to Canadians that the nurse practitioner is worthy of their support and communicates to potential students that it is worthy of their considerable investment—with little evidence that the issues that have surrounded nurse practitioners for decades have been or will be solved.

■ ANALYZING THE ISSUE: WAYS OF UNDERSTANDING

An analysis of the nurse practitioner movement opens us to understandings of what makes this a significant issue for nurses, for nursing, and for Canadians seeking health care. In part, the complexity of the issue lies with the discordance between the imagined benefits from the installation of nurse practitioners in Canada's health care system and the realities of what is really possible or probable within the context of our current political, educational, and regulatory worlds. On the surface, we have the impression that the realization of the nurse practitioner movement could address significant gaps in the system of health care delivery, bene-fiting the health care of Canadians; facilitate the autonomous functioning of nurses in practice, expanding the professional practice of individual nurse practitioners; and provide an opportunity for the discipline of nursing to support and enact the Canada Health Act by improving access to the provision of primary health care. The intention of the analysis, and, we would suggest, the reason behind the urgency of such an analy-sis, is to move below the surface impressions of the nurse practitioner movement and to open to question-ing and understanding the conditions and realities that will shape the future of nurse practitioner practice in Canada.

Understanding the Issue Historically

The point is to write about and to render historical what has hitherto been hidden from history.

Joan Scott, 1992

A historical analysis raises questions for consideration in relation to the origin and evolution of the issue. In the case of the nurse practitioner movement, this includes the conditions surrounding the issue and, importantly, how those conditions have changed over time. The significance of this analysis is that rather than merely recounting history as it has been recorded, a historical analysis opens to question our taken-for-granted understandings of the issue. If we draw on the work of feminist historians such as Scott (1992), we come to realize that histories are written from particular perspectives. A historical analysis reminds us that the issues of advanced nursing practice that we are currently facing have their origins in the past and have continued salience for the future of nurse practitioner practice.

The way a topic such as the nurse practitioner movement is understood historically contributes to the way issues on that topic get articulated. For example, the history of nurses practising beyond their scope of practice (i.e., in addition to what they have been educated and authorized to perform) has been fraught with problems for nurses.

Part of Canada's nursing history includes the reality that nurses have acted in a nurse practitioner–like role, often in rural and remote regions, and frequently where physicians were unavailable or unwilling to practice. The expanded scope of practice for these nurses evolved in response to conditions where physician-delivered health care was unavailable. Despite the significant contribution these nurses have made to the health of Canadians, the formal recognition of such a role has "historically been sporadic and inconsistent, especially with respect to role title, scope of practice, licensure requirements or continuing competence requirements. Over time, different provinces and territories have developed a hodgepodge of approaches to these key concerns" (Canadian Nurses Association, 2003b, p. 2).

The 1970s was a time of great promise and excitement in the nurse practitioner movement in Canada. Pilot projects were under way in several Canadian provinces. In Newfoundland, a 9-month expanded-role nursing education program was offered jointly by the school of nursing and the faculty of medicine at Memorial University (Chambers & West, 1978). Graduates of this program were engaged as family prac-tice nurses (FPN) attached to urban medical practices. Although this pilot project was deemed to be suc-cessful, "when federal government project funding terminated, hesitation by the provincial government and the fee-for-service physicians to plan for the future of the FPNs led to the dissolution of the urban attachments after the initial one year period" (Chambers & West, 1978, p. 459). Similarly, a pilot project for nurse practitioners in rural areas of Saskatchewan was announced in 1973. One of the purposes of this pilot project was to evaluate how a nurse–physician team would be accepted by physicians and by community members seeking care (Cardenas, 1975). Although 302 door-to-door interviews with community members were held, in which individuals were reportedly "enthusiastic about the arrival of nurse practitioners in their towns" and indicated "that they would make use of any health care services the nurse could provide" (p. 715), "as has been reported in many other projects, physicians vary widely in their ability to accept with confidence the competence of nurse practitioners" (p. 719). In her analysis, Cardenas further points out that "where the physician has seen the practitioner role as an extension instead of a complement of his [sic] own, episodic medical care has resulted in place of more comprehensive individual care" (p. 719). The nurse practitioners found over time that they had "a unique dimension to add to health care services" (p. 719).

During this same era, nurses were being prepared as nurse practitioners at McMaster University. The reflective article "The Nurse Practitioner—What Happened?" documents an interview held with Dorothy Kergin, who was instrumental in founding this first family nurse practitioner program in Canada in 1970. Kergin (LeFort & Kergin, 1978, p. 15) reports that the Ontario Ministry of Health, like many governments, *was convinced that demonstration projects and research in the primary care field were worth doing. A big factor too was the number of what they termed medically underserviced areas. The Ministry was interested in having nurses as providers of primary care in some of those underserviced areas. Our provincial funding for 1970 and subsequent federal funding centered on providing care in these underserviced areas.*

In the same published interview (LeFort & Kergin, 1978, p. 16), Mona Callan, director of the Educational Program for Nurses in Primary Care, relates the following:
In 1970 there was a shortage of physicians . . . so the nurse practitioner wasn't a threat, she was an asset. Now, there is a surplus of physicians and people are perceiving the situation in a different way. Some physicians acknowledge that nurse practitioners make important contributions to primary care but they are unable to employ them because of the lack of reimbursement for their services under provincial health insurance plans.

The landmark research from this era, "The Burlington Randomized Trial of the Nurse Practitioner" (Spitzer et al., 1974), was undertaken by a team of nurses and physicians. Although the results of this randomized control study, conducted to assess the effects of substituting nurse practitioners for physicians in primary care, found "that a nurse practitioner can provide first-contact primary care safely and effectively, with as much satisfaction to patients, as a family physician" (p. 255) and is "cost effective from society's point of view, the new method of primary care was not financially profitable to doctors because of current restrictions on reimbursement for the nurse-practitioner services" (p. 251).

A decade later, in the article "The Nurse Practitioner Revisited: Slow Death of a Good Idea," Spitzer (1984, p. 1050) laments, "The promise that the nurse-practitioner movement held in the early 1970s for better quality and more balanced primary care, better access for the disadvantaged, containment of health-service costs and a more rational deployment of health manpower is largely unfulfilled." In this article, a year after the closure of the last educational program for nurse practitioners in Canada at McMaster University, Spitzer reflects on his earlier optimism for the nurse practitioner movement in Canada. "In 1978, I wrote that the experiment with nurse practitioners seemed to be off to a promising start, but the final verdict was not yet in. I [now] judge the verdict to be clear in Canada. The programs, the opportunities for practice, and concrete plans for the future are dead" (Spitzer, 1984, p. 1050). Although Spitzer goes on to say that the future for nurse practitioners in the United States is less clear, he points out that "the most important factor in the economic viability of the nurse practitioners in the United States will be the level of their remuneration," citing two studies where nurse practitioners are "increasingly disillusioned with their role because of low pay and their inefficient use as a resource" (Spitzer, 1984, p. 1050).

It is important to point out that for several decades nurses have been participating in educational programs to prepare themselves to practice beyond the scope of a registered nurse, and these nurses have faced problems that we have yet to resolve. Historically, nurses have faced the reality that, after completing very challenging and expensive educational programs, the positions open to them through pilot projects have been discontinued and many of the opportunities to work in primary care have been located in very rural and remote parts of the country.

Although the closure of the McMaster Family Practice Nurse Program (later called Educational Program for Nurses in Primary Care) may have marked the end of an era of the nurse practitioner movement in primary care, the recurrence of a physician shortage less than a decade later led to yet another strategy for the use of nurse practitioners, this time with an acute care focus:

In the 1990s, acute care hospitals in Ontario witnessed a reduction in the number of medical residents and an increase in the number of admissions for patients who were acutely ill, and required complex and comprehensive care. The hospitals introduced Acute Care Nurse Practitioners (ACNPs) as qualified health care providers to effectively and efficiently meet these changes (Sidani et al., 2000, p. 6).

However, these practitioners were different from their earlier counterparts in primary care in that "they do not work in isolation and do not replace physicians or residents; they are an integral member of the health care team" (Sidani et al., 2000, p. 12).

Although the barriers to the implementation of the role of ACNPs are significant and include a lack of knowledge of and a perceived lack of support for the role by other health care team members and absence of mentorship for new ACNPs in clinical practice (van Soeren & Micevski, 2001), their contribution to "*outcome* achievement is yet to be determined" (Sidani et al., 2000, p. 12; italics added).

As the emerging role for nurse practitioners in acute care settings continues, we see once again the re-emergence of educational and practice initiatives for nurse practitioners in primary health care. For example, the Strengthening Primary Care Initiative in Nova Scotia, launched in 2000, was funded by the provincial and federal governments and included the introduction of primary health care nurse practitioners working in collaboration with one or more family physicians. The project findings suggest that some of the difficulties with this initiative rest with the realities that "not only were the nurse practitioners new and unfamiliar in the province, [but that] the nature of the practice configuration historically was not based on a collaborative practice model" (Martin-Misener et al., 2004, p. 42). In commenting on this report, Gallagher (2004) identifies structured, unstructured, and policy-driven barriers for collaborative interdisciplinary projects. Among these barriers are legislation, fee-for-service frameworks, and dated policies that privilege physician authority. Added to these structural barriers are relational issues, intolerance for the unpredictable and the unknown, and "insufficient political will for change" (Gallagher, 2004, p. 46).

Recounted in this history of the nurse practitioner movement in Canada is the notion that educational programs and positions created to address political agendas can be easily replaced by new agendas, and the cost for individual nurses, for the profession, and for health care is high. So, how can nurses convince governments to move past the idea of short-term problem intervention to recognize the need for long-term planning and policy development that will address the health care needs of Canadians? How is it that time and time again nurses have been complicit in the short-term solutions to the problems of care delivery that impede or avoid resolution of the issues?

Understanding the Political Nature of the Issue

Politics is often talked about as the art of influencing another person. Although some nurses claim they are not political, others insist that there is no escaping politics. In the history of the nurse practitioner movement, one can identify multiple decisions that have been politically motivated and influenced by the multiple stakeholders, including governments, nurses, and other health care provider groups. A political analysis asks about the relationship of knowledge and power in a particular situation, including who gets to decide what counts as knowledge and whose knowledge counts as important. When individuals and groups with disparate values enter into decision making, politics shapes the content of what is discussed and the decision-making process itself. In this analysis, we raise the questions about how important decisions related to the nurse practitioner movement get made, who makes these decisions, and by what authority; this analysis is not to establish whether the nurse practitioner movement is good or bad.

One of the central questions in this analysis is who has the authority to decide what nurse practitioner practice will look like (CNA, 2003a). Multiple groups want to influence the decisions of what constitutes nurse practitioner practice, including nurse educators, provincial/territorial regulatory powers, government bodies, and the medical community. In the case where the provision of nurse practitioner practice responds to a political agenda, the interests of particular governments will be served. Typically, the medical community has more influence on governmental decision making than other health care providers. This implies that those seeking to influence governmental decisions will have to lobby and gain the support of other groups that hold power and influence with the government. What is perhaps most surprising is that the recipients of health care have such little influence on governmental decisions.

Closely linked to the topic of power and influence, and to the circumstance that underpins the questions of who has the authority to decide, is the allocation of economic resources. Educational institutions, in particular, are inextricably tied to governmental agendas as they negotiate for funds for nurse practitioner educational programs.

Economic Understandings

An economic analysis of this issue is complex, in part because it explores the allocation of resources in the lives of individuals, educational institutions, and governments. In many situations, an economic analysis looks at ideas of supply and demand. In the case of the nurse practitioner movement, however, governments are providing considerable funds to increase the supply of nurse practitioners across the country, without any clear indication of whether these positions will be funded federally or provincially/territorially. In other words, there is a supply being generated that is driven by something other than a demand for these positions. We would suggest that the economics that underpin the nurse practitioner movement are motivated by a particular political agenda rather than an agenda that addresses the health care needs of Canadians.

Throughout the history of the nurse practitioner movement, questions have been raised about the economic benefits of use of nurse practitioners in Canadian health care delivery. Although there is research evidence over a 25-year period that indicates "patients are more satisfied with nurse practitioner care than physician care and that there are no differences in terms of patient health status in the two types of care" (Shortt, 2004, p. 8), the research exploring the economic benefits of nurse practitioners is merely speculative. In a systematic review of research literature conducted in 2002, Horrocks and associates found that "it was not possible to conduct a robust economic analysis of the costs of care from nurse practitioners compared with doctors...the lack of good evidence about the economic impact of substituting nurse practitioners for doctors needs to be addressed in future research, otherwise changes may be introduced that are thought to be efficient when they may not be so" (Horrocks, Anderson, & Salisbury, 2002, p. 822). It would seem that the most significant barrier to a comprehensive economic analysis of the use of nurse practitioners is the disparity between the methods of remuneration; for example, the majority of nurse practitioners would be in salaried positions whereas most physicians work on a fee-for-service payment schedule.

We have some sense from this analysis of what underlies the political agenda to expand the nurse practitioner movement. The resounding question, however, is, given the historical and political realities, what compels individual nurses to pursue nurse practitioner practice and education? Is it the belief of nurses that, given the opportunity and resources, nurse practitioners might offer a different health care service leading to improved health for Canadians?

Social and Cultural Understandings

Cultural ideas about gender are inherent in claims about what constitutes skill or what counts as knowledge, and these often unexamined assumptions create boundaries shaping what we are able to see and perhaps more importantly, what we don't see when we look to understand nursing.

Ronnie Steinberg, 1990

Important questions that contribute to our understandings of the social and cultural context explore the prevailing attitudes, the values and priorities, and the privileging of the dominant culture and the influences of these on a particular issue. Given the uncertainty that surrounds this movement, and the question we have raised of what compels individual nurses to pursue nurse practitioner practice and education, we look to social and cultural attitudes and values to extend our understanding. We would like to suggest several possibilities that underlie nurses' participation in the nurse practitioner movement, drawing on nurses' position as members of society as well as on their informed access to the realities of the current health care system. As members of society, many nurses internalize the prevailing attitudes of society that highlight the value of medical practice over nursing practice. Nurses are understandably influenced by the status ascribed to the expanded scope of nurse practitioner practice, which includes diagnosing, ordering investigative procedures, and prescribing a full range of pharmaceuticals and treatments. It is not surprising that many nurses who have been carrying out these functions with varying degrees of supervision or autonomy under the cover of physicians' orders would welcome the opportunity to extend their knowledge base and practice independently.

In addition to being members of society, nurses have a particular view of the inadequacies of the current health care system and a vision of how a nurse practitioner might attend to the health care needs of the significant portion of society whose needs are not well addressed in the current system. It is important to say that, in embracing the nurse practitioner movement, nurses envision improved health care not only for people who are living in rural and remote regions of the country but for underserved people in urban settings as well as for countless Canadians whose needs are poorly served in the current physician-driven model of health care. Nurses, as informed consumers of health care, are in a position to see the current reality and how it could be otherwise. Also, nurses working in the current system experience the daily frustrations of a system moving away from addressing health care toward a business model of health care delivery that makes nursing practice as they originally envisioned it almost impossible. Thus, it is easy to see why nurses would respond to an opportunity to practice differently.

Critical Feminist Understandings

A feminist analysis helps us to understand the views and the effects of the views that others hold about nurses' abilities and realities. It also makes us more aware of how we as nurses—most of us women—participate in perpetuating these views. Put another way, a feminist analysis helps us to understand our own complicity in sustaining structures and ideologies that foster misinterpretation of women's and nurses' experiences. A feminist analysis of a nursing issue is useful because it increases our knowledge and awareness of relevant power structures and thereby positions us effectively to participate in changing them. The discourses that define nurses are more than merely "ways of thinking": They are ways of constituting the knowledge, practices, subjectivities, and relations of power that together make up the meanings of nursing (Weedon, 1999). The term *discourse* as it is used here pertains to "the social practices, values and cultural beliefs that prevail in a given culture or subculture at a specified historical moment, and shape the collective view of what is right, proper, worthwhile and valuable" (Thorne, McCormick, & Carty, 1997, p. 2).

In the situation of the nurse practitioner, a critical feminist analysis asks how this issue is influenced by power inequities and the hierarchical structures within the health care system. For example, we might consider the power inequities in remuneration between nurse practitioners and physicians. On the one hand, it would seem plausible, even reasonable, that nurse practitioners and medical practitioners performing the same work would be compensated similarly. The reality to date, however, is that it appears unlikely that nurse practitioners will even qualify for the same model of remuneration as physicians. Another question that this raises is whether governments and employers, who may see nurse practitioners performing the same work as physicians for less remuneration, expect a savings to the system. It could be said that the argument for nurse practitioners as "cost effective" to the system really means that (1) the expectation is that nurses would do the same work for less and that (2) nurse practitioners will take up the care of less prestigious populations and carry out that work in less than ideal conditions. In spite of the apparent expected inequities that nurse practitioners will face in practice, we cannot help but wonder if the elevated status of the work of medicine over the work of nursing is the impetus for some nurses to pursue nurse practitioner practice.

Ethical and Legal Understandings

An ethical-legal analysis of the nurse practitioner movement considers questions of regulation and who will have the authority to define the scope of nurse practitioner practice. Like the health care system itself, tensions generated by differences between national and provincial/territorial legislation result in significant and important distinctions in what constitutes nurse practitioner practice across the country. Although an in-depth discussion of these difference can be found in Chapter 9, it should be noted that there are significant differences across provinces and territories regarding what nurse practitioners can do, the degree of autonomy nurse practitioners can have, what nurse practitioners are called, and whether the title "nurse practitioner" is protected by legislation in the way that "registered nurse" is protected and regulated.

■ BARRIERS TO RESOLUTION

One of the most important strategies for moving an issue toward resolution is identifying barriers that may impede the resolution process. Once the barriers are identified, chances for resolution through mediation, collaboration, or negotiation increase. What makes identifying barriers so useful in issue resolution is that we may lack awareness of the taken-for-granted assumptions that sustain an issue and obstruct its resolution. Nowhere is this truer than for the issues surrounding the nurse practitioner movement.

The first barrier is that, despite a well-developed theory base dating back to the 1960s that distinguishes the professional practice of nurses from that of other disciplines, many educational programs and nurse practitioners themselves have been hesitant to make the theory base central to their professional practice. Instead, the dominant conceptualization has been that of nurse practitioner practice as roles and competencies rather than as a dimension of professional nursing practice that is informed by the advanced nursing knowledge that graduate level education provides. Competencies and roles make clear what it is that nurse practitioners are able to do, which accounts in part for professional practice. However, this conceptualization fails to account for the need for an articulation of advanced knowledge that underpins the competencies. The appeal of conceptualizing nurse practitioner practice as roles, competencies, and standards lies in the ease with which they can be demonstrated, measured, and tested. Although this model appeals to the provincial/territorial professional organizations whose concern it is to regulate practice, a tension is created for educators, employers, and nurses in that it accounts for part but not all of professional nurse practitioner practice. For example, Baer (2003, p. 51), in her chapter on the philosophical and historical bases of advanced practice nursing, states that "nursing's focus on people: its blend of medical, behavioral and social science expertise; and its commitment to caring, teaching and counseling and supporting patients are the characteristics of nursing that make nurses so uniquely qualified to provide advanced practice and primary health care services to the public." Baer (2003, p. 47) also draws on the classic work of Donaldson and Crowley in their discussion of the discipline, noting

nursing's recurrent themes and focus on the wholeness of people, the interaction between people and their environment, and nursing's management of people and environment to enhance comfort, quality of life, and general well being during, and beyond, illness. In fact, and with irony, it must be noted that this very breadth of background is what makes nursing so clearly suited to the primary health care provider role.

We would suggest that this conceptualization of nursing knowledge provides a theoretical understanding of and an underpinning for advanced nursing practice far beyond the scope of competencies and roles.

A second barrier is the lack of consistency about what constitutes nurse practitioner practice across the country. There is, among provinces and territories, a wide variation in the requirements of entry to practice for nurse practitioners. In some provinces, you can become a nurse practitioner with a diploma in nursing, experience, and a certificate in nurse practitioner practice. In other provinces, a baccalaureate degree with experience and a certificate will suffice. Several other provinces require a master's degree in nursing as part of the nurse practitioner preparation. Added to this inconsistency is the fact that there are many registered nurses already in practice across the country who identify themselves as nurse practitioners because of extensive practice and/or additional course work. Eighteen educational programs prepare nurse practitioners, with more seeking approval, all of which are accountable only to their provincial/territorial professional associations. Despite the Canadian Nurses Association's (CNA) efforts to standardize nurse practitioner preparation at the graduate level, provincial/territorial professional associations, influenced by differing provincial/territorial legislation, have yet to implement national standards. In addition to the provincial/territorial differences surrounding educational preparation and entry to practice, there are significant differences in the scope of practice for nurse practitioners across the country. In some locations, nurse practitioners will have autonomy to diagnose, treat, and prescribe a full range of pharmaceuticals. In other provinces/territories, nurse practitioners can perform the same functions but only in collaboration/supervision with medical practitioners. Some jurisdictions set limits on the types of pharmaceuticals that nurse practitioners can prescribe. The consequences of this high degree of variability between provinces and territories include limiting the mobility of nurse practitioners between provinces and interfering with the understanding of nurse practitioner practice by both other health care practitioners and health care consumers.

A barrier that is closely related to the variability of entry to practice is the difference among educational programs for nurse practitioner practice. At least in part, this variability is driven by the connection between educational institutions and government funding. Regardless of the programs that educators might imagine would benefit the health care system, they rely on government funding, which is directly linked to political agendas. That is, governments faced with primary care physician shortages are willing to fund nurse practitioner programs to alleviate this shortage, whereas nursing programs not linked to political agendas are underfunded. In this way, political agendas serve as barriers to health care agendas. We might also add that the teaching resources in educational institutions are likely to follow the funding, meaning that teaching resources are diverted to the politically motivated nurse practitioner agenda. As a consequence, other nursing programs within faculties and schools of nursing, such as plans for doctoral education in some institutions, have been put aside while the nurse practitioner agenda takes precedence. The nurse practitioner movement, an initiative in response to a political agenda, has been instituted at a time when graduate programs across the country have been concerned with the long-term goals of preparing nurse leaders to participate in and direct health care reform.

There is a lack of definitive information about nurse practitioner employment across the country. If governments would have educational institutions graduate increasing numbers of nurse practitioners, it would seem reasonable that governments would also allocate sufficient funding within health care budgets for institutions to be able to hire these graduates. However, anecdotal evidence suggests that employers cannot foresee hiring new nurse practitioner graduates until they receive funds to cover the additional costs that remuneration to nurse practitioners would require. This leaves nurses in the position of entering a nurse practitioner program with no actual prospects for employment. In some cases where positions have been created or plans for positions are under way, employers, when asked, were unable to say what a fair remuneration for a nurse practitioner position would be. Given that at least part of what these nurses would be doing has until now been considered medical practice, it seems clear that the fee-for-service remuneration model, which applies to most physicians, is not being considered for nurse practitioners. An additional complexity with the barrier of remuneration centers on the inclusion or exclusion of nurse practitioners from the collective bargaining process. The argument for inclusion of nurse practitioners in the collective bargaining process suggests that nurse practitioners would benefit from protection against changing political agendas and shifting "solutions" put forth by employers. On the other hand, some suggest that professional nurse practitioner practice would benefit from being outside the agenda of nursing unions. This may arise, in part, from the inherent contradiction in a role that includes the functions of both medical practice and nursing practice, a notion that could be problematic for union supporters.

A related barrier is that, regardless of what we imagine nurses might be able to do in "collaborative practice," nurse practitioner practice relies on the good will and tolerance of individual medical practitioners. The CNA document titled *Helping to Sustain Canada's Health System: Nurse Practitioners in Primary Health Care* reports that there are "concerns about collaborative practice expressed by the medical community" (CNA, 2003b, p. 2). On the one hand, it would seem that unless we have the full cooperation of the medical community, the nurse practitioner movement will not be able to progress in the way that has been imagined. On the other hand, the cost of obtaining that cooperation might mean less autonomy than we had first imagined for nurse practitioner practice or, even more disturbing, that nurse practitioner autonomy would be at the discretion of individual medical practitioners.

■ STRATEGIES

After the articulation, analysis, and discussion of barriers to resolution of a nursing issue, strategies for resolution must be generated. Although there are a wide variety of effective strategies to choose from, a complex issue such as the nurse practitioner movement calls for particular strategies for resolution. As the analysis of issues surrounding the nurse practitioner movement in this chapter has clearly shown, long-term strategies are most important in moving this issue toward resolution. Given the political nature of this issue, the strategies will be directed toward uncovering the political agenda of the nurse practitioner movement and will challenge those points that might suggest that this could be otherwise.

The first strategy, then, is for us to acknowledge the political nature of this movement and that, as such, many of the strategies that will need to be in place to move these issues to resolution depend on political agendas and political power. This acknowledgment includes the reality that we are working amidst diverse provincial/territorial political agendas. This is not to say that we are powerless in addressing these issues but to suggest that much of the energy that is driving these issues lies outside of nursing. Thus, our strategies as nurses must include a vocal critique of the political nature of the movement so that what does unfold across the country serves not the political agenda but professional nursing practice and thereby the health of Canadians.

Although no one can argue about the differences across provinces and territories and the influences those differences must have on the way the nurse practitioner movement is unfolding, deans and directors of educational institutions and presidents and executive directors of professional nursing organizations and colleges must work to support the development of national standards for professional nurse practitioner practice. At the time of the writing of this chapter, several strategies have been undertaken: On June 2, 2004, a draft of a Core Competency Framework to direct the development of a national blueprint for a Canadian Nurse Practitioner Examination was approved by the CNA Forum on Nurse Practitioner Assessment. In September 2004, representatives from all provinces and territories met in Ottawa as part of the CNA Forum on Nurse Practitioners and completed a blueprint for the first national examination. This examination is developed using the same model as the registered nurse examination. The first offering of this examination is scheduled for June 2005. As positive as the sense of accomplishment around this development is, we cannot underestimate the need for continued strategies to move each of the provinces and territories to require that their nurse practitioners qualify to take—and pass—this examination.

Likewise, strategies to move us toward a common curriculum in educational preparation for nurse practitioner practice, including master's level education, are necessary. A working group of the CNA developed core competencies and position statements for nurse practitioners, clinical nurse specialists, and those in advanced nursing practice. Educators are able to draw on both of these national documents to inform the development of nurse practitioner curriculum. It is, in fact, strategic for all developing educational programs to align themselves with the framework of the CNA.

The CNA, funded by the federal government, has formed the Canadian Nurse Practitioner Initiative (CNPI), whose overall goal is to "collaboratively develop mechanisms and processes to support the implementation of the Nurse Practitioner role in Canada." The CNPI is organized around five broad mandates:

1. *Educational preparation*—Develop recommendations for educational preparation of nurse practitioners, including prior learning assessment, continuing education, and re-entry.
2. *Practice and evaluation*—Articulate appropriate and consistent practice guidelines, and develop a framework to support full integration of nurse practitioners into primary care health settings.
3. *Government legislation and professional self-regulation*—Develop recommendations related to legislative framework, including a common definition of the role(s), and related to professional regulation of nurse practitioners, including a national examination.
4. *Change management, social marketing, strategic communications*—Foster a collaborative environment in which governments, health professionals, employers, and academics integrate the nurse practitioner role into Canada's health care system. This will also require gaining public acceptance of a new model of care that includes the nurse practitioner role as well as promoting the role as a desirable nursing career choice.
5. *Health human resource planning and primary health care*—Develop usable models so that provinces and territories can determine current and future demands for nurse practitioners as well as develop recommendations to increase the nationwide pool of nurse practitioners.

■ SUMMARY

The issues surrounding the nurse practitioner movement are complex and multilayered. This chapter highlights some of the issues that the nurse practitioner movement presents for educators, regulators, and potential employers, not to mention the dilemmas posed for potential nurse practitioners. Of particular concern to us, the authors, and to educators is our implied complicity in a movement that communicates to Canadians that the nurse practitioner is worthy of their support when, in our assessment, the movement is being driven by a political rather than a health care agenda.

In our analysis, in which we open the issues to multiple understandings, a number of barriers to the resolution of the issues emerge. Among these is the obstacle that is created when we conceptualize advanced practice based on roles and competencies rather than on professional nurse practitioner practice that is underpinned by advanced nursing knowledge. The potential implementation of the nurse practitioner movement will have to negotiate significant obstacles created through the variability and inconsistency across the country regarding scope of nurse practitioner practice, entrance to practice requirements, educational approaches and entry requirements, and the absence of definitive employment opportunities and a commitment on the part of physicians to practice collaboratively with nurse practitioners. Because of the complexity and the breadth of these barriers, it is neither possible nor desirable to move to a position of problem solving the issues. To bow to a political agenda that views these issues as merely problems to be solved obscures both the historical contribution that nurses have made and the potential for the development of a viable, sound, nationally coherent nurse practitioner practice.

Rather than a premature and politically driven launch of the movement, our analysis suggests that the health care of Canadians would be well served if the stakeholders in this issue, including nurse educators, regulators, employers, physicians, and governments, engage in dialogue that addresses the barriers as outlined in this chapter. At the time of writing this chapter, the CNA and provincial and territorial organizations and colleges are in the beginning stages of these dialogues. The political nature of the nurse practitioner agenda, driven by government funding and aimed at addressing physician rather than nursing shortages, has accelerated the nurse practitioner movement beyond the supporting organizations' and institutions' sustainability.

Online Resources

Add to your knowledge of this issue:

Canadian Health Services Research
   Foundation

www.chsrf.ca

Canadian Nurses Association

www.cna-nurses.ca

Canadian Provinces and Territories Links

www.canada.gc.ca/othergov/prov_e.html

Centre for Health Services and Policy
   Research

www.chspr.ubc.ca

Government of Canada

www.gc.ca

Health Canada

www.hc-sc.gc.ca

Parliament of Canada

www.parl.gc.ca

REFLECTIONS on the Chapter . . .

1. What information would influence your decision to pursue nurse practitioner education and practice?

2. Given what has been discussed in this chapter, take a stance on the educational level required for nurse practitioner practice and support your position.

3. Locate the Web site for the professional nursing organization within your province or territory and answer the following questions: What is the scope of practice for nurse practitioners in your area? Are nurse practitioners regulated in your province or territory? What is the educational requirement for nurse practitioner licensure in your province or territory?

4. What are the strengths and the limitations of national competencies and standards for nurse practitioner practice?

5. What other barriers to and strategies for resolving this issue can you identify?

6. What other readings or resources have assisted you in understanding this complex issue?

■ GLOSSARY OF TERMS

Adapted from the Canadian Nurses Association. (2002, April). *Advanced nursing practice: A national framework.* Ottawa: Author.

Advanced Nursing Practice (ANP)

ANP is an umbrella term. It describes an advanced level of nursing practice that maximizes the use of in-depth nursing knowledge and skill in meeting the health needs of clients (individuals, families, groups, populations, or entire communities). In this way, ANP extends the boundaries of nursing's scope of practice and contributes to nursing knowledge and the development and advancement of the profession.

Basic education

Education required for entry into the profession; this may be a diploma or a baccalaureate degree in nursing, depending on the requirements of the provincial or territorial registering body.

Certification

A voluntary and periodic process (recertification) by which an organized professional body confirms that a registered nurse has demonstrated competence in a nursing specialty by having met predetermined standards of that specialty.

Clients

Individuals, families, groups, populations, or entire communities.

Clinical nurse specialist (CNS)

A CNS is a registered nurse who holds a master's or doctoral degree in nursing and has expertise in a clinical nursing specialty. An expert practitioner, the CNS provides direct care, education, and consultation to clients as well as education and consultation to the health care team.

Competencies

The specific knowledge, skills, judgment, and personal attributes required for a registered nurse to practise safely and ethically in a designated role and setting.

Expert practice

Expert practice is characterized by the ability to assess and understand complex client response in a particular practice area; to have a significant depth of knowledge and intervention skills, often acquired informally; and to possess strong intuitive skills in the practice area.

Graduate education

Education beyond a baccalaureate degree level, extending from the master's to the doctoral and postdoctoral levels.

Nurse practitioner

A nurse practitioner is an advanced practice nurse whose practice is focused on providing services to manage the health care needs of individuals, families, groups, and communities. The nurse practitioner role is grounded in the nursing profession's values, knowledge, theories, and practice and is a role that complements rather than replaces other health care providers. Nurse practitioners have the potential to contribute significantly to new models of health care based on the principles of primary health care.

Protected title

A title protected by legislation and, therefore, not to be used by others.

Scope of nursing practice

The activities nurses are educated and authorized to perform, as established through legislated definitions of nursing practice and as complemented by standards, guidelines, and policy positions issued by professional nursing bodies.

Standard

A desirable and achievable level of performance against which actual performance can be compared.

References

Baer, E. (2003). Philosophical and historical bases of advance practice nursing roles. In M. Mezey, D. McGiven, & E. Sullivan-Marx. *Nurse practitioners: Evolution of advanced practice* (4th ed., pp. 37–53). New York: Springer.

Canadian Nurses Association. (2000). *Position statement: The nurse practitioner*. Ottawa: Author.

_____. (2002a). *Fact sheet: Cost effectiveness of the nurse practitioner role*. Ottawa: Author.

_____. (2002b). *Fact sheet: Financing nurse practitioner services*. Ottawa: Author.

_____. (2003a) *Fact sheet: Legislation, regulation, and education of the nurse practitioner in Canada*. Ottawa: Author.

_____. (2003b). *Helping to sustain Canada's health system: Nurse practitioners in primary health care*. Ottawa: Author.

Cardenas, B. D. (1975). The independent NP: Alive and well and living in rural Saskatchewan. *Nursing Clinics of North America, 10*(4), 711–719.

Chambers, L. W., & West, A. E. (1978). Assessment of the role of the family practice nurse in urban medical practice. *Canadian Journal of Public Health, 69*(6), 459–468.

Donaldson, S. K., & Crowley, D. M. (1978). The discipline of nursing. *Nursing Outlook, (26)*2, 113–120.

Fagin, C. (2003). Primary care as an academic discipline. In M. Mezey, D. McGiven, & E. Sullivan-Marx (Eds.), *Nurse practitioners: Evolution of advanced practice* (4th ed., pp. 65–83). New York: Springer.

Gallagher, S. (2004). Commentary: Nurses lead the way . . . . *Canadian Journal of Nursing Leadership, 17*(2), 45–46.

Horrocks, S., Anderson, E., & Salisbury, C. (2002). Systemic review of whether nurse practitioners working in primary care can provide the equivalent care to doctors. *British Medical Journal, 324*, 819–823.

LeFort, S., & Kergin, D. (1978). The nurse practitioner—What happened? An interview. Part I. *Canadian Nurse, 74*(4), 14–17.

Martin-Misener, R., McNab, J., Sketris, I. S., et al. (2004). Collaborative practice in health systems change: The Nova Scotia experience with the Strengthening Primary Care Initiative. *Canadian Journal of Nursing Leadership, 17*(2), 33–45.

Scott, J. (1992). Experience. In J. Butler & J. Scott (Eds.), *Feminists theorize the political*. (pp. 22–40). London: Routledge.

Shortt, S. (2004). Reflection on continuity in contemporary Canadian primary care. *Canadian Journal of Nursing Research, 36*(2), 7–10.

Sidani, S., Irvine, D., Porter, H., et al. (2000). Practice patterns of acute care nurse practitioners. *Canadian Journal of Nursing Leadership, 13*(3), 6–12.

Spitzer, W., Sackett, D., Sibley, J., et al. (1974). The Burlington randomized trial of the nurse practitioner. *New England Journal of Medicine, 290*(5), 251–256.

Spitzer, W. O. (1984). The nurse practitioner revisited: Slow death of a good idea. *New England Journal of Medicine, 310*(16), 1049–1051.

Steinberg, R. (1990). Social construction of skill: Gender, power and comparable worth. *Work and Occupations, 17*(4), 449–482.

Thorne, S., McCormick, J., & Carty, E. (1997). Deconstructing the gender neutrality of chronic illness and disability. *Health Care for Women International, 18*(1), 1–16.

van Soeren, M. H., & Micevski, V. (2001). Success indicators and barriers to acute nurse practitioner role implementation in four Ontario hospitals. *AACN Clinical Issues: Advanced Practice in Acute and Critical Care, 12*(3), 424–437.

Weedon, C. (1999). *Feminism, theory and the politics of difference*. Malden, MA: Blackwell.

Critical Questions

As a way of engaging with the ideas in this chapter, consider the following:

1. What views do you hold of the Canadian health care system and how have you come to hold those views?

2. What are your thoughts about how the health care system structures nursing practice?

3. In what ways does the health care system support the health of Canadians?

4. In your view, what is the major challenge facing those who manage the health care system?

CHAPTER

3

Janet Storch

Canadian Health Care System

Nurses find more meaning and reward in their work when they can care for their patients as professionals and when the conditions of work support the scope of practice gained through education and experience. Used with permission, Faculty of Nursing, University of Calgary.

After completing this chapter, you will be able to:

1. Understand how and why Canada's health care system differs from other systems of health care.

2. Recognize the history in our current challenges in health care.

3. Understand the system's impact on Canadian nursing and on the work of individual nurses.

4. Recognize the need for nursing leadership in maintaining all that is good about health care and making changes to correct deficiencies.

5. Identify future possibilities for nurses in the health care system.

Nurses' practice is influenced by social, cultural, and historical realities worldwide, and Canadian nursing practice is no exception to this. These influences underlie the context within nurses' practice, a context that affects their everyday lives as nurses.

Therefore, nurses need to understand how social, cultural, and historical influences, along with economic and political forces, have shaped Canadian health services and the systems in which nurses work. Such understanding includes the philosophical framework for Canadian health care, the values that underlie a mainly public health insurance system, and key policy decisions that established the national programs. By gaining greater awareness of how social and cultural values influenced the development, financing, and delivery of health care, nurses can appreciate the nature of the value conflicts that underlie current health care debates. Further, through such understanding, nurses can better understand their practice environments and take an informed political advocacy role to continue shaping health care for the benefit of patients.

This chapter aims to provide nurses with an understanding of the health care system in which they work to equip them for the challenges involved in preserving the best of the system while making changes and improvements to health care. Specifically, the chapter invites nurses to focus on how the system affects the nursing profession and how nurses have attempted to influence the system and their own work. The reader is encouraged to consider nursing's involvement in the health care system (past and present) and the nursing leadership needed to make a difference in this complex system.

■ HEALTH CARE IN THE GLOBAL CONTEXT

Comparing Canada's approach to health care to that of other countries is important in establishing its context and in assessing the challenges and potentials of our collective approach to health care. How and why health care systems differ is a function of multiple influences, which may include societal values and beliefs, sociocultural climate, the state of the economy, political realities, geographic density, international influences, historical accident, established practices and programs, and other factors. As we consider how Canada's system developed, it is clear that several of these factors were at play at different points in time. The same is true for countries around the world.

One way to think about system differences is to consider that all Western countries provide for health care in a variety of ways, all of which involve variable combinations of private or public funding of services and delivery of services (Health Canada, 2002). The typologies that follow show the degree of public involvement in financing health services and the essential role envisioned for the health care system (Najman & Western, 1984; Table 3.1).

In the first type (type I) of health care system, private approaches to health services predominate, wherein both physician or other caregiver (such as midwife) and patient have maximum autonomy. This means that those who can afford private health insurance, or who simply can pay for their health care directly, choose their care providers and receive health services. Those who cannot pay do not have choice or benefit. In the purest form of type I, there would be no option other than to pay for service. In reality,

| TABLE 3.1 | Types of Health Care Systems in the Western World | | |

TYPE I	TYPE II	TYPE III	TYPE IV
Private health insurance	National health insurance	National health service	Socialized health system
Primary goal: preserve autonomy	Primary goal: egalitarian	Primary goal: egalitarian	Primary goal: essential service
Secondary effect: acceptance of social differences	Secondary effect: preserve autonomy	Secondary effect: public management	Secondary effect: physicians as state employees

From Najman, J. M., & Western, J. S. (1984). A comparative analysis of Australian health policy in the 1970s. *Social Science and Medicine, 18*(1), 949–958, with permission.

most countries have adopted a mix of system types. For example, although the United States has mainly a private pay system of health care, there are some publicly funded programs to assist elderly and poor people. Even with these programs, it is estimated that 42 million Americans have no health insurance and, therefore, are limited in their ability to access health care.

The polar opposite of type I is type IV. This type of health care system focuses on keeping people healthy so they can contribute to society and the economy. Health care is considered an essential service, not necessarily driven by compassionate motives for those who are ill as much as by motives of productivity. Physicians are considered agents of the state whose job it is to keep others working efficiently. In former Communist countries, this was the role of the physician. In Canada, the military establishment runs a similar system, as do most hockey and other sports teams.

Between the two extremes are two other types of health care systems. Type III is a health care system funded and operated by the government. This would have been typical of the health care system in Great Britain some years ago. There, the state-operated and state-funded health services were based on an egalitarian value. Public management of each service was considered key to efficient and effective operation.

Finally, type II is a hybrid of types I and III, wherein egalitarian values are high while autonomy of practitioner and patient is preserved to the maximum extent possible, thereby reconciling the two often-conflicting values. Type II health care systems use tax dollars to pay for health services through health insurance available from a nonprofit agency (e.g., government), and each health service is operated more or less autonomously by others: municipalities, citizen groups, or physicians or physiotherapists in private offices, group practices, or other modes. All services rendered to patients are then paid from the central pool of health insurance funds created through taxation. This distinctly Canadian approach embodies collective sharing of burdens and benefits while allowing a degree of autonomy in delivery (Storch, 1996).

Before moving on, it is important to underscore several qualifying points. First, the term *health care system* is a misnomer. In Canada, health services are far from being integrated systems of care, yet the ideal of an integrated and coordinated system of health services is important. Second, the four types noted do not include those found in a group of Third World countries that cannot afford the type of health care enjoyed in Canada. Yet many of these countries have developed primary health care systems that are not as institution dependent as those in Canada. Primary health care includes preventive health care as well as first point of contact and continuing care. In some cases, these preventive systems have been undermined by the influence of Western countries promoting high technology and institutionalization. Finally, even within the countries that finance health insurance through tax dollars, there are variations in services provided: For example, some fund home care whereas others do not, and some provide coverage for prescription drugs while others do not.

To appreciate how Canada's health care policies and modes of delivery influence nursing, one needs to consider how the health care system developed. As you reflect on the origins and development of Canada's health care system, identify the multiple factors influencing development and how that development led to patterns of care that are commendable and to others that are less than ideal.

■ HISTORY AND BACKGROUND: CANADA'S HEALTH CARE SYSTEM

For some, history can be a tedious subject. With that in mind, the following focuses on the key historical necessities for understanding Canada's health care system and its legacy, that is, individuals who took leadership at particular points in time to create, sustain, reform, or challenge the health care services system as we know it today. These individuals, who provide mental images of real people who influenced health care, include a lay nurse and hospital administrator named Jeanne Mance; a group of leaders known as the Fathers of Confederation; a visionary physician named J. W. McIntosh; an ambitious graduate student named Leonard Marsh and a bored politician named Ian MacKenzie; Tommy Douglas, a young boy stricken with osteomyelitis; a prime minister from Saskatchewan, John Diefenbaker; a French Canadian health minister, Monique Begin; two provincial premiers, Ralph Klein and Mike Harris; an actress named Shirley Douglas; an ex-premier, Roy Romanow, and a senator, Michael Kirby; and Nelia Laroza and Tecla Lin, two nursing heroes.

Jeanne Mance and the Period Before Confederation

In the late 1600s and up until the late 1800s, the new territory eventually named Canada was being settled. It was a time characterized by very limited government involvement in any social or health services. The colony was largely a rural society, and the limited collective health efforts needed centered on communicable diseases, epidemics, and other concerns that were beyond the helping capacity of neighbors or lay workers. For example, historical accounts focus on the need for better care for the mentally ill, referring to the need for "lunatic asylums" or "institutions for the feeble-minded," noting that these facilities were badly overcrowded and that preventive work was underdeveloped (Cassidy, 1947). Charitable organizations and religious orders, the latter particularly in Quebec, were essential in providing care.

Jeanne Mance was the first lay nurse in North America and the first to arrive in Canada. Her task of building the first hospital in Mont Royal (Montreal) and her negotiation with benefactors in France to bring more nurses to Canada (Ross Kerr, 1996) was a mark of her commitment to the new colony. Following her lead, the Grey Nuns of Montreal, a "uniquely Canadian order of nuns," formed. They were visiting nurses as well, and the order was instrumental in serving pioneers in western Canada (Ross Kerr, 1996). Ross Kerr also notes that the French influence in early Canadian nursing was important because it allowed Canada to escape some of the effects of the regressive period of nursing rampant in the United Kingdom at the time. As the colony that was to become Canada approached confederation in 1867, there were isolated actions involving government regulation (e.g., for selling meat, for managing epidemics), but, for the most part, this was generally a time of *ad hoc* decision making in health care.

The Fathers of Confederation

The Fathers of Confederation are notable mainly for what they did not know—and what they could not have known—about health care needs. When these leaders set out the terms of the British North America (BNA) Act of 1867, which continues to form a part of our current Constitution Act, they had no idea how trends in industrialization and urbanization would affect health care needs (Cassidy, 1947; Hastings & Mosley, 1980; Wallace, 1950). Thus, they wrote of what they knew and outlined very basic responsibilities of the federal government, leaving wide room for the provinces to be the key players in the provision of health care and believing that individuals could and should be self-reliant.

The federal responsibilities were seen as follows (Van Loon & Whittington, 1976):

Sec. 91—taking of the census, . . . collecting statistics (birth, marriage, death), establishing quarantine regulations and hospitals for those in quarantine, and taking responsibility for Canada's native peoples.

For the provinces, a clause was developed that proved to be inclusive of almost all types of health services (Van Loon & Whittington, 1976):

Sec. 92 (7)—The Establishment, Maintenance and Management of Hospitals, Asylums, Charities, and Eleemosynary Institutions in and for the Province, other than Marine Hospitals.

This division of federal and provincial responsibilities created permanent tension between the federal government, who collected most of the taxes, and the provincial governments, who saw their mandate for the provision of health services growing each year (Lindenfield, 1959).

Before being too critical of the Fathers of Confederation, however, one must note that the philosophical basis of the Canadian constitution they developed establishes that the federal government is responsible for making " . . . Laws for the Peace, Order and good Government of Canada" (Van Loon & Whittington, 1976, p. 480). In contrast to the U.S. Constitution, which centers on individual liberties and freedoms, Canada's set the stage for enacting legislation emphasizing the common, or collective, good.

A Visionary Thinker

Between the signing of the BNA Act in 1867 and World War II, the young country of Canada underwent profound change. Immediately after confederation, a number of charities were formed to address growing unmet needs. These charities included several that involved Canadian nurses to a substantial degree, such as the Red Cross, the Victorian Order of Nurses, and the Canadian Mental Health Organization (Meilicke & Storch, 1980). Canada was urbanizing as well. With the series of economic depressions that befell the new country, it became evident that reliance on self and family often was insufficient; many needed social assistance and health services (both prevention and curative). Because there were no federal structures to facilitate the development of health services and no provincial structures yet in place, local municipalities were forced to take significant responsibilities in providing health care (Cassidy, 1947)—even though they had limited resources available to help them do so. The unmet health needs of Canadians were never more apparent than when many of Canada's young men volunteered to fight in World War I and were found unfit for combat because of poor health.

Just before World War I, the president of the Vancouver Medical Society, J. W. McIntosh (1914), delivered a paper at the Royal Sanitary Conference in Vancouver on the topic of the interrelationship of physician, citizen, and state to public health. He provided a conceptual framework to describe the disabilities affecting many Canadians, classifying them as hereditary, personal or self-imposed, or environmental— "the gift of our neighbors and surroundings." Years later, his framework would resonate with the writing of a federal civil servant named Laframboise (1973). Laframboise wrote an article that was the basis of a prominent Canadian report known as the Lalonde Report (1974), named after the minister of health during whose tenure this report was released, Marc Lalonde. The Lalonde Report, entitled "A New Perspective on the Health of Canadians," marked Canada as a leader in formulating a four-point policy framework that considered heredity, environment, lifestyle, and health services as critical to health. Although McIntosh was visionary in his views, his ideas for implementation may have been traditional, as reflected in the concluding comments of his speech: "Of good omen is the welcome announcement from Ottawa, that shortly, the government will create a Public Health Department and appoint a member of the Cabinet—a trained medical man—as Minister of Public Health" (McIntosh, 1914, p. 454).

Between World War I and World War II, public health activities increased significantly in an attempt to address deficiencies in health services, and public health nursing expanded (Hastings &

Mosley, 1980, pp. 149–150). This growth threatened many physicians because "... these nurses worked semi-independently in the community" (Coburn, 1988, p. 443). Physician concern about nursing independence continues to be prevalent in Canadian nursing today. Yet it must also be recognized that there was a degree of support and cooperation between the two professions. Further, even as many nurses attempted to gain professional recognition, there was division within nursing ranks about whether nursing should pursue this independence as an important goal, just as there was division within medical ranks about nursing aspirations (Kinnear, 1994). This same diversity of opinion characterizes nursing and medical–nursing relationships in the 21st century.

A Bored Politician and an Ambitious Graduate Student

By the time Canada entered World War II, health care needs continued to exceed the supply of any type of comprehensive health care. Infant and maternal mortality rates were high, and morbidity and mortality from communicable diseases were of grave concern (Taylor, 1987). One third of the men who were examined for military service were unfit for service, with one third of that group rejected because of "psychiatric disorders" (Cassidy, 1947, p. 51).

As World War II began, a young politician by the name of Ian MacKenzie was minister of defense. The demands of his position were not seen as particularly challenging until the time for real engagement in the war began. At that point, his boss, Prime Minister Mackenzie King, moved Ian MacKenzie from the Department of Defense to what was considered a less demanding role in the Department of Pensions and National Health. Despite being excluded from the main focus of government attention and action (i.e., the war), MacKenzie was not content to remain idle. In 1939, he wrote to Prime Minister King "urging that unemployment and health insurance be introduced as war measures," suggesting that the demand for a national health system was inevitable (Taylor, 1987, p. 16). Over time, he managed to present a convincing case by suggesting that Canada owed such services to its returning troops, noting that other countries were developing these types of programs as well and thereby heightening his moral persuasion.

Meanwhile, a young graduate student in economics at London University, Leonard Marsh, participated in research for Lord William Beveridge (Bliss, 1975; Taylor, 1987), a British author famous for the Beveridge Report, which advocated social insurance in Great Britain. Marsh subsequently relocated to Canada and became director for social research at McGill University. There, he directed a program of research on employment and produced several major studies on Canadian social conditions. In this and later posts, he was a consultant to the federal government and gradually became involved with the Committee on Postwar Reconstruction in 1944–45. Meanwhile, Ian MacKenzie commissioned Director of Public Health Services Dr. J. J. Heagerty to develop proposals for health insurance. In doing so, he urged Dr. Heagerty to consult with provincial counterparts and establish an Inter-Departmental Advisory Committee on Health Insurance. Heagerty did so, and he produced a massive report at the same time Marsh was completing his "Report on Social Security for Canada." Marsh's report is now regarded as the single most important document in the historical development of the welfare state in Canada and a key document in the development of postwar social security programs, the Canadian equivalent of the Beveridge Report. Marsh's report included a comprehensive package of social programs for Canadians (Rice & Prince, 2000) and recognized that all are deserving of adequate social supports for living.

The reports of Marsh and Heagerty in 1943 became a key part of the documentation for discussions on postwar reconstruction, and they were tabled together at the Postwar Reconstruction Conference by Ian MacKenzie on August 6, 1945. They reflected a postwar idealism fostered by international influences, such as the freedoms outlined in the Atlantic Charter (Marsh, 1975; Taylor, 1973). As told so dramatically by Malcolm Taylor, these reports and proposals were comprehensive, and the agenda for the meeting at which they were to be discussed was hailed by Prime Minister King as likely the "most important Canadian conference since Confederation" (Taylor, 1987, p. 50). But a hiatus in proceedings occurred when news of the bombing of Hiroshima was received. The meeting's adjournment and rescheduling left room for those considering economic priorities rather than philosophical and humanitarian commitments to defeat this comprehensive plan for health and social security. (Note that this type of tension in world views is not dissimilar from current opposing positions in health care today.) Nevertheless, over the next 20 years, the plans set out by Marsh and Heagerty served as something of a blueprint for the development of health insurance and social insurance in Canada.

A Young Boy From Saskatchewan

Much of the difficulty encountered in the acceptance of the Proposals for Postwar Reconstruction was also related to who had the legal authority for health care. The BNA Act's division of federal and provincial responsibilities was high in the minds of those proposing less federal interference and more provincial autonomy—a theme that continues to dominate debates in Canadian health care today. However, in the province of Saskatchewan, a different mentality was at play. In many respects, the rural and isolated population in this prairie province did not mind as much who offered the programs to combat, in the words of Lord Beveridge, "Want, Disease, Ignorance, Squalor, and Idleness" (Taylor, 1987, p. 34) as that programs be available to all.

Saskatchewan had a long history of working collectively to solve practical problems of everyday living. And when it came to health care, the province united in the significant step of using public tax dollars to pay a physician a retainer to ensure medical care would be available to all in the municipality. This plan, called the Municipal Doctor System, was implemented in 1916 and was followed shortly thereafter by collective action to develop hospitals through pooling municipal monies (Gelber, 1966).

As a result, in 1945, Saskatchewan was positioned to benefit from whatever federally funded programs the government would offer. When the federal government's decision to move ahead with the recommended programs was aborted, Saskatchewan determined that it would go ahead on its own. Because the hospital construction had been planned and was under way, this province was ready for the federal program funding hospital construction, a program the federal government was able to salvage from the aborted postwar reconstruction proposals of 1945 (Taylor, 1987). In addition, with these matched funds, Saskatchewan was ready to introduce a hospital insurance program in 1947, at least 10 years before the introduction of hospital insurance in most of the other provinces. Key architects of this planning and development were members of the Co-operative Commonwealth Federation (CCF), a predecessor of the New Democratic Party (NDP). Soon, Tommy Douglas emerged as a leader.

Having suffered with disease and disability as a child, Douglas understood the importance of good health care covered by health insurance and the need to make it available to all (Margoshes, 1999). Douglas became both premier and health minister at one point, helping to bring about his vision of a comprehensive health insurance program. Other provinces in Canada had also engaged in various programs and strategies to make "insurance against sickness" a reality (including the British Columbia Legislative Assembly's resolution of 1922 to urge the federal government to "give early consideration to legislation providing for an adequate system of insurance against sickness" and Alberta's adoption of initiatives similar to those in Saskatchewan). Saskatchewan's leadership became a model for the rest of Canada (Gelber, 1966). In fact, Saskatchewan, under Douglas, became the "laboratory" of pilot projects for what eventually became national health insurance programs involving hospital insurance and medical insurance. Table 3.2 outlines this history.

Although hospital insurance was greeted by almost all with appreciation and relief when it was introduced in Saskatchewan in 1946–47, the same could not be said about medical care insurance when it was introduced in 1961–62. The introduction of the Medicare program was radically opposed by physicians, who took strike action to protest what they regarded as a slip into socialized medicine. Their relative pleasure with hospital insurance is understandable. After World War I, and particularly after World War II, many of the new medical technologies discovered and advanced during the war years were introduced in North America. The average physician could not afford the new diagnostic and treatment technologies for the individual office. Therefore, hospitals became the logical place for doctors to access these new tools of their trade. As early as the 1920s, medical and surgical procedures previously performed at home had moved to

TABLE 3.2	Saskatchewan as a Laboratory for Federal Programs: Key Legislation	
YEAR	**PROVINCE OF SASKATCHEWAN**	**GOVERNMENT OF CANADA**
1916	Rural Municipality Act; Union Hospital Act	
1944		The Department of National Health and Welfare Act
1947	Hospital Insurance Act	Provincial grants, including public health grants and a grant for hospital construction
1956–57		Hospital Insurance and Diagnostic Services Act, with provision for in-patient insurance and testing
1962	Medical Care Insurance Act	
1967–68		Medical Care Act

hospitals. Hospital holdings of x-ray machines and laboratory equipment increased dramatically in the 20-year period following. By the early 1950s, hospitals had been transformed (Hastings & Mosley, 1980; Torrance, 1987).

The effect on nurses and nursing was equally dramatic. No longer were most nurses working relatively independently, caring for patients in homes. By 1948, about 65% of nurses were working in hospitals or nursing schools, as compared with 25% in 1930 (Coburn, 1988). This change in service venue created a significant shift in how nursing was practised and how it was valued. Stinson (1969), in describing and comparing the model nurse of the 1920s with the model nurse of the 1960s in terms of professionalization and deprofessionalization, observed that the private duty nurse of the 1920s was a "near-paragon of solo practice" (p. 333): She was not supervised by other nurses, was rarely supervised by physicians, and was quite autonomous. However, she had little authority over anyone but herself and, to some extent, the patient and the family. Stinson noted that the nurse of the 1960s had far more responsibility but less autonomy in her hospital-based and technology-laced practice. Further, this 1960s nurse had many "masters," including the doctor, the hospital administrator, the nursing supervisors, and possibly the patient and family (Stinson, 1969).

A Prime Minister From Saskatchewan

The final plank of Canada's health care system, a national Medicare program, was put in place in the mid-1960s. It would seem natural that the battle for Medicare fought in Saskatchewan would pave the way for a relatively easy introduction of a similar program in Canada. However, such was not the case. Many provinces had already established systems of private medical insurance they believed were superior to any national plan. At least three provinces, for example, paid all or part of the costs of health insurance for those considered poor risks while leaving the majority of the population who could afford voluntary insurance to the private sector (Taylor, 1987).

With the popularity of private medical insurance plans (particularly in the eyes of physicians and business leaders), and with hospitals now available for use, Prime Minister Diefenbaker, as leader of the Progressive Conservative government, was reluctant to hurry to introduce the long-promised medicare program. Instead, he chose to take the advice of the Canadian Medical Association (CMA) to appoint a Royal Commission on Health Services (1964, 1965) to study the matter. This commission was chaired by Justice Emmett Hall, and neither the prime minister nor the CMA would have believed that this commission would strongly recommend a national Medicare program. Yet when the commissioners considered the total package of health care services needed by a Canadian family, they rejected the extra costs of creating a means test for eligibility for these services and recommended that it was cost-effective to subsidize the 10 health insurance programs in Canada (Taylor, 1973).

Further, public support for a comprehensive health insurance system was evident. By the time this program came into being, a new government had been formed under the leadership of Prime Minister Lester B. Pearson, who could at last fulfill the longstanding Liberal election promise, the introduction of Medicare. As in Saskatchewan, this national program was controversial and politically costly. However, it served to complete the general blueprint proposed in the Marsh and Heagerty documents even though the final programs were not nearly as comprehensive nor as farsighted as the 1945 proposals.

So how did the federal government manage to succeed in introducing these federal programs when the BNA Act gave primary responsibility for health care to the provinces? This is a particularly germane question given that, in the late 1930s, another royal commission had been appointed to examine the matter of federal–provincial responsibility (Lindenfield, 1959). The commission's findings reaffirmed the provincial authority for health care as established in the BNA Act. The breakdown of the Postwar Reconstruction Conference reinforced the federal government's powerlessness to establish national programs. Yet the federal government was able to overcome these obstacles to develop national programs. How?

First, they compromised some of the blueprint for federal programs by developing a single-payer (the public) system utilizing the tax base to pay (health insurance) for health services that would be supplied by autonomous or semiautonomous "private" providers, such as physicians and hospitals (Fuller, 1998).

Next, ingenious ways were found to influence national standards in health care, approaches that continue to be the vehicle for such federal interventions today. One way was to amend the BNA Act. This was rarely used, and it was only used once for social security reasons—to introduce old-age pensions, so the provinces welcomed this without controversy. Another way was to give the provinces specific grants, because nothing could stop one government *giving* to another. The cost of taking the grant was that "rules" prescribed the way in which each specific grant (e.g., a grant for venereal disease control, for tuberculosis control, for hospital construction) had to be used. In fact, the federal government offered numerous grants to the provinces with a particular emphasis on public health, thereby establishing priorities and setting standards. These conditional grants offered in 1946–47 formed the basis of public health departments and programs within the provinces for many years (Defries, 1962), thereby fulfilling the objectives of the federal government without breaching constitutional mandates.

A third way to influence national standards in health care was to establish cost-shared programs, whereby the federal government would give any province roughly 50% of the cost of a program if that province paid the other 50% and agreed to a set of principles. The principles of Medicare included that the programs be universally available, comprehensive in coverage of services, portable across the provinces, and operated on a nonprofit basis. This particular strategy for developing national programs was used to introduce hospital insurance and diagnostic services in the late 1950s and again to introduce Medicare in the late 1960s. It frequently took several years before all provinces bought into either program, but most could not afford to forego the 50% funding offered. Both programs were difficult for the Quebec government to accept, with the consequence that citizens of Quebec were late beneficiaries of these programs. In Quebec, the longstanding tradition of Catholic charity (Cassidy, 1947), ties to the "Old World," a commitment to maintaining an identity, and a lag in industrial development (Lindenfield, 1959) were some of the barriers that precluded easy adoption of these and other federal programs.

Once these major federal–provincial programs were in place, both federal and provincial governments conducted extensive studies to determine the effectiveness of the established system. A theme of many of these studies was that costs were rising and were out of control. Consumers and politicians alike wanted to know how much is too much. All countries were facing rising health care costs, and there was tension in the allocation of resources regarding how much should go to the health care system and how much should go to the rest of society (Evans, 1984).

One federal study in the late 1970s was the second Hall Commission, which examined the existing system to determine its effectiveness (Hall, 1980). The Canadian Nurses Association (CNA) was quick to respond to its request for input. Their submission to the Health Services Review '79, entitled "Putting Health Back into Health Care" (CNA, 1980), represents positions nurses continue to take up with the federal government. Its recommendations included the following:

- That the existing legislation underlying the hospital and medical insurance programs be revised to allow the emergence of a health insurance program that would stimulate the development of primary health services, permit the introduction of new entry points, and promote the appropriate utilization of qualified health personnel
- That provincial legislation be revised to enable qualified nurses and other prepared health personnel to undertake activities currently defined as medical acts
- That remuneration of all health personnel be by salary
- That Health Services Review '79 strongly support the initiation of better preventive, diagnostic, and ambulatory care programs through various community-based points of entry
- That the federal and provincial governments, together with relevant nongovernmental organizations, develop criteria to ensure that the underlying principles of the Canadian health insurance system are being upheld
- That a health sciences research council be established to focus on the study of health services, the system of delivery, and its effectiveness
- That the federal government be requested to reinstitute a national health survey which would provide the necessary information on which to build and evaluate a health care system to meet the needs of the people
- That all governments and health profession organizations be urged by Health Services Review '79 to adopt, as a priority, better and broader health education programs to sensitize consumers to the cost of acute care services

Not surprisingly, the second Hall report, "A Commitment for Renewal: Health Services Review '79," was strongly supportive of the health programs implemented, and it was open to recommendations, such as those offered by CNA. This overall support of the health care system strengthened the federal government's conviction about the need to maintain these programs. Yet even with that conviction, both the federal government and the provinces were reluctant to tackle long-standing traditions in health care, such as moving physicians toward salary or capitation payment and away from fee-for-service payment, and implementing the types of recommendations for primary health care put forward by Canadian nurses. This includes care provided in an accessible health care system focused on health promotion and illness prevention with public participation, appropriate use of technology, and intersectoral cooperation (CNA, 2000b).

Enter Health Minister Monique Begin

In particular, the various government reports published between the mid-1960s and mid-1970s indicated grave concern about rising costs of medical care; indeed, costs did rise in the first few years of Medicare's introduction. Payments to doctors increased because doctors were now being paid to care for patients they had previously served without pay when those patients could not afford payment. Suddenly, reimbursement was available to physicians. But those mounting costs soon settled to a reasonable level before rising again as a function of a growing medical technology and changing demographics. During this time as well, the federal and provincial governments renegotiated the cost-sharing arrangements for health care and postsecondary education. Rather than continue on the roughly 50–50 basis of cost sharing, which left the federal government with a serious problem of predicting health care expenditures, the federal government transferred taxation points to the provinces in exchange for payment of a lower cash transfer to them (Van Loon, 1978). At the time, the provinces were delighted; the country's economy was good, and they stood to benefit from the additional taxation power. Yet political opposition to these federally sponsored programs continued.

Concerns about rising costs, about socialized medicine interfering with doctor–patient relationships, and about any number of other reasons were put forward for the need to increase the private operation of health services. In Alberta in particular, physicians moved to bill patients extra for the care they received based on the premise that limited Medicare funds restricted their right to adequate compensation for services. This practice, known as *extra billing* or *balance billing*, set the stage for a national drama as the federal health minister, Monique Begin, took a highly public stance against the Alberta government on this issue. With the transfer of tax points to the provinces, the federal government had lost some leverage in its insistence that the provinces adhere to the national standards for Medicare. The outcome was the passage of a new federal act meant to enforce the principles of Medicare.

Thus, the Canada Health Act was introduced in 1984 to affirm the four principles of Medicare and to add a fifth, "access to care" (Table 3.3). The act also replaced the Hospital Insurance and Diagnostic Services Act and the Medical Care Act, and it banned extra billing (Rice & Prince, 2000). The penalties for provinces that allowed extra billing involved withholding cash transfer payments, dollar for dollar, to those provinces. The residual effect of this action on the provinces has been strained relationships with the federal government and continual accusations of reduced funding. Although reduced funding is a reality, what the provinces seldom acknowledge is the provincial benefit of the tax point transfer they agreed to in 1977. This tax money, now collected by the provinces, was intended to be used for health services; where these funds are now being directed is not always clear to the public.

TABLE 3.3	Canada Health Act (1984): Principles of "Medicare"

Principle/Criterion/Condition	Definition
Public administration	The province's health care insurance plan must be administered and operated by a public authority accountable to the provincial government. Provincial governments determine the amount spent.
Comprehensiveness	The plan must insure all medically necessary services, i.e., services "for purposes of maintaining health, preventing disease, or diagnosing or treating an illness or injury, or disability" must be covered.
Accessibility	The plan must provide for all Canadians to have reasonable access to insured hospital and physician services without barriers. Additional charges to insured patients for insured services are not allowed. No one can be discriminated against on the basis of income, age, health status, etc.
Universality	The plan must entitle 100% of the insured population (i.e., eligible residents) to insured health services on uniform terms and conditions. This also means that Canadians do not have to pay an insurance premium in order to be covered through provincial health insurance programs.
Portability	The plan must ensure that Canadians are covered by their provincial plan when they move from province to province, or when they travel within Canada or abroad. There may be some limits on coverage for services provided outside Canada, and prior approval for nonemergency out-of-province services may be required.

From Health Canada (2002). *Canada's health care system*. Health Canada Web site and Canadian Nurses Association (2000a) fact sheet on the Canada Health Act, also on the CNA Web site, with permission.

The Klein and Harris Governments (Alberta and Ontario)

By the late 1980s, the economic downturn began to threaten seriously Canada's federal–provincial health care programs. The political climate of the Western world was strongly influenced by the dominant neo-conservative ideology of political leaders in England, the United States, and Canada (Prime Minister Brian Mulroney). The development of large corporations, a concentration of wealth, and free trade were outcomes of this ideology, which included adopting a business model for health care delivery, identifying people as deserving and undeserving, and growing attempts of governments to withdraw from involvement in comprehensive public programs and to promote private sector providers. In Alberta, Premier Ralph Klein took the lead in downsizing health care through sudden and severe budgetary cutbacks. For those who were involved in Premier Klein's health care roundtables, it was not difficult to see parallels between a book published in New Zealand called *Unfinished Business* and the tactics employed by the premier. Although participants in his roundtables urged Klein to implement changes over a period of several years to preserve the best of the systems in place, he was determined to act quickly. His use of the phrase that he "would not blink" seemed a sure sign that *Unfinished Business* had become his bible for health care reform. *Unfinished Business* included 10 "principles," and these seemed to take effect in Alberta (and later, in Ontario, when Premier Mike Harris followed Alberta's lead). These included recommendations to implement reform in quantum leaps, to regard speed as essential because it is almost impossible to go too fast, to ensure that momentum once started does not stop, to strive for consistency and credibility to create confidence, and to remember "not to blink" because public confidence rests on your composure (Douglas, 1993).

Thus began massive layoffs of hospital workers—particularly nurses. Although layoffs were occurring in other Canadian provinces as well, Klein's confidence in the rightness of the government's actions and the support he was enjoying from prominent business leaders gave impetus to the continued and often merciless dismissals of staff nurses and senior nurse leaders. Included in these cutbacks was the removal of one or two levels of nurse managers from the system, an action that ensured no one was there to advocate for professional nursing care. The effects of these actions are most evident today in the serious nursing shortages, the low morale in nursing, and the absence of clinical nurse leaders to mentor and support nurses entering practice and those changing practice settings (Broughton, 2001; Canadian Nursing Advisory Committee, 2002; Shamian & LeClair, 2000).

Part of the downsizing strategy included a push toward health care reform that promoted health care as just another "business" and promoted the regionalization of health services. Regionalization involved the rationalizing of services with some potential for good outcomes. However, when this approach was put in place too rapidly, limited attention was given to preserving the good elements of the system. The result has been that, in many areas, regionalization has been more destructive than constructive. Further, there has rarely been a good explanation as to how the effect of hospital closures would improve services (or even save money). In regionalization, the downsizing of the provincial health departments was also a consequence because centralized policies and services are no longer needed. The loss of intellectual ability, experience, and wisdom in public sector management and in health care policy development cannot be measured.

Although there is no question that some of these changes may have led to improved services, the cost to the morale of the health professionals, most of whom were excluded from decision making, has been monumental (Shamian & LeClair, 2000). Although considerable restructuring has occurred, actual health reform is not readily apparent.

Many regions also implemented program management, an approach adopted from the business world that is built on product-line management strategies. The goal in program management is the integration of care through "seamless systems" that would be devoted to one similar focus of care, such as heart health, to include the spectrum from prevention to tertiary care (Leatt, Lemieux-Charles, & Aird, 1994). However, adopting this business way of thinking overlooks the unique aspects of health care, including the fact that patients, for example, do not fit into neat categories like product lines such as shoes or cars. This might be described as the "false simplification of human life" (Saul, 1995). Although there is a cry for evidence-based practice, the evidence to support removing many good systems that were put in place to promote high-quality care is lacking.

In the midst of this conundrum, some parts of the health policy framework suggested by McIntosh (1914), Laframboise (1973), and Lalonde (1974), and by the CNA's response to the second Hall Commission Report (1980), began to resurface. In September 1994, the Meeting of Health Ministers received a report entitled *Strategies for Population Health: Reinvesting in the Health of Canadians*, which called for governments to address the entire range of factors that determine health rather than focus on risks and clinical factors related to particular diseases. The report also urged a focus on collective health rather than on individual health only. Its framework for action included attention to the social, economic, and physical environments, personal health practices, individual capacity and coping skills, and health services (Frank & Mustard, 1994; *Strategies,* 1994). Embedded in all of these strategies was healthy child development. As with the 1974 Lalonde Report, there was considerable discussion about the sensibility of such an approach with limited action taken. This was followed by a rapidly decreasing level of interest by provincial governments, who likely could see only an expanded mandate in health care when their key desire was for a reduced one.

In 1994, the federal government established a National Forum on Health Care (1997) to make recommendations about the "crisis in health care." This eight-member committee studied various aspects of health care and came out in strong support of the merits of current Canadian health programs, adding to them the need to enhance home care services as well as to improve coverage of pharmaceutical costs. Most of the forum's (1997) recommendations have yet to be implemented as other political agendas shift the emphasis in health care reform. Many Canadians doubt that the promise of regionalization has been fulfilled; many see it as a way for provincial governments to shed their responsibility to regional boards, who lack the funding to effect needed changes in service offerings but who will be blamed for service deficiencies.

In 1999, the federal and provincial governments signed the Social Union Agreement, the purpose of which was to define the principles "for the design and development of social policies and programs" (CNA, 2000a). The principles include citizen engagement and accountability, and the agreement reconfirmed the conditions (principles) of the Canada Health Act of 1984.

Yet regional variations in availability and caliber of services remain problematic within each province. Further, data released by the Canadian Institutes for Health Information indicate mounting evidence of wide gaps in health care benefits across the provinces. In May 2001, for example, the press reported on a survey suggesting that the likelihood of surviving a heart attack varied from 9% mortality during a hospital stay in Alberta to 18% in Newfoundland. Further evidence of regional variation is seen in the erosion of the principle of portability of the Canada Health Act. For example, the experience of those attempting to coordinate benefit programs for employees of nationally based voluntary organizations leads one to conclude that variations in health services covered in each province are increasingly detrimental to a comprehensive national health insurance program that has portability as one of its principles.

Enter Shirley Douglas, Actress and Advocate

In the fall of 2000, Alberta's Premier Klein chose to use his political power to assert provincial responsibility for health care. He made clear his plan to make legal provision in Alberta for the increasing involvement of private for-profit health services delivery. He did this by developing Bill 11, a bill that made provision for using public health care funds to subsidize private for-profit acute care hospitals, private imaging clinics, and other private for-profit services (Alberta Association of Registered Nurses [AARN], 2000).

The AARN was among the groups most actively opposed to this bill. In other provinces as well, there were protests about Alberta's Bill 11 by those who regarded it as destructive to Canada's health programs. In British Columbia, many nurses joined the march against this bill, and these protests were led by Shirley Douglas, actress, advocate for Medicare, and daughter of the late Tommy Douglas, the boy from Saskatchewan.

A Committed Ex-Premier and a Senator

In early April 2001, a former premier of Saskatchewan, Roy Romanow, was commissioned by an Order in Council of the federal government

to inquire into and undertake policies and measures respectful of the jurisdictions and powers in Canada required to ensure over the long term the sustainability of a universally accessible, publicly funded health system, that offers quality services to Canadians and strikes a balance between these investments in prevention and health maintenance and those directed to care and treatment (Commission on the Future of Health Care in Canada, 2002, p. iii).

By November 2002, Romanow tabled his report after one of the most extensive public consultations in Canadian history. Through these consultations he was able confirm that

- Canadians remain attached to the values at the heart of the system
- Medicare has served Canadians extremely well
- The system is as sustainable as Canadians want it to be
- Canadians want and need a truly national health care system
- Canadians want and need a more comprehensive health care system
- Canadians want and need a more accountable health care system
- The Canadian system is based on values (Commission on the Future of Health Care in Canada, 2002, p. xvi-xix)

Romanow offered numerous recommendations in his 356-page report, almost all supported by strong research evidence secured through commission staff and commissioned papers. His key recommendations centered on the need for an infusion of funds into health care with calls for a dedicated health transfer payment to the provinces; a Canada health care covenant; modernizing the Canada Health Act; a home care transfer for post-acute, palliative, and mental health care; a catastrophic drug transfer; and a rural and remote access fund. He also recommended the formation of a Health Council for Canada, reminiscent of the Dominion-Provincial Health Council formed in the 1940s, and he advised against for-profit delivery of health services.

Meanwhile, the Senate of Canada was also busily engaged in parallel activity by authorizing a committee led by Senator Michael Kirby to examine the fundamental principles on which Canada's publicly funded system is based, its historical development, the pressures and constraints on the system, and the role of the federal government in Canada's health care system. Kirby recommended no change to the Canada Health Act, set funding priorities on service-based funding for hospitals, and urged that greater responsibility be given to regional health authorities for delivering or contracting out publicly insured health services. As priorities, he recommended primary health care reform, a health care guarantee, coverage of catastrophic prescription costs, and home care. Kirby did not address Canadian values, and he left the door open to more private sector involvement. As Roberge (2003) observed,

One of the ironies of the current crisis and the nature of the debate is that it was the desire to ensure access that led to the creation of public health insurance in Canada in the first place. Now it appears that a desire to ensure access is being used as an argument to move away from a public system. Public health insurance was designed to shift the burden from the individual to the collective through government funding. Now the financial burden of health care on governments has led to reduced access and there is pressure to shift the burden, at least in part, back to the individual (p. 14).

Whereas Romanow's findings were based on public consultation with over 40,000 Canadians, Kirby could only boast 400 voices.

Some argue that portraying Kirby as the proponent of privatization and Romanow as the champion of a public system creates a false polarity (Chodos & MacLeod, 2004), but both Kenny (2004), an ethicist, and Deber (2004), an economist, disagree. Kenny suggests that the difference lies in Kirby's suggestion to let the market decide for itself, while Romanow sees health care as a moral enterprise and not a business venture. Deber concludes that very limited benefits are likely to arise from an increase in the delivery of for-profit clinical services. She suggests that

This does not mean that they should not be outlawed, or that one should be comfortable with the status quo. But neither does it present any reason why they should be encouraged.... Improving care delivery, particularly more careful attention to best practices, communication and coordination, appears essential (pp. 59–60).

The Canadian Health Services Research Foundation (2004) has pointed out that drawing money from another source does not make the system more affordable because Canadians still have to pay for it. Further, sustainability is not only about money. Included in measures to sustain the system are changes that must be made in the system, and normally changes that have been resisted, such as a greater focus on primary health care, better home care services, more focused preventive services, more interdisciplinary teamwork, and salaried physicians. Sinclair (2004, p. 69) quotes Tommy Douglas, who had stated:

When we began to plan medicare [in the mid-forties], we pointed out that it would be in two phases. The first phase would be to remove the financial barrier between those giving the service and those receiving it. The second phase would be to re-organize and revamp the delivery system—and of course that is a big item. It's the big thing that we haven't done yet.

As Kenny (2002, p. 29) points out, if these and similar recommendations to sustain the system are "eminently sensible and obviously necessary for maximum efficiency, why have they not been implemented? Who benefits from the status quo?"

In part as a consequence of these two reports, in February 2003, a Health Care Renewal Accord was passed by the First Ministers' conference to reaffirm their commitment to the five principles of health insurance in Canada. In this accord, they called for a standard of care that would include

- Access to a health care provider 24 hours a day, 7 days a week
- Access to diagnostic procedures and treatments
- Reduction in duplication of patient histories and testing for every provider they visit
- Access to quality home and community care services
- Access to quality care no matter where they live
- A health care system that is efficient, responsive, and adapting to changing needs (Health Care Renewal Accord, 2003).

To reach these goals, the federal government agreed to establish a long-term Canada Health Transfer (CHF) to include a portion of the current cash and tax points corresponding to provincial expenditures and with predictable annual increases. An election call in the ensuing months and a federal election on June 28, 2004, resulted in a Liberal minority government with many matters yet undecided and many actions in limbo. However, in the campaigns of three major political parties, improving health care for Canadians was a very strong election platform, and, by July, Prime Minister Paul Martin had made arrangements to meet with the premiers to "hammer out a deal" for health care. Whether this "deal" will address restoring public health resources remains to be seen.

Nelia Laroza and Tecla Lin: Nursing Heroes

In Spring 2003, Toronto was rocked by the outbreak of sudden acute respiratory syndrome, commonly known as SARS. As a result of that outbreak, two nurses lost their lives on the frontlines of caregiving. Nelia Laroza, who worked at the North York General Hospital, was the first nurse to contract the disease and die of SARS. She was 51. Tecla Lin contracted SARS during her work at Toronto's West Park Healthcare Centre's interim SARS unit, where 14 infected staff members from Scarborough Hospital had been transferred. She was 58. Her husband also died from SARS (Canadian Nurses Foundation, 2004). Although details of the tragedy of SARS and its aftermath in Asia and in Canada, particularly the lack of attention to the voices of nurses that may have prevented the second Toronto outbreak, are not the substance for this particular chapter, Laroza and Lin are heroes. Their legacy is having exposed the inadequacies of the public health system in Canada and should include a focus on fixing these serious threats to the life and health of Canadians.

Over the past two decades, it has become increasingly clear that cutbacks to the public health system have created a high degree of vulnerability for all Canadians. In the mid-1990s, the quality of the water supplies in many cities and towns, particularly in Walkerton, Ontario, was found to be faulty. As the years have progressed, many municipalities have had to put their citizens on an unsafe water supply alert for a temporary period. The advent of mad cow disease (bovine spongiform encephalopathy [BSE]), the West Nile virus, and many other threats to public health have found the system wanting. As some of the earliest advances in maintaining health and preventing disease in early Canadian history had to do with improving water supply, sanitation, and conducting meat inspections, it is somewhat alarming to think that we may have returned to situations somewhat akin to pre-confederation days. When basic pillars for health promotion and preservation are removed from the health system, there are bound to be serious threats to health. Public health measures such as these have been taken for granted by most Canadians, and the warnings are clear: A public health system cut to the bone is not able to safeguard the health of Canadians.

The outbreak of SARS was another sign that systems had broken down. Commissions appointed to examine the problems found "serious disconnects" at all levels (Gottlieb, Shamian, & Chan, 2004)

...between governments and public health departments; between public health departments and hospitals; among and within hospitals; between hospital administrators and hospital units; and among public health units, government and the media. There was a disconnect between those making the policies and issuing directives and those needing directives to follow—directives that in fact did not fit the realities of the frontline.

In short, systems for dealing with outbreaks or epidemics have been so minimized as to be ineffective. The tragedy is that since the SARS outbreak, there seems to be limited action across the country to avoid and minimize similar outbreaks, and recommendations of reports released from the various SARS commissions have yet to be taken up (Office of Nursing Policy, 2003). The long-term effect on peoples' lives and health of, for example, the SARS outbreak is profound (McGillis Hall, Angus, Peter, et al., 2003).

■ RECURRING POLITICAL AND ECONOMIC THEMES IN HEALTH CARE: IMPACT ON NURSING

For more than two decades, Evans (1984) and his colleagues in health economics provided sound evidence to show the effect of rising costs when public and private for-profit systems coexist. They found that duplicate administrative costs and for-profit practices increase costs without an accompanying increase in quality health care. They also found that socially and economically disadvantaged patients' access to health care is affected by for-profit health services delivery. Further, they highlighted the lack of evidence to support the claim that introducing competition into health care with private for-profit systems will provide better and less expensive care.

John Ralston Saul (1995) spoke about the corporatist society, urging that people be alert and react to false consciousness, stating "...we live in a corporatist society with soft pretensions to democracy. More power is slipping every day over to groups [sic, corporations]. That is the meaning of the marketplace ideology and of our passive acceptance of whatever form globalization happens to take" (pp. 34–35). Andre Picard (1999) added a note of caution to this matter in stating that free trade may be boosting corporate profits, but it is systematically undermining public health measures and leading to poorer health for Canadians.

Canada does, in fact, have a mix of public and private for-profit care, but the private for-profit element is normally linked to certain sectors of care. Roughly 70% of total health expenditures in Canada are paid by public sector funding, with 30% financed privately through supplementary insurance, employer-sponsored benefits, or direct out-of-pocket expenditures (Health Canada, 2002). For example, dental and orthodontic care falls outside the publicly funded health services in most provinces. There are also numerous private for-profit nursing homes because these fall outside the acute care and medically oriented emphasis of Canada's health programs, and complementary medicine is not normally covered.

What is different about initiatives in Alberta, Ontario, and some other provinces is that private for-profit care, subsidized by government, would be offered as a service competing with the publicly funded service. What does this do to integration and coordination of care? Will this eventually lead to patients with better finances routinely jumping waiting lists to pay for their surgeries and other services, thereby creating even longer waiting times for those unable to purchase a place at the top of the queue? Might it lead to a competition for health professionals if a for-profit service offers significantly better salaries and benefits to doctors and nurses, thereby creating a two-class system of care? Should private profit through public funds be permitted in health care?

In June 2001, the Organization for Economic Cooperation and Development reported that 29.4% of Canada's health care spending was in the private sector, which is twice the rate of the United Kingdom and Sweden, and that Canada's health care ranking had dropped (National Post, 2001). This 29.4% estimate stands in sharp contrast to Evans' estimate of 15% as the for-profit share of health care expenditures in the early 1980s (1984, p. 209).

■ PAST AND CURRENT IMPLICATIONS

In reflecting on the way health services unfolded in Canada, it can be helpful to think about all the "what-ifs." How would the current situation be different if different choices had been made?

The What-Ifs of Health Care

What if we had paid more attention to socioeconomic and environmental influences on health in the early 1900s? What if that emphasis had continued to be strong throughout the decades? What if nurses had been able to continue to take a greater role in public health services and in institutional care, similar to their more independent role between the 1920s and the 1940s? What if medical care insurance had been introduced before the building of hospitals and before the passage of the Hospital Insurance and Diagnostic Services Act? What if Klein in Alberta, and Harris in Ontario, had proceeded more slowly with their health reforms and had involved health professionals in thinking through how to move toward goals of integration and coordination of care? What if the CNA's (1980) recommendations to the second Hall Commission had been implemented when they were offered? Why, despite some visionary thinkers and planners dating as far back as the early 1900s, do power dynamics within the health care system seem so little changed?

Our Heritage in Health Care

Despite all its flaws, Canada's system of health care is well-worth saving. While respecting its limitations, one can make a few general statements about the system's virtues. People in Canada do not have to be as fearful about their access to care nor about the devastating costs of an illness or surgery as do many in the United States. And Canadian patients have considerably more choice in the selection of their doctors—and even their hospitals—than many of their neighbors to the south. Many managed care plans in the United States, for example, offer extremely limited choices to the consumers, reserving considerable choice for the managers of the plans whose goal is to purchase the most cost-efficient services for their patient groups.

Physicians in Canada have freedom to choose their practice locations without restriction, and they can set their work pace and manage their scheduling. Canadian national programs have also allowed for an enviable collection of data about hospital stays, patients' conditions, and physician services. And the programs still have the support of the majority of the public.

The serious pressures on the system in the 21st century need to be carefully considered both in relation to our historical legacy and to the wider context of international capital in which our health care system and other countries' health care systems are embedded (Coburn & Rappolt, 1999). Problems arising from this legacy are our failure to develop a comprehensive system of care and our failure to re-create, re-energize, and renew our systems based on known evidence. These problems also represent our failure to change traditional practices, to move to primary health care, and to utilize all health professionals well. All of these problems might well be included in what Coburn and Rappolt (1999) describe as the "logic of medicare."

So what has our history, our heritage, told us about our current situation in health care and the need and potential for change?

1. We continue to operate under the terms of the BNA Act provisions (now incorporated into the Constitution Act) for determining federal and provincial responsibilities in health care. This means that we operate with the same division of federal and provincial responsibilities in health care as seemed timely in 1867. Such a division of responsibility leaves room for provinces to assert their authority when it suits their particular situations, and it forces the federal government to work through three main alternate approaches to influence health care. More importantly, it leaves room for each level of government to blame the other for failure to take action (e.g., in areas such as pollution or home care) and to leave the public waiting (and often lobbying) for the impasse to be overcome.

2. We continue to talk about social determinants of health but have yet to deal with those determinants in a comprehensive and committed way. Governments and the public are both responsible for the lack of attention to these matters, yet conditions like full employment, a guaranteed annual income, stamping out poverty, and other such fundamental health-related conditions could have a significant effect on improving the health status of all and decreasing expenditures on tertiary health care.

3. Medicare continues to enjoy a high level of public support, although that level is slipping as corporate claims of better, more efficient care by for-profit medicine woo the public to their way of thinking. This is often accomplished by scare tactics, which distort the facts about current and projected public health care spending. As a prominent U.S. medical ethicist stated some years ago, "Today's exigencies are created less by scarcity of resources than by a disinclination to share them" (Pellegrino, 1975, p. 49).

4. As our history shows, in implementing federal and provincial programs, we have continued to compromise on what should be included and how the systems should operate. In the mid-1940s, we did not adopt a comprehensive approach to health and social security as had been suggested by Marsh and Heagerty. Instead, we chose to implement publicly appealing programs selectively (Armstrong, Armstrong, Bourgeault, et al., 2000). This had the effect of setting us up for rising costs because many of these programs were oriented toward high-technology medicine (e.g., the hospital insurance and diagnostic services program) and took the focus away from holistic patient care. Further, these programs excluded funding for many services, such as nursing homes, home care, and pharmaceutical coverage, and thereby disadvantaged elderly and poor people. Later during the introduction of Medicare, Saskatchewan first and the federal government second abandoned the concept of all-on-a-salary and gave in to doctors' demands for fee-for-service payments instead. This also paved the way for cost increases for health care and closed the door to a more level playing field in power relationships among physicians, nurses, and other health professionals. This has had a serious effect on women and on nursing.

5. The majority of nurses work in hospitals or other institutions where their autonomy is more limited than that of their counterparts working in the community. Relationships between physicians and nurses are not ideal, and this does not create the best environment for high-quality care.

6. The promise of health reform has yet to be realized; in fact, reforms such as regionalization may have added to the shortfall in comprehensive care as different regions make different decisions about what services they are prepared to offer.

7. Canada has failed to manage the growth of medical technology in a rational way. We have been unable to set limits to professional desires and public expectations.

8. The CNA's recommendations to the second Hall Commission continue to be as necessary today as they were in 1980. However, we have yet to develop primary health care services, to make legislative provision for new entry points to the system, or to promote better use of qualified health personnel. Health promotion and disease prevention are key recommendations critical to current population needs.

■ WHAT CONSTRAINS FUNDAMENTAL CHANGES IN THE HEALTH CARE SYSTEM?

Many health care policy experts agree that fundamental health care system problems have either not been addressed or have been dealt with marginally, often by throwing money at them. Leatt and colleagues (2000, p. 32) noted that "in comparison to other countries, Canada has a relatively static healthcare system. Many providers are organized and paid in the same ways as when Medicare was implemented in the 1960s." Many policymakers, past and present, continue to identify concerns and offer worthwhile suggestions, but they may still constrain their perceptions of what could be by thinking "within the box" of health care; there is a pressing need to think "outside the box."

To think "outside the box," for example, would be to question whose interests are being served in keeping the system relatively unchanged since the 1960s. We need to ask what effect free trade and increased moves to globalization have had on maintaining a system characterized by medical dominance, an emphasis on technology without limits, unequal access to care, and marginalization of many health professionals and patient groups. It is also necessary to ask what effect ideologies of individualism and egalitarianism have had on our inability to see the socioeconomic barriers that prevent patients from taking personal responsibility for their health (Anderson & Reimer-Kirkham, 1998).

Joan Anderson, a nursing professor at the University of British Columbia (UBC), and her colleagues from various academic disciplines have engaged in thinking outside the box. They suggest that the rhetoric that emerges from assumptions of individuals' equal opportunities to maintain good health, for example, are embedded in some of the finest government policies about health promotion. This rhetoric blinds us to the actual barriers to health care (e.g., clinic hours from 9 to 5, uncomfortable waiting rooms, inadequate financial assistance for healthful diets). These researchers stressed the importance of understanding and acknowledging assumptions in our health institutions today so we can move toward fundamental changes in the health care system. Recognizing the context of our "medical–industrial system," they believe, would allow us to see that the capitalist world system drives the economic realities of health care (Anderson & Reimer-Kirkham, 1998).

This thinking is like that of John Ralston Saul (1995) and others who urge us to not be complacent and accepting of the way things are. Saul suggests that readily agreeing that health care costs are out of control and unaffordable is a false consciousness. As noted previously, there is no question about the need to work toward greater coordination and efficiencies in health care, as in any line of work. But, at the end of the day, the questions remain: Where else is the money going? What other corporate demands are driving health care? Who is profiting by maintaining the status quo in health care?

Within health care, recent media attention has, once again, been directed at the extremely high and rising costs the pharmaceutical companies are imposing on the health care dollar and the government dollars the Canadian government is investing in these private firms. The promised return on this investment was to have been job creation in Canada. Yet according to media sources (Robinson, 2001), there was minuscule job creation as a result, and generic drug companies were limited in their ability to reduce the cost of drugs by recent federal legislation. Another media report began to surface in late spring 2004, when the case of *Jacques Chaoulli et al. v. Attorney General of Quebec* raised the issue of "whether there is an infringement of Charter rights that occurs when the public system is unable to provide timely access to needed services while simultaneously prohibiting individuals from purchasing these services using their own resources" (Chodos & MacLeod, 2004, pp. 24–25). This case, currently being considered in the Supreme Court of Canada, could have far-reaching implications for the future of health care in Canada.

■ WHAT WILL DRIVE THE HEALTH CARE SYSTEM IN THE 21ST CENTURY?

Several analysts (Armstrong et al., 2000; Coburn & Rappolt, 1999) provide insights for understanding the context of health care today and prospects for tomorrow. They suggest that the gradual rise in medical dominance over the past decades in Canada and the implementation of Medicare by the governments in Canada were the last keys in the welfare state. In their analysis, Coburn and Rappolt (1999) see this as representing the triumph for labor and for the state (the government). However, they suggest that the gradual decline of medical dominance in health care and a decline in government involvement in health care has occurred as a result of a "...major transformation of national and international political economies towards the internationalization of capital" (p. 142). This has led to an increase in business power and a decrease in the relative autonomy of the state.

Coburn and Rappolt (1999) suggest that the "...welfare state, and particularly anything to do with labour market policy, is brought under fierce attack from a newly united right and its international and national agents in the business community, in neoliberal international institutions such as the International Monetary Fund, in national neoconservative policy institutions and think tanks, as well as the conservatively skewed media" (p. 152). Labeling this relatively recent phenomena as the "internationalization of capital" or "global capitalism," Coburn and Rappolt note how the International Monetary Fund, the World Bank, and the new ideologic unity between large and small business have had substantial influence on domestic business interests. This has enhanced the power of business with Canadian governments (both federal and provincial) and has particularly strengthened the hand of American influences on governments. Thus, free trade agreements are viewed as inevitable costs of keeping Canada competitive, even though they have the potential to undermine Canadian social programs.

The potential scenario here is that governments' gradual undermining of social programs causes the public to see these programs as inadequate or outdated for 21st-century needs. One has only to cut costs to particular services for so long before the public comes to believe that there must be no more money and, therefore, there is "no choice" except to welcome private for-profit health care services. The effect has been one of transformation with new "...structures of class, state, welfare state, health care, health profession interaction [taking] one form under the particular dynamics of monopoly capitalism and [assuming] a new form under the somewhat different structure of global capitalism" (Coburn & Rappolt, 1999, p. 160). The overall impact has been designed "...to produce powerlessness...making citizens powerless within their own countries" (p. 160).

Yet when Coburn and Rappolt (1999) examine how "global" globalization really is, they point out that within the three major trading blocs in the world, the greatest influence on Canada is from the United States; the effect in health care is that we are harmonizing downward toward this partner (p. 161). (This strong U.S. influence has become even more apparent since the September 11, 2001, terrorist attacks on the World Trade Center in New York, as many cherished Canadian policies in areas outside of health care, such as border guards carrying firearms in Canada, changed because of U.S. demands.) By altering the balance of power in Canada, the Free Trade Agreement (the agreement between the United States and Canada for free trade) and NAFTA (the North American Free Trade Agreement that includes Mexico) have far-ranging consequences for Canada's social fabric and its social policies (p. 161). But even Coburn argues that there are "...degrees of freedom and openings for resistance to neoliberal doctrines" (p. 160). To suggest that there is no choice left and that we cannot expect our social programs to continue is to adopt a fatalistic view that flies in the face of the power of individual and collective action to make a difference. A documentary called *The Corporation*, which was shown in theaters across the country in 2004, makes this point most clearly.

■ NURSES LEADING TO INFLUENCE CHANGE

If nurses are to be effective leaders in influencing change both individually and through collective action, some homework is needed. Nurses need to understand the history and structures of the health care system in Canada, to educate themselves to the needs of their patients, and to set goals and work together to achieve those goals.

What Nurses Need to Know

Individually, there is a need for nurses to know about the history of Canadian health care, or at least to be aware of basic programs and structures that have been put in place over time. This includes some understanding of the historical ideologic debates and how those same debates continue to play out in health care today. This knowledge and understanding should not only give nurses confidence in stating their case but also ensure that they are not susceptible to being silenced by others' rhetoric. Additionally, nurses must be clear about some of the international and national pressures on the health care system and be ready to push against the perceived inevitability of a greater uptake of the business orientation that can diminish the effectiveness of health care delivery.

Second, nurses need good—and updated—information. This includes keeping up to date with public debates in the media and elsewhere and also digging deeper to uncover reliable facts and other viewpoints. Professional nursing associations, educational institutions, public libraries, and the Internet can be helpful resources for nurses.

Other information needed by nurses includes keeping abreast of the influence of trade agreements on health care and professional practice as well as on basic needs for the public's health, such as an adequate supply of clean water, clean air, security, and other essentials of life. The knowledge of ethics in nursing practice is critical to reflection on these issues (Storch, Rodney, & Starzomki, 2004). Nurses also need to know about their professional associations, including the freedom and responsibilities of self-regulation and the importance of collective action.

What Nurses Need to Be

Above all, nurses need to be well-educated, good listeners, and sensitive caregivers. Nurses need to see and respond to the many people who are marginalized in society—aboriginal peoples, immigrants, different ethnic groupings, women and particularly single mothers and their children living in poverty, poor elderly people, and so forth. We also need to see and critically think about the dominant players in health care and seek to understand their views as well as direct attention toward ways to broaden and influence their thinking (e.g., Pauly, 2004; Varcoe, 2004). Despite the difficulties nursing faces today in regard to being valued, we need to keep on caring without regard for race, color, creed, religious persuasion, or political alignments. In short, we need to continue to be role models of caring practices.

What Nurses Need to Do

Collectively, nurses need to be willing to work together to reach good outcomes for their patients and for themselves. Canada has fine examples of nurses involved in collective action to make a difference. The push toward Direct Access to Care in Alberta, led by the AARN in the early 1990s, is one example of such collective action to influence the types of issues nurses continue to strive for (AARN, 1993). Similar activities are part of other provincial nursing association agendas, including specific focuses during provincial and federal elections, such as the Registered Nurses Association of Ontario (RNAO, 1999), and in the activities of individual nurses (e.g., Wilson, 1996).

Nurses also need to use the knowledge gained through nursing education and nurse–patient relationships to focus attention on the determinants of health. Frank and Mustard (1994), and many before them, demonstrated the relationships between illness and socioeconomic factors. In addition to noting how the job hierarchy influences health, these authors suggested that "…an individual's sense of achievement, self-esteem, and control over his or her work and life appears to affect health and well-being" (p. 9). As nurses come to know their patients, they see the effects of these variables on patient well-being and on their own health. That is important knowledge to be utilized in dialogue with politicians or bureaucrats.

Working collectively toward the goal of primary health care for all is also critical work for nurses today (Rodger, 1993). The evidence is in: Nurses in advanced nursing practice make a difference to patient care and can improve the health system overall. Unfortunately, attempts to implement advanced nursing practice are often thwarted by physician, government, or business interests who see a loss of power for their own interests if they collaborate with nurses in practice or support nurses' independence to practise. Such is the case of the nurse practitioner movement in Ontario, wherein family health networks failed to use the full range of services nurse practitioners could offer (Mackie, 2001). However, the persistence of nurses in moving toward these patient-centered goals continues to make a difference within specific areas, and has a spillover effect over time (Pauly et al., 2004).

Individually, nurses can also be ready to speak, to question, and to spread hope (Broughton, 2001). As nurses, we may not have all the answers, but we do know most of the questions. With regard to information about the political economy discussed earlier in this text, an individual nurse may not have complete knowledge but can ask politicians, government bureaucrats, as well as other civil servants, neighbors, friends, and colleagues questions to make them think and potentially to influence their actions however large or small they may be. This is to move against a place of powerlessness.

The history and current status of Canadian health care make it clear that many of the important ideas and services in health care came about through struggle and persistence. A commitment to change is a commitment to engage in a political struggle that accompanies the change (Anderson & Reimer-Kirkham, 1998; Rodney et al., 2002; Storch et al., 2002).

■ SUMMARY

Nurses need to clarify what drives today's health care system, particularly in regard to the underpinnings of Medicare, the international economic manipulation of resources available for health care, and related disempowerment of health care professionals.

The same value conflicts that we see today were inherent in the development of Canadian policies and programs since their inception: a focus on individual responsibility and self-reliance versus collective responsibility; a free market system versus more socially oriented collective policies and programs in health care (the privatization debate); an emphasis on scientific discovery and technologic imperatives versus humanism and care for the disadvantaged; and those who believe that all have equal opportunities to health care versus the reality that gender, race, and class differences affect the way in which health care is delivered.

These are some of the influences that keep Canada's health care system focused on primary care as opposed to primary health care: "*Primary care* is a medical concept referring to a situation wherein the physician provides diagnosis, treatment, and follow-up for a specific disease or problem" (CNA, 2000b). *Primary health care*, as adopted by the World Health Organization in 1978 as the basis for the delivery of health services, most effectively involves both "a philosophy and an approach" to the way health services are delivered. It includes health promotion, disease prevention, curative services, rehabilitative care, and supportive or palliative care (CNA, 2000b). Primary health care involves a shift from traditional practices and power dynamics in health care to a system in which all health professionals are utilized to their maximum potential to effect good patient outcomes in care. Nurse practitioners, advanced practice nurses, and staff nurses alike are able to practise to their full scope of practice in this model.

This is the model of care Canadian nurses have sought for almost three decades, and it continues to be a model worth pursuing. In fact, it is one of the CNA's two key goals in the new millennium; the other goal is achieving improved quality of work environments for nurses.

Nurses can influence change by attending to the history, current status, and future projections for health care; by being listening and caring caregivers; and by taking action individually and collectively to influence greater attention to social determinants of health and better health care provision for their patients.

As nurses, we need to be clear about our own values and opinions and able to stand by them so our voices can help shape better approaches to health care. If we are not prepared to do so, nursing and nurses will have little to say in the health care system of tomorrow.

Online Resources

Add to your knowledge of this issue:

Canadian Nurses Association   www.cna-nurses.ca
Health Canada   www.hc-sc.gc.ca

REFLECTIONS on the Chapter . . .

1. In what ways do you think the Canadian health care system would have been different and less subject to political influence if the Fathers of Confederation had chosen to assign principal responsibility for health care and education to the federal government rather than to the provinces?

2. If medical care insurance had been introduced before the introduction of hospital insurance, what differences might we have seen in the formation of health facilities? What contributions do you think this might have made in controlling the costs of technology? Would primary health care likely have become the norm?

3. Do you believe that health care costs are out of control? Why or why not?

4. In reflecting on what you know about nurses' individual or collective actions to influence better health care, what types of knowledge have they utilized to influence change?

5. To what degree have you felt powerless or powerful against business interests in health care? Why have you felt that way?

ACKNOWLEDGMENTS

The author acknowledges, with gratitude, the helpful contributions of Bernadette Pauly and an anonymous reviewer, which brought greater clarity to several sections of this chapter.

References

Achbar, M. (Producer/Director), Abbot, J. (Director/Editor), & Simpson, B. (Producer). (2003). *The Corporation*. [Motion Picture]. Canada: Big Picture Media Corporation.
Alberta Association of Registered Nurses (AARN). (1993). Direct access to services provided by registered nurses: A nursing perspective. *AARN Newsletter, 49*(1), 15–17.

_____. (2000). AARN action on Bill 11. The health care protection act (HCPA). *Alberta RN, 56*(5), 6.

Anderson, J., & Reimer-Kirkham, S. (1998). Constructing nation: The gendering and racializing of the Canadian health care system. In V. Strong-Boag, S. Grace, A. Eisenberg, et al. (Eds.), *Painting the maple: Essays on race, gender, and the construction of Canada* (pp. 242–261). Vancouver: UBC Press.

Armstrong, P., Armstrong, H., Bourgeault, I., et al. (2000). *"Heal thyself": Managing health care reform.* Aurora, Ontario: Garamond Press.

Bliss, M. (1975). A preface. In L. Marsh, *Report on social security for Canada.* Toronto: University of Toronto Press.

Broughton, H. (2001). *Nursing leadership: Unleashing the power.* Ottawa: Canadian Nurses Association.

Canadian Health Services Research Foundation. (2004). *Myth: For profit, ownership of facilities would lead to a more efficient health care system.* CHSRF: Ottawa.

Canadian Nurses Association. (1980). *Putting "health" back into health care*: Submission to the Health Services Review '79. Ottawa: Author.

_____. (2000a). *The Canada Health Act.* Ottawa: Author.

_____. (2000b). *The primary health care approach.* Fact sheet. Ottawa: Author.

Canadian Nurses Foundation. (2004, Spring). Nursing heros. *Foundation Focus,* 1–2.

Canadian Nursing Advisory Committee. (2002). *Our health, our future: Creating quality workplaces for nurses.* Final report. Ottawa: Health Canada.

Cassidy, H. M. (1947). The Canadian social services. *The Annals of the Academy of Political and Social Sciences, 253*(September), 190–201.

Coburn, D. (1988). The development of Canadian nursing: Professionalization and proletarianization. *International Journal of Health Services, 18*(3), 437–456.

Coburn, D., & Rappolt, S. (1999). The "logic of medicare": Variants of capitalism and medical dominance. Contextualizing profession-state relationships. In D. Coburn, S. Rappolt, I. Bourgeault, et al. (Eds.), *Medicine, nursing and the state* (pp. 139–167). Aurora, Ontario: Garamond Press.

Chodos, H., & MacLeod, J. J. (2004). Romanow and Kirby on the public/private divide in healthcare: Demystifying the debate. *HealthcarePapers, 4*(4), 10–25.

Commission on the Future of Healthcare in Canada. (2002). Commissioner R. J. Romanow. Ottawa: Health Canada.

Deber, R. B. (2004). Cats and categories: Public and private in Canadian healthcare. *HealthcarePapers, 4*(4), 51–60

Defries, R. D. (1962). *The federal and provincial health services in Canada* (2nd ed.). Toronto: Canadian Public Health Association.

Douglas, R. (1993). *Unfinished business.* Auckland, New Zealand: Random House.

Evans, R. (1984). *Strained mercy: The economics of Canadian health care.* Toronto: Butterworths.

Frank, J. W., & Mustard, J. F. (1994). The determinants of health from a historical perspective. *Daedalus,* Fall, 1–19.

Fuller, C. (1998). *Caring for profit: How corporations are taking over Canada's health care system.* Vancouver: New Star Books.

Gelber, S. M. (1966). *The path to health insurance. Canadian Public Administration, 9*(June), 156–165.

Gottlieb, L. N., Shamian, J., & Chan, S. (2004). Lessons from SARS: Challenges for the international nursing research community. *Canadian Journal of Nursing Research, 36*(1), 3–7.

Hall, E. M. (1980). *Canada's national–provincial health program for the 1980s: A commitment for renewal.* Justice E. M. Hall, Special Commissioner. Ottawa: Department of National Health and Welfare.

Hastings, J. E. F., & Mosley, W. (1980). Introduction: The evolution of organized community health services in Canada. In C. A. Meilicke & J. L. Storch (Eds.), *Perspectives on Canadian health and social services policy: History and emerging trends* (pp. 145–155). Ann Arbor, Michigan: Health Administration Press.

Health Canada. (2002). Canada's health care system. Available at http://www.hc-sc.gc.ca/

Health Care Renewal. (2003). First ministers accord on healthcare renewal. Available: http://www.hc-sc.gc.ca/english//hca2003/accord.html

Kenny, N. (2002). *What good is health care?* Ottawa: CHA Press.

_____. (2004). Value(s) for money? Assessing Romanow and Kirby. *HealthcarePapers, 4*(4), 28–34.

Kinnear, J. L. (1994). The professionalization of Canadian nursing, 1924–1932: Views in the CN and the CMAJ. *CBMH/BCHM, 11,* 153–174.

Laframboise, H. L. (1973). Health policy: Breaking the problem down into more manageable segments. *Canadian Medical Association Journal, 108*(February), 388–393.

Lalonde, M. (1974). *A new perspective on the health of Canadians.* Ottawa: Information Canada.

Leatt, P., Lemieux-Charles, L., & Aird, C. (1994). *Program management and beyond: Management innovations in Ontario hospitals.* Ottawa: Canadian College of Health Service Executives.

Leatt, P., Pink, G. H., & Guerriere, M. (2000). Towards a Canadian model of integrated healthcare. *HealthcarePapers, 1*(2), 13–35.

Lindenfield, R. (1959). Hospital insurance in Canada: An example in federal–provincial relations. *Social Services Review, 33,* 148–160.

Mackie, R. (2001, July 9). Project not helping ease MD shortage. *The Globe and Mail,* p. A7.

Margoshes, D. (1999). *Tommy Douglas: Building the new society.* Montreal: XYZ Publishing.

Marsh, L. (1975). *Report on social security for Canada 1943.* Toronto: University of Toronto Press.

McGillis Hall, L., Angus, J., Peter, E., et al. (2003). Medial portrayal of nurses' perspectives and concerns in the SARS crisis in Toronto. *Journal of Nursing Scholarship, 35*(3), 211–216.

McIntosh, J. W. (1914). Inter-relation of physician, citizen and state to public health. *The Public Health Journal, 5*(July 14), 451–455.

Meilicke, C. A., & Storch, J. L. (Eds.). (1980). *Perspectives on Canadian health and social services policy: History and emerging trends.* Ann Arbor, Michigan: Health Administration Press.

Najman, J. M., & Western, J. S. (1984). A comparative analysis of Australian health policy in the 1970s. *Social Science and Medicine, 18*(1), 949–958.

National Forum on Health Care. (1997). *Canada health action: Building the legacy.* Ottawa: Health Canada.

National Post. (2001, June 29). 29% of our health care private.

Office of Nursing Policy, Health Canada. (2003). *Report of the national advisory committee on SARS and public health.* Ottawa: Author.

Pauly, B. (2004). Shifting the balance in funding and delivery of health care in Canada. In J. Storch, P. Rodney, & R. Starzomski (Eds.), *Towards a moral horizon: Nursing ethics for leadership and practice* (pp. 181–208). Toronto: Pearson Education Canada.

Pauly, B., Schreiber, R., MacDonald, M., et al. (2004). Dancing to our own tune: Understandings of advanced nursing practice in British Columbia. *Journal of Nursing Leadership, 17*(2), 47–57.

Pellegrino, E. (1975). The Catholic hospitals: Options for survival. *Hospital Progress, 56*(2), 49.

Picard, A. (1999, November 9). Free trade agreement no boon to health care, U.S. conference told. *The Globe and Mail.*

Registered Nurses Association of Ontario (RNAO). (1999). *Putting nurses back into health care: Who will respond?* Toronto: Author.

Rice, J. J., & Prince, M. J. (2000). *Changing politics of Canadian social policy.* Toronto: University of Toronto Press.

Roberge, G. (2003). A four part paper on health policy and management implications of the Romanow and Kirby reports. Unpublished paper. Faculty of Human and Social Development, University of Victoria, Victoria, British Columbia.

Robinson, J. (2001, April 27). Prescription for high prices. *National Post.*

Rodger, G. L. (1993). Success and nurses: Its influence on society. *AARN Newsletter, 49*(1), 17–18.

Rodney, P., Varcoe, C., Storch, J. L., et al. (2002). Navigating towards a moral horizon: A multisite qualitative study of ethical practice in nursing. *Canadian Journal of Nursing Research, 34*(3), 75–102.

Ross Kerr, J. (1996). Nursing in Canada from 1760 to the present: The transition to modern nursing. In J. Ross Kerr & J. MacPhail (Eds.), *Canadian nursing: Issues and Perspectives* (3rd ed., pp. 11–22). Toronto: Mosby.

Royal Commission on Health Service (Vols. I, II). (1964, 1965). Justice E. Hall, Commission Chair. Ottawa: Queen's Printer.

Saul, J. R. (1995). *The unconscious civilization.* Concord, Ontario: Anansis.

Shamian, J., & LeClair, S. J. (2000). Integrated delivery systems now or . . . ? *HealthcarePapers, 1*(2), 66–75.

Sinclair, D. G. (2004). The big thing we haven't done yet. *HealthcarePapers, 4*(4), 69–73.

Stinson, S. M. (1969). Deprofessionalization in nursing. Unpublished dissertation. Columbia University, Health Sciences.

Storch, J. L., Rodney, P., & Starzomski, R. (2004). *Towards a moral horizon: Nursing ethics for leadership and practice.* Toronto: Pearson Education Canada.

Storch, J. L., Rodney, P., Pauly, B., et al. (2002). Listening to nurses' moral voices. *Canadian Journal of Nursing Leadership, 15*(4), 7–16.

Storch, J. L. (1996). Foundational values in Canadian health care. In M. Stingl & D. Wilson (Eds.), *Efficiency vs. equality: Health reform in Canada.* Halifax: Fernwood Publishing.

Strategies for population health: Investing in the health of Canadians. (1994). Prepared by the Federal, Provincial and Territorial Advisory Committee on Population Health for the Meeting of the Ministers of Health, September 14–15.

Taylor, M. G. (1973). The Canadian health insurance program. *Public Administration Review, 33*(January-February), 31–39.

_____. (1987). *Health insurance and Canadian public policy* (2nd ed.). Montreal: McGill Queens University Press.

Torrance, G. M. (1987). Hospitals as health factories. In D. Coburn, C. D'Arcy, G. M. Torrance, et al. (Eds.), *Health and Canadian society* (2nd ed.). Markham, Ontario: Fitzhenry & Whiteside.

Van Loon, R. J. (1978). From shared cost to block funding and beyond: The politics of health insurance in Canada. *Journal of Health Politics, Policy and Law, 2*(Winter), 454–478.

Van Loon, R. J., & Whittington, M. S. (1976). *The Canadian political system: Environment, structure and process* (2nd ed.). Toronto: McGraw-Hill Ryerson.

Varcoe, C. (2004). Widening the scope of ethical theory, practice, and policy: Violence against women as an illustration. In J. Storch, P. Rodney, & R. Starzomski (Eds.), *Towards a moral horizon: Nursing ethics for leadership and practice* (pp. 414–432). Toronto: Pearson Education Canada.

Wallace, E. (1950). The origins of the social welfare state in Canada, 1867–1900. *Canadian Journal of Economics and Political Science, 16*, 383–393.

Wilson, D. (1996). Where do we go from here? The 72 billion dollar question. In M. Stingl & D. Wilson (Eds.), *Efficiency vs. equality: Health reform in Canada.* Halifax: Fernwood Publishing.

Critical Questions

As a way of engaging with the ideas in this chapter, consider the following:

1. Drawing on your own experience in nursing practice and education, how do you understand leadership in nursing and its impact on the broader health care system?

2. Specifically, what qualities and abilities might be important to enable a nurse leader to effectively influence health care reform?

CHAPTER

4

Deborah Tamlyn
Sandra Reilly

Innovation and Contemporary Nursing Leadership

Deborah Tamlyn (center), during her tenure as dean of the Faculty of Nursing, University of Calgary, among faculty and staff. Photo by Ken Bendiktsen. Used by permission from the Faculty of Nursing, University of Calgary.

Chapter Objectives

After completing this chapter, you will be able to:

1. Analyze proposed changes pertaining to the role of nurses in the delivery of health care.
2. Describe the implications for nursing leadership associated with the transformation of the health system.
3. Suggest alternatives to the current health care delivery system.
4. Formulate questions related to the leadership role of nurses in the Canadian health system.
5. Discuss the importance of innovation as it relates to leadership in the health care delivery system.
6. Discuss the competencies now required of nursing leaders.

The premise of this chapter is that health reform demands that Canadian nurses adopt a new style of leadership (Chow, Coffman, & Morjikian, 1999) to participate in reshaping the delivery of health care. Certainly, most agree that rapid changes in the 1990s irrevocably transformed the Canadian health delivery system. As this transition continues, nurses can expect to assume significantly different leadership competencies. How they meet these challenges will determine the quality of health care now and in the future.

Many words and phrases describe what has happened to the health care system in Canada. Terms such as *reshape*, *reform*, and *restructure* are used to describe the changes taking place. Useful in drawing attention to what has happened, these terms provide little, if any, information about how nurses can contribute to the process of health care change.

For their part, nursing leaders have to help nurses prepare for their new roles as knowledge workers (Drucker, 1999). In 1959, Drucker coined the term *knowledge worker* to describe the emerging class of new workers in postindustrial America (1994). Unlike the earlier industrial worker, this new worker requires significant "formal education and the ability to acquire and to apply theoretical and analytical knowledge" (p. 62). For the knowledge worker, the operative words are *acquire* and *apply*.

Nurses certainly have to "acquire" new knowledge throughout their careers. As practice scientists, nurses have to learn continuously in fields where knowledge doubles every 18 to 24 months.

Nurses, like their counterparts in medicine, understand that knowledge has the most value when you "apply" it to help unravel problems. Consequently, nursing, as a practice science, focuses on evidence-based outcomes.

You usually find that knowledge workers function best on teams. That is, the demand for more applied education to resolve complex problems leads to more specialization among workers. Typically, as workers learn more and more about less and less, they increasingly depend on others for those skills outside their scope of knowledge. As such, several kinds of knowledge workers are often found on a team within a knowledge-intense organization.

Nurses lead not only as administrators but also as clinicians, researchers, and educators. In all of these roles, nurses recognize that change, which represents the *sine qua non* of contemporary society, demands nothing less. Change calls for innovation, which requires leadership. As change occurs, the system needs new procedures and practices. All nurses can expect in the course of their professional careers to have opportunities to become innovators and, by necessity, leaders. Whether they choose to do so is ultimately a personal decision.

As will soon become evident, this chapter takes an asset-based approach to the role of leadership. Those curious about an alternative approach can read Goldsmith, Morgan, and Ogg (2004); they take more of a deficit-based outlook that examines the common frustrations associated with many leadership roles. Of necessity, their approach discusses the negative conditions that undermine innovation: inertia, ignorance, jealousy, elitism, isolation, concealment, and pride.

An asset-based approach, however, focuses on the attributes and skills of successful leaders. Besides its inherent civility, such an approach accentuates the positive qualities that innovative leaders bring to changing work environments. Certainly, Porter-O'Grady and Malloch (2002) as well as Wheatley (2002) believe as much. In his or her way, each believes that in any discussion of the future the emphasis belongs on its promise not on its inherent risks and uncertainties. Individuals, like the organizations where they work, flourish in positive, healthy environments.

This is not to suggest that conflict is avoidable. Conflict management remains integral to the leadership process. The successful leader knows how to heal injuries and maintain or build a healthy environment. Goleman, Boyatzis, and McKee (2002) make this point quite emphatically in their discussion of emotional intelligence, with its emphasis on compassion, accountability, and personal satisfaction.

This chapter takes up the idea that nursing leaders have a twofold responsibility: They endeavor to develop structures suitable to the organization's purpose, and they build teams of stakeholders interested in devising innovative responses to changing health systems (Giuliani, 2002).

■ HISTORICAL CONTEXT OF NURSING LEADERSHIP

Like their colleagues in medicine, psychology, pharmacy, and social work, to name a few, nurses at the turn of this century find themselves without their traditional sense of purpose and autonomy (Storch & Stinson, 1988). Efficiency too often replaces effectiveness as a standard of practice. For example, many nurses now come under the direct authority of business managers with financial agendas. In these circumstances, nurses find themselves measured against outcomes that bear little resemblance to the profession's ideologic values. The accompanying loss of purpose and autonomy has untoward consequences on the quality of care and delivery of services.

We are not the first to recognize that the current situation in nursing calls for attention (Nunn, 2001). Nevertheless, unless these problems are addressed, patient care suffers as nurses become demoralized by a pervasive sense of mistrust in the system. This mistrust likely accounts "for decreased commitment and job performance" (Corey-Lisle, Tarzian, Cohen, et al., 1999, p. 36). Regrettably but understandably, the consequence is that fewer nurses seem willing to assume leadership roles. In other words, at the same time nursing faces significant challenges, it lacks a cadre of leaders ready to provide direction to the largest group of well-educated professionals in the entire health care system.

Changing Health Care Landscape

Changes to the Canadian health care system became commonplace in the 1990s. Many practicing nurses still remember how, as students, they received their training in a hospital system with expressed religious and paramilitary overtones. Supported by the scientific management principles of Frederick Taylor (1947), training emphasized the command–control practice model, which employed a strict hierarchical approach and invested all authority in physicians. By the 1990s, memories of these practices became increasingly distant. And it seems the paradigm shift from such linear, top-down, deterministic thinking has only just begun.

Sometime after World War II, North America began changing from an industrial to a service economy. This change, with its emphasis on meeting human needs, began a transformation that questioned the century-old conviction in measuring human success solely by scientific, industrial, and material progress. Instead of extolling reason and order, society began, certainly by the 1960s, to place increasing importance on the rights and needs of individuals.

Social commentator Alvin Toffler (1980) believes that the self-help and wellness movements represent tangible evidence of how these changes have affected the practice of health care. Instead of behaving strictly as passive consumers of health care, individuals now behave as active "prosumers," which Toffler describes as a combination of producer and consumer. According to his logic, as patients assume more responsibility for their own care, we can expect a decrease in paternalistic, authoritative, physician-centered thinking (Bulger, 1999).

Certainly, as patients gain a greater role in decisions about their care, they often turn to alternative providers. The emergence of nurse practitioners testifies to a public willingness for nurses to expand their scope of practice. Because patients often perceive nurses as social and economic equals, nurses enjoy special access in helping patients become informed consumers and managers of their health. Of course, this access extends to entire communities where public health nurses have a long history of working with diverse population groups.

Nurses can reasonably expect that the transformation of society and the health care sector will present increased opportunities and challenges to provide more comprehensive care for patients. In such an environment, nurses can expect their traditional job titles, with their well-defined scopes of responsibilities, to disappear as health care systems devise new, multiskilled teams (Spitzer, 1998).

The changes facing nursing reflect those occurring in the wider society, which appears ready to change the essence of health care delivery. Albeit challenging, the question is simple enough: How can the Canadian health care system operate efficiently and effectively, especially when an aging population, with heightened expectations of health care, makes greater demands of a system with limited resources?

Nursing Leadership and Reform of the Health Care System

In many ways, the situation for nurses is emblematic of the system-wide problems in health care. Better educated and increasingly expected to increase their effectiveness and efficiency, nurses face restrictions that hinder their efforts. Without innovative models for alternative kinds of practice, nurses likely face the ongoing dilemma of how to actualize the self-care and wellness movements. For example, consider the challenge that nurses face in educating policymakers and the public that a comprehensive health care system includes not only health protection but also health promotion. Heavily invested in a hospital system, organized around body parts and diseases, governments appear reluctant to challenge the traditional medical approach. In short, nursing leaders have to divest policymakers of the belief that health care means sickness care.

Health care is extraordinarily complex and requires that providers simultaneously pay attention to the person, the environment, and the system. Regrettably, the system remains highly compartmentalized and too often unresponsive. Yet unless the professions address this failure, they face uncertain futures. According to Spitzer (1998, p. 168), any profession that fails to redefine itself during this transformation "can be consumed, reduced, transformed or expelled out of the system as it reorganizes and adapts."

A recognized nursing leader and past president of the Canadian Nurses Association (CNA), Ginette Lemire Rodger looks at this crisis as vindication for all the reforms asked for by nurses over the past 20 years. These reforms include

- Concentrating on "health, not just health care"
- Arranging for more "health services in the community, not just in hospital"
- Developing "multidisciplinary networks of practitioners, educators, researchers, and managers, not just solo players" with something to offer patients
- Welcoming "public participation in shaping the system, not just public consultation"
- Focusing on "inter-sectoral health, not just health care"
- Using "appropriate technology, not just 'high tech'"
- Directing attention to "ecology, not just environment" (Hibberd & Rodger, 1999, p. 261)

To repeat the obvious, the current health care system begs for innovative nursing leadership. Nevertheless, according to Porter-O'Grady and Krueger-Wilson (1995, p. 298), nursing, like other health professions, lacks a "ready and able group of leaders waiting in the wings...[and] institutions of higher education are just barely changing their curriculums to fit the new reality."

Some universities take the matter seriously. For example, doctoral students enrolled in the Faculty of Nursing at the University of Calgary examine leadership as the critical element in health care reform. They understand that leadership roles are important not only in administration but also in clinical and research areas. One particular course, "Contemporary Issues in Health Care," required of all doctoral students, many of whom participate by videoconferencing and audioconferencing from across Canada, invites national leaders to discuss health care reform issues from multidisciplinary perspectives. The syllabus for this course reminds students that (Reilly & Tamlyn, 2000, pp. 2–3):

> [T]he last decade of the twentieth century witnessed a revolution in health care. Largely driven by fiscal constraints, policymakers...downsized the health care system. In time, consumers accepted shorter hospital stays, postponements for specialized diagnoses and treatments, and more technologically elaborate home care programs. Noticeably, the system provided few opportunities for consumers to engage with practitioners in revamping the system.
>
> As eventually became evident, the imposition of budgetary constraints alone has limited usefulness. It too easily focuses on achieving efficiencies at the expense of ensuring and improving outcomes. And because health care ultimately concerns matters of life and death, such oversights affect more than quality of life issues. Downsizing, without adequate strategic thinking, raises questions about standards of care. In the face of these "realities," health care practitioners have to reexamine how they can collaborate with consumers to redesign the delivery of care. If they do any less, they effectively deny their expertise to consumers and fail to provide "leadership" to their colleagues.
>
> In addition to fiscal constraints, other changes, more social than economic, require reexamination of the health care system. Delegated and narrowly defined roles, with carefully proscribed responsibilities, dominated by strict hierarchical relationships characterized the modern era. Today, as part of an ongoing paradigm shift from the modern to the postmodern era, rationality and centrality no longer dictate organizational behavior. In the postmodern era, roles have become interdependent and flexible. Consumers, policymakers, and practitioners expect to share responsibility in setting the agenda for new multidisciplinary health teams, sometimes organized on an ad hoc basis.

■ NEW RELATIONSHIP BETWEEN PROFESSIONALS AND POLICYMAKERS

Whatever transformations result from health care reform, the movement toward more people-centered health care will undoubtedly continue. This, in turn, will lead to other innovations. According to Porter-O'Grady and Krueger-Wilson (1995), the transformation of health delivery services will likely proceed along several lines. Services will become more integrated, with the development of more structures that provide a continuum of care. Nurses, like other professionals, will recognize the social reality of the self-help and wellness movements and enter new partnerships with various communities.

There is evidence that some organizations appear ready to accept such innovative thinking by abandoning hierarchical, expert-driven ways of thinking. For example, consider the seemingly innocuous decision by the Calgary Regional Health Authority (CRHA), after only 7 years since its inception, to rename itself. In June 2001, it became known as the Calgary Health Region.

According to a press release, members of the staff helped prompt the decision when they requested a more collaborative nomenclature. By omitting "Authority," with its emphasis on hierarchical thinking, from its title, the Calgary Health Region now permits "individual sites, portfolios, and programs" to identify themselves in all their correspondence (http://www.crha-health.ab.ca/frontlines/issue41_1.htm, 2001). Accordingly, "The [revised] name Calgary Health Region...is a much better reflection of the collaboration between hospitals, community care providers, physicians, nurses and a wide range of other care providers and partners in the community" (p. 2).

This thinking extends to the organization's new logo. Whereas the previous one (Figure 4.1) symbolized a linear system that promoted a power relationship between the organization and the community, the

CRHA
Calgary Regional Health Authority

FIGURE 4.1 The earlier logo, with the word *Authority*, suggests a hierarchical relationship between the provider and the community.

new logo (Figure 4.2) expresses a "caring, accessible and integrated" delivery system that recognizes how all human activity integrates "people, growth and the cycle of life" (p. 2).

The obvious differences between the two logos emphasize the transformations associated with health reform. The previous logo and the prominence given to the word *Authority* in its title presumed a hierarchical relationship between the provider and the community. It implied the organization functioned in a stable environment with predictable problems and routine responses. From this, it followed that power rested in the vertical relationship between professionals and patients. In this system, professionals had strictly defined roles, supported by intractable relationships among different specialties or disciplines. The new logo opens the organization to change and innovation. Highly suggestive of an organization ready to adapt and even introduce new systems, the new logo has a dynamic quality. It suggests fluidity, participatory decision making, and openness to innovation. With a more horizontal arrangement of power, the new logo implies a nonlinear decision-making process more in keeping with complex, multifaceted, systemic health problems in the 21st century.

These changes in the Calgary Health Region make another important point about contemporary work-life in health organizations: Workers can affect policy—when they choose to do so.

The changes at the Calgary Health Region inform us that the system has begun to change, but they also tell us much about the role of knowledge workers in these organizations. Health care organizations represent the ultimate learning environments. According to Sorrells-Jones (1999), organizations in which 40% or more of the workers use information to solve problems, as well as to generate ideas and services, rank as knowledge-intense environments. Their workers perform "nonroutine, unpredictable, nonlinear, multidisciplinary, nonrepetitive activities in a long time frame with evolving goals" (Beyerlein, Johnson, & Beyerlein, 1995, p. x).

In such organizations, human capital represents the most important asset. Their workers represent more of a resource than an expense because human capital has as much, if not more, importance to the organization's mission as its property or equipment. To succeed, these organizations purposefully strive to attract the right kind of people and provide them with "flat, agile structures, open information, power that moves to expertise, and systems that create knowledgeable employees" (Lawler, 2001, p. 17) who want nothing less than to devise innovative options to practical problems.

This leads to one inescapable conclusion. In knowledge-intense organizations, knowledge workers have a substantive, if largely undefined, role in formulating policies and practices. That is, the organizations, if they seek credibility with their workers, want to include their workers' input and innovative ideas.

FIGURE 4.2 The current logo suggests a dynamic organization that is adaptable and open to change.

For their part, knowledge workers in the health care organizations, who certainly include nurses, require new kinds of motivation. In addition to their compensation, they seek new kinds of rewards and recognition. They want meaningful work, which makes use of their abilities and provides opportunities for successful outcomes.

■ CALL FOR A NEW KIND OF NURSING LEADERSHIP

Successful organizations, like their workers, embrace change. Yet as world-renowned authority on corporate management Peter Drucker (1999, p. 73) tells us, "one cannot manage change. One can only be ahead of it." If one accepts his reasoning, it then follows that organizations or professions require leaders who can remain in front of change. Or, in the words of Hibberd & Rodger (1999), "nursing requires visionaries, who see the future in terms of its possibilities."

The call for nursing visionaries seems a daunting quest but actually describes much of what many, though certainly not all, nurses do already. Does anyone doubt that nurses regularly study every product, service, and process in terms of its usefulness? If it fails this utilitarian assessment, they abandon it. However, abandonment does not necessarily mean obsolescence. Redesign can enliven a product, service, or process. The changing role of professional nurses demonstrates that nursing continually abandons some services or processes only to replace them with more useful, evidence-based endeavors. Such change, to use Drucker's expression, represents a kind of "organized improvement" because it purposefully increases efficiency and effectiveness by staying ahead of change.

Nursing history also serves to teach us that challenges, albeit daunting, are not insurmountable. About 40 years ago, nursing leaders, who long ago recognized the dangers of routinizing nursing practice, envisioned nursing practice as more collaborative. They advocated abandoning the 100-year-old hospital-based training system, with its adherence to the militaristic principle of obedience to authority. In its place, they proposed that a baccalaureate education become the entry point for nursing. These leaders faced serious opposition, and the struggle continues, as demonstrated by recent efforts of some provincial legislators to propose the reopening of hospital diploma nursing programs. Nursing requires visionaries who understand the importance of advanced education in preparing nurses for expanded responsibilities in reshaping the health care system.

Challenge Facing Nursing Leaders

By their own account, Canadian nurses believe that they are underutilized and undervalued by the health care system. They state as much in two Canadian reports.

Health Canada (Office of Nursing Policy, 2001) reports that nurses suffer from a lack of appreciation and recognition in the workplace. Indeed, more than any group of health care workers, nurses report "lower levels of autonomy, poorer relationships with physicians and less job satisfaction" (p. 5), which apparently contribute to job-related stress.

In another report, the Registered Nurses Association of Ontario (2000) attributes inappropriate "workloads and the lack of professional development opportunities" to "fragmented patient care and the disillusionment of nurses with their profession" (p. 8). The report goes on to make 89 recommendations for improving nursing practice. Generally divided into two categories, the recommendations focus on providing more educational opportunities for nurses and ensuring that nurses exercise more responsibilities in keeping with their abilities.

If a sense of undervaluation and underutilization lies at the center of nurses' dissatisfaction, it also represents the major challenge facing nursing leaders. As one nursing leader questioned, how can the system reinvent itself so as to re-establish trust with nurses so that they become meaningful partners in the Canadian health care system (Shamian, 2000)?

Attributes of Contemporary Nursing Leaders

As practical scientists in knowledge-intense organizations, nurses require leaders capable of devising and disseminating innovation. Whether their work takes them to the clinical, research, educational, or administrative areas, this leadership requires certain attributes.

According to Hibberd and Rodger (1999), leadership requires four primary attributes. Successful leaders display an ability to translate a *vision* into reality; they possess the *knowledge* and the *confidence* to deal with uncertainty; and, at the same time, they demonstrate a commitment to maintain their *visibility* as nurses. Goleman (1997) refers to these attributes as characteristics of emotionally intelligent individuals. Highly pragmatic and relational, they work very well with teams of knowledge workers.

Translating Vision Into Action

Successful nursing leaders demonstrate vision when their ideas successfully bond the mission of the organization with the larger purposes of society and the ideals of the profession. That is, nurses expect a high order of satisfaction from their work. Successful nursing leaders take their insights and create a vision that compels the participation of others. In so doing, nursing leaders actually stimulate innovation because of their ability to envision what will happen in the long run.

Knowledge

For the transformation of the health care sector to occur with minimal disruption, successful nursing leaders also have to possess comprehensive knowledge about the larger society as well as about different areas of the health care system. In doing so, these nursing leaders first perceive nurses and their organizations within these new paradigms and then help others to do the same. They have the skills to organize activities without polarizing other team members along professional, departmental, or specialty lines. Such knowledge obviously goes beyond mere understanding; it includes the appreciation of what constitutes the essence of the new paradigm inherent in the information age.

Confidence

Confidence represents the most personal and least tangible of the attributes associated with successful leadership. According to Hibberd and Rodger (1999, p. 264), "nursing needs confident leaders who have self-esteem and are able to live with insecurity." Not only do they think outside the box but they also possess the fortitude to express ideas that run counter to the prevailing wisdom. For example, although public participation represents a fundamental tenet of the "new public health," consultation between communities and providers largely represents an unrealized goal. A successful nursing leader challenges traditional practices and helps the system make the necessary adjustments so that system can interact with the community.

Visibility

An equally important attribute of successful nursing leadership is visibility. Here we have one of those paradoxes so typical in this period of transformation. At the same time that health care reforms have downgraded the role of professionals (Storch & Stinson, 1988), the complexity of health care tells us that professionals consistently play an essential role and that they require the support of health care organizations. It is ironic then, as Hibberd and Rodger (1999, p. 265) remind us, that health care organizations continue to eliminate "nursing positions at the policy and senior-management levels of health-care agencies." Although nurses still hold management portfolios, now they more often function as health care leaders, not necessarily as nursing professionals. This omission of their professional credentials from the administrative work of nurses has serious consequences. For certain, nursing runs the risk of becoming "invisible and disposable." And this diminished profile of nursing can lead to unnecessary fatalities because of lower standards of care.

The aforementioned situation raises a substantive problem. By "making assumptions about the nature of the [clinical] task, [hospital] reformers make assumptions about the nature and role of professionalism" (Southon & Braithwaite, 1998, p. 26). They assume that clinical protocols can predict clinical problems and that individual needs are reducible to classification. Whether one agrees that such changes devalue professionals, it seems obvious that professional assessments—at least for individual patients—count for less. This conundrum raises another important question for nursing leaders: How does the system deliver health services efficiently without compromising the effectiveness of these services?

■ SHARED LEADERSHIP

Tamlyn (2004), in her inaugural speech as president of the CNA, noted the importance of fostering a shared leadership approach. Leadership is not so much about what one nurse will do but what a group of nurses can do together. Through shared leadership, we need to build a legacy that outlasts our individual contributions in place and time.

■ CIRCUMSTANCES THAT PROMOTE INNOVATION

Innovation is one of those familiar words that requires study to discern its meaning (Mintzberg, 2002). Certainly, most human experiences appear largely repetitive and rarely unique. Few experiences rate as innovative. For whatever reason, people usually resist change unless compelled by circumstances or persuaded by a leader who willingly shares responsibility for it.

Drucker (1998), one of the first to write on this subject, discusses how events initiate and promote the innovative process and how they refer indirectly to leadership. In "The Discipline of Innovation" (1998), Drucker assigns a critical, if largely unspecified, role to the vision and knowledge required of change leaders. In several places, he makes it clear that innovation occurs only when a change leader takes a highly visible position on changes as they take place. Without trivializing the process by which innovation occurs, Drucker implies that innovation occurs because the right person is in the right place at the right time.

Drucker believes that innovation represents a critical function of any organization, whether a multinational corporation, a public service institution, or a family business. Indeed, only through innovation can an organization develop practical solutions in an environment of rapidly changing markets and technologies. He characterizes these changes as opportunities, in the belief that change is inevitable and that successful leaders actually welcome such developments.

Drucker organizes all innovation around various kinds of opportunities, which he divides into two classes or sources. One, internal sources, refers to opportunities that arise within an organization. The other, external sources, considers opportunities that turn up outside it.

Internal Sources of Innovation

Internal sources of innovation arise within an organization, and workers are first likely to recognize them. Unlike external sources of innovation, internal sources are more symptomatic than causal. As such, they require little effort to put into practice.

Unexpected Sources of Innovation

Sometimes innovation is fickle. It arrives unannounced and occurs in the most unlikely places. When it occurs serendipitously, organizations sometimes see it as anomalous and even label it as "unsound, unhealthy, and obviously abnormal" (Drucker, 1998, p. 38). Why do people mistrust innovation of this kind? Maybe they have an inherent suspicion of anything unfamiliar. Or maybe they believe that change suggests incompetence. Or maybe they wonder if change in one area will prompt other organizational changes that risk offending special interests or dominant groups.

Drucker (1998) tells the story of the inventor of procaine (Novocain), who refused to market his discovery to dentists. Throughout his life, he remained committed to his original idea that procaine belonged exclusively to surgeons, who, he stubbornly believed, needed a new form of anaesthesia. For years, he traveled to dental schools criticizing dentists' use of his invention. Obviously, he lacked the perspicacity to evaluate his discovery for what it offered humankind.

Similarly, organizations often lack the tools with which to appreciate success, especially qualitative success. To redress any lack of "vision, knowledge, and understanding" (Drucker, 1998, p. 41), organizations continuously have to ask themselves the question, "What basic changes are now appropriate for this organization in the way it defines . . . [itself]?" (p. 42).

Incongruities

Drucker (1998, p. 57) defines an incongruity as "a discrepancy, a dissonance, between what is and what 'ought' to be, or between what is and what everybody assumes it to be." Like other sources of innovation, incongruities invite change. Unlike other sources of innovation, however, incongruities are solely qualitative and clearly definable within specific industries, markets, or processes. They are divided into four kinds:

- *Incongruity between economic realities.* Sometimes economic incongruities prompt innovation. One example from the health care sector makes the point quite nicely. In the United States, families without medical insurance rely on hospital emergency rooms (ERs) for their primary care. Whatever the complaint, the ER is their first choice because the law entitles everyone to emergency treatment. The resultant expense of treating so many uninsured families forced some ERs to close and caused some patients to wait unconscionably long times at others. Staff knew this but, mired in traditional practices, did nothing about it. Eventually, financial considerations prevailed. A combination of expediency and new management practices gave rise to emergent care centers outside of hospitals, where nonemergency cases receive attention around the clock.
- *Incongruity between assumptions and reality.* If people make false assumptions, even successful innovations will ultimately fail. For example, after a decade of success in reducing HIV/AIDS transmission among homosexuals, health promotion efforts stalled because policymakers reduced health education programs, assuming that the homosexual population knew everything about the prevalence and transmission of the disease. Only after the incidence of the disease began to increase did the system renew its health education program for this population. Although the jury is still out, early results look promising.
- *Incongruity between perceived and actual values and expectations.* Of all the incongruities, those between organizations and their clients occur most frequently. That is, it is not unusual for organizations erroneously to perceive what their clients actually want. The very nature of the relationship between the organization and the client fosters such misperceptions. Consider health care, especially obstetrics, palliative care, geriatrics, and pain management. Physicians and nurses typically presume that they know the meaning of health care for patients in these specialties. They usually define it in absolute terms and apply it equally to every patient. Yet in the case of obstetrics, as the increasing popularity of doulas makes evident, expectant mothers want something more than the traditional obstetric experience.
- *Incongruity within the rhythm or logic of a process.* People within an industry or market often know when something is "out of sync" in a process or in the way things are done. They come to this understanding by way of their experiences. In this regard, because of the continuity of care they provide patients, nurses have the benefit of knowing more about the operations of an organization than other groups. In a regular column, "Nurse(s) to Know," which first appeared in 1998, the *Canadian Nurse* profiles one nurse each month who has produced an innovation. For example, one nurse became an agent for an internal source of innovation when, working in an overcrowded maximum-security jail, she realized that bureaucratic bungling and malfeasance interfered with the delivery of nursing care. She

consulted with other professionals and prepared a report that led to the complete review of the situation. Ultimately, her innovative action led to improved services to a highly marginalized population.

Need

A major source of innovative opportunity, "process need," begins with a job that needs doing. The innovator focuses on a task and "perfects a process that already exists, replaces a link that is weak, redesigns an existing old process around newly available knowledge" (Drucker, 1985, p. 69). This highly successful kind of innovation comes in response to a problem everyone in the organization knows about but has never paid much attention to correcting. The innovation, once designed, is immediately accepted because it is obviously called for. Examples of this kind of innovation abound in the health care system and certainly include the role of auxiliary personnel to assist nurses, pharmacists, and social workers.

Industry and Market Changes

Although their size appears to indicate otherwise, markets or industries are fragile entities with limited life spans. They disintegrate and reinvent themselves more quickly than most people imagine.

The *Canadian Nurse* provides another example of how a nurse became a source of innovation in her practice. The graduate of a diploma program, she returned to school for her baccalaureate and master's degrees and created a role for advanced practice nursing in cardiology when it had yet to exist in her province. To establish her credentials as a practitioner, she took it upon herself to complete a medical school course in physical assessment. In the same innovative manner, she went on to establish a preadmission program for assessing cardiac patients about to undergo catheterization. In effect, at a time when the system had only begun to make adjustments to increase the effectiveness and efficiency of its operations, she had already exhibited leadership ability.

Another example concerns the practice of medicine. Not so long ago, almost all physicians had their own practices. Today, most work along with partners in group practices or have salaried positions in health care organizations. This happened because the complexity of health care services requires a more elaborate management system, which individual medical practitioners find too expensive.

External Sources of Innovation

Sources outside the organization also prompt innovation. Although less reliable and predictable than the internal sources of innovation, these external sources do have certain advantages. Because they arise from within the environment, they are highly visible and often have greater consequence.

Demographics

For many policymakers, demographics provide the most predictable, unambiguous, and transparent source information about innovation. Consider how population data, including gender, live births, occupation, and income distribution, tell us about what to expect in the future. For example, what we know about family life—that women marry later, have fewer children, and likely work outside the home—certainly deserves consideration before policymakers propose any innovation in the delivery of health care.

Besides the obvious effects of an aging population, what other demographic events will influence nursing services? Consider the recruitment and retention of nurses. Within a decade, a worldwide shortage of nurses will decrease the number of professional nurses by more than half. Besides increasing the number of graduates, what other measures are available to policymakers?

Perceptual Changes

A highly qualitative matter, perception concerns how individuals interpret facts. In other words, do they see the glass as half full or half empty? Many North Americans, despite the remarkable advances in medical technology, seem obsessed with aging or with the disabilities ordinarily associated with growing old. What demands will this aging population, with heightened expectations of the health care system, make on society and their own families? Some pharmaceutical companies have already decided: They focus their product research on products that reduce or eliminate incontinence, maintain sexual potency, or reduce hair loss.

Knowledge-Based Changes

Innovation also occurs as the result of scientific or intellectual accomplishments. These accomplishments differ from all other sources of innovation primarily because of the lead-time, failure rate, predictability, and challenges inherent in such work. For example, even when pharmaceutical companies receive permission for fast-tracking "miracle drugs," the time between development and large-scale production extends to a decade or more, and the diffusion of intellectual innovation usually takes even longer. Although the Internet promises faster dissemination of ideas, especially with the emergence of English as the primary global language, societies are reluctant to change how they think. For this reason, change leaders of knowledge-based innovation have to possess a clear focus, comprehend the scope of the changes, know how to sell their ideas, and correctly anticipate the subsequent outcome.

■ DIFFUSION OF INNOVATION

Innovation seems synonymous with health care. How innovation is shared or diffused in such a knowledge-intense system has critical importance.

Over 80 years in development with about 4,000 publications on the topic (Rogers, 1995), diffusion of innovation theory provides the most comprehensive framework for understanding the communication process whereby participants "create and share information with one another to reach a mutual understanding" (p. xvi).

Everett Rogers' model for the diffusion of innovation traces an S-shaped curve. To contextualize it with what we already know about Drucker's seven sources of innovation, we amalgamate both in Figure 4.3. This representation agrees with what management and communication sciences teach us. First, according to Drucker, innovation occurs in response to various internal and external environmental sources. Second, as Rogers points out, once introduced, innovation takes a diffused path as it makes its way from one person to another. The conceptualization in Figure 4.3 represents how Drucker's sources of innovation hypothetically interrelate with Rogers' diffusion theory.

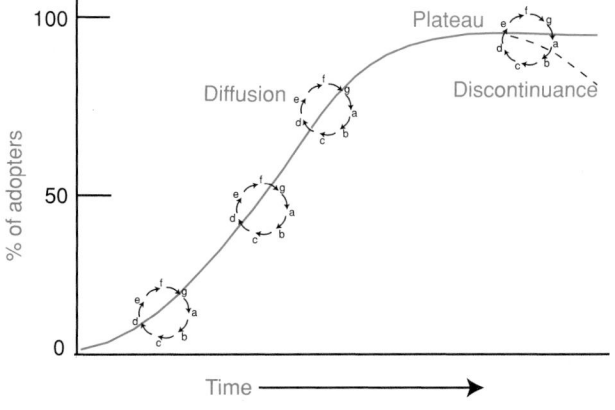

FIGURE 4.3 The relationship between the sources of innovation (Drucker, 1985) and the diffusion of innovation (Rogers, 1995). Key: (a) Unexpected outcomes; (b) Incongruities; (c) Process needs; (d) Industry and market changes; (e) Demographics; (f) Changes in perception; (g) New knowledge.

Remembering what Drucker tells us about the sources of innovation, we can now concentrate on how change leaders win over others to their innovative products, services, and processes. According to Rogers, diffusion of innovation consists of four elements: *innovation*, *communication channels*, *social systems*, and *time*.

Innovation

An innovation is completely circumscribed by its newness. That is, to qualify as an innovation, the idea, practice, or object has to appear new to the individual. The individual can know about the idea, practice, object beforehand, but it remains innovative if he or she never formed any judgments or considered it for adoption previously. In effect, innovations are not necessarily original; they are only new to the individual. He or she judges the innovation in terms of other ideas, practices, and objects previously accepted or adopted. If anything, the decision of whether to adopt an innovation likely depends on its usefulness.

Communication Channels

The diffusion of or communication about an innovation is "a process in which participants create and share information with one another in order to reach a mutual understanding" (Rogers, 1995, p. 35). Because this sharing, or channeling, is highly subjective, homophily plays an important part in the effectiveness of any communication. Defined as the degree to which individuals share the same attributes, homophily includes factors such as social status, education, and the like. Rogers believes that an increase in homophily comes about with an increase in communication.

Social Systems

According to Rogers (1995), a social system is "a set of interrelated units that are engaged in joint problem-solving to accomplish a common goal" that includes "individuals, informal groups, organizations, and/or subsystems" (p. 23). Within the social system, the diffusion of information largely depends on the social relationships or communication networks among members. Some members, labeled "opinion leaders," have leadership positions because they regularly succeed in influencing the attitudes and behaviors of others. These opinion leaders earn and maintain their positions by reason of "technical competence, social accessibility, and conformity to the system's norms" (Rogers, 1995, p. 27). Because they exemplify the best in the system, these opinion leaders usually occupy privileged positions within the communication network. Linked to other individuals within the social system, they appear more knowing and innovative.

Time

The fourth element in the process, time, plays an essential part in diffusion. That is, insofar as the diffusion of innovation represents an information gathering and processing activity, time becomes critical.

Rogers (1995) divides the diffusion process into five steps. *Knowledge* comes about when an individual or any decision-making (organizational) unit begins to evaluate an innovation. *Persuasion* occurs when an individual or unit forms an opinion about the innovation. *Decision* happens when an individual or unit undertakes activities in support or rejection of an innovation. *Implementation* happens when the individual or unit applies the innovation. Finally, *confirmation* occurs when the individual or organizational unit looks for others to reinforce the earlier decision to implement the innovation.

The period of time required to complete a successful diffusive process describes the slope of the S curve (Figure 4.3). That is, if the quantity (distribution) of individuals or units that adopt an innovation is plotted against the vertical line and the required time is plotted against the horizontal line, then the rate of a successful diffusive process typically appears as an S curve. In other words, as more individuals or units adopt an innovation, the diffusion curve climbs to a point where the trajectory of adoption levels off on a plateau, when fewer and fewer individuals or units, who have not adopted the innovation, remain.

As Figure 4.3 makes clear, the discontinuance of an innovation can also occur. Certainly, given the vibrant and dynamic character of the various internal and external sources of innovation identified by Drucker, discontinuance likely occurs more frequently than not. That is, individuals can always discontinue a previously accepted innovation. They can replace it with another, more suitable innovation. Then again, other innovations are rejected because of disenchantment; individuals or units become dissatisfied with the outcomes associated with the innovations. It matters little whether this results because of a failure to consider all the consequences of adopting particular innovations or because long-term outcomes differ markedly with short- or intermediate-term outcomes. Remember that pragmatism drives the diffusion of innovation and that any innovation deserves discontinuance if it no longer has any perceived advantage.

■ RELATIONSHIP OF INNOVATION TO NURSING LEADERSHIP

Apropos of any discussion of how innovation relates to the reform of health care are the accomplishments of Canadian nursing leaders. Unfortunately, nurses typically do not share their innovations with the wider community, so nurses who closely work with small groups of colleagues seldom receive the wider recognition that they deserve (Beason, 2000).

Fortunately, for nearly 38 years, the government of Canada, through the office of the governor general, has recognized the outstanding achievements and lifetime contributions of those Canadians, including many nurses, who have made significant contributions to our society. Created in 1967, the Order of Canada lies at the center of Canada's system of honors. Divided into three levels, the Order of Canada includes, in ascending order: Members, Officers, and Companions. Of the nurses who received the Order, 36 are Members, 13 are Officers, and 1 is a Companion (Table 4.1).

The only recipient of the highest level of the Order of Canada is Dr. Helen K. Mussallem. Her accomplishments make her emblematic of the innovative contributions of all the nurses who have received the Order. Highlighting only some of those instances in which Dr. Mussallem had the distinction of being first or truly innovative makes the point that nurses have made sizeable and innovative contributions to health care.

Dr. Mussallem stands as the first Canadian nurse to earn a doctoral degree in nursing. Her published dissertation, from Teachers College, Columbia University, provided the impetus for subsequent significant innovations in Canadian nursing education. In addition, she holds the distinction of being the first nurse to address the Annual Assembly of the Canadian Medical Association. She also conducted a survey for the Royal Commission on Health Services (Hall Commission) and a national survey of Canadian schools of nursing. She served as chair (and the only Canadian) on both the World Health Organization Scientific Group on Research in Nursing and on the Economic Council of Canada. She worked on the formation of the Commonwealth Nurses Foundation and received a Commonwealth Lectureship. She also completed international assignments in 37 developing countries under the auspices of the World Health Organization, the Pan American Health Association, the Commonwealth Foundation, and the Canadian International Development Agency (CNA, July 23, 2001).

Other leaders have received national recognition. They include recipients of the Ethel Johns Award (Table 4.2), given by the Canadian Association of University Schools of Nursing (CAUSN), and the prestigious Jeanne-Mance Award (Table 4.3), given by the CNA.

Today's nurses have a plethora of opportunities to introduce innovation into the health care environment. Porter-O'Grady (2000) classifies these innovative opportunities into three categories of change: knowledge-based, perceptual, and unexpected.

TABLE 4.1   Nurse Leaders Who Are Recipients of the Order of Canada (1969–2003)

Name	Date Appointed	Name	Date Appointed
Moyra Allen, **O.C.**	1986	Dorothy A. Macham, **C.M.**	1980
Myra M. Bennett, **C.M.**	1973	Louise Y. Maheu, **C.M.**	1992
Barbara Bromley, **C.M.**	2000	Edith E. Manuel, **C.M.**	1990
Susan Calne, **C.M.**	2001	Helen McArthur, **O.C.**	1971
Rae Chittick, **C.M.**	1975	Maura McGuire, **O.C.**	1967
Christina Cole, **C.M.**	1991	Marvelle McPherson, **C.M.**	1994
M. Dorothy Corrigan, **C.M.**	1978	Cécile J.G. Montpetit, **C.M.**	1990
Lyle Creelman, **O.C.**	1971	Helen K. Mussallem, **C.C.**	1992
Beverly Witter Du Gas, **C.M.**	2001	Margaret Ruth Page, **C.M.**	1997
Josephine Gibbons, **C.M.**	1992	Evelyn Agnes Pepper, **C.M.**	1996
Alice Girard, **O.C.**	1968	Margot Phaneuf, **C.M.**	2003
Helen Preston Glass, **O.C.**	1988	Edith B. Pinet, **C.M.**,	1979
Jean Goodwill, **O.C.**	1991	Edith May Radley, **C.M.**	1978
Patricia T. Guyda, **C.M.**	1992	Helena F. Reimer, **C.M.**,	1974
Margaret Hillson, **C.M.**	2003	Vera Roberts, **C.M.**	1986
E. Prudence Hockin, **C.M.**	1980	Margaret Sinn, **C.M.**	1976
Margaret M. Hunter, **C.M.**	1984	Harriet (Halle) Sloane, **C.M.**	2003
Jane L. Hutchings, **C.M.**	1972	Verna Huffman Splane, **O.C.**	1995
Audrey Jakeman, **O.C.**	1968	Juliette A. St.-Pierre, **C.M.**	1976
Jean Cecilian Leask, **O.C.**	1973	Shirley Stinson, **O.C.**	2002
Denise Lefebvre, **O.C.**	1983	Margaret M. Street, **C.M.**	1976
Marie Lemire, **O.C.**	1969	Constance Alexa Swinton, **C.M.**	1987
Clara Yee Lim, **C.M.**,	1979	F. Elva Taylor, **C.M.**	1991
Millicent Loder, **C.M.**	1982	Eveline Tremblay, **C.M.**	2000
Kathleen Mary Jo Lutley, **C.M.**	1986	D. Ethel Williams, **C.M.**	1984

Legend:

C.M.   **Members of the Order of Canada** are recognized for distinguished service in or to a particular group, locality, or field of endeavor.

O.C.   **Officers of the Order of Canada** are recognized for national achievement and merit of a high degree.

C.C.   **Companions of the Order of Canada** are recognized for outstanding achievement and merit of the highest degree, especially service to Canada or humanity at large.

TABLE 4.2   Nurse Leaders Who Received the Ethel Johns Award (1988–2004)

Date	Name	Date	Name
1988	Dr. Dorothy Kergin	1998	Dr. Susan E. French
1990	Professor Joan Gilchrist	1999	Dr. Helen Glass
			Dr. Marilyn Wood
1992	Sister Jeanne Forest	2000	Dr. Shirley Stinson
1993	Professor Marie France Thibaudeau	2001	Dr. Carol Jillings
1994	Dr. Moyra Allen	2002	Edith Côté
			Louise Chartier
1996	Dr. Alice Baumgart	2003	Dr. Peggy Anne Field
1997	Dr. Denise Alcock	2004	Dr. Janet Storch

TABLE 4.3	Nurse Leaders Who Received the Canadian Nurses Association Jeanne-Mance Award (1971–2004)		
Date	**Name**	**Date**	**Name**
1971	Dr. Helen McArthur	1986	Dr. Dorothy Kergin
1974	Dr. Lyle Creelman	1988	Dr. Maria Rovers (posthumous)
	Dr. Alice Girard	1990	Dr. Shirley Stinson
	E.A. Electa MacLennan	1992	Dr. Helen Glass
1977	Dr. Rae Chittick	1994	E. Louise Milner
1979	Moyra Allen	1996	Margaret Neylan
	Dr. Huguette Labelle	1998	Peggy Anne Field
1980	Dr. Helen K. Mussallem	2000	Dr. Dorothy Pringle
1982	Dr. Verna Huffman Splane	2002	Dr. Janet Rush
1984	Dr. Florence Emory	2004	Dr. Ginette Lemire Rodger
	Sister Denise Lefebvre		

Knowledge-Based Changes

The first source of innovative opportunity arises from outside an organization. Porter-O'Grady (2000) thinks of technologic innovations as limitless opportunities that will significantly increase the independence of patients, who will function more as prosumers. With increased home care, outpatient services, day surgery, and effective health promotion programs, he expects a decrease in the number and size of hospitals. He advocates that nursing leaders reject all patient services that warehouse the chronically challenged or economically marginalized. The ongoing task for nursing is not to fill beds but to reframe the notion of long-term care so individuals devise more ingenious solutions to chronic care. In this way, patients become more responsible, and nurses receive more recognition for improving the effectiveness and efficiency of health care services.

Perceptual Changes

Whatever nurses think about the newfound importance of economic outcomes in health care, managerialism now drives health care services. Nurses and other professionals have to grow accustomed to this change (Reilly & Tamlyn, 2001). Targets and outcomes have come to replace goals and plans as costs and resource allocations have come to enjoy new prominence in health care jargon. The challenge that waits the next generation of nurses is how to devise strategies whereby nurses exercise "responsible autonomy." Unlike the traditional professionalism to which nurses are accustomed, this new way of doing things holds out considerable promise if nursing leaders devise more innovative approaches to health care. Only then do nurses become more like knowledge workers, who function outside a strict hierarchical system.

Unexpected Changes

Porter-O'Grady (2000) speaks of a new foundation for health care when he describes the diminution of an overbuilt hospital system. In this new era in which human capital counts for as much as buildings, equipment, and real estate, nursing leaders have to recognize this event as yet another unrealized opportunity to restructure health care delivery. They have to devise innovative responses to enable nurses to expand their scope of responsibilities beyond the hospital structure. If nurses are to fulfill society's expectations of them, they have to assist in moving health services out of the hospital and into the community. They have to share their vision that health promotion is as important as health protection. They have to embrace educational opportunities to increase their competencies so they can become more accountable.

■ SUMMARY

This chapter examines nursing leadership as an important factor in health care reform and in the diffusion of innovation. Consideration is first given to the changing health care environment and to the leadership role played by nurses in health care reform. Regrettably, nursing, like other knowledge-intense occupations, currently lacks a sufficient cadre of visible and vocal leaders required to develop innovative strategies to address these challenges.

Described as visionary, knowledgeable, confident, and highly visible, these leaders must possess the special ability to promote innovation. They must also know how to diffuse innovative ideas within an organization. In so doing, they can influence others on the health care team to implement new strategies that increase the effectiveness and efficiencies of the system.

Online Resources

Add to your knowledge of this issue:

Calgary Health Region's *Frontlines*	**www.crha-health.ab.ca/frontlines**
Canadian Association of Schools of Nursing	**www.causn.org**
Health Canada	**www.hc-sc.gc.ca**
Order of Canada	**www.gg.ca/honours/order_e.asp**
The Peter F. Drucker Foundation for Nonprofit Management/Leader to Leader Institute	**drucker.org**
Registered Nurses Association of Canada	**www.rnao.org**

REFLECTIONS on the Chapter . . .

1. Select from among your student experiences an example of how nurses introduced an innovation. Identify the sources of the innovation and critical steps in the innovation process.

2. From your most current clinical practicum, suggest some innovative ways to increase effectiveness or efficiency. Describe the leadership attributes or competencies called for in the innovation process.

3. This chapter discusses the changing health care environment in terms of nursing leadership. How can a new graduate prepare for such a role?

4. The four attributes of leadership, according to Hibberd and Rodger, are meant to apply to one individual. Provide examples of how different nurses, whom you have observed, displayed one of these attributes.

References

Beason, C. F. (2000). Advancing innovative nursing practice. *Nursing Clinics of North America, 35*(2), 569–577.

Beyerlein, M. M., Johnson, D. A., & Beyerlein, S. T. (Eds.). (1995). *Advances in interdisciplinary studies of work teams.* Vol. 2: Knowledge work in teams. Greenwich, CT: Jai Press.

Bulger, R. J. (1999). What will health care look like in the future? In E. J. Sullivan (Ed.), *Creating nursing's future issues, opportunities and challenges* (pp. 14–31). St. Louis: Mosby.

Calgary Health Region. (2001). A (slightly) new name and a new look for the region. Available at: http://www.crha-health.ab.ca/frontlines/issue41_1.htm.

Canadian Nurses Association. (2001). Communication Services, July 23. Ottawa: Author.

Chow, M. P., Coffman, J. M., & Morjikian, R. L. (1999). Transforming nursing leadership. In R.W. Gilkey (Ed.), *The 21st century health care leader* (pp. 290–298). San Francisco: Jossey-Bass.

Corey-Lisle, P., Tarzian, A. J., Cohen, M. Z., et al. (1999). Healthcare reform: Its effects on nurses. *Journal of Nursing Administration, 29*(3), 30–37.

Drucker, P. (1985). *Innovation and entrepreneurship: Practice and principles.* New York: Harper & Row.

_____. (1994, November). The age of social transformation. *The Atlantic Monthly*, pp. 53–56, 59, 62, 64, 66–68, 71–72, 74–78, 80.

Drucker, P. F. (1998). The discipline of innovation. *Harvard Business Review, 76*(6), 149–157.

_____. (1999). *Management challenges for the 21st century.* New York: Harper Business.

Giuliani, R. (2002). *Leadership.* New York: Miramax Books.

Goldsmith, M., Morgan, H., & Ogg, A. J. (2004). *Leading organizational learning.* San Francisco: Jossey-Bass.

Goleman, D. (1997). *Emotional intelligence.* NY: Bantam Books.

Goleman, D., Boyatzis, R., & McKee, A. (2002). *Primal leadership.* Boston: Harvard Business School Press.

Hibberd, J. M., & Rodger, G. L. (1999). Contemporary perspectives on leadership. In J. M. Hibberd & D. L. Smith (Eds.), *Nursing management in Canada* (pp. 259–277). Toronto: W. B. Saunders.

Lawler, E. E. (2001). The era of human capital has finally arrived. In W. Bennis, C. M. Spreitzer, & T. G. Cummings (Eds.), *The future of leadership* (pp. 14–25). San Francisco: Jossey-Bass.

Mintzberg, H. (2002). Managing to innovate. In F. Hesselbein, M. Goldsmith, & I. Somerville (Eds.), *Leading for innovation* (pp. 141–152). San Francisco: Jossey-Bass.

Nunn, K. (2001, February). *What about nursing leadership? A discussion paper for the nursing leadership conference.* Paper presented at the Nursing Leadership Conference, Ottawa.

Office of Nursing Policy, Health Canada. (2001). Healthy nurses, healthy workplaces. *Proceedings of the National Stakeholder Consultation Meeting.* Ottawa: Author, Health Policy & Communications Branch.

Porter-O'Grady, T. (2000). Visions for the 21st century: New horizons, new health care. *Nursing Administration Quarterly, 25*(1), 30–38.

Porter-O'Grady, T., & Krueger-Wilson, C. (1995). *The leadership revolution in health care: Altering systems, changing behaviors.* Gaithersburg, MD: Aspen.

Porter-O'Grady, T., & Malloch, K. (2002). *Quantum leadership: A textbook of new leadership.* Gaithersburg, MD: Aspen.

Registered Nurses Association of Ontario. (2000). *Ensuring the care will be there: Report on nursing recruitment and retention in Ontario.* Toronto: Author.

Reilly, S. M., & Tamlyn, D. (2000). *Nursing 769: Contemporary issues in health care* (pp. 2–3). Calgary: Faculty of Nursing, University of Calgary.

_____. (2001). The function of health knowledge teams in building a learning environment. *Proceedings of the 2nd International Conference on Researching Work and Learning* (pp. 485–492). Calgary: Faculty of Continuing Education, University of Calgary.

Rogers, E. M. (1995). *Diffusion of innovations.* New York: The Free Press.

Shamian, J. (2000). On the heels of Florence Nightingale: Re-energizing hospital care. *Reflections on Nursing Leadership, First Quarter*, 24–26.

Sorrells-Jones, J. (1999). The role of the chief executive in the knowledge-intense organization of the future. *Nursing Administration Quarterly, 23*(3), 17–25.

Southon, G., & Braithwaite, J. (1998). The end of professionalism? *Social Science & Medicine, 46*(1), 23–28.

Spitzer, A. (1998). Nursing in the health care system of the postmodern world: Crossroads, paradoxes and complexity. *Journal of Advanced Nursing, 28*(1), 164–171.

Storch, J. L., & Stinson, S. M. (1988). Concepts of deprofessionalization with applications to nursing. In R. White (Ed.), *Political issues in nursing: Past, present and future* (Vol. 3, pp. 33–44). Chichester, NY: John Wiley & Sons.

Tamlyn, D. (2004, September). New president's vision. *Canadian Nurse, 100*(7).

Taylor, F. (1947). *Scientific management.* New York: Harper & Row.

Toffler, A. (1980). *The third wave.* New York: William Morrow.

Wheatley, M. J. (2002). We are all innovators. In F. Hesselbein, M. Goldsmith, & I. Somerville (Eds.), *Leading for innovation* (pp. 11–21). San Francisco: Jossey-Bass.

Critical Questions

As a way of engaging with the ideas in this chapter, consider the following:

1. What comes to mind when you think about nursing policy? Consider one health or nursing policy that influences nursing practice.
2. What do you anticipate might influence or shape policy?
3. Which nurses are most effectively positioned to influence policy?
4. What do you imagine is the link between nursing/health policy and the delivery of health care?

Public policy forms a basis for emerging institutional, nursing, and organizational policies.

CHAPTER
5

Heather Clarke

Health and Nursing Policy: A Matter of Politics, Power, and Professionalism

University of Victoria School of Nurse Practitioner students speak with a Ministry of Health representative.

After completing this chapter, you will be able to:

1. Appreciate the real and potential contributions of nurses to health and nursing policy.
2. Understand types of policy.
3. Understand the policy process and the significance of contextual factors.
4. Identify roles, responsibilities, and opportunities for nurses in the policy process.
5. Identify challenges to nurses' involvement.
6. Determine strategies required for successful involvement.

This chapter discusses health and nursing policy and nurses' responsibilities and roles within the policy process. Policy is introduced as a process, as a product, and as an instrument. Relevant contextual and infrastructure requirements for nurses' involvement in policy are also discussed and illustrated with examples of nurses' influence in health and nursing policy.

The importance of nurses understanding policy—its development, implementation, and evaluation—cannot be overemphasized. Public policy decisions directly affect the health care of everyone as well as the practice of nursing. Nurses can and should become more involved with the policymaking process to ensure that decisions benefit the public at local, provincial/territorial, and national levels. Nursing leadership in the public policy arena will give nurses the best opportunities for putting forth agendas that will accomplish health goals that are in the public's interest.

■ POLICY, POLITICS, POWER, AND PROFESSIONALISM

Health policy, nursing policy, and institutional policy are all significant types of public policies that call for nursing involvement. A policy—a broad goal statement—has been defined as "the principles that govern action directed towards given ends" (Titmus, 1974, p. 23).

Policy

Public policy is whatever governments choose to do or not to do (Dye, 1978). It is a conscious choice of action directed toward an end, it is based on a commonly held value, and it gives direction for action (e.g., rules, laws).

Health policy, one aspect of public policy, includes the directives and goals for promoting the health of the public. Health policy may include policy related to population health goals, such as provincial health goals; health care system principles, such as the Canada Health Act; and service priorities and accountabilities, such as the Saskatchewan Health Performance plan. (Refer to the Online Resources section at the end of this chapter for more information.)

Nursing policy may be an aspect of, and influenced by, public policy (e.g., provincial and territorial nursing acts, free trade agreements) as well as a component of institutional policy (e.g., clinical practice guidelines, care maps, and critical paths). Nursing policy also includes organizational policy of the nursing association (e.g., policy and position statements, nursing practice and education standards).

Organizational policies, such as those of professional nursing associations, are the rules governing and the positions taken by an organization. Some organizational policies may be determined by public policy (e.g., registered nursing acts, scope of practice), whereas others are association specific (e.g., education standards, registration requirements).

Institutional policies, such as those of a hospital or health care agency, comprise the rules governing workplaces. Some institutional policies may be grounded in public policies (e.g., policies governing responsibility and accountability of health authorities), whereas others, such as mission, vision, and core value statements, are institution specific.

The difference between public policies, such as health policy, and institutional, nursing, and organizational policies is that government does not necessarily have the policy responsibility for the latter types. The responsibility belongs to the professional regulatory body, governance board of an agency, or managerial staff of a department. However, there is interplay and influences between these types of policies, as each type of policy is shaped by politics and power.

Distinguishing Policy From Politics

In determining how to participate in shaping any type of policy, one needs first to distinguish between political strategies and policy agendas. *Policy* deals with *shoulds* and *oughts*. *Politics* deals with *conditions* and sometimes impedes or accelerates the policy process. Politics involves using power to influence, persuade, or otherwise change—it is the art of understanding relationships between groups in society and using that understanding to achieve particular outcomes. As a phenomenon, politics is often reactive. Policy, on the other hand, is based in values, goals, or principles, even when those values may represent idiosyncratic biases (Table 5.1). Policy is more proactive, involving give-and-take in negotiation (Solomon & Roe, 1986).

Policy development is a value-laden process, beginning with what problems become policy issues and concluding with who decides how a policy will be evaluated. When values are in conflict, as they often are in the health and nursing policy arenas, politics necessarily comes in to play. When individuals and groups with disparate values enter into the policy process, politics, a major determinant of health policy, shapes the content and process of policy development (Mason, Talbott, & Leavitt, 1993).

People perceive politics in different ways. For some, the term evokes images of smoke-filled rooms, devious dealings, or power in the hands of a few. For others, the images have a different and more generic meaning (Ross Kerr & MacPhail, 1996). Whatever the perception, politics can be viewed as the art of influencing another person. There is no escaping politics in any arena. Many nurses recognize the importance of developing political skills, realizing that these skills are as important on the nursing unit as they are in

TABLE 5.1	Policy and Politics: Some Comparisons

Policy	Politics
Deals with shoulds and oughts	Focuses on conditions
Based on values, goals, and principles	Uses power to persuade and influence
Frequently proactive—negotiable	Primarily reactive—nonnegotiable
Stages of development from formation of the problem through adoption of the policy, implementation, and evaluation	Political process is the way policy is developed—requires identification of true issues and stakeholders and their goals and interests
Objective is to be evidence based (e.g., using research, epidemiology, databases in health information, surveys)	Foundation is philosophical—party oriented (e.g., liberal, conservative, socialist)
The chosen theoretical perspective with its values and principles determines details of the policy process	Shapes the content for the policy and the policy process

other spheres of social activity where decisions must be made. For this reason, the Registered Nurses Association of Ontario initiated a Nursing Policy Summer Institute in 2004. In both the policy and political processes, individuals require the following skill and qualities:

- Analytical thinking
- Visionary perspective—future and goal oriented
- Force of commitment
- Communication of goals
- Reliability and integrity

Power

The concept of power is not generally associated with nursing. The media, public at large, and other opinion makers refer to the power of major corporations, politicians, trade unions, medical associations, and male-dominated organizations; seldom are the nursing profession and nurses considered powerful (Ferguson, 1993). However, today's idea of empowerment replaces yesterday's notion of power (Barnum & Kerfoot, 1995), and nurses are demonstrating significant empowerment in all contexts of practice. Instead of the capacity one has to influence others to accomplish something they would not normally accomplish, empowerment is authority purposefully shared with others to increase the total amount of nurses' influence in the organization. Nurses, like anyone else, fulfill their mission better when they are empowered to work to their full capacity. The Canadian Nurses Association (CNA) facilitates this empowerment among nurses. Sources of empowerment include the following:

- Expanded expertise and restructured practice that aim to use each nurse's skills and knowledge level
- Nurses who are valued as scarce resources and knowledgeable workers who cannot be spared to do lower-level tasks
- New legal powers that legitimize various nurse roles, such as nurse practitioner, and public acceptance of these roles integrated into the health care system
- New roles, such as clinical nurse specialist, that provide clinical expertise as well as contribute to system-level responsibilities, such as quality assurance, research, and evidence-based practice
- Changed self-perception—accepting one's own ideas or the ideas of one's leader over those imposed by others who would create limitations (Barnum & Kerfoot, 1995)

Why should nurses pay attention to power and empowerment? Ferguson (1985) notes that:

- Nurses must be able to get things done on behalf of the people they serve—they are advocates.
- Nurse educators and nurse administrators need to make course content in schools of nursing and activities in service settings of interest and applicable to students.
- Nurses' power base is expanded as nurses encourage and support nurse candidates for political office and professional organization lobbying efforts.
- Knowledge is power. As such, it confers authority on the possessor. Knowledge, then, may be nurses' greatest source of power.

Nurses find that a number of strategies and skills increase their ability to influence policy (Grohar-Murray & DiCroce, 1997; Loveridge & Cummings, 1996). These include the following:

- Enhanced skills and knowledge—being well informed and current—are the basis for attaining credibility.
- Good working relationships with all coworkers are essential and include networking and consultation.
- The ability to convince others of the appropriateness of one's views is based on providing logical arguments and proposing positive solutions.
- Being visible and in a position to speak with groups and individuals is the basis for influencing those groups and individuals.

The new enabling legislation allowed nurses and health professionals other than physicians to be fully used in a reformed health care system inspired by primary health care. The primary health care approach is both a philosophy of health care and an approach to providing services (World Health Organization [WHO], 1978; WHO, 1986). Primary health care embraces five types of care, which are based on principles of accessibility, public participation, appropriate technology, and intersectoral cooperation. The five types of care are promotive, preventive, curative, rehabilitative, and supportive/palliative. Since then, the national, provincial, and territorial professional nursing associations have been clarifying their positions on primary health care, a major thrust of nursing, and recommending strategies to attain health for all (CNA, 2003a; Rodger & Gallagher, 2000).

Primary health care demonstration projects (e.g., Comox Valley Nursing Centre in British Columbia, Saskatchewan's Beechy Collaborative Practice Pilot Project, Nova Scotia's Cheticamp Primary Health Care Project), position statements, briefs, and meetings with politicians and bureaucrats have been developed and implemented by nurses since the mid-1980s. The CNA (2000a) states that "the goal of nursing practice is to improve the health of clients. In working to that goal, nurses must apply the five principles of the primary health care approach. This is true for nurses involved in direct care, in education, in research, in administration, or in policy roles."

More recently, the nursing profession has been successful in obtaining legislation and education for nurse practitioners (NPs) as a strategy for increasing primary health care in Canada (CNA, 2003b). The CNA recommends that stakeholders (e.g., policymakers, governments, regulatory bodies) work together to achieve a national, coordinated framework (i.e., policy foundation for a coordinated approach) as NPs have the potential to contribute significantly to new models of health care based on the principles of primary health care (CNA, 2003c).

Today, the policy work of nurses is more important than ever. Federal, provincial, and territorial governments are recognizing the need to have senior nurses at the policy table. In creating the Office of Nursing Policy, federal health minister Alan Rock stated, "The new position is a positive step towards finding ways to better utilize the remarkable knowledge and expertise of nurses in strengthening the health of all Canadians" (cited in Shamian, 2000). Since then, Health Canada also created in the First Nations and Inuit Health Branch an Office of Nursing Services with an executive director. Several provincial governments and the health regions/authorities have also instituted offices or positions for nursing policy and strategic planning, and others are in the process of doing so. The proactive work of professional nursing associations and unions is increasingly recognized as an important component of public policy work.

Historical Significance of Policy

Policies determine the context in which nurses provide and clients receive care, whether it is in an institutional or community setting, whether care is privately or publicly funded, which individuals and groups are entitled to receive care, and which resources are allocated to fund services. Policies influence nurses' roles at a number of levels: provincial/territorial, professional associations, health care organizations, units within organizations, and individuals. Although nurses are generally knowledgeable about policies that guide specific nursing practices (e.g., use of restraints, incident reporting), they have less understanding of public policy (e.g., health and nursing) and its relationship to their work (i.e., practice and work environment). Yet the relationship between nursing practice and public policy is crucial when we consider that nurses' daily working lives and clients' daily lives are defined and controlled by this policy.

The CNA states that "nursing is a political act . . . a natural extension of the essence of nursing—of caring" (CNA, 2000b, p. 4). Health care privatization, increasing poverty, environmental pollution and destruction, and escalating violence all have clear repercussions for health and nursing.

Regardless of the policy context—government, association, workplace—involvement of all nurses is needed to address health and nursing policy and strategic planning priorities, which include the following:

■ Nursing-related human resource planning and deployment
■ Safe, healthy, and professionally supportive work environments

- Scope and models of nursing practice grounded in primary health care principles
- Utilization and involvement of nurses in decision making and policymaking as well as in leadership roles
- Nursing data requirements in clinical and administration health information systems and electronic health records
- Education for lifelong learning, including undergraduate, graduate, postdoctoral, and continuing professional education

Theoretical Perspective

Conventional wisdom holds that elected governments make health policy; that federal and provincial cabinets approve programs and policies on the advice of their minister of health; that ministers of health are advised by professional public servants working in their departments; and that Canada's parliament and provincial legislatures then formally make health policy by passing laws governing the health system (Decter, 2001). This conventional wisdom can be applied to nursing policy development at government, association, or local levels. In reality, however, the policy process is more complex and messy and is shaped and influenced by public strategies, media reports, interest groups and stakeholders, academics, and policy consultants. The policy process is not always the same or as rational and linear as logic and democratic beliefs suggest (Brooks, 1998).

Several theories, or theoretical perspectives, have been developed in an attempt to bring more logic and understanding to the policy process. A theory offers an explanation of why things happen the way they do. With respect to the policy process, theories, or theoretical perspectives, provide a map that directs our attention to particular features of the world or issue. Depending on the theoretical perspective, our attention focuses on different features of the situation we seek to understand, different stakeholders and players who will be involved, different priorities to set, and different goals to identify (Brooks, 1998). Major theoretical models include the pluralistic, public choice, and Marxist models.

Pluralistic Model

A pluralistic model of policymaking in democratic societies views the process as a competition among elites. Powerful groups influence policymakers to have their wishes applied to all (Brooks, 1998). Such groups as physicians, unions, and policy consultants have influenced health policy in the past. More recently, professional nursing associations and consumer groups have become more powerful and influential in the process, advocating for issues related to health promotion (e.g., tobacco legislation), injury and disease prevention (e.g., bicycling helmet regulations), and choice of health care practitioners (e.g., nurse practitioners).

Public Choice Model

The public choice model, concerned with economics and individual positions, grounds the policy process in strategic behaviors of individuals. Individual politicians and bureaucrats act on the basis of rational self-interest, often under conditions of imperfect knowledge (Brooks, 1998). Politicians and board members seek to be elected and, once elected, to maintain themselves in power, while bureaucrats and staff seek promotion and more control of their work environments (Brooks, 1998). Policy influence is primarily at the individual-to-individual level. Thus, new government chief nurse positions are important for exerting influence on a one-to-one basis as well as within groups, bringing forward nursing issues, perspectives, and evidence-based knowledge.

Marxist Model

The Marxist model is based on the belief that antagonistic relationships exist between different social and economic classes of people. This antagonism is the central factor of politics and policies (Brooks, 1998).

The capitalist class, considered supreme, is the determinant of public policy decisions. The private versus public health care system policy debate exemplifies the Marxist model. Influencing this policy process perspective may be difficult if the issue is not framed as a social or economic class issue.

Understanding the Complexity of Policy

No one theoretical perspective is consistently taken in the policy process. The perspective differs depending on a variety of factors, including the specific policy issue, timeframe for resolution, political agenda, and power relationships. What is important for nurses to understand and learn is how to become part of the process and use their knowledge and expertise to enlighten and influence specific policy processes, regardless of the theoretical perspective taken.

Policy development involves a conscious choice that leads to deliberate action or inaction. The conscious choice of selecting a particular goal requires a plan of action—or the means for achieving the goal—to be developed and put into effect. Policy goals may be actualized in such products or instruments as laws, regulations, policy or position statements, briefs, taxes, or fines.

Spheres of Nurse Involvement

"Our challenge is to exercise our power and influence and use the political process to help bring about a major change in the delivery of nursing services to society" (Rodger, 1993, p. 25). Professional nursing holds significant and plausible solutions to current crises in health care.

Nurse leaders are increasingly aware that all health issues, no matter how seemingly remote from nursing, will have an impact on the direction of health policy and thus eventually on nursing. For example, today's nursing shortage is the result of policy decisions made in the mid-1990s to reduce the number of hospital beds and at the same time reduce the number of students accepted into nursing schools. Other policy decisions, such as regionalization, reduction in funds for certain services, scopes of practice, and decreased funding for equipment, have direct effects on nurses' professional practice in direct care, education, administration, and research.

Workplace: The Health Care Institution

At an institutional level, evidence-based policy is required not only to address management and financial issues (e.g., health and human resource deployment, health information systems) but also to make critical interdisciplinary clinical decisions (e.g., practice guidelines for prevention and treatment of pressure ulcers, care maps) and develop work environments supportive of quality care and professional nursing practice. Clinical practice is a political endeavor because nurses must effectively influence the allocation of scarce resources, collaborate in evidence-based clinical decision making, work in the interest of other parties (e.g., clients or clients' families), and facilitate development of health resources and supports for groups and communities. Involvement in the policy process may be related to clinical practice guidelines specific to nursing care, care maps and critical paths for interdisciplinary care, or system-wide quality assurance initiatives, for example. Nurses in clinical and administrative practice frequently lead interdisciplinary care teams in development, implementation, and evaluation of evidence- and outcome-based policies and guidelines as well as in advocating for practice environments supportive of quality care. The international interdisciplinary study on hospital characteristics and client and nurse outcomes has contributed to our understanding of critical relationships between the work environment and outcomes and notes areas where changes in policy are required (Clarke et al., 2001). In addition to adequate resources, nursing leadership at middle management and executive levels is crucial to improving client and nurse outcomes.

A health care agency's or an institution's mission, vision, and core values are the foundations for operational policy and decision making as well as strategic planning. Nurses have a responsibility to contribute to the development of their institution's policy foundations and to the philosophy of nursing and client care at both institutional and unit levels. It is the role of nurse leaders and senior executive nurses to ensure that a process is in place to facilitate nurses carrying out this responsibility. Nursing practice councils are one structure that has been used to encourage and support nurses' participation in these institutional policies.

Nurses also need to be aware of their institutions' key policies: the organizational charts with their lines of communication and responsibility (i.e., power); mission statements, goals, and objectives (i.e., organizational culture); and policy and procedure manuals (i.e., expectations). Additionally, all health care institutions and agencies have an informal life not bound by a formal chain of command, board of directors, or committee structure. Nurses who want to influence an institution should take stock of the informal structure and processes. Those with formal titles usually have power and authority; however, others who do not have such formal titles can also wield power and influence. It is important for nurses to know where all the sources of power and influence lie.

Policies in health care institutions are profoundly influenced by policies and politics of government as well as by changes in the workforce and client populations and by economic and social changes within communities and professional organizations. In turn, workplace policies influence learning experiences for students, new employees, and nurses with new or different responsibilities. Important opportunities, such as mentoring, preceptoring, organizing orientations, and promoting professional development, are directly affected by clinical and institutional policies. Empowered nurses and students can influence such policies and their implementation.

Government

An understanding of political, demographic, epidemiologic, and other forces shaping health care now and in the future is necessary if nurses are to ensure that workplace policies promote the health of the public and foster a supportive environment in which health care is provided—health care that spans the continuum of care from health promotion and illness and injury prevention to rehabilitative and palliative care. One of the most pressing policy issues facing all societies today is the nurse shortage and how to plan for and maintain relevant health resources, with an appropriate mix and optimal utilization of these scarce resources.

Although nursing is a self-regulating and self-governing profession, government provides society with a legal definition of nursing and what is within its scope of practice. Nursing associations and individual nurses advocate with government to ensure that nursing legislation and subsequent rules are in the best interest of the public—that they facilitate and support the full participation of nursing practice to achieve the goal of safe and appropriate health care.

Government also determines who will get what kind or level of health care (e.g., needle exchange sites, medications). Canadian nurses have been influential, locally and globally, in advocating for health care policy that promotes health and prevents illness in addition to curing disease, rehabilitating, and providing palliative care. Canadian nurses have also exerted influence to ensure that quality care is accessible, universal, and equitable and is supported by qualified, professional health care providers who are publicly accountable. The CNA's advocacy role in federal policy and politics has been increasingly evident at the turn of the century, as has its involvement of individual members and provincial and territorial nursing regulatory and professional associations (Box 5.2).

BOX 5.2 Strengthening the Voice: The Ninth Decade of the Canadian Nurses Association

Looking back throughout each decade in its history, the Canadian Nurses Association (CNA) has made a significant impact on the advancement of the nursing profession and the promotion of quality, accessible health care for Canadians. The document identified below by its online address is a retrospective of the period 1990 to 1999, the ninth decade since the creation of the CNA.

Canadian Nurses Association. Retrieved August 20, 2004, from http://206.191.29.104/_frames/aboutcna/aboutusframe.html

In recent years, governments have once again recognized the need to provide infrastructure aimed at increasing nurses' input into the health and nursing policy process. At both federal and provincial levels, positions and offices are once again being created for senior nurse executives. The first federal principal nursing officer, Verna Huffman Splane, was appointed in 1968 (Splane & Splane, 1994); in 1938, Laura Holland was the first appointed nurse advisory to the British Columbia Ministry of Health (Paulson, Zilm, & Warbinek, 2000). Multiple-stakeholder federal, provincial, and territorial nursing committees and studies are also being instituted to advise government ministers and senior staff. It is absolutely critical that nurses support both these current initiatives by contributing their expertise to the policy work to be undertaken.

Through its funding priorities, government can influence which health problems will be researched and targeted for government funding and support. Without nurses' unfaltering involvement in research policy and sharing their nursing knowledge and evidence, research-funding agencies would not recognize the value of supporting nursing research. In turn, nurses would not be able to make significant contributions of knowledge to improve the health of the public. The Nursing Research Fund within the Canadian Health Services Research Foundation (CHSRF) and the recently established Nursing Care Partnership Program are the result of lobbying by Canadian nurses and demonstrate the power of nursing knowledge (Box 5.3).

Professional Organizations and Unions

Professions exist at the pleasure of society and address specific human needs (Joel, 1993). Out of respect for the complex and learned nature of its work, the public allows a high degree of internal regulation by the profession and recognizes the complexity of professional practice and looks to the profession as a collective to define its standards of safety and competence. Until the 1973 Supreme Court decision *Service Employees International Union v. Saskatchewan Registered Nurses Association* (SRNA), collective bargaining was a function of the professional association. The Supreme Court decision agreed with the union's contention that the SRNA could not legally represent staff nurses in Saskatchewan because of management domination. Since then, there has been a separation of professional associations and unions (Rowsell, 1982).

Today's professional organizations' decision-making bodies develop policy to meet their public mandates, move strategic plans, direct the associations' resources, and guide implementation. It is important for their policies to target both nursing and health issues and to provide clarity about the point beyond which there is no compromise. The professional associations of Canadian nurses have the potential to influence the nursing profession, health policy, and client care.

BOX 5.3   **The Nursing Research Fund**

The Nursing Research Fund was created as an answer to concerns raised by nursing organizations and others representing nursing interests. The CNA and other major nursing voices lobbied the federal government extensively for funding to develop nursing researchers and to support research on nursing recruitment, retention, management, and the issues emerging from health-system restructuring. In 1999, the federal government responded by providing the foundation with enough funds to support research personnel, research dissemination, and research projects on nursing management, organization, and policy at a level of $2.5 million per year for 10 years. The fund supports the production of research with health-system decision makers in mind, as well as training and personnel support. Nursing leadership, organization, and policy are themes of the open grants competition. In 2003, the CHSRF granted the Canadian Nurses Foundation a 5-year renewable award of $2.5 million for the administration of the Nursing Care Partnership Program (NCP) to support clinical nursing.

Canadian Health Services Research Foundation, Nursing Research Fund. Retrieved August 20, 2004, from http://www.canadiannursesfoundation.com/nursecare.htm; http://www.chsrf.ca/nursing_research_fund/index_e.php

Professional nursing organizations are instrumental in shaping nursing practice. They develop standards for nursing practice, education, ethical conduct, and continuing competence. They lobby for progressive changes in the scope of nurses' practice and play a role in collective action that influences workplace policies. Whether the issue of concern is primarily nursing or health care, nurses have responsibilities to use their political skill and nursing expertise to contribute to their associations' leadership role in public policy development—policy that aims to improve the health of communities and to ensure the provision of high-quality nursing care.

Unions representing nursing are primarily concerned with the development of legally binding agreements that regulate staff nurses' salaries, working conditions, and other negotiable benefits. However, unions also advocate for health and nursing policy related to other issues (e.g., scope of nursing practice, primary health care). Nurses may be involved in union policy work—its development and implementation as well as monitoring contractual agreements. Such involvement is essential to the promotion of work environments supportive of nurses' practice and their health.

Professional organizations and unions have some common goals, including the welfare of members and the improvement of their working conditions. They share a concern for professional ethics, although it is the professional organization that is responsible for ensuring that the standards of professional conduct reflected in the codes of ethics are practised. Although they do have common interests, professional organizations and unions are different in many ways, with different responsibilities and perspectives on public policy, including that related to health and nursing. When relevant, professional nursing organizations and unions work together to influence policy affecting the professional practice of nursing and the health of the population. Such collaboration was evident in identifying workplace issues affecting nurse retention and recruitment; enabling employment of student nurses outside their educational requirements; addressing mentor–preceptor issues; working on the Canadian Nursing Advisory Committee, which has culminated in a final report and recommendations, *Our Health, Our Future: Creating Quality Workplaces for Canadian Nurses* (Canadian Nursing Advisory Committee, 2002); and participating in the Nursing Sector Study, *Building the Future: An Integrated Strategy for Nursing Human Resources in Canada* (Nursing Sector Study Corporation, 2004).

Educational Institutions

Both faculty and students have opportunities and responsibilities to be involved in public education policy. Such involvement may be with government-level policy (e.g., initiatives with respect to legislation, funding, scholarships and bursaries, quality of education); within the institution level (e.g., with respect to mission, vision, curriculum, learning opportunities); and with associations (e.g., Canadian Association of Schools of Nursing, Canadian Nursing Students' Association, professional specialty associations) and their policies, positions, standards, and the like (Box 5.4).

Community

As members of a community, nurses have a responsibility to promote the welfare of the community and its members. The community's resources can be invaluable assets for health promotion and health care delivery. Nurses' contributions through community development and participation in community initiatives provide another credible and trusted voice in the policy process. Outcomes of nurses' contributions can be witnessed in the sustainability of demonstration and pilot projects, such as nursing and community health centers in a number of Canadian provinces and territories.

Nurses working with First Nations communities are especially aware of the need to work with the community to incorporate aboriginal values, beliefs, and practices into health care and nursing policies. Reaching community health goals can only be achieved with true partnerships, with nurses contributing their expertise while at the same time listening to and understanding the priorities and preferences of First Nations people. The Nuu-chah-nulth Community and Human Services Community Health Nurses on Vancouver Island received the Advocacy for Health Award from the Registered Nurses Association of

| BOX 5.4 | Professional Nursing Educational Associations: CASN and CNSA |

The Canadian Association of Schools of Nursing (CASN) was formed to promote desirable standards of education and research and to support the development of future university schools of nursing. CASN, the official accrediting agency for university nursing programs in Canada, is a voluntary association representing all universities and colleges that offer undergraduate and graduate programs in nursing. CASN participates in a national network for discussion of issues in higher education:
www.casn.ca/casn/mission.htm
The Canadian Nursing Students' Association (CNSA) is the national voice of Canadian nursing students in diploma and baccalaureate registered nursing programs. The aim is to increase the legal, ethical, professional, and educational aspects that are an integral part of nursing. The association is dedicated to an active and positive promotion of nurses and the nursing profession as a whole.
www.cnsa.ca

British Columbia for their advocacy in providing culturally sensitive nursing care to the people of the communities (Moore, 2001). The community health nurses have not only developed a nursing framework that defines their relationship with their clients, setting the parameters of a health partnership that recognizes Nuu-chah-nulth traditions and values, but they have also developed nursing program strategic directions, with client-focused objectives, outcomes, and measurable indicators.

■ CONCEPTUALIZING THE POLICY DESIGN PROCESS

Policymaking, a dynamic and cyclical process, can be conceptualized as a model of systematic and functional activities (Anderson, 1990) aimed at exploring the causal links between problems and solutions. Shamian and colleagues (2003) describe an eight-phase cycle to move from issue to policy. Although a model is useful, one must also remember that policymaking is messy, often with multiple iterations of some of the stages. There are also power differentials to take into consideration in the policy process. Some current powerful influencers of policy include characteristics of the economy and society and the recent globalization of information availability. The latter has both competition and cooperation potential because of unequal access to information technology within the country. Also, there are differential power relationships between governments (e.g., federal and provincial governments regarding federal contributions to provincial health care funding) as well as between governors and the governed (e.g., the professional regulatory organization and its members regarding continuing competency requirements for registration). These differences bring with them opportunities for negotiation and revisions to a proposed or existing policy.

Identifying Issues

Policy problems are identified through situations that produce needs or dissatisfaction for which relief is sought (Anderson, 1990). Policy problems must be brought to the policymakers' attention. Once there, the policy issues and theoretical perspective to policymaking are influenced by many factors (Brooks, 1998). The strengths of political and cultural influences are often determined by geographic location (e.g., rural, urban), language (e.g., English, French), ethnicity (e.g., majority, minority), and values and principles (e.g., public, private). Problem definition develops as values, beliefs, and social attitudes toward a concern are delineated and policy approaches are considered.

Setting Priorities: The Policy Agenda

Ideally, policymaking involves interested parties coming together to formulate ideas and solutions to given circumstances or problems. In reality, however, struggles for power are, and always have been, principal factors in motivating change (Hart, 1994). At provincial and federal levels, commissions have been formed to help identify policy issues, priorities, and strategies. In recent years, many provincial governments have also established health care commissions to address issues related to health care systems and the health profession. The 2001 Federal Commission on the Future of Health Care in Canada, commissioned to make recommendations on sustaining a publicly funded health system that balances investments in prevention and health maintenance with those directed to care and treatment, released its final report, *Building on Values: The Future of Health Care in Canada* (Romanow, 2002). Although such commissions provide information for decision making and priority setting, they are frequently linked to politics and the political party of the time. Thus, findings and recommendations are often not acted on because of change in government or political priorities. However, with policy advocacy from many stakeholders, including nursing organizations, Romanow's recommendations for a Health Care Renewal Accord was signed by Canada's First Ministers and a Health Council was established.

Policy issues and priorities may also arise from research. However, historically, there has been a gap between research and policy—having the evidence available for policymakers when it is required, researching issues of current interest to policymakers, and having policymakers focus on evidence in decision making. More recently, attention has been given to encouraging a closer link between policymakers and researchers. Granting agencies, such as the CHSRF, promote and fund management and policy research in health services and nursing to increase the quality, relevance, and usefulness of this research for health system policymakers and managers and work with health system decision makers to support and enhance their use of research evidence when addressing health management and policy challenges (Brokering Program, 2004).

Besides gaps between researchers and policymakers and the re-examination of issues through commissions, challenges to nurses' consistent and meaningful involvement in setting policy agendas are related to the following:

- Dominance of the medical profession
- Culture, values, and structures of predecessor health care systems
- Invisibility of nursing
- Stability of the "iron triangle" of civil servant (bureaucrat), politician, and physician (Hart, 1994)

Uncovering the Evidence

Discovering reasons for policy involves discovering the data on which policies are based (Solomon & Roe, 1986). However, sometimes there are no data, just someone's idea of what should be. Although this situation can be found at the level of public policy as politics, it is also evident at the clinical level, where many practices have become policy for less than rational reasons.

Ideally, policy depends on data—data gathered from existing information and summarized and synthesized with a particular question in mind. Existing sources of data used in the policy process include published and unpublished reports, briefs, and research as well as public, stakeholder, or member communication. Thus, it is critical for nurses to pay attention to the development of data-gathering systems (e.g., health information systems, nursing workload and classification systems) and to learn how to make clinical knowledge and wisdom accessible and meaningful to the policy process.

During data analysis—a systematic description and explanation of causes and consequences of action and inaction—conversation among researchers and scientists and among politicians and stakeholders or advocates should be maintained (Anderson, 1990). The role of nurses in data analysis is part expert advisor and part advocate in providing their unique professional nursing perspective for policy decisions.

Choosing Instruments for Policy Formulation

The successful attainment of policy goals depends on the choice of instruments for achieving them (Brooks, 1998) and is influenced by values and the theoretical perspective taken (pluralist, public choice, Marxist). Instruments may include passage of a law or regulation, the expenditure of money, an official speech, or some other observable act. In general, carrots (incentives) are less intrusive than sticks (commands and prohibitions) and are more likely to be preferred by those decision makers predisposed toward smaller governance structures and greater scope for individual choice. In deciding how best to accomplish a policy goal (or set of related goals), policymakers consider a number of factors, such as the following:

- Political considerations
- Past experiences
- Bureaucratic or staff preferences
- Random factors, like personal values of key decision makers
- Measures most likely to achieve the goals
- How the goals can be accomplished at the least cost

Some of the policy instruments or products particularly relevant to nurses, but also used in other public policies, are the following:

- Endorsed positions (e.g., CNA Code of Ethics for Registered Nurses by other nursing jurisdictions)
- Briefs, position statements, official messages (e.g., CNA response to the Health Services on Health Care in Canada, *Putting "Health" Back Into Health Care* [CNA, 1980])
- Strategic policy (e.g., mission, vision, core values, priorities)
- Procedures (e.g., clinical practice guidelines)
- Standards (e.g., practice standards, care and accreditation standards)
- Rules and regulations (e.g., communicable disease control)
- Legislation (e.g., nurse registration acts)

Adopting and Implementing the Policy

Adoption of the policy, or enactment of legislation, occurs before implementation of the policy. Consideration must be given to ensuring that stakeholders are aware of the policy. For example, most professional nursing organizations publish new or revised position and policy statements, practice expectations, and standards in a form that all members receive. Although it is the responsibility of the policymaker to communicate the policy, it is the responsibility of those affected, the stakeholders, to recognize and take note of any new policy and its enactment.

Implementation is about doing: accomplishing a task, achieving a goal. Policy implementation is the process of transforming the goals associated with policy into results (Brooks, 1998). However, goals established by policymakers may be extremely vague, relying on words whose meanings are ambiguous and open to interpretation. Policymakers do not always know exactly what they want; consequently, their instructions are sometimes imprecise or even conflicting (Brooks, 1998). Thus, goals must be set, well articulated, understood, and translated in programs with budget and funding appropriations. Programs are vehicles by which policies are implemented and ideally have input from those who have a stake in the issue—policymakers, interest groups, professional associations, and others (Anderson, 1990). Once a legitimate authority approves the program, it can be implemented.

Implementation involves such activities as applying the rules, interpreting regulations, enforcing laws, and delivering services. Ideally, at this time, evaluation criteria are set for determining whether a program meets policy goals and objectives. Program development and implementation are usually the responsibility of staff of an organization or government.

Communicating the Policy

Communication is tremendously important; it is a vital link between goals and implementation. Without clear and concise communication about the policy—what it means and how it is to be implemented—policy goals will never be accomplished. Furthermore, implementation and communication problems may be related to coordination within and between organizations. Virtually all programs depend on some level of joint action. As the number of separate decisions that must be made increases, the likelihood of successful implementation decreases (Brooks, 1998).

Recognizing Barriers to Implementation

Other issues confound the implementation of policy. These include the following:

- Attitudes and beliefs of program administrators
- Territorialism and reluctance to give up that which is considered to be one's own
- External stakeholders' interests
- Political culture

Evaluating the Outcome

A feedback or monitoring process should be included from the beginning of any policy program development. Planned evaluation should be carried out at specified intervals throughout the process to monitor the impact of the policy (outcomes evaluation) and to be certain that the policy deals with the identified needs, issues, and goals (Glass & Hicks, 2000). How do we know when a program works or whether the policy has achieved its goal? How can we be sure that the results achieved have been accomplished as efficiently as possible? Although difficult, evaluation is an important part of policy and its implementation. Successful strategies involve early partnerships among evaluators/researchers, policymakers, and program implementers as well as the identification of appropriate, measurable outcome indicators. The primary difficulties to overcome include:

- Realizing that quantity does not necessarily mean quality
- Accepting that policy goals may be nebulous and use language such as "promoting, protecting, improving" something
- Learning that some politicians have an interest in hard numbers, and others have an interest in ambiguous, or soft, data

Revising the Policy

Findings from the evaluation phase should identify whether a program has satisfactorily met the original concerns and should be continued. Segments of the original policy goals may remain unmet, or new issues may surface, indicating that the policy process cycle needs to start again with further clarification of the policy problem.

Given the complexity and barriers within the policy process, it is not unreasonable that nurses and others are skeptical about the actualization of policy intents or goals. However, this only emphasizes the need for nurses to be involved in all stages of the policy process. Whether one is a student, new graduate, seasoned expert, or leader, all nurses can play important roles in the policy process.

■ IMPACT ON NURSING: THE RELEVANCE OF A NURSING PERSPECTIVE

A policy perspective for nurses must be one that assumes professional nurses pay attention to what clients need and deliver that service (Solomon & Roe, 1986). That means health and nursing policy are part of the practice of nursing. Nurses need to shape policy in a variety of ways and in a variety of places, not the least of which are the places where they work (Mason et al., 1993). Nursing perspective and expertise are required in government and professional association policy work. Nurses who understand the institutions in which they work, the professional associations they belong to, their community organizations, and the government structures are more likely to be able to participate in the policy process effectively.

Professional associations need the energy, expertise, and vision of all nurses, from students to renowned leaders. Support and influence for professional nursing organizations' policies and involvement in public policy can be expressed in many ways, including the following:

- Active membership
- Submission of resolutions
- Membership on task forces or committees
- Identification of issues
- Candidacy for or membership on board of directors
- Membership or leadership in a professional specialty group
- Support of lobbying efforts with letters, telephone calls, networking, and the like

■ FUTURE IMPLICATIONS: CHALLENGES AND STRATEGIES

What is often thought of as a challenge frequently takes on the characteristics of an opportunity requiring particular strategies. Changing one's perspective from challenge to opportunity requires a vision and a belief in one's self and the nursing profession. Thus, the challenges that follow can be thought of as nothing more than opportunities to change what existed in the past and what can exist in the future.

Challenges

Nurses often have the experience of not being listened to or not finding a suitable channel through which their voices will be heard and their contributions to policy valued. Sometimes change occurs and that change is to the detriment of nurses who have not known what the full consequences of change would be. Change also occurs when nurses feel powerless, when they believe any resistance or any attempts to effect change on a specific issue would be hopeless. This most often occurs when nurses lack the empirical evidence on which to make their cases.

Yet the clinical knowledge and expertise of nurses are their greatest assets in the policy process. Expert power is actualized in the increasing number of well-educated and degreed nurses. There is also recognition of nursing as a learned profession with the capacity for independent as well as collaborative practice and all the attendant and inherent rights, responsibilities, and accountabilities that go along with that status.

Nurses need to feel empowered with the authority commensurate with this knowledge and expertise as caregivers closest to clients and proportionate to their numbers. They need power to ensure their ability to provide competent, humanistic, and affordable care to people; power to help shape health policy and alter the disproportionate leverage of physicians; and power to ensure that nursing is an attractive career option for women and men who expect to influence and improve nursing, health care, and health policy (Ferguson, 1993).

The fundamental source of empowerment is self-confidence—the projection of a powerful image that emanates from a sturdy self-image. The key to acquiring this lies, to a great extent, in the hands of nursing leaders and managers in decision-making roles who actualize nurses' legitimate power and the authority to bring about change (Ferguson, 1985). The role of the governing structures in institutions and government is important in establishing and maintaining organizational and professional arrangements by which nurses control their practice and professional affairs. The workplace must be committed to ensuring that nurses have accountability for decisions affecting nursing.

Some groups are more adept at exploiting the policy process and are better placed to do so. This can pit the interest not only of one occupational group against another but also of individuals within a particular group, such as nursing. An example of this can be found in the increased number of hospital nurses at a time when primary health care policies and directions dictate that more resources and nursing personnel be directed into community nursing. "There can be little doubt that one of the primary problems facing nurses is actually identifying what their best interests are and then arriving at strategies for advancing them" (Hart, 1994, p. 184). Not being a homogeneous group endlessly complicates the policy-influencing process, as does nurses' general position in the health care system pecking order. The closer nurses in all contexts of practice work together to advance policies that will improve the health of the public, and the more collaboration there is between nursing professional associations and unions, the greater will be the voice and influence of nursing in the policy process.

Strategies for Involvement

Nurses need to be sensitive to the political process. Experience shows that positive results are most often obtained by working with the system, not against it (Glass & Hicks, 2000). Working with the system requires an understanding of the political process, of the global perspective of the health system, and of issues in the local community. It is essential for nurses to be knowledgeable about current policy directions, to be aware of the expected outcomes of the programs, and to participate in the development of policy in the many sectors influencing health and nursing.

Some strategic guidelines for influencing the policy process include the following:

- Educate yourself about the issue, the decision makers, and other stakeholders.
- Vote for policymakers who support humanistic policies. Get to know your representatives personally at various levels—local, tribal/band, provincial, territorial, federal.
- Participate in your professional nursing association's work; this communicates your message to the appropriate people. Hold an office. Be on a committee.
- Join a professional organization with goals and philosophies you can identify with and support in working to shape nursing and health care.
- Work with colleagues to transform the places in which health care is provided or nursing is taught.
- Involve those directly affected by an issue in planning and carrying out strategies.
- Enlist allies; mobilize a group of colleagues to address a policy issue in government.
- Participate in improving neighborhoods, schools, and communities.
- Speak from your experience as a nurse; learn how to communicate your ideas effectively using examples, analogies, and history.
- Create public support for an issue; develop the important socialization and networking skills to convey your points to the policymakers.
- Use the media (e.g., local newspaper, association newsletter); cultivate relationships with media personnel you believe will be sympathetic to your issue.
- Learn the arts of compromise and tact; sometimes, it is more advantageous to reach half your goal than lose the entire fight. See others' points of view so you understand where the opposition is coming from. Plan your strategy and reach compromise without sacrificing your beliefs.
- Volunteer to serve as a member of a local health or nursing advisory committee (CNA, 2000b; Mason et al., 1993; Ross Kerr & MacPhail, 1996; Vance, 1993).

"Walking the corridor," meeting with departmental heads in informal ways, and contributing to policy-making and decision making through telephone calls and conversations are approaches to policy influence that need to be better developed and more readily available to nurses (Hart, 1994). Nurses are beginning to learn the benefits of collective action, mutual support, and interdependence (Beck, 1982) not just in labor issues but also in other issues that affect their ability to provide safe and effective care. Individual nurses increase the power of all nurses when they acknowledge their own expertise and that of their peers. Nurses who participate in interdisciplinary groups with consumers of health care services and in organizations, associations, and boards beyond nursing achieve personal growth and help others understand nurses and nursing better.

Knowledge is a strategic resource that confers authority on its possessor. Nurses who view themselves as lifelong learners will have a more potent effect on deliberations and the ultimate decision-making process than nurses who fail to devote time to their formal and informal continuing education.

In a dynamic environment, where conditions change rapidly and power and influence take on new forms, the continued acquisition of knowledge and skills is essential. Power and empowerment are gained, maintained, and expanded as nurses give sustained attention to perfection of practice, education for practice, research to improve practice, and administrative activity to enable practice (Ferguson, 1993). As nurses compete for increased participation in management, governance, planning, and policy development in the health care system, they must value scholarship and continually apply it.

■ SUMMARY

Reconceptualizing nursing and the nursing role as a political act will promote a new understanding of the role and its relationship with policy. Such reconceptualizing will need to defend and expand knowledge in the fields of clinical practice, management, education, research, and policy as well as challenge the power structures that seek to devalue nurses' roles.

Nurses have gradually gained understanding of the processes and skills involved in influencing others, thereby becoming more powerful and exercising more control of the factors that influence their working lives. The nursing profession's history of political action and policy influence is something of which every nurse can be proud. Yet many more challenges in the 21st century require the policy expertise of nurses—expertise that requires political savvy and power.

Nursing and policy, with its adjuncts of politics and empowerment, are as congruent to nursing practice as are diagnosis and intervention—both require acute problem-solving and decision-making skills. Nurses are part of the policy solution to health care and public health problems. Nursing's history, both recent and remote, is filled with examples of nurses who have understood the inherent political and policy nature of nursing. Our challenge is to continue that legacy.

Online Resources

Add to your knowledge of this issue:

Canada Health Act	laws.justice.gc.ca/en/C-6/index.html
Chair of the Health Council and 25 Councillors Announcement	www.hc-sc.gc.ca/english/media/releases/2003/ 2003_97.htm
First Ministers' Accord on Health Care Renewal (2003)	www.hc-sc.gc.ca/english/hca2003/accord.html
Health Goals for British Columbia	www.healthservices.gov.bc.ca/pho/hlthgoal/ goals.html
Saskatchewan Health Performance plan	www.health.gov.sk.ca/mc_dp_perfplan.pdf

REFLECTIONS on the Chapter . . .

1. Nurses' policy roles and responsibilities may vary throughout their careers. As a senior student or new graduate, identify opportunities to enact a policy role in clinical practice, through student affairs, or in a professional association. Discuss ways in which you could fulfill the responsibilities of that policy role.

2. One of the major challenges to nurses influencing the policy process is the invisibility of nursing as a political force. How might individual nurses and the nursing profession address this challenge?

3. Identify a public policy—health or nursing—that has been developed at a government or professional association level. Determine how the policy process unfolded from issue identification to outcome evaluation.

4. From your clinical or educational experience, identify and select an issue that concerns you and that you think requires a new or revised policy. Compose a letter to an appropriate decision maker to propose a policy change.

5. Review resolutions submitted to the recent annual meeting of your professional association. For one of the resolutions, critique the background, rationale, and recommendations for policy implications and the feasibility of developing a policy.

6. Consider ways in which you have been influenced by a health or nursing policy—whether as a citizen, student nurse, or graduate nurse. Determine where in the policy process you could have been influential and what strategies you could have used to exert such influence.

References

Allemang, M. M. (2000). Development of community health nursing in Canada. In M. J. Stewart (Ed.), *Community nursing: Promoting Canadian's health.* (2nd ed., pp. 4–32). Toronto: W. B. Saunders.

Anderson, J. E. (1990). *Public policymaking.* Boston: Houghton Mifflin.

Barnum, B. S., & Kerfoot, K. M. (1995). *The nurse as executive* (4th ed.). Gaithersburg, MD: Aspen.

Beck, C. T. (1982). The conceptualization of power. *Advances in Nursing Science, 8,* 1–2.

Brokering Program. (2004). Canadian Health Services Research Foundation. Available: http://www.chsrf.ca/brokering/index_e.php

Brooks, S. (1998). *Public policy in Canada: An introduction.* Toronto: Oxford University Press.

Brown, D. J. (2000). *The challenge of caring: A history of women and health care in British Columbia.* British Columbia: Ministry of Health and Ministry Responsible for Seniors, Women's Health Bureau.

Canadian Nurses Association. (1980). *Putting "health" back into health care.* Submission to the Health Services Review '79. Ottawa: Author.

_____. (2000a). Primary health care approach. Fact Sheet. Available: http://206.191.29.104/_frames/policies/policiesmainframe.htm

_____. (2000b). Nursing is a political act: The bigger picture. *Nursing Now: Issues and Trends in Canadian Nursing, 8,* 1–5. Available: http://206.191.29.104/_frames/issuestrends/issuestrendsframe.htm

_____. (2003a). Primary health care–The time has come. *Nursing Now: Issues and Trends in Canadian Nursing, 16.* Available: http://www .cna-nurses.ca/_frames/issuestrends/issuestrendsframe.htm

_____. (2003b). Legislation, regulation and education of the nurse practitioner in Canada. Fact Sheet. Available: http://206.191.29.104/ _frames/policies/policiesmainframe.htm

_____. (2003c). The nurse practitioner. Position Statement. Available: http://www.cna-nurses.ca/_frames/issuestrends/issuestrendsframe.htm

Canadian Nursing Advisory Committee. (2002). Our health, our future: Creating quality workplaces for Canadian nurses. Health Canada. Available: http://www.hc-sc.gc.ca/english/pdf/Office-of-NursingPolicy.pdf

Clarke, H. F., Lashinger, H. S., Giovannett, P., et al. (2001). Nursing shortages: Workplace environments are essential to the solution. *Hospital Quarterly, 4*(4), 50–57.

Decter, M. (2001). Who makes health policy? *Health Policy Forum, 3*(3), 2.

Dye, T. (1978). *Understanding public policy* (3rd ed.). Englewood Cliffs, NJ: Prentice-Hall.

Ferguson, V. D. (1985). Power, politics and policy in nursing. In R. R. Wieczorek (Ed.), *Power, politics, and policy in nursing* (pp. 5–15). New York: Springer.

_____. (1993). Perspectives on power. In D. J. Mason, S. W. Talbott, & J. K. Leavitt (Eds.), *Policy and politics for nurses* (2nd ed., pp. 118–125). Philadelphia: W. B. Saunders.

Glass, H., & Hicks, S. (2000). Healthy public policy in health system reform. In M. J. Stewart. (Ed.), *Community nursing: Promoting Canadians' health* (2nd ed., pp. 156–170). Toronto: W. B. Saunders.

Grohar-Murray, M. E., & DiCroce, H. R. (1997). *Leadership and management in nursing.* Stamford, CT: Appleton & Lange.

Hart, C. (1994). *Behind the mask: Nurses, their unions and nursing policy.* London: Bailliere Tindall.

Joel, L. A. (1993). Contemporary issues in nursing organisations. In D. J. Mason & S. W. Talbott (Eds.), *Policy and politics for nursing* (2nd ed., pp. 539–548). Menlo Park, CA: Addison-Wesley.

Krampitz, S. D. (1985). Historical overview of nursing and politics. In D. J. Mason and S. W. Talbott (Eds.), *Political action handbook for nurses* (pp. 10–22). Menlo Park, CA: Addison-Wesley.

Loveridge, C. E., & Cummings, S. H. (1996). *Nursing management in the new paradigm.* Gaithersburg, MD: Aspen.

Mason, D. J., & McCarthy, A. M. (1985). Politics of patient care. In D. J. Mason & S. W. Talbott (Eds.), *Political action handbook for nurses* (pp. 38–52). Menlo Park, CA: Addison-Wesley.

Mason, D. J., Talbott, S. W., & Leavitt J. K. (1993). *Policy and politics for nurses* (2nd ed.). Philadelphia: W. B. Saunders.

Moore, G. (2001). Advocates for culture, advocates for health. *Nursing BC, 33*(4), 18–22.

Nursing Sector Study Corporation. (2004). *Building the future: An integrated strategy for nursing human resources in Canada.* Available: http://www.buildingthefuture.ca/e/study/

Paulson, E., Zilm, G., & Warbinek, E. (2000). Pioneer government advisor: Laura Holland, RN, RRc, CBE, LLD (1883–1956). *Canadian Journal of Nursing Leadership, 13*(3), 36–39.

Pringle, D. M., & Roe, D. I. (1992). Voluntary community agencies: VON Canada as example. In A. J. Baumgart & J. Larsen (Eds.), *Canadian nursing faces the future* (2nd ed., pp. 611–626). St. Louis: Mosby Year Book.

Rodger, G. L., & Gallagher S. M. (2000). The move toward primary health care in Canada: Community health nursing from 1985 to 2000. In M. J. Stewart (Ed.), *Community nursing: Promoting Canadian's health* (2nd ed., pp. 33–55). Toronto: W. B. Saunders.

Rodger, L. M. (1993). Nurses and the political process. *AARN Newsletter, 49*(2), 24–25.

Romanow, R. J. (2002). *Building on values: The future of health care in Canada.* Available: http://www.hc-sc.gc.ca/english/care/romanow/hcc0086.html

Ross Kerr, J., & MacPhail, J. (1996). Political awareness in nursing. In J. Ross Kerr & J. MacPhail (Eds.), *Canadian nursing issues and perspectives* (pp. 208–215). St. Louis: Mosby.

Rowsell, G. (1982). Changing trends in labour relations: Effects on collecting bargaining for nurses. *International Nursing Review, 29*(5), 141–145.

Shamian, J. (2000). Office of Nursing Policy comes to Ottawa. *Registered Nurse, 12*(5), 5–6.

Shamian, J., Skelton-Green, J., & Villeneuve, M. (2003). Policy is the lever for effective change. In M. McIntyre & E. Thomlinson, (Eds.), *Realities of Canadian nursing–Professional, practice, and power issues* (pp. 83–104). Philadelphia: Lippincott Williams & Wilkins.

Solomon, S. B., & Roe, S. C. (1986). *Integrating public policy into the curriculum.* New York: National League for Nursing.

Splane, R. B., & Splane, V. H. (1994). *Chief nursing officer positions in national ministries of health: Focal points for nursing leadership.* San Francisco: University of California.

Titmus, R. M. (1974). *Social policy: An introduction* (p. 23). New York: Pantheon Books.

Vance, C. (1993). Politics: A humanistic process. In D. J. Mason, S. W. Talbott, & J. K. Leavitt (Eds.), *Policy and politics for nurses* (2nd ed., pp. 104–117). Philadelphia: W. B. Saunders.

World Health Organization. (1978, September 6-12). *Declaration of Alma-Ata International Conference on Primary Health Care,* Alma-Ata, USSR. Available: http://www.who.int/hpr/NPH/docs/declaration_almaata.pdf

_____. (1986, November 17–21). *Ottawa Charter for Health Promotion: An International Conference on Health Promotion.* Retrieved July 20, 2000. Health Canada, Population Health Approach. http://www.hc-sc.gc.ca/hppb/phdd/docs/charter/

Critical Questions

As a way of engaging with the ideas in this chapter, consider the following:

1. What are your assumptions about what makes effective policy?
2. What do you assume to be the link between policy and research?
3. What do you already know about the influence of political agendas on policy development?
4. How do you understand the influence of policy on change?

CHAPTER
6

Judith Shamian
Judith Skelton-Green
Michael Villeneuve

Policy: The Essential Link in Successful Transformations

The power of representation is illustrated in political action. Here, nurses confer with Ginette Lemire Rodger (center), former president of the CNA, to begin the process for change that will protect the health of Canadians and the nursing profession. Photo by Tony Fouhse. Used with permission from the Canadian Nurses Association.

Policy sets
the direction
for *action*

Chapter Objectives

After completing this chapter, you will be able to:

1. Describe the relationship between research and policy.

2. Explain why quality research is insufficient to effect policy change.

3. Identify and explain the key components of effective research–policy linkages.

4. Apply a basic change formula to analyze and plan for change.

5. Identify the steps in the policy cycle and give examples of how the various steps might play out with a real-world issue of nursing concern.

6. Describe the connection between political acumen and policy influence.

7. Identify ways in which political acumen may be leveraged in the advancement of nursing policy.

P olicy "involves the application of reason and evidence to problem solving, whether in public or private settings. It connects basic scientific knowledge to practice....Policy incorporates both a process of decision-making and the product of that process" (Helms, Anderson, & Hanson, 1996, p. 32). In *Health Policy and Politics: A Nurse's Guide*, the term *public policy* is defined as the "directives that document government decisions...the process of taking problems to government agents and obtaining a decision or reply in the form of a program, law, or regulation" (Milstead, 1999, p. 1). *Health policy* has been defined as "the principles, plans and strategies for action guiding the behaviour of organizations, institutions and professions involved in the field of health, as well as their consequences for the health-care system" (West & Scott, 2000, p. 818).

Policies exist as part of the everyday practice of nursing. They are found in many forms:

- Governmental laws and regulations
- Organizational policies
- Union contracts
- Nursing unit procedures

At the most basic level, policies guide "the way things are done around here," particularly when they are explicitly stated. Policies are often equated with rules. And policies may even be found to be limiting, as in "You can't do that for your patient because it is the policy here that we don't allow...." Indeed, Cheek and Gibson (1997) caution that the unrestrained generation of policy—particularly at the organizational level—can actually serve to limit and control negatively the practice of nursing.

Why should nurses be concerned with health policy? Clinical care can be improved either by focusing on the work of individual caregivers or by focusing on the systems in which they work. A clinical policy may guide nurses at the point of care, for example, by suggesting at what age a child should receive a certain vaccination or how often a tubing should be changed in a critical care unit. At the systems level, broader health policy will dictate how many hospital beds and community health centers will exist in the system to provide those services—and what will be the number and mix of caregivers employed to deliver them. The organization of health care services, the culture of health care organizations, and the quality of worklife are as important to quality patient care as are the clinical policies that drive nurse–patient encounters (West & Scott, 2000). Health policy is an important vehicle for influencing and changing the environments in which nurses practise. As limiting as policy can be at times, it is certain that if ideas aren't translated into policy, they won't be translated into action.

This chapter illustrates the reasons that compelling research findings—often demonstrating clearly what nurses need in their work environments to optimize their contributions to society—do not always result in the changes that are needed in nursing practice environments. This chapter also proposes ways to overcome such barriers by recognizing that effective influence of policy occurs when five levers are utilized:

- High quality evidence or research
- Effective research–policy linkages
- An understanding of change management
- An understanding of the policy cycle
- Political acumen

Ultimately, this chapter aims to help the reader understand and use each lever, to provide examples of how others have done so, to examine lessons learned, and to encourage every nurse to think about and become involved, in some way, in influencing health policy.

■ THE CHALLENGE: AVOIDING CRITICAL SITUATIONS

North America is experiencing a nursing shortage that threatens to worsen considerably in the next 10 years if left unchecked. Given all of the studies of nursing workplace satisfiers that occurred in the 1980s and 1990s, it seems reasonable to expect that we would have learned lessons to help us avoid yet another critical situation. For a number of reasons, this hasn't happened. First among those is the reality that, as health economist Robert Evans has said so simply, "policy is possible." Policy decisions taken in the 1990s to reduce the number of nursing graduates had their intended effect. Between 1990 and 2000, the number of registered nurse (RN) graduates dropped by some 40% at the same time as Canada's population increased by 15%. There were actually less RN graduates in 2000 than in the mid-1960s, and, of course, the existing nursing workforce continued to age and move toward retirement. Over just a decade, the balance has shifted such that the number of exits from nursing threatens to be greater than the number of new nurses coming into the profession. So the appearance of shortages of nursing services in the early part of this century is a result of deliberate policy choices; they are not a mystery.

Shortages

So, what to do about shortages that are now before us? The actions taken to address historical "boom and bust" cycles of nursing shortages and surpluses have too often been short-sighted, providing interim relief but long-term residue. During the shortage of the 1980s, many organizations introduced unregulated health care workers to deliver some aspects of patient care. Research now shows that patient care outcomes may have been negatively affected by this decision (McGillis Hall et al., 2001). Alternately in Canada, during the period of fiscal restraint and health care system restructuring of the mid-1990s, thousands of nurses across the country were laid off or accepted offers of early retirement. Thousands more underwent job changes in the bumping that followed. In Quebec, the government-appointed Clair Commission concluded that these departures and changes contributed to weakening the level of expertise within the system and negatively affected the team environment (Commission d'étude sur les services de santé et les services sociaux, 2000). The short-term solutions in both of these circumstances had long-range consequences that were not anticipated—and might have been avoided.

It is not a sufficient excuse that health care leaders and policymakers did not know, or could not have predicted, what the long-term consequences of these decisions might be. Research suggesting a correlation between levels of RN staffing and patient morbidity and mortality had begun to emerge well before many of the policy decisions impacting patients and nurses were taken in the 1990s (Aiken, Smith, & Lake, 1994; Hartz et al., 1989; Knaus et al., 1986; Prescott, 1993).

Second, policymakers, managers, and others have generally done a poor job of translating research into actions. Despite increasingly robust research defining what nurses need to optimize the effectiveness of their work environments and to balance that with the demands of their personal lives, nurses have not always been very effective at influencing those who make the decisions that affect their practice.

Kimball and O'Neil (2001) suggest that several major developments have contributed to the unique and overwhelming nature of the current nursing crisis: a changing demography, a changing health care system, changing social values, and an alteration in the nature of work. They indicate that the size and complexity of these changes are so significant that strategies to deal with past nursing shortages will be inadequate for today's crisis. Recent evidence suggests that Canada's looming shortage threatens to rival only that of the United States as the worst of all the member nations of the Organization for Economic Cooperation and Development (OECD, 2004), and most of the member countries report worrying shortages. By about 2011 in the United States, for example, as the population continues to grow, the number of new RN licenses issued will, for the first time, be less than the number of retirees. By 2016, the RN shortage in Canada is predicted to be in the 30% range unless drastic countermeasures are taken immediately and are sustained over the next decade. We face a loss of as much as 28% of the Canadian RN workforce by 2006 alone, based on a typical retirement of nurses at age 55 (O'Brien-Pallas, Duffield, &, Alksnis, 2004). Furthermore, the OECD work gives every indication that the demand for nursing services will continue to grow.

Actions to Ameliorate Shortages

Kimball and O'Neil (2001) describe a continuum of the kinds of actions needed to address shortages in the nursing workforce. They make a convincing case that for long-lasting, positive impact, solutions that use and respect the nurse as a valued asset and professional partner will be most effective. The four kinds, or stages, of actions follow.

Stage 1: Scramble

In the early stage of a workforce shortage, there is a "scramble"—a flurry of short-term actions that are unilaterally initiated by providers of care. Examples include colorful recruitment brochures, international headhunting visits, sign-on bonuses, accelerated placement on the wage scale, and other activities focused on monetary incentives. These kinds of actions treat the nurse as a commodity that will respond to traditional market incentives. In the scramble stage, little attention is paid to changing nursing education, the nature of work, or the structure of the profession.

Stage 2: Improve

Once the reality and the seriousness of the shortage are clear, employers begin to recognize that nurses have particular wants and needs, after which the employers begin to approach nurses as customers. Interventions focus on increasing choice, reducing stress, and improving safety. Examples of improve-stage responses are improved clinical experiences in nursing programs, scholarships and loans, Internet-based distance learning, flexible benefits and scheduling, and preceptorship and mentorship programs—activities designed to make longer-term investments in people to cultivate their loyalty. In this stage, there is still minimal structural change to the professional aspects of nursing.

Stage 3: Reinvent

As the challenge of providing high-quality care with fewer professional nurses continues to mount, it becomes clear that there is a need to rethink the ways professional nurses are recruited and trained, how they are integrated into the system, and how they are challenged and rewarded. In the reinvent stage, new roles are developed that blur the traditional boundaries between nursing roles. Examples of reinvent-stage responses include shared governance models, specialty internships, the adoption of magnet hospital values, and incentive rewards for sustained clinical outcomes improvement. The role of the professional nurse in the delivery of high-quality, patient-centered care is not only recognized but also leveraged by the employer as a valued asset. The employer, in turn, is rewarded with improved patient clinical outcomes and satisfaction.

Stage 4: Start Over

At the far end of the response continuum are interventions in which nurses are viewed as professional partners practising at the upper limits of their professional licenses and respected by consumers as patient advocates, information resources, and teachers and supporters of self-care. Examples of start-over actions include new systems of care delivery and professional practice that cross traditional care boundaries, such as academic nursing schools' establishment of community-based, primary-care clinics staffed by nurse practitioners.

At the time of writing of this chapter, stage 2 probably best characterizes where we find ourselves, overall, in response to shortages that began to appear about 6 years ago. We have seen a variety of improvement mechanisms put into place that do make aspects of working life more tolerable for some nurses, but we have not moved to a serious rethink of the way nurses are educated, integrated, and utilized. Early efforts in that direction are under way, but we are not to stage 3 just yet.

The key question is this: How can nursing recruitment and retention be managed in a more predictable, thoughtful, and stable fashion than in the past? In particular, how can policymakers move beyond short-term, knee-jerk scramble and improve strategies to longer-term reinvent and start-over strategies?

This shift will require more deliberate and more carefully managed approaches to the problem, with policy being the key that unlocks the door to these higher-level solutions; it is only with the introduction of significant, broad-based policy change that substantive solutions will have staying power. If nurses want to influence successfully the formulation of appropriate and relevant policy, they must learn to utilize a number of levers, including the following:

- High-quality evidence or research
- Effective research–policy linkages
- Change management
- Policy cycles
- Political acumen

■ HIGH-QUALITY EVIDENCE

Evidence-based decision making has become a growing expectation in health care since the 1990s not only for clinical aspects of health care but also for management and policy formulation. Along with this expectation, nursing research funding and initiatives have increased dramatically.

Essentially, two basic kinds of information or evidence are needed to make meaningful changes in nursing recruitment, retention, and role optimization:

1. *Information about nurses themselves.* What are the demographics of today's nurses? What will attract the right candidates into the profession? What is it that nurses need to perform their work most effectively? What is required to keep them in the workforce?
2. *Information about the context within which nursing is practised.* What are the health and health care needs of Canadians? What are the most significant determinants of health? What changes are occurring and anticipated in the Canadian health care system? What can be learned from what is happening elsewhere in the world? What are the plans, initiatives, and political agendas of those in power?

Progress is being made in both areas of research. The information to answer the first set of questions is becoming more plentiful and more robust. Provincial nurse registries now track the demographics of their members on a number of key dimensions. Numerous studies have been published that clearly point out the conditions that will attract, retain, and satisfy nurses. These studies have been cited in other parts of this chapter and in other chapters in this book. In late 2001, the Canadian Institute for Health Information (CIHI) released a paper summarizing what we know and what we do not know about factors affecting the supply, demand, education, health, and worklives of the health care providers in Canada (CIHI, 2001b). Much of the information to answer the second set of questions is also available, although the data are somewhat more elusive and certainly less well known and less frequently accessed by nurses.

If the necessary evidence regarding nursing practice is growing, why is it that those in decision-making positions are not acting on the information? First, the timing may not be right. Policy windows open and close at their own pace, having more to do with election cycles, public opinion, and fiscal years than with the quality of research findings. Even when a study has been directly commissioned and competently performed, it will have to compete for attention with other priorities and influences at the time that it is completed.

Second, although some of the data may be in, the facts are not always clear. Jonathan Lomas, executive director of the Canadian Health Services Research Foundation (CHSRF), cautions us that with recent increases in research funding come risks. Rather than research supporting and informing practice changes, a gap may emerge between researchers and decision makers (Lomas, 2000). On the one hand, researchers' bias for methodologic purity can limit the practical utility of their findings; on the other hand, managers' push for speed and output can compromise the quality of the research. The CHSRF has developed a unique linkage-and-exchange approach to its work, which it hopes will offset both risks. This approach is in keeping with Davis and Howden-Chapman's (1996) conclusions that research is more likely to be translated into policy if researchers, policy analysts, managers, and politicians negotiate the language and frame of reference before research is undertaken.

Finally, the pace at which evidence is being developed has surpassed our knowledge of how to most effectively use research findings to influence policy. Chunharas (2001) suggests that although high-quality research on policy-relevant issues, with well-packaged and well-targeted products, may succeed in informing decision-making processes, the linkages between policy and research will only be optimized through an understanding of the key components of their interface.

■ EFFECTIVE RESEARCH-POLICY LINKAGES

Chunharas (2001) identifies five key components of effective research–policy linkages:

- Interface between the dual processes of research and policy development
- Sensitivity to the context in which they both operate
- Appreciation for the attitudes of the stakeholders involved
- Astute use of the research outputs
- Role of mediators

Interface Between Research and Policy Development

Chunharas (2001) emphasizes the importance of building linkages between all steps of the research and decision-making processes, from the definition of research questions and policy priorities to the dissemination of research results and policy or program implementation. He argues that both processes will be richer for the interaction.

Sensitivity to Context

Chunharas uses the word *context* to mean the social, political, and economic environment surrounding the research and decision-making processes. He emphasizes the need to consider deep-seated values, practices, and traditions as well as prevailing decision-making climates and mechanisms and the influence of mass media.

Appreciation for Stakeholders' Attitudes

Chunharas identifies three main stakeholders in the research–policy interface: researchers, decision makers, and members of the community. He suggests that decision makers would be more likely to use research results if researchers involved them in formulating questions and problems. Researchers, on the other hand, may be more interested in conducting needed research if they were consulted about the appropriate approach and methodology, Finally, members of the community—the putative subjects and targets of research and decision making and who are often intimidated by both researchers and decision makers and are forgotten in the processes—can contribute much to both the issues that need investigating and the appropriate application of results.

Astute Use of Research Outputs

One of the critical requirements in using research outputs effectively is the ability to tease out from complex research methods and findings a limited number of clear, concise, and relevant messages.

West and Scott (2000) suggest that research ideas (and, we would suggest, messages) related to the "great themes of our times," and those that offer solutions to current problems, are more likely to be taken up and implemented than ideas that are not currently high on the political agenda. This assertion emphasizes the importance of knowing the popular themes and priorities as well as the importance of making the connection between "our findings" and "their priorities." To ensure that important research comes to the attention of policymakers, West and Scott suggest publishing summaries of scientific papers in journals that policymakers are likely to read and including *health policy* as key words in academic publications.

Even more basic is the fact that the key policy-relevant messages in research papers are often difficult to locate. From their study of what got the attention of policymakers in presentations by tobacco control advocates, Montini and Bero (2001) advise that advocates present science in a format that is well organized and easily absorbed. Gebbie and associates (2000), in a study of 27 American nurses active in health policy, suggest that researchers write findings in a style that can help policymakers draw conclusions and include in every study (including clinical studies) a clear and deliberate discussion of policy ramifications.

Role of Mediators

The differences between the priorities, time constraints, languages, and cultures of researchers and policy decision makers have been acknowledged, described, and likened to the existence of two communities that prohibit successful communication. A number of authorities (CIHI, 2001a; Crosswaite & Curtice, 1994; Feldman, Nadash, & Gursen, 2001) argue the case for skilled mediators or research-knowledge brokers who can bridge the gaps. Research brokers have been described as individual specialists with effective communication skills, the ability to educate and report, and familiarity with differing approaches and research methods—a hybrid of journalist, teacher, and researcher (Crosswaite & Curtice, 1994). Although Chunharas (2001) recognizes that the mediator role can be critically important, he also emphasizes that researchers themselves must develop skills of communication and advocacy as well as an understanding of how decision makers make resource allocation decisions and how policymakers develop, implement, and monitor policies. Nurses may argue that nurses and the nursing profession can act in a brokering role, strengthening the linkages among research, decision making, and policy formulation.

■ CHANGE MANAGEMENT

In a presentation to federal and provincial/territorial policymakers in Ottawa in 2001, Gina Browne, founder and director of the System-Linked Research Unit on Health and Social Service Utilization, stated, "I don't think we should ever fund another study on the efficacy of nurse practitioners. Every piece of research for 30 years has shown the effectiveness of the role. Why have we not been able to translate all those robust findings into action?" Browne went on to answer her own question this way: "I really don't think any more that we have a serious knowledge development problem. We have a serious research dissemination and transfer problem." In other words, leaders and policymakers in the health care system generally haven't been very good at making and managing change.

Dannemiller and Jacobs (1992) describe a basic change formula that is very useful both for diagnosing a situation and for developing interventions in change situations. The formula is as follows:

$$D \times V \times F > R$$

Dannemiller and Jacobs state that change can and will only occur when the product of discomfort or dissatisfaction (D) with the present situation, a vision (V) of what is possible or desired, and the concrete first steps (F) toward reaching the vision are greater than the resistance (R) to the change. It is important to understand that it is the product of the factors on the left side of the equation with which one must be concerned. If any one of these variables (D, V, or F) is zero or near zero, the product of the three will also be zero or near zero, and the resistance cannot and will not be overcome.

Consider this example: Many hospitals have attempted to implement self-scheduling on their nursing units. The appeal (vision, V) of nurses managing their own schedules is clear, and it fits with their ideals of nursing autonomy and work–life balance (let's give the V 1 out of 1). The steps needed to implement self-scheduling are carefully thought out and put into place (first step, F, gets 0.8 out of 1). About a third of the staff is quite unhappy with the current scheduling system and keen to try the new system along with the manager. Some staff members are indifferent, and some are reluctant (let's say dissatisfaction, D, is initially 0.4, and resistance, R, is 0.2). At the outset of the change effort, the formula looks favorable, if not overwhelmingly so:

$$D\ (0.4) \times V\ (1.0) \times F\ (0.8) = 0.32$$

R, however, is only 0.2.

Nonetheless, implementing the new scheduling practices proves awkward; it creates tensions among staff members, and some individuals do not get as many of the "preferred" shifts as they had hoped. Grumbling breaks out, along with accusations of favoritism or breaking the rules. Some of the original proponents even become disillusioned (resistance, R, grows to 0.5; dissatisfaction, D, falls to 0.2). Eventually, those responsible for adequately staffing the ward (whether front-line staff volunteers or the manager) become discouraged, and the staff votes to discontinue the plan. This can be explained by the fact that the change equation has shifted, and now looks like this:

$$D\ (0.2) \times V\ (1.0) \times F\ (0.8) = 0.16$$

Here, R is 0.5.

What was missing in this change situation was that not enough staff members were unhappy enough with the old schedule to carry the change momentum through the difficult adjustment period. Spending more time at the outset getting people "on board" and really wanting to replace the "old, unsatisfactory" scheduling practices with new ones could have enhanced the likelihood of success.

The applications to the research–policy links are clear. One can think of examples of situations in which research data have been the primary driver of health policy change—for instance, seatbelt and bicycle helmet legislation. In these cases, one might argue that the resistance to the policy change was low, and thus the dissatisfaction quotient did not play out as a large factor. On the other hand, there are other situations—like tobacco and gun control in the United States—in which organized resistance has been strong, and the absence of strong dissatisfaction with the status quo has hindered necessary policy change.

In summary, credible research may provide the data that underpins a vision of a better world for nurses. A robust and detailed plan may even be proposed to act on the research. However, if there is not sufficient dissatisfaction with the status quo to overcome any resistance that may be encountered, the desired policy changes may not occur.

■ POLICY CYCLE

Milstead (1999) elaborates on four major stages of the policy process: agenda setting, legislation and reg-ulation, program implementation, and program evaluation. Agenda setting is concerned with identifying a problem and bringing it to the attention of government; legislation and regulation are the formal responses to the problem; program implementation is the execution of programs designed to enact the legislation; and program evaluation is the appraisal of the program's performance. Milstead emphasizes that "the policy process is not necessarily sequential or logical. The definition of a problem, which usually occurs in the agenda-setting phase, may change during legislation. Program design may be altered significantly during implementation. Evaluation of a policy or program (often considered the last phase of the process) may pro-pel onto the national agenda (often considered the first phase of the process) a problem that differs from the original" (Milstead, 1999, p. 21).

Of particular concern in this chapter are the first two of Milstead's four stages. The federal Office of Nursing Policy (ONP) has promoted understanding of a conceptual framework (adapted from Tarlov, 2000) that explains the way in which nurses can move matters onto the policy agenda and how they can move that agenda forward into action. Figure 6.1 illustrates the eight-step policy cycle of (1) values and cultural beliefs, (2) emergence of problems or issues, (3) knowledge and development of research, (4) public aware-ness, (5) political engagement, (6) interest group activation, (7) public policy deliberation and adoption, and (8) regulation, experience, and revision.

The actions taken by the ONP to move the issues surrounding nurses' health and working conditions in the settings where nurses practise onto the country's policy tables illustrate how the cycle works. The policy cycle has two distinct phases, each of which is anchored by a particular step in the cycle. The first

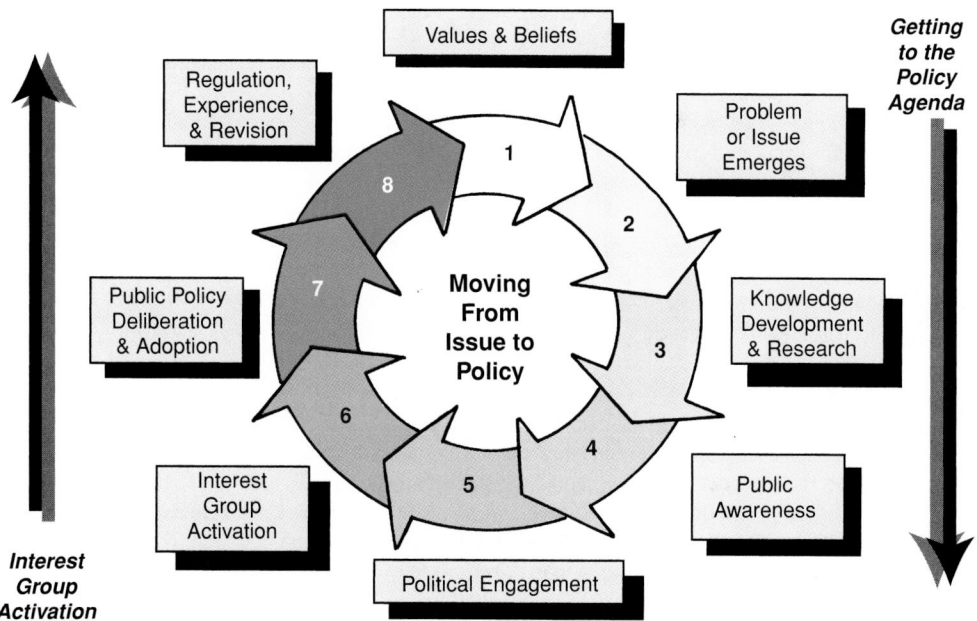

FIGURE 6.1 The policy cycle (adapted from Tarlov, 1999, 2000).

phase, getting to the policy agenda, is anchored by beliefs and values. If society and its representative structures do not value and believe in the issues that are put forth in the policy arena, the issues will have no oxygen to feed them and they will die on the floor.

The second phase, moving into action, is anchored by political engagement. To advance an issue to policy and then to action, political engagement is required. Without the engagement of political sponsors, policy issues can be "out there" and acknowledged by various stakeholders, but they will not result in policy change.

Values and Cultural Beliefs

Action on any policy issue must be firmly grounded in a supportable set of values and cultural beliefs. In the case of the *Healthy Nurses, Healthy Workplaces* agenda, four basic—yet powerful—beliefs or values were dominant:

- Canadians are firmly in support of the principles of the Canada Health Act.
- Nurses are an essential part of the health care delivery system.
- To offer both access and quality, the health care system needs nurses.
- The public trusts nurses.

Identification, validation, and articulation of these basic values were important not only at the outset of the initiative (to ensure that the agenda was value based) but also in moving forward (to connect others who share those values).

Emergence of Problem or Issue

Kingdon (1995) makes the point that an issue can come from anywhere and that in some ways its source or origin does not matter. Rather, it is essential that the issue lands on fertile soil and is nurtured. That is to say, it is not sufficient for an issue just to exist; it must have some urgency. It must be a problem that is visible and important to others, not just to those affected. Kingdon (1995, p. 167) also points out that "policy windows open infrequently and do not stay open long." It is important, therefore, for those who wish to advance policy initiatives to be alert to opportunities.

For years, nurses complained that aspects of their workplaces were negatively affecting not only their productivity and performance but also their personal health. More recently, they were vocal in articulating the effects of organizational downsizing and restructuring on their workloads. They related that the situation was becoming intolerable and that it was leading to increased absenteeism, increasing job dissatisfaction and low morale, and high illness rates. Most importantly, by noting that shortages and high workloads were chipping away at the vigilance function that lies at the heart of excellent nursing care, some nurses began to tie their working conditions to patient outcomes and patient safety. In 2000, the frustration boiled over, with highly emotional and visible job action surrounding labor contract negotiations in many provinces.

Knowledge and Development of Research

Once the issues are clear and pressing, one must ask whether research and solid evidence exist to support the anecdotal perceptions. In the case of nurses' health, the answer is a resounding "yes."

Data from the Statistics Canada Labour Force Survey showed that in 2002, the rate of RN illness- and injury-related absenteeism stood at 8.6%, up from 5.9% in 1987. That figure translates to the equivalent of paying 10,808 full-time nurses to stay off the job for a full year (Canadian Labour & Business Centre, 2003). Although statistics were not available for licensed practical nurses (LPNs) or registered psychiatric nurses (RPNs), RNs had a rate of temporary absences due to illness and injury that was 83% higher than the Canadian average in 2002, exceeded only by the group that includes nurse-assisting occupations such as orderlies. That rate has climbed slowly and steadily each year since 1987, with no signs of slowing (Canadian Labour and Business Centre, 2002).

It is not only the absenteeism rate that is climbing. Looking again at 2002, 26% of RNs worked overtime *each week*—considerably higher than the rate of 15.3% in 1997 and higher than the average of 22.5% reported among all other workers. The Canadian Labour and Business Centre (2002) estimated that the number of nurses working overtime more than doubled between 1997 and 2002. To fill that demand for nursing services, 8,643 full-time RNs would have had to be hired across Canada in 2002 alone.

Previously documented correlations between overtime and absenteeism seem to be borne out in these findings. The impact of the RN overtime and absenteeism situation—not only on costs to the health care system but on quality of patient care—is significant and unsustainable. It is especially a concern during a time of shortage to note that dropping the rate of RN absenteeism just to the Canadian average would return thousands of full-time job equivalents to the system.

The relationship between nursing and patient outcomes has also become increasingly well established, through, for example, the magnet hospital studies (Aiken et al., 1994) and the International Study of Nurse Staffing and Patient Outcomes (Aiken et al., 1998). Recent evidence suggests that, as a result of hospital bed cuts in Ontario, more patients have to compete for both fewer beds and fewer nurses. Long wait times threaten patient health and safety, and growing demands on nurses and other caregivers still in the system play out as increased work pace and rising workloads. In the light of those kinds of findings, it is even more compelling to note the growing body of research demonstrating that patient health outcomes are significantly better in settings that have more favorable nurse-to-patient ratios and higher proportions of registered and practical nurses on the care team. These studies have indicated that a higher number and proportion of RNs are associated with reduced risk-adjusted mortality, a lower risk of medical complications, a higher nurse-assessed quality of care, and a shorter length of stay (OECD, 2004).

And finally, multiple studies and reports—from the late 1970s (Slavitt et al., 1978), 1980s (Blegan & Mueller, 1987; Price & Mueller, 1981), and 1990s (Irvine & Evans, 1992), more than two decades of magnet hospital research (Scott, Sochalski, & Aiken, 1999), through to the most recent studies of Ontario's Nursing Health Services Research Unit (Clarke et al., 2001; O'Brien-Pallas & Shamian, 2003; O'Brien-Pallas et al., 2001; O'Brien-Pallas et al., 2004), and *Commitment and Care*, a synthesis paper commissioned by the Canadian Health Services Research Foundation (Baumann et al., 2001)—have clearly, consistently, and repeatedly described the conditions that make a difference to nurses' satisfaction with the quality of their workplaces.

Although additional research might prove valuable, it was more important to make the messages about the existing results accessible and compelling. The ONP set out to do just that, creating tight, succinct, emotionally engaging messages (based on facts such as absenteeism statistics) that could be easily articulated, easily repeated, and easily reported. Speaking engagements for the executive director were used as opportunities to present these messages. To add emphasis and credibility to the case, the many sources supporting the key messages were cited.

Public Awareness

The next phase in the policy cycle is the creation of broad-based awareness—both of the issue and of the solution or strategy for addressing it, as identified in the research. In this quest, it is important to identify as many potential supportive audiences as possible and to customize the message for each audience. When customizing the message, one needs to think as the target group thinks, identifying how they would benefit from change. The various publics targeted by the ONP for the *Healthy Nurses, Healthy Workplaces* message included nurses and nursing organizations, other care providers, employers, unions, politicians (both government and opposition), and the general public. Of course, it was also important to include both the broadcast and print media: Radio, television, newspapers, and magazines such as *Chatelaine* and *Macleans* picked up articles about the health of nurses and the impact of healthy workplaces.

Political Engagement

Kingdon (1995) says that for an issue to be placed on a political agenda, it must have been "softened up." The softening-up process refers to the fact that people have to get used to the idea so that support and acceptance for the proposed solution or strategy can be built. This process of political engagement should be designed to initiate a ripple effect that can grow into a wave of support for the proposed strategy. In planning for political engagement, it is critically important to accomplish the following:

■ Know the government structure, committees, caucus, and key members of Parliament (those in power, those in opposition, and the nonelected players who have informal power).
■ Target individuals with interest, information, passion, or influence regarding your topic.
■ Utilize carefully considered, person-to-person contacts.
■ Customize the message for each contact person.
■ Keep these individuals regularly updated regarding your activities, your progress, and your specific needs for ongoing support.

Milstead (1999) emphasizes the importance of personal stories gained from professional nurses' experiences. These stories provide real-world anchors for altruistic conversations and forge an emotional link that is important in connecting the targets with the proposed strategies. In building support, it is also wise to encourage complementary initiatives that might be undertaken by other individuals or organizations.

Interest Group Activation

Once public awareness and political engagement have been sparked, it is important to exploit deliberately every opportunity to repeat the message and, if possible, to build the ripples of interest into a tidal wave. Actions taken by the ONP to engage other interest groups in the agenda included the following:

■ Direct mail from the office ("Here is the basic message; please spread and respond; please send input regarding any activities happening on the ground in your locale")
■ Publications (the ONP electronic newsletter, and editorials and columns in other nursing and health publications—both regular and by special request)
■ Word of mouth (speeches, regional visits, interviews, and formal and informal gatherings and meetings)
■ Bringing key people together (e.g., a National Policy Forum was hosted by the ONP in February 2003 immediately following the First Ministers' meeting and release of Health Accord 2003)
■ Direct dialogue with nursing organizations (e.g., the Canadian Nurses Association, the Canadian Practical Nurses Association, Registered Psychiatric Nurses groups, Canadian Federation of Nurses Unions) and other health care organizations (e.g., Canadian Council on Health Services Accreditation, Canadian Healthcare Association).

Public Policy Deliberation and Adoption

When the wave of interest and support is great enough, the agenda needs to be deliberately moved to the tables where it can be debated and policy can be formulated. Kingdon (1995) says that once an issue is on the political agenda, it must meet five criteria if it is going to survive: technical feasibility, value acceptability within the policy community, tolerable cost, anticipated public agreement, and a reasonable chance for elected officials to be receptive to it.

At the time this chapter was written, the policy cycle for the *Healthy Nurses, Healthy Workplaces* agenda had progressed to this stage. The issue had appeared on public and government agendas, including the First Ministers' meeting (February 2003), in the national level health system reviews conducted by Kirby and Romanow, and in similar reviews conducted in each of the provinces and territories. A final report of Nursing Strategy for Canada (2000) was released in 2003, and its offspring, the Canadian Nursing Advisory

Committee, issued its final report in 2002. The establishment of a national Canadian Nursing Advisory Committee (CNAC)—the first recommendation of the Nursing Strategy for Canada—represented an important step forward in the policy cycle. The CNAC offered 51 recommendations to improve quality of nursing work life, further strengthening the positioning of nurses and nursing in the health and human resources policy agenda.

As a result of those cumulative efforts, health human resources (HHR) was built into the federal/provincial/territorial Health Accord 2003, which included a specific focus on national HHR planning, recruitment and retention, healthy workplaces, and interprofessional education for collaborative clinical practice. Nearly $90 million has been targeted for 2004–2008 to strengthen Canada's HHR, and nurses had a strong voice at the table when that aspect of the Health Accord was shaped.

Still ahead lie the challenges of monitoring the health status of nurses, but a national survey of nurses' health is in development and will be conducted from 2005 to 2006. Mechanisms should be put in place to provide accurate, ongoing information about nurses' health, absenteeism, and overtime to update the nursing and policy communities and to supplement—in greater detail—the Labour Force Survey.

Regulation, Experience, and Revision

In the final stage of the policy cycle, the proposed action becomes a formal policy, law, or regulation. This, in turn, becomes a new cultural value or norm, which is routinely experienced and revised until the next issue comes along. During this phase, program implementation and program evaluation take place, and these processes may, in turn, generate new information to continue the cycle. For example, new workplace quality indicators have been developed by the Canadian Council on Health Services Accreditation and are now being tested. These indicators will become part of the standards used to assess accreditation of health care settings across the country and force employers to think about and address working conditions and their impact on employees and patients. Health Accord 2004 puts in place accountability mechanisms that will require provinces and territories to report on access to health professionals by the public to reduce waiting times and "lead to better care for patients, more efficient health care, and greater public confidence in Medicare" (Health Accord 2004). Putting that plan in place will continue to position the importance of HHR and the need to complete the work plan laid out in Health Accord 2003.

■ POLITICAL ACUMEN: THE DRIVE BEHIND POLICYMAKING

It is important to keep in mind that policymaking is not always—in fact, it is seldom—the rational, step-by-step process portrayed in the previous discussion. It is rarely driven by factual data or logical process. Rather, it is more often a value-driven, dynamic, and at times chaotic cascade of influence and decision-making behavior. It is a process of social influence involving activities of persuasion, attitudinal change, decision making, and compromise (Mittelmark, 1999; Taylor, 1997). This is why the final requisite for influencing policy is political acumen.

Florence Nightingale perhaps stands out as the ultimate role model for nurses' use of political skill to influence policy for the benefit of patients. Milstead (1999) traces the current recognition of the importance of the links among nursing, politics, and policy to the 1960s and 1970s, when the explosion of social programs and the raising of social consciousness alerted nurses to the value of political activity. Since that time, increasing numbers of nurses have realized that to control practice and to move the nursing profession forward as a major player in the health care arena, nursing and nurses need to become politically involved in influencing and formulating policy. Nursing colleagues in the United States have historically been more organized and more deliberate about this initiative than have Canadian nurses. For example, in 1992, the American Nurses Association (ANA) realized that decisions that affected nurses and their patients were made in Washington, DC, so it moved its national headquarters to that city. The ANA also accomplished the following:

- Created political action committees that developed processes for endorsing public officials
- Created a department of governmental affairs that employed registered lobbyists who developed ongoing relationships with elected and appointed officials and their staffs and undertook significant fundraising to support these activities
- Educated nurses about the political process through continuing education programs
- Created senate and congressional district coordinators—nurses who volunteered to create relationships with their senators and representatives and served as liaisons between legislators and organized nursing
- Created the Nurses Strategic Action Team (N-STAT), a grassroots network of nurses throughout the country who were informed when immediate action was needed and who responded quickly to their legislative representatives
- Promoted political appointments of nurses to key positions in government (Milstead, 1999)

The Canadian Nurses Association (CNA) has undertaken similar targeted political activities through the 1990s, including Action 301, aimed at ensuring that across Canada, nurses are actively engaging politicians on issues in each federal riding. The CNA executive board meets regularly with senior federal officials including the health minister and, on some issues, collaborates strategically with partners such as the Canadian Medical Association and Canadian Healthcare Association in its lobbying efforts. Groups such as the Canadian Practical Nurses Association (CPNA) and the Canadian Federation of Nurses Unions (CFNU) have also widened their activities to include more education of their members around policy and politics, and the CFNU has adopted a more evidence-based approach to its lobbying efforts on behalf of nurses. In other words, evidence suggests that nurses and nurse leaders are rapidly awakening to the notion that the message and the timing really are as important as the content. According to Haylock (2000, p. 76), "for nurses to gain acceptance in health policy arenas, individual nurses and groups of nurses must become expert in assessing the environment, the interpretation of cues, and the development and implementation of realistic strategies targeting priority health policy and legislative issues." To these suggested areas of expertise may be added the use of social networks, rhetoric, and the media. This section of this chapter discusses these means to enhance nursing's political acumen.

Helms and colleagues (1996) emphasize the need to understand how the environment of policymaking shapes both the substance of policy change and the strategies needed for political adoption. They advise that both the health care sector and the health care policy agenda are large, complex, and profoundly affected by current organizational behavior. They offer a number of tips for nurses and nurse leaders to increase their chances of successfully influencing policy in this environment, three of which are offered here:

- Become "insiders" within the halls of policy formulation so you can identify and capitalize on opportunities of timing and design. This idea gets to one of the principles often talked about in the Office of Nursing Policy—"you want to be at the table, not being *talked about* at the table."
- Learn to formulate policy options with greater potential for adoption within the range of available resources and controllable variables. Understand what can be done, not just what should be done.
- Do not try to formulate specific policy objectives too broadly. Rather, strive to nudge policy forward in smaller ways that can incrementally improve the health of the population and the role of nurses.

West and Scott (2000) highlight the importance of social relationships in the policymaking process. They describe *policy networks* as formal or informal groups of politicians, civil servants, policy analysts, experts, and professionals that use their relationships to influence the formation and implementation of policy. Boundaries around the policy networks create "insider" and "outsider" roles, wherein insiders are needed by government for advice or cooperation to advance an item on the policy agenda. Nurses must maneuver to be included in policy networks as insiders; they can be successful in achieving this status on the basis of either their specialized knowledge or their ability to promote or thwart the aims and objectives of the policymakers.

Hewison (1999) argues that if nurses become skilled in the art of rhetoric and combine this with a thorough understanding of the policy process, they can be more effective in shaping policy. *Rhetoric* is defined as communication with the objective of persuading or identifying with an audience to influence attitudes and behavior. Hewison points out that language does more than simply reflect that which it attempts to describe; the act of labeling something plays a significant role in how that thing is acted toward. Therefore, if nurses become skilled at using rhetoric, they will become more effective in influencing and modifying policy that never makes it onto the policy tables, even though there are people who feel and speak passionately about them. Rather, there exists a complex agenda-setting process, which is an ongoing competition among the proponents of a set of issues, to gain the attention of media professionals, the public, and policymakers. Problems, these authors suggest, require exposure—coverage in the mass media—before they will be considered public issues and thus of sufficient importance to be addressed through policy. The Centre for Advancement of Health (2001) suggests the following tips for researchers in interacting with the media:

- Get their attention (be strategic!).
- Write an engaging news release.
- Think like a reporter.
- Prepare for and conduct successful interviews.

The CNA has published several useful documents for nurses wishing to enhance their knowledge and skills in the political arena, for example, *Getting Started: A Political Action Guide for Canada's Registered Nurses* (1997) and *Nursing Is a Political Act: The Bigger Picture* (2000). Similar publications are available from a number of provincial RN and LPN associations as well as from unions and other bodies. A good example is the Alberta Association of Registered Nurses' (AARN's) MLA Mentorship Program, which encourages registered nurses to engage and interact with elected representatives to promote understanding of AARN's positions and increase the individual nurse's understanding of ways that nurses can influence public health policy.

In 1996, several Centres of Excellence for Women's Health (CEWH) were established across Canada, with the goal to improve women's health. The CEWH research bulletin from the summer of 2001 investigates the influence that the centers have had on policy. Several of the articles describe mechanisms to "get the word out" and to ensure that research findings become part of policy debates. Processes used include media events, research symposia, Web sites, policy road shows, a dedicated research chair, and women's health awards. For example, the Montreal Centre hosted a symposium with caregivers' associations from various parts of the province of Quebec and then took this information, along with 5 years of research experience on women caregivers and a coalition of interested groups, into public consultations to change policy at the local community-health level.

■ OVERCOMING BARRIERS: LESSONS FROM THOSE WHO HAVE WALKED BEFORE

In countless situations, nurses have been involved with change in general and the policy cycle in particular. Examples that illustrate many of the points made in this chapter follow.

Success Abroad

Aitken and coworkers (2001) describe the successful creation of a bill to fund a nurse home visitation program for high-risk mothers in Arkansas. In summarizing what allowed them to be successful in this policy initiative, the authors noted six factors:

1. Realistic time commitment
2. Community needs assessment, data assimilation, and review of existing resources

3. Identification and incorporation of stakeholders
4. Narrow focus on the area of greatest need
5. Backing of political partners
6. Favorable opportunities to advance child health issues

Valentine (2000, pp. 45–46) shares policymaking and political lessons learned in the course of a partially successful crusade to upgrade the chief nurse position in the U.S. Veterans Health Administration (VHA). Her insights and words of advice include the following:

1. Advocacy for a decision-making role in an organization requires stamina and commitment and takes time, effort, and passion.
2. Changing organizational culture takes time and requires the involvement of senior-level champions.
3. Never underestimate the value of non-nurse advocates.
4. Never underestimate the value of turnover among one's adversaries.
5. Nurses are right most of the time, but not all of the time—we need to listen to criticism more carefully.
6. Benchmarking is important, but it may not be sufficient to call the question.
7. There is no such thing as overnight success. The keys are hard work and never giving up.

Success at Home

Nurses do not have to look south of the border for examples. Professional nurses and nursing organizations across Canada have been successful in influencing policy change in several different venues. Take the following examples:

1. Across the country, provincial and territorial governments are putting in place regulatory mechanisms and legislation that will facilitate increased opportunities for the employment of nurse practitioners (NPs). Although NPs are sometimes able to practise only in underserviced areas, the new legislation will permit employers to engage the services of NPs wherever there is felt to be a need. That outcome reflects the culmination of a careful, collaborative process spearheaded by the Canadian Nurses Association, its members, and its partners over many years. In 2004, CNA received $8 million in funding from Health Canada to integrate and sustain the role of the NP in primary health care by undertaking initiatives across the country in educational preparation, practice, policy, legislation, government and professional self-regulation, health human resource planning, change management, social marketing, and strategic communication. This project was given life within an environment of growing advocacy for primary health care—specifically, one in which the NP role in primary health care delivery was recognized as perhaps the most important initiative in health reform. For example, the Alberta Association of Registered Nurses recognized the opportunity and timing and led the policy lobby in Alberta while governments worked collaboratively and enabled legislative changes, employers agreed to provide the actual employment and contractual arrangements, and nurse educators implemented the requisite NP programs—all serving as a prime example of nurse-led policy change that took perfect advantage of timing, stakeholder interest, and political will.
2. In Quebec, the Ordre des infirmières et infirmiers du Québec (2000) actively used its political clout to obtain government adoption of a regulation enabling second-year nursing students to be hired as "externs" for summer and holiday season vacation relief work. This regulation, which benefits both the nursing students and employers, resulted in nearly 1,200 students being hired by 50 institutions in its second year of operation.
3. In the late 1980s, in response to research and lobbying by nursing associations for nurses to have greater participation in the decisions that affected them, the Ontario minister of health introduced a new regulation to the Public Hospitals Act, mandating the seating of elected staff nurses and (s)elected nurse managers on all hospital committees dealing with administrative, financial, operational, and planning matters (Skelton-Green, 1996).

4. In Saskatchewan, the "Band-Aid" campaign, led by student nurses and supported by the Saskatchewan Registered Nurses Association (SRNA), was significantly influential in forcing the provincial government to backtrack on an announced policy change that would have caused nursing education to revert from the baccalaureate degree to the diploma. In January 2000, the provincial government had said it could not support the SRNA's position on baccalaureate education as entry to practice for RNs and was going to look again at diploma programs. Backed by SRNA, the student nurses sent postcards to every member of the legislative assembly and to the premier and appeared in person on the steps of the legislature, asserting that reverting to diploma education was a "Band-Aid" solution that would do nothing for nursing recruitment and retention in the long term. Eventually, the government dropped its plan and has since supported the SRNA in its position on the minimal education for RNs.

5. In 1998, a nursing task force was established to address concerns regarding the future supply and retention of RNs and registered practical nurses in Ontario. In 1999, in response to one of the two key recommendations of the task force, the minister of health and long-term care (MOHLTC) created a $375 million Nursing Enhancement Fund (NEF). Over the next 2 years, the NEF supported more than 12,000 new nursing positions in the province (Joint Provincial Nursing Committee, 2001) and the rate of full-time work has increased (Joint Provincial Nursing Committee, 2004). As of June 2003, a total of 164 advanced clinical/practice fellowships had been awarded and 123 completed. Development of a broad slate of best practice guidelines is under way with funding through the MOHLTC, Health Canada, and the Registered Nurses Association of Ontario.

6. At the federal level, it was the successful lobbying of nurses, nursing organizations (such as the CNA), and individual nurse leaders that led to the creation of the ONP and revival of the notion of a chief nurse for Canada. The same now holds true across the country: Senior nurses have been appointed in the governments of nearly every province.

These are just a few among dozens of success stories that were provided to the ONP in response to a request for instances where nurses have influenced policy change. Clearly, nurses can make a difference!

■ OVERCOMING BARRIERS AND INITIATING ACTION

Nurses and the nursing profession are at the center of public health issues that are of tremendous and long-lasting importance—issues such as who has access to what providers and what makes a difference in quality and cost-effectiveness of care. There are also issues crucial to the future of the nursing profession, such as who will be the gatekeeper in primary care and what is the appropriate scope of practice for RNs, LPNs, and RPNs across various service sectors. As Milstead (1999) says in *Health Policy and Politics: A Nurse's Guide*:

Nurses are articulate experts who can address both the rational shaping of policy and the emotional aspects of the process. Nurses cannot afford to limit their actions to monitoring bills; they must seize the initiative and use their considerable collective and individual influence to ensure the health, welfare, and protection of the public and health care professionals (p. 23).

She also says the following:

The opportunity to sustain an ongoing, meaningful dialogue with those who represent [us]…and those who administer public programs is ours to initiate. Nurses must become indispensable to elected and appointed officials (p. xi).

Milstead contends that nurses who have been reluctant to become "political" cannot afford to do so any longer. She emphasizes that "each nurse counts, and collectively, nursing is a major actor in the effort to ensure the country's healthy future" (Milstead, 1999, p. 34). Gebbie and coauthors (2000) suggest several strategies that individual nurses can use to influence policy formulation:

■ Cultivate and maintain relationships with knowledgeable and influential people.
■ Become knowledgeable about current developments on policy-relevant issues.
■ Join professional nursing organizations.
■ Develop network strategies to mentor political neophytes.
■ Share the "how to" success stories of individual nurses and nursing organizations in the policy arena.
■ Create linkages between nursing research and political and policy-related activity.
■ Develop clear, well-informed, jargon-free communication when interacting with policymakers.
■ Capitalize on the positive views that communities have of the nursing profession by being visible at forums and other community meetings.

If individual nurses can do this much, organized nursing groups can accomplish even more. For example, Gebbie and coauthors (2000) suggest that representatives from nursing organizations could develop an annual national institute for policy to bring nurses' best research into the policy arena. Professional nursing organizations could set aside time at national meetings to allow nurses to converse about health policy strategies and activities and include planned discussions of ways nurses can effectively influence health policy at individual and organizational levels. Individuals in these organizations should become experts in interacting with the media and positioning their work to draw media attention.

The perspective of nurses in shaping health policy is essential. Together, RNs, LPNs, and RPNs account for more than a third of the health workforce (CIHI, 2001b, p. 10) and exert an enormous influence on the health of this nation. Nurses know about health and health care; they know about communities and people. It is the knowledge and experience of nurses that shaped much of the public health history of this country and contributed significantly to the state of health that makes Canadians the envy of most of the world. It is the vigilance of nurses in hospitals, nursing homes, and long-term care facilities that continues to shepherd patients safely through their health challenges and transitions. The presence of nurses comforts, prevents disease, and improves health. And we know now that when the system creates conditions that result in too few nurses, the impact of work overload and fatigue on patients, families, and nurses themselves can be catastrophic. Nurses' voices must be heard as health and social policy is developed. And so, this chapter concludes with a challenge to all nurses to think about ways in which they can positively influence health policy, both individually and collectively and wherever they practise.

■ SUMMARY

Effective policy is best linked with research findings. In health care, an example of what happens when policy does not factor in research is the recurrent cycle of nursing shortages.

Research indicates what nurses want and need in their work environments to optimize their contributions to health care, but these findings went unheeded when policymakers implemented workforce cutbacks.

A variety of levers can be used to effect change and influence health care policy. They include conducting good research, making effective links between research and policy, understanding how to initiate and manage change, understanding the policy cycle, and being politically savvy.

Research is more likely to be translated into policy if researchers, policy analysts, managers, and politicians negotiate the language and frame of reference before any research is undertaken.

Keys to effecting change are appreciation and an understanding of the policy cycle, which includes agenda creation, legislation and regulation, program implementation, and program evaluation. Behind the development of policy are values and cultural beliefs from which certain problems or issues emerge. Ideally, interested parties then build knowledge and research related to the problems or issues; they bring the knowledge to the attention of the public, become politically active in various arenas, and participate in the activation of interest groups. Public deliberation and adoption of policy related to the issues ensue, and ongoing regulation, revision, and refinement of the policy follow. A component of most successful policies is political acumen, a process of social influence involving activities of persuasion, attitudinal change, decision making, and compromise.

Valuable tools and tactics for successful policymaking include maintaining ongoing positive relationships with knowledgeable and influential people; being interested in and understanding current developments in policy-relevant issues; promoting activity in professional nursing organizations; networking and mentoring; sharing success stories and previously successful strategies; creating links between nursing research and political and policy-related activity; communicating clearly and intelligently with policymakers; and capitalizing on nursing's positive aspects and image in the community.

Online Resources

Add to your knowledge of this issue:

Canada Health Infoway	www.infoway-inforoute.ca
Canadian Institute for Health Information	www.cihi.com
Canadian Patient Safety Institute	www.cpsi-icsp.ca
First Ministers' Accord on Health Care Renewal (2003)	www.hc-sc.gc.ca/english/hca2003/accord.html
First Ministers' Meeting on the Future of Health Care (2004): A 10-year plan to strengthen health care	www.hc-sc.gc.ca/english/hca2003/fmm/index.html
Health Council of Canada	www.hcc-ccs.ca
Institute of Medicine (U.S.)	www.iom.edu
National Forum for Health Care Quality Measurement and Reporting	www.qualityforum.org
The Organisation for Economic Co-operation & Development	www.oecd.org
Patient Safety Institute (U.S.)	www.ptsafety.org
Statistics Canada	www.statcan.ca
World Health Organization	www.who.int/en

REFLECTIONS on the Chapter . . .

1. Think of an existing health care policy that you consider successful. What kind of research, if any, do you think is linked to this policy? What factors do you think make the policy successful?

2. Alone or with a group of classmates, select a problem or an issue that you have encountered in your own experience as a nursing student or in a related situation. What kind of action plan do you think would be effective in building a policy to address the issue(s)?

References

Aiken, L. H., Salmon, M., Shamian, J., et al. (1998, April). *An international study of the effects of the organization and staffing of hospitals on patient outcomes.* Presentation at Outcomes/Indicators Session, WHO, CCNM, Korea.

Aiken, L. H., Smith, H. L., & Lake, E. T. (1994). Lower Medicare mortality among a set of hospitals known for good nursing care. *Medical Care, 32*(8), 771–787.

Aitken, M. E., Rowlands, L. A., & Wheeler, J. G. (2001). Advocating for children's health at the state level: Lessons learned. *Archives of Pediatrics and Adolescent Medicine, 155*(8), 877–880.

Baumann, A., O'Brien Pallas, L., Armstrong-Stassen, M., et al. (2001). *Commitment and care: The benefits of a healthy workplace for nurses, their patients and the system. A policy synthesis.* Ottawa: Canadian Health Services Research Foundation & the Change Foundation.

Blegen, M. A., & Mueller, C. W. (1987). Nurses' job satisfaction: A longitudinal analysis. *Nursing and Health, 10,* 227–237.

Browne, G. (2001, October 24). *Key findings from the System-Linked Research Unit on Health and Social Service Utilization.* Presented to the Advisory Committee on Health Human Resources' Working Group on Nursing & Unregulated Healthcare Workers. Ottawa.

Canadian Institute for Health Information. (2001a). An environmental scan of research transfer strategies. *Canadian Population Health Initiative,* February. Ottawa: Author.

_____. (2001b). *Canada's health care providers.* Ottawa: Author.

Canadian Labour and Business Centre. (2002). *Full-time equivalents and financial costs associated with absenteeism, overtime, and involuntary part-time employment in the nursing profession: A report prepared for the Canadian Nursing Advisory Committee.* Ottawa: Author.

Canadian Nurses Association. (1997). *Getting started: A political action guide for Canada's registered nurses.* Ottawa: Author.

_____. (2000). Nursing is a political act: The bigger picture. *Nursing Now. Issues and Trends in Canadian Nursing, 8.* Ottawa: Author.

Centre for the Advancement of Health. (2001). *Communicating health behavior science in the media: Tips for researchers.* Washington DC: Author.

Centres of Excellence for Women's Health. (2001, Summer). *Research Bulletin 2*(1).

Cheek, J., & Gibson, T. (1997). Policy matters: Critical policy analysis and nursing. *Journal of Advanced Nursing, 25*(4), 668–672.

Chunharas, S. (2001). Linking research to policy and action. In N. Neufeld & N. Johnson (Eds.), *Forging links for health research: Perspectives from the Council on Health Research for Development.* Ottawa: International Development Research Centre.

Clarke, H. F., Lashinger, H. S., Giovannetti, P., et al. (2001). Nursing shortages: Workplace environments are essential to the solution. *Hospital Quarterly, 4*(3), 50–55.

Commission d'étude sur les services de santé et les services sociaux. (2000). *Les solutions émergentes: Rapport et recommendations.* Québec: Gouvernement du Québec. ISBN 2-550-36958-0.

Crosswaite, C., & Curtice, L. (1994). Disseminating research results: The challenge of bridging the gap between health research and health action. *Health Promotion International, 9*(4), 289–296.

Dannemiller, K. D., & Jacobs, R. W. (1992). Changing the way organizations change: A revolution of common sense. *Journal of Applied Behavioral Science, 28*(4), 480–498.

Davis, P., & Howden-Chapman, P. (1996). Translating research findings into health policy. *Social Science and Medicine, 43,* 865–872.

Feldman, P. H., Nadash, P., & Gursen, M. (2001). Improving communication between researchers and policy makers in long-term care: Or, researchers are from Mars; policy makers are from Venus. *The Gerontologist, 41*(3), 312–321.

Gebbie, K. M., Wakefield, M., & Kerfoot, K. (2000). Nursing and health policy. *Journal of Nursing Scholarship, 32*(3), 307–315.

Hartz, A. J., Krakauer, H., Kuhn, E. M., et al. (1989). Hospital characteristics and mortality rates. *New England Journal of Medicine, 321,* 1720–1725.

Haylock, P. J. (2000). Health policy and legislation: Impact on cancer nursing and care. *Seminars in Oncology Nursing, 16*(1), 76–84.

Helms, L. B., Anderson, M. A., & Hanson, K. (1996). "Doin' politics": Linking policy and politics in nursing. *Nursing Administration Quarterly, 20*(3), 32–41.

Hewison, A. (1999). The new public management and the new nursing: Related by rhetoric. Some reflections on the policy process and nursing. *Journal of Advanced Nursing, 29*(6), 1377–1384.

Irvine, D., & Evans, M. (1992). *Job satisfaction and turnover among nurses: A review and meta-analysis.* Toronto: Quality of Worklife Research Unit, University of Toronto.

Joint Provincial Nursing Committee (JPNC). (2001). *Good nursing, good health: A good investment. First progress report on the Nursing Task Force recommendations.* Toronto: Ministry of Health and Long-Term Care.

_____. (2004). *Good nursing, good health: Progress report November 2003.* Toronto: Ministry of Health and Long-Term Care.

Kimball, B., & O'Neil, E. (2001). The evolution of a crisis: Nursing in America. *Policy, Politics, & Nursing Practice, 2*(3), 180–186.

Kingdon, J. W. (1995). *Agendas, alternatives, and public policies.* New York: HarperCollins College Publishers.

Knaus, W. A., Draper, E. A., Wagner, D. P., et al. (1986). An evaluation of outcome from intensive care in major medical centers. *Annals of Internal Medicine, 104,* 410–418.

Lomas, J. (2000). Using "linkage and exchange" to move research into policy at a Canadian foundation. *Health Affairs (Chevy Chase), 19*(3), 236–240.

McGillis Hall, L., Irvine Doran, D., Baker, G. R., et al. (2001). A study of the impact of nursing staff mix models and organizational change strategies on patient, system and nurse outcomes. Toronto: University of Toronto.

Milstead, J. A. (1999). *Health policy and politics: A nurse's guide.* Gaithersburg, MD: Aspen.

Mittelmark, M. B. (1999). The psychology of social influence and healthy public policy. *Preventive Medicine, 29*(6, Pt. 2), S24–S29.

Montini, T., & Bero, L. A. (2001). Policy makers' perspectives on tobacco control advocates' roles in regulation development. *Tobacco Control, 10*(3), 218–224.

O'Brien-Pallas, L., Duffield, C., & Alksnis, C. (2004). Who will be there to nurse: Retention of nurses nearing retirement. *Journal of Nursing Administration, 35*(6), 298–302.

O'Brien-Pallas, L., & Shamian, J. (with Buchan, J., Duffield, C., Hughes, F., et al.). (2003, February 13). An international examination of the cost and impact of turnover on patient safety and nurse outcomes: Preliminary findings. *Fifth Joint National Conference on Quality in Health Care,* Toronto.

O'Brien-Pallas, L., Thomson, D., Alksnis, C., et al. (2001). The economic impact of nurse staffing decisions: Time to turn down another road? *Hospital Quarterly, 4*(2), 42–50.

Ordre des infirmiéres et infirmiers du Québec. (2000). *Le financement et l'organisation des services de santé et des services sociaux.* Mémoire présenté á la Commission d'étude sur les services de santé et les services sociaux. Montréal: Author.

Organization for Economic Cooperation and Development (OECD). (2004). *Resolving nurse shortages in OECD member countries.* Human Resources for Health Care Nursing Project. Paris, France.

Prescott, P. A. (1993). Nursing: An important component of hospital survival under a reformed health care system. *Nursing Economics, 11,* 192–199.

Price, J. L., & Mueller, C. W. (1981). A causal model of turnover for nurses. *Academy of Management Journal, 24*(3), 543–565.

Scott, J. G., Sochalski, J., & Aiken, L. (1999). Review of magnet hospital research. *Journal of Nursing Administration, 29*(1), 9–19.

Skelton-Green, J. M. (1996). The perceived impact of committee participation on the job satisfaction and retention of staff nurses. *Canadian Journal of Nursing Administration, 9*(2), 7–35.

Slavitt, B. B., Stamps, P. L., Piedmont, E. G., et al. (1978). Nurses' satisfaction with their work situation. *Nursing Research, 27,* 114–120.

Tarlov, A. (1999). Public policy frameworks for improving population health. *Annals of the New York Academy of Sciences, 896,* 281–293.

_____. (2000, August 10–13). *The future of health in Canada: "The art of the possible."* Proceedings of the 69th Annual Couchiching Summer Conference, Geneva Park, Orillia, Ontario.

Taylor, C. (1997). The ACIDD test: A framework for policy planning and decision-making. *Optimum, the Journal of Public Sector Management, 27*(4), 53–62.

Valentine, N. M. (2000). The evolving role of the chief nurse executive in the Veterans Health Administration: Policy and leadership lessons. *Policy, Politics, & Nursing Practice, 1*(1), 36–46.

West, E., & Scott, C. (2000). Nursing in the public sphere: Breaching the boundary between research and policy. *Journal of Advanced Nursing, 32*(4), 817–824.

REGULATORY POWER

Critical Questions

As a way of engaging with the ideas in this chapter, consider the following:

1. How might a historical perspective contribute to our understanding of the International Council of Nurses (ICN)?

2. Who are the members of the ICN?

3. What are your assumptions about the role and the purpose of the ICN?

4. Consider how an international organization such as the ICN might influence health care delivery or health care policy.

CHAPTER

7

Geertje Boschma
Barbara Brush
Meryn Stuart

The International Council of Nurses: A Historical Perspective

Delegates register at the 1997 ICN Congress held in Vancouver, B.C., Canada (with permission from the Lynaugh Collection, Bryn Mawr, PA; in Brush, B.L., Lynaugh, J.E., Boschma, G., et al. [1999]. *Nurses of all nations: A history of the International Council of Nurses, 1899–1999.* Lippincott Williams & Wilkins).

Chapter Objectives

After completing this chapter, you will be able to:

1. Reflect on the history of the ICN.

2. Identify selected roles and objectives of the ICN.

3. Understand the ICN's relationship to world health.

4. Discuss some of the current issues facing the ICN and analyze strategies put in place to address them.

This chapter presents a historical perspective of the development of the International Council of Nurses (ICN) and discusses its current objectives in the broader historical context of the evolution of organized nursing. Specifically, this chapter reviews the history of the ICN in relationship to its contributions to world health and its initiatives to support national regulation of the nursing profession within the ICN membership countries. Some examples of current issues facing the ICN and the ICN responses to them are also discussed.

■ THE ICN: A HISTORICAL PERSPECTIVE

In 1999, at the ICN Centennial Conference in London, England, the ICN celebrated its 100th year as an international organization for nurses. For more than a century, the ICN has sustained its place as an important and meaningful organization for nurses around the world. The overall goal of the ICN is to unite nurses worldwide by forming a confederation of national nursing organizations while supporting national nursing organizations in their efforts to influence national health and nursing policy. Throughout the years, motivation, commitment, and enthusiasm banded nurses together despite turbulent social and economic changes, hardships of war, and profound cultural differences. Currently, the ICN represents national nursing organizations from more than 120 countries and has more than 1 million members. Yet the ICN started out as a small organization in the broader context of the women's movement. It was founded in 1899, upon the initiative of the British nurse and suffragist Ethel Gordon Manson, later Mrs. Bedford Fenwick, a prominent leader of the British Nurses Association (BNA).

Early Goals

From the outset, the professional welfare of nurses, the interests of women, and the improvement of the people's health were intertwined goals for the founders of the ICN. A small group consisting primarily of British, American, Canadian, Scandinavian, and German nurses, the ICN intended to unite nurses worldwide through an international organization. Nursing as a respected, paid, professional occupation for middle-class women was a new phenomenon at the end of the 19th century.

Health care profoundly changed as a result of industrialization and urbanization. Hospital reform and modern hospital development were important goals throughout Europe and North America at the time, and the foundation of hospital schools to train nurses followed in their wake. The women's movement sprung in part from the desire of middle-class women to make themselves more socially useful and to carve out respectable work opportunities in areas deemed appropriate for women, thereby extending women's traditional roles in the family, such as caring for the sick, teaching, and performing social work. The founding members of the ICN were part of the growing number of women who were active in social and health care reform and who simultaneously sought to improve women's social position and to obtain the right to vote.

On July 1, 1899, Fenwick attended the Annual Conference of the Matron's Council of Great Britain and Ireland in London, where 200 women and nurses from around the world had gathered. At this meeting, she proposed organizing an international council of nurses, modeled after the International Council of Women

FIGURE 7.1 Founder and charter members of the ICN (left to right): founding President Ethel Gordon Fenwick (Britain), Secretary Lavinia L. Dock (U.S.), and Treasurer Agnes Snively. (Photos of Ethel Gordon Fenwick reproduced with permission from Dock, L.L. [1912]. *History of nursing* [Vol. 3]; of Lavinia Dock, from Lynaugh Collection, Bryn Mawr, PA; of Agnes Snively, from Bridges [1967]. *History of the International Council of Nurses*; in Brush, B.L., Lynaugh, J.E., Boschma, G., et al. [1999]. *Nurses of all nations: A history of the International Council of Nurses, 1899–1999*. Lippincott Williams & Wilkins.)

(ICW). The next day, she instituted a provisional committee to draft a constitution. Among the founders were Lavinia L. Dock, a nurse and activist in the women's movement from the United States, and Agnes Snively, an influential Canadian nurse, as well as various representatives from Australia, Denmark, the Netherlands, New Zealand, and the Union of South Africa. A year later, the constitution was approved, with Fenwick elected as president, Lavinia L. Dock as secretary, and Agnes Snively as treasurer (Figure 7.1).

The ICN held its first meeting in 1901 in Buffalo, New York, at the Pan American Exposition, and it met again 3 years later in Berlin in conjunction with the congress of the ICW. This time, German nurses, inspired by nurse leader Agnes Karll, joined the group as well.

Aware of the need to establish their independence as a predominantly female professional group and to run their own affairs free from hospital, medical, or state control, the early leaders envisioned the ICN as a federation of national nurses' organizations, headed by a nurse, representing nurses only. However, at that time, nurses in most countries had not organized on a national level. At the 1904 meeting, only Germany, Great Britain, and the United States were ready for confederation.

In many ways, the ICN requirement that only self-regulated bodies of nurses could join stimulated the formation of independent national nursing organizations. For example, Canadian nurse leaders were organized jointly with their U.S. colleagues until that time. After the Berlin meeting, however, Snively, who served as director of the influential Toronto General Hospital School of Nursing from 1884 until 1910, helped form the Canadian National Association of Trained Nurses, later the Canadian Nurses Association (CNA, 1968). Canada joined the ICN at its next congress, held in 1909 in London, as did the Netherlands, Finland, and Denmark.

As nurses organized, their commitment to creating an international body of nurses became evident. Indeed, influenced by their involvement in the women's movement, the founding leaders believed that an international organization of nurses would improve their professional standing and unite their efforts to develop a firm basis for nursing education and practice. They argued that if nursing practice met universal standards and was protected by state regulation, nurses, as women, could make crucial contributions to social progress and improve people's health. The examples of professional nursing already developed in North America and western Europe inspired the founding leaders. In a sense, their ideas reflected Western cultural dominance typical of international politics at the time. The early ICN leaders—all from American and western European backgrounds—were strongly committed to spreading the international idea of nursing.

Early Impact of Organized Nursing: Developments in German Nursing

The establishment of the German Nurses Association (*Berufsorganisation der Krankenpflegerinnen Deutschlands*), and its involvement with the ICN during the early decades, exemplify the significance of international relationships for the development of nursing within diverse national contexts (Boschma, 1996). Agnes Karll (1868–1927), the influential president of the German Nurses Association, energetically sought to change contemporary conditions of nursing by creating opportunities for a respected, independent, paid career for German nurses. Their situation illustrates the wider social and political impact on nursing around the time of World War I.

The work opportunities and social position for German nurses changed profoundly at the turn of the 20th century as a result of rapid population growth, industrialization, changing health needs in the population, and, in response, a changing role for women. By 1900, Germany was one of the largest industrial powers of Europe. Religious and charitable nursing orders provided most nursing care to the sick in Germany, and the situation was comparable to that in Canada, where the Grey Nuns were among the leaders in establishing modern nursing (Paul, 1994). Roman Catholic orders had flourished in Germany since the early 19th century, and eventually, Protestants followed the Catholic example and revived the function of the deaconess. The most famous deaconess institute was in Kaiserswerth and was established by Theodor Fliedner in 1836. Organized in a motherhouse, or convent, structure, the institute enabled deaconesses to pursue a socially accepted public role. However, by the early 20th century, with its rapidly changing social context, the motherhouse system was unable to meet the increasing demand for nurses. Especially in the cities, many nurses separated themselves from motherhouses and began to work either in private duty or in municipal hospitals. A new generation of nurses sought economic independence and an autonomous life. Yet the "free" nurses, as those who had separated themselves from motherhouses were called, risked their reputations and remained vulnerable because they were largely unprotected and prone to exploitation. Moreover, in the urban hospitals, work conditions were harsh. Many nurses experienced poor physical or mental health at early ages (Lungershausen, 1964; Bischoff, 1984).

With the founding of the German Nurses Association in 1903, Agnes Karll sought to change the situation of the independent nurses. She had obtained training in nursing at the Clementinen House in Hannover, a Red Cross motherhouse, and then worked in private duty nursing in Berlin. But by 1901, the hard work had weakened her physical condition and, at the age of 33, she was forced to abandon private duty. Thereafter, Karll devoted herself to the betterment of nurses' social conditions. Through her connections with the women's movement, she gradually envisioned an avenue toward self-organization for nurses and arranged for the founding meeting of the German Nurses Association in Berlin. One of the association's key functions was to create an employment bureau to actively protect and mediate the placement of nurses in private duty.

Karll's efforts attracted the interest of the ICN leaders and led to their accepting the German Nurses Association into the ICN at the 1904 Berlin meeting. The connection with international colleagues was a valuable resource for Karll. She perceived the accomplishments of American and British colleagues as a model for German nurses, and she corresponded regularly with Lavinia L. Dock, ICN secretary, to discuss German nursing affairs.

In 1909 in London, England, at the second quinquennial ICN Congress, Karll was elected president. The congress strongly supported women's suffrage and recommended that each national group advocate for state regulation of nursing practice. Although the ICN did not retain a regulatory function itself, it supported the establishment of state regulation through its member organizations. Upon an invitation by the German nurses, the ICN held its next congress in Cologne, Germany, in 1912. There, the urgency of improving nurses' social welfare and working conditions was widely discussed; the keynote speech addressed the effects of physical strain and fatigue on nurses' health. In addition, the objectives of suffrage, nurses' expanding role in social progress and public health, and improving nurses' work conditions preoccupied the minds of the ICN delegates. Delegates also discussed the need for common standards of nursing and for clear ICN-admission criteria.

Finding common working ground and bridging the diverse national contexts of nursing took considerable effort by the ICN members (Brush & Stuart, 1994). Despite the enthusiasm for the nursing cause, stability within the ICN was threatened by unstable international politics before the beginning of World War I. In Cologne, delegates elected American Annie Goodrich, inspector of nurse training schools in New York, as the ICN's fourth president and decided to have their next meeting in San Francisco in 1915. However, growing political tension soon disrupted this plan.

The Interwar Years

World War I abruptly interrupted the innovative initiatives of the ICN. Because of the devastating war situation, which mobilized many nurses for war service, the 1915 congress never happened. With members suddenly on opposite sites of the world conflict, the ICN's deliberate neutral stand toward national politics was compromised. At the much smaller meeting that was held in 1915, delegates elected Henny Tscherning from war-neutral Denmark as the new president, marking the beginning of a more prominent northern European presence among the ICN leadership in the interwar years. Tscherning, a founding member and president of the Danish Council of Nurses, was instrumental in connecting nurses in the northern European countries, and in 1920, she cofounded the Northern Nurses Federation (Wingender, 1995). Tscherning and the Scandinavian national organizations provided continuity in turbulent times and kept the ICN going.

The ICN members did not meet again until 1922, when the fourth regular ICN meeting was held in Copenhagen, Denmark. Tscherning's leadership facilitated a gradual shift away from the strong dominance of Anglo-American leadership in the ICN: The unity of the Nordic nurses probably strengthened the role of northern European leaders. In Copenhagen, another Scandinavian nurse, Sophie Mannerheim of Finland, was elected president. She was one of the early presidents of the Finnish national nurses' association, founded in 1898, and she played a central role in international nursing activities for more than 25 years. Christiane Reimann from Denmark became secretary, replacing Lavinia L. Dock, who had been in the position for 22 years.

In assuming this role, Reimann also became the first paid ICN secretary. She traveled frequently to facilitate the establishment of national nursing councils and often contributed from personal funds to maintain the ICN activities and publication of the *ICN Bulletin*. What started as a small newsletter regularly sent to all members gradually evolved into a professional international nursing journal. Today, the *International Nursing Review* is the official journal of the ICN and is published four times per year.

By 1922, the ICN represented 15 countries, including China. Prior contact with Anglo-European nursing influence and direction was a key feature in many countries' successful linkage with the ICN. Russia, unlike China, for example, never joined the ICN. However, Western powers controlled China at the time and facilitated the establishment of a Western health care system there, even though traditional Chinese medicine did not disappear (Chen, 1996). Along with the creation of Western hospitals, training schools for nurses were opened in China and were often directed by American or European nurses. In 1914, a Chinese national nurses organization was founded; it joined the ICN in 1922.

Sophie Mannerheim turned out to be the right leader to navigate the ICN through complex post–World War I nursing politics. Revolutions spread over Europe at that time, and intense nationalism characterized international politics. Economic malaise and political unrest created complex problems. Tuberculosis and high infant mortality threatened public health. The Red Cross established many new schools of nursing in eastern European countries to meet the pressing demand for qualified nurses. Many times, British or North American nurses headed these schools and formed linkages with the ICN. Red Cross standards of nurse training, however, did not necessarily match the ICN ideal of a 3-year nurse training program, and this created considerable debate within the ICN. To meet demands for military nursing, the Red Cross had instituted many short training programs, which exacerbated tension over standardization of nurse training and the legal regulation of nursing practice. At that time, various European countries that were not ICN members founded the European Council of Nursing Education (ECNE), whose perspective on nursing education also varied from that of the ICN. Mannerheim, participating in both the Red Cross and the ICN, was an excellent mediator in these politics and ensured the role of the ICN in international health affairs.

The ICN and World Health

From the time of its founding, the ICN was strongly committed to the improvement of world health. In the early decades of the 20th century, contagious diseases and high infant mortality had a devastating impact in the industrializing Western world. The ICN's initial dedication to furthering social progress and public health assumed new meaning in the aftermath of World War I. Wartime devastation prompted the expansion of public health services, especially in child welfare and tuberculosis care, and set a new public health agenda. The Red Cross and the League of Nations facilitated the preparation of qualified nurses for public health activities, but philanthropic foundations, such as the Rockefeller Foundation, also funded the training of public health nurses.

The Rockefeller Foundation considered nurses essential for postwar public health service. Through their International Health Commission, the Rockefeller Foundation supported public health programs throughout the world, either by founding or by cooperating with existing medical and nursing schools. Foundational support often involved and facilitated linkages with the ICN because American and European nurses led most of the foundation's projects. The Rockefeller Foundation profoundly influenced tuberculosis control in France, for example, and financed the establishment of training schools for nurses and health visitors in several French cities. In the process, the foundation helped establish the French Central Nursing Bureau in 1925. In that same year, France joined the ICN under the leadership of Leonie Chaptal, a long-standing leader in French public health nursing and the founder of an independent professional organization for French nurses (Boschma & Stuart, 1999).

In Helsinki at the 1925 ICN meeting, Bulgaria, Cuba, France, Irish Free State, and Poland became part of the confederation, increasing membership countries to 20. American Nina Gage, representing the Chinese nursing association, was elected president. Meanwhile, ICN board members decided to move the ICN headquarters to Geneva, Switzerland. Viewed as politically neutral and stable, Geneva became the center of an increasing number of international organizations.

During the 1929 ICN meeting in Montreal, Leonie Chaptal was elected ICN president. Massive changes in public health nursing dominated the agenda. Acceptable standards and conditions for general and public health nursing education provoked much debate. The Nursing Education Committee, headed by Isabel Stewart from Teacher's College of Columbia University (New York), presented its report on nursing education. The powerful presence of Teacher's College graduates in the ICN influenced the ICN's thinking that science and research in nursing should be promoted as a way to strengthen the nursing profession. For most membership countries, however, this novel idea had limited immediate relevance, although the issue would never disappear from the ICN agenda.

Effect of Worldwide Depression on Nursing

By the time the ICN regained some stability in the 1930s, the worldwide economic depression had had an impact on nursing. Discussing the unemployment rate of nurses was high on the agenda of the ICN Paris–Brussels Congress in 1933, and debates on dues and monetary exchange rates also reflected difficult financial times. At that meeting, Austrian Princess Anna Schwarzenberg became the new executive secretary and Alicia Lloyd Still from Great Britain was elected president. The ICN counted 30 member countries, growing increasingly diverse in cultural and political backgrounds, which gradually confuted the dominance of Western countries in ICN affairs. Soon however, threat of war once again determined the ICN's leaders' action. The rise of national socialism in Germany ended the independence of the German

Nurses Association, which dissolved into the Reich's Union of German Nurses and Nursing Assistants in 1939. In that same year, World War II broke out as Hitler overran Poland.

Effie Taylor, elected the ICN president in 1937 in London, made sure that ICN records and office materials, which had just been moved to new headquarters in London, were transported to the United States. She temporarily established an ICN office at her own workplace at Yale University in New Haven, Connecticut. The London ICN offices were destroyed by bombs in 1941; all ICN meetings were postponed.

■ ROLES, OBJECTIVES, AND SCOPE OF THE ICN AFTER WORLD WAR II

In 1947, the ICN was able to meet in Atlantic City, New Jersey, for the ninth ICN Congress. More than 40 countries participated, and Gerda Hojer from Sweden was elected president. Delegates decided to return the ICN headquarters to London, and, within 2 months, the ICN opened new offices at the site of the British College of Nurses at 19 Queens Gate—a building undergoing repairs because of war damage. By 1948, Daisy Bridges, former president of the National Council of Nurses of Great Britain and Northern Ireland, was appointed as executive secretary. Bridges would serve the ICN for the next 13 years, moving its work increasingly into the international field.

Alice Sher, former president of the International Nurses Screening Board, became the ICN's assistant general secretary. Sher's prior role was to oversee the Displaced Persons (Nurses) Register, which the ICN had taken over from the International Relief Organisation. The board of this organization determined the professional status of nurses who had lost their credentials during the war. Sher was instrumental in helping thousands of displaced nurse refugees continue their professional careers.

The disruption, destruction, and political realignments of the two world wars resulted in profound social change and ultimately changed the postwar identity of the ICN. The organization struggled to regain normalcy as many member associations had changed, others no longer existed, and some rejoined under new circumstances. However, still inspired by its commitment, the ICN regrouped and set a new, ambitious agenda at its 1947 meeting. Two years later, the ICN celebrated its 50th anniversary at a conference in Stockholm. Three member associations whose activities had been suspended during the war years— Australia, Germany, and Japan—were reinstated. Five new national organizations joined—Haiti, Italy, Korea, South Rhodesia, and Turkey.

The ICN and World Health After World War II

After World War II, international initiatives to make health care accessible for all gained momentum. The powerful advent of antibiotics and medical technology on a wider scale generally increased confidence that world health could be improved and should be considered a basic human right. In 1948, the newly established World Health Organization (WHO) declared that "health is a state of complete physical, mental and social well-being and not merely the absence of disease or infirmity" (Howard-Jones, 1981, p. 472).

In many ways, the 1949 ICN conference in Stockholm marked the ICN's voice—and thus nurses' voice—among other international players all working toward the common goal of world health. Gradually, the ICN carved out the right to speak for nursing in an ever-wider sphere of influence. In the 1950s, the ICN assumed a more activist role, linking with other international organizations, such as the United Nations and the WHO. The ICN implemented a new, global agenda, addressing economic, racial, religious, and gender issues that continued to complicate the professional development of nursing in many countries.

To carry out its many new international responsibilities, the ICN raised its dues and staff members undertook a series of visits to national organizations to strengthen international ties. In response to postwar changes, the initial voluntary approach to international organization gave way to a professional way of running ICN affairs. Gradually, the ICN's board put in place more adequate staff and facilities, hiring professionally trained and qualified staff to carry out its growing number of programs and activities, and reflecting a more prosperous situation.

The ICN's "official relationship" status with the WHO gave the ICN new privileges and responsibilities. The ICN was also on the mailing list of the UNESCO, the United Nations Educational, Scientific, and Cultural Organization; the Economic and Social Council; and UNICEF, the United Nations Children's Fund. These developments furthered recognition of the ICN as the international voice of nursing. In 1949, Olive Baggallay, formerly the secretary of the Florence Nightingale International Fund (FNIF), became the first nursing consultant to the WHO. In the early 1950s, the ICN also strengthened its relationship with the International Labour Organization (ILO) and began to officially represent nurses on employment issues. During this time, the ICN developed the International Code of Nursing Ethics, translated it into numerous languages, and then updated it in 1973 (International Council of Nurses, 1973). It provides national nurses associations with a valuable resource to address ethical nursing issues. Up until the 1980s, the CNA, for example, relied on the ICN ethical standards for its own code of ethics.

The ICN Vision Affirmed

Some issues, on the agenda since the beginning of the ICN, remained after World War II: educational standards of professional nurses; the meaning of national nursing representation; and financial matters. On the definition of nursing, a certain consensus was reached. The powerful statement on the unique function of the nurse formulated by Virginia Henderson (Figure 7.2) became the basis for the ICN's vision statement on nursing. Henderson's influence was largely due to her leadership status in U.S. nursing. A longtime faculty member of the department of nursing at Teachers' College, Columbia University, Henderson moved away from detailed descriptions of separate nursing tasks to a comprehensive perspective on the goals of nursing: "The unique function of the nurse is to assist the individual, sick or well, in the performance of those activities contributing to health or its recovery (or to a peaceful death) that he would perform unaided if he had the necessary strength, will or knowledge" (Lynaugh & Brush, 1999).

FIGURE 7.2 Virginia Henderson (with permission from American Journal of Nursing Collection; in Brush, B.L., Lynaugh, J.E., Boschma, G., et al. [1999]. *Nurses of all nations: A history of the International Council of Nurses, 1899–1999.* Lippincott Williams & Wilkins).

FIGURE 7.3 More and more nurses from more and more nations joined the delegates arriving at the ICN Congress of 1965, held in Frankfurt (with permission from the American Journal of Nursing Collection; in Brush, B.L., Lynaugh, J.E., Boschma, G., et al. [1999]. *Nurses of all nations: A history of the International Council of Nurses, 1899–1999*. Lippincott Williams & Wilkins).

Later, the ICN definitions of nursing and restatements of its vision would remain faithful to this early work. At the occasion of its 60th anniversary, at the ICN meeting in Helsinki in 1959, the ICN board approved Henderson's publication *Basic Principles of Nursing Care* as a core publication on behalf of the ICN Nursing Service Division. Within 5 years, the booklet had been translated into 12 languages. Eventually it would become a classic nursing text and be translated into more than 30 languages.

A new internationalism in the 1950s gradually displayed a shift in the ICN leadership away from Anglo-European control. Much of this shift coincided with the introduction of new member associations from a broader contingency of nations. Better economic circumstances and conditions for women's work, for example, enhanced nurses' ability to create organizations in Africa, Asia, South America, and Latin America. In 1957, more than 3,000 nurses from 57 countries attended the congress in Rome. The national nurses associations of Barbados, Colombia, Ethiopia, Iran, Israel, Liberia, Malaysia, Panama, and Uruguay were admitted, and Yugoslavia rejoined. Cold War–barriers, however, prevented membership in Eastern European countries, Russia, and China (Figure 7.3).

In 1966, the ICN relocated its headquarters again to Geneva, reflecting the importance of the ICN's growing external relationships. At that time, Canadian Alice Girard (Figure 7.4) was president of the ICN (1965–1969). She was the founding dean of the Faculty of Nursing Education at the Université de Montreal and the first bilingual president of the CNA (1958–1960). In the 1980s, the ICN and the League of Red Cross and Red Crescent Societies (RCRCS) collaborated in preparing a teaching kit on human rights and the Geneva Convention, and it continued to work with the WHO, UNICEF, and the ILO toward world health.

Increasing Activism: Position Statements

The increasingly activist role of the ICN impacted its political course. At the international meetings, the ICN began to adopt position statements that publicly articulated the membership's point of view on nursing and health matters such as "the nurse's role in family planning" or "smoking and health." Also, more political statements were accepted on topics such as "activities of war and their influence on personality development of children and adolescents" (International Council of Nurses, 2004a). Position statements had political implications; the aim was that national nursing organizations would strive to implement the suggestions made in the statements within their countries. In doing this, nurses at the

FIGURE 7.4 Canadian nurse Alice Girard *(left)* was president of the ICN from 1965 to 1969. Here, she takes time for tea and talk with colleague Helen Nussbaum, who was the ICN's general secretary from 1961 to 1967. (Photo courtesy of ICN Collection; in Brush, B.L., Lynaugh, J.E., Boschma, G., et al. [1999]. *Nurses of all nations: A history of the International Council of Nurses, 1899–1999.* Lippincott Williams & Wilkins.)

national level would be better able to influence national health policy and to develop strategies for nursing action.

However, an increasing political course created new dilemmas. Although the ICN claimed neutrality in the national affairs of its member countries, a profound internal conflict arose within the ICN over the membership of South Africa. The South African Nurses Association (SANA) adhered to its country's apartheid directives, inhibiting nonwhite membership into the organization. Faithful to the ICN standpoint on racial matters, some member organizations insisted that SANA open up membership to all nurses irrespective of racial background or national law. Eventually the Dutch and Swedish national organizations moved that the ICN accept a resolution to expel South Africa from membership; the resolution was passed in 1974. By declaring itself against racism, the ICN also disapproved of the internal politics of one of its member associations. As a consequence, the ICN lost one of its earliest members (Rafferty & Brush, 1995). Today, a newly integrated South African national nursing organization, the Democratic Nursing Organisation of South Africa (DENOSA), is an active ICN member (Box 7.1).

The ICN's scope widened after World War II. By 1985, the ICN represented 97 countries, and national nurses associations paid dues based on their number of individual members. "ICN membership grew 18% between 1980 and 1985, from 862,123 to 1,056,066 members" (Brush et al., 1999, p. 169). Despite the ICN's increasing diversity, however, 11 ICN countries (Japan, United States, Canada, United Kingdom, Sweden, Denmark, Australia, Spain, Finland, Norway, and Switzerland) accounted for 86% of its members. The agenda of industrialized countries importantly influenced policy directions within the ICN. However, the political point of view of the ICN changed from the past and now represented a more multinational vision. During the 1970s and 1980s, the ICN clearly spoke out against human rights violations and political suppression; the ICN considered health a basic human right for all.

BOX 7.1	ABCs of Who's Who

The following list identifies various nursing and other organizations referred to by acronyms or abbreviations in this chapter.

ANA	American Nurses Association
BNA	British Nurses Association
CNA	Canadian Nurses Association
CNR	Council of National Representatives
DENOSA	Democratic Nursing Organisation of South Africa
ECNE	European Council of Nursing Education
FNIF	Florence Nightingale International Fund
ICN	International Council of Nurses
ICW	International Council of Women
ILO	International Labour Organization
NNA	National Nurses Associations
NNF	Northern Nurses Federation
RCRCS	Red Cross and Red Crescent Societies
SANA	South African Nurses Association
UNESCO	United Nations Educational, Scientific, and Cultural Organization
UNICEF	United Nations Children's Fund
WHO	World Health Organization

■ CURRENT THINKING: ISSUES FOR THE ICN AND THE INTERNATIONAL COMMUNITY*

Many concerns facing the ICN in the 1990s had been issues throughout the organization's history, including professional service issues, economic stability, international relations, and global nurse representation. In the 1990s, the ICN sought new ways to address these familiar problems. As the century drew to a close, more than 4,500 nurses from every region of the world gathered with joy and pride at the ICN Centennial Conference in London, where they accepted a new vision to lead the ICN and nursing into the 21st century.

Regulating Nursing

With the many new national nurses associations joining the ICN in the 1970s and 1980s, regulation of nursing again became an agenda of the ICN. Many national associations facing difficult legal and cultural circumstances often called on the ICN for help in dealing with these complex matters. To assist leaders of national nurses associations (NNAs) to develop and implement national nursing regulatory systems that would meet international ICN guidelines, the ICN held six "Nursing Regulation: Moving Ahead" project workshops between 1988 and 1991. Through this project, the ICN helped prepare 161 nurses from 99 NNAs and 62 governments to take an active role in assessing and revising national regulations and laws controlling nursing practice and care delivery in their countries. At its 1995 meeting, the Council of National Representatives (CNR) approved continued international examination of national

---

* This section is adapted from Brush, B.L. (1999). Leading nurses to a new century: ICN during the 1990s. *International Nursing Review, 46*(5), 151–155, with permission.

nurse regulation. The W.K. Kellogg Foundation provided the ICN with funding for a 3-year nursing regulation study to be conducted by ICN nurse consultant Fadwa Affara.

Korean Mo-Im Kim, elected ICN president in 1989, played an essential role in increasing political activities in regard to nursing regulation. Kim, who had previously served as the president of the Korean Nurses Association and as a member of the Korean Parliament (1981–1985), was keenly aware of the urgency for all nurses to become more politically involved in defining nursing's place in their countries' health care systems. Without an official position on international regulation of nursing practice, she argued, the ICN and its member associations were vulnerable to the *ad hoc* decisions of local government officials. Nurse education and practice varied widely among nations, which enhanced opportunities for politicians to create nurse practice acts based on their own political agendas rather than on professional nursing standards.

Standardization and Credentialing

After these initiatives, in 1999 at the Centennial Conference, the CNR proposed to expand nursing's role in professional standard setting and quality assurance in health care. The CNR believed it was time to develop a framework and criteria for international standardization and credentialing procedures for nursing and health care as a way to assure health care recipients of the competency of nurses and other health professionals.

Regulation became one of the key program areas of the ICN, in addition to professional practice issues and the socioeconomic welfare of nurses. The ICN's long-standing goal to enforce standards for nursing education and practice provoked a renewed effort to develop universal guidelines for basic and specialty practice. In this way, the ICN sought to assist NNAs dealing with expanding roles of nurses, new educational standards, and the evolution of nursing specialties.

After World War II, membership countries faced the increased use of auxiliary and unlicensed personnel in a rapidly expanding health care system, making clear definitions and explication of boundaries of nursing practice all the more urgent. The ICN's recent involvement in an advisory and supporting role in credentialing is part of its strategy to respond to changing practice demands. The ICN's position on these issues and its effort to collect reliable data on nursing help NNAs to effectively represent nursing within national health policy debates and governmental politics (International Council of Nurses, 2004b). Recently, the ICN established a Web-based resource, Registry of Credentialing Research, to make research findings on credentialing available to researchers and nurses, thus assisting NNAs with their credentialing processes (International Council of Nurses, 2004c).

Global Shortage of Nurses

The urgency of addressing issues related to regulation, credentialing, and classification of nursing care in the 1990s provoked immediate ICN strategies. However, critical nursing shortages emerging around the world compromised these initiatives at the same time.

In its 1989 report to the 42nd World Health Assembly, the ICN urged the WHO member states to develop strategies to:

- Recruit, retain, and educate nurses and midwives
- Elevate nurses to senior leadership and management positions
- Support nursing research
- Adopt policies to include nurses in primary care activities

Factors that influenced decreasing numbers of nurses in many industrialized nations included declining lengths of hospital stays, increased nursing workloads through the use of technology and higher patient acuity, shift work, and attrition through marriage and childbirth. Low wages and layoffs resulting from health reform in the 1990s also played a role. Canada, for example, facing severe budget cuts in health care in the early 1990s and, consequently, layoffs in nursing, saw many of its qualified nurses cross the borders to better-paying nations. Simultaneously, however, nurses from developing countries were attracted to

Canada. To balance their demand for nurses, many developed nations recruited nurses from developing countries: Higher salaries and better working conditions, coupled with high-powered recruitment strategies, attracted nurses to the United States, Canada, Great Britain, Australia, Israel, and other industrialized nations. A case in point is the Philippines, which faced a severe "brain drain" of its qualified nurses in the 1980s. In 1989, about 65% of the country's 13,000 new nurse graduates emigrated abroad, mostly to the United States and Middle Eastern countries, leaving many of the health care facilities in the Philippines short of staff (Brush, 1999b). Beverly Malone, general secretary of the Royal College of Nurses in the United Kingdom, recently commented on the ethical dimensions of international recruitment, emphasizing the importance for governments, employers, and nurses alike of maintaining responsible recruitment and hiring strategies (Malone, 2003).

African nations suffered severe shortages of nurses because of the increased demand for nursing and preventive care in the face of a rapidly spreading AIDS epidemic. In 1991, in sub-Saharan Africa, 7 million individuals were reported to be infected with HIV/AIDS. Despite widespread need for nursing care, only an estimated 2.5 nurses per 10,000 individuals were available in this area. In Europe, reports on nursing short-ages varied. The Nordic countries had the highest nurse-to-population ratio in the world, at approximately 85 to 87 nurses per 10,000 individuals. Other members of the European community, however, such as Italy, Germany, Britain, and the Netherlands, reported increasing national shortages of nurses. The United States and Canada reported similar problems. Nurse migration compromises local and international efforts to improve short-term nurse recruitment and retention as well as long-term personnel planning. The ICN seeks to assist member associations in studying nursing personnel needs and resources, sharing information per-taining to nursing's worldwide employment status, and continuing discussions of the international impact of nurse shortages (Brush, 1999b).

Furthering Nursing Practice

A key problem with global nurse regulation is the dearth of data about *what* constitutes nurses' work and *how* it is shaped by health care service payments. In response, in 1989, the American Nurses Association (ANA) proposed a council resolution urging national nurses associations to develop nation-specific classi-fication systems for nursing care. The initiative may have been triggered by a difficult situation the ANA was confronted with when the American Medical Association proposed introducing a new health care worker in the United States. The ANA, which successfully lobbied against such a decision, argued that the nursing profession must name its distinct contribution to health care to be recognized in worldwide health care planning and financing. The ANA offered to collect, document, and share data on nursing practice across countries, clinical settings, and patient populations to assist national associations in planning types and amounts of nursing needed, in determining skill mixes for various care settings and patient groups, and in evaluating clinical efficacy and cost.

Responding to the ANA resolution in 1990, the ICN board of directors invited June Clark (UK) and Norma Lang (U.S.) to develop a feasibility study for an International Classification for Nursing Practice (ICNP). Margretta Madden Styles, who was chair of the Professional Services Committee and elected ICN president in 1993; nurse consultant Fadwa Affara; and Denmark's Randi Mortenson and Gunnar Nelson completed the team. From 1990 to 1997, they consulted with nurses and classification experts to collect, group, and rank nursing phenomena, interventions, and outcomes, with the ultimate goal of creating a uni-versal nursing language (Brush, 1999b). In 2000, the ICN made ICNP an official program and continued to update and revise the classification system (International Council of Nurses, 2004d). In that same year, the ICN published an updated version of its Code of Ethics for Nurses to provide nurses with a continuous resource to help maintain ethical practices worldwide (Fry, 2002).

Another pertinent issue that arose in the 1990s was advancing nursing practice to respond to expanding primary health care demands and changing conditions of specialty nursing care. The ICN established an International Nurse Practitioner/Advanced Practice Nursing Network with the view to provide international resources for nurses practising in these roles and to allude policymakers and health planners to the essential

This chapter provides an overview of the role of the Canadian Nurses Association (CNA) and the context in which it exercises its role and functions. Various examples highlight the complexity of the issues, including the tensions or contradictions inherent in bringing about social change and success. The structure and the governance process of the CNA are described, the current priorities and challenges are discussed, and the areas of representation and self-regulation are featured as well.

■ ROLE OF PROFESSIONAL ORGANIZATIONS

The role of professional organizations is derived from the need of professions to interface with society. This social reality can be described either generically or specifically for the profession of nursing.

Professional Organization: Characteristics of Professions

Many people have offered definitions of a professional association or organization. Several of the definitions are conditioned by the context in which the professional organization exists. For example, Dalton and colleagues (1994) focused on the role of a professional association in two parts: one related to educational standards and licensing fulfilled by the Boards of Nursing in the United States, and one related to influence and focus on protection of the public and improvement of practice fulfilled by the state associations, which are nursing unions. Dollinger (2000) focused on the role of the professional association in speaking to the public on behalf of nursing and exerting political influence as a moral duty of professionals. These roles are related to protecting the public and include developing standards of practice, granting licenses to practise, setting educational standards, acting as nursing advocates, and protecting the nurse, which involves negotiating collective agreements and advocacy in the workplace.

In his seminal work, Merton (1958) focused on the nature of the professional association. "The professional association is an organization of practitioners who judge one another as professionally competent and who have banded together to perform social functions which they cannot perform in their separate capacity as individuals" (p. 50). Each individual professional cannot speak on behalf of his or her profession unless mandated by the collective to represent the profession. Paradoxically, the behaviors of individual professionals reflect on their professions and contribute to the public image of a profession. A profession is recognized by several characteristics that have evolved over the years and most frequently include the following:

- Specialized body of knowledge
- Code of ethics
- Competent application of knowledge

- Standards of practice
- Self-regulation
- Tradition of public service
- Autonomy
- Accountability
- Professional association (Hawthorne & Yurkovich, 1994; Registered Nurses Association of British Columbia [RNABC], 1999; Styles, 1983).

Of the various characteristics, one is the existence of a professional association. Merton (1958) recognized that, despite diversity, associations essentially perform functions that are related to the individual practitioners, the profession as a whole, or society in general. These functions are not mutually exclusive. For example, a specific professional association or organization like a nursing union exists to ensure the protection of the individual nurse by negotiating contracts, promoting healthy workplaces, advocating for patient safety, providing educational support, and speaking out about the health care system. Similarly, a professional association or college exists to ensure the protection of the public by establishing standards of practice and education, determining competencies and licensure requirements, monitoring the quality of the workplace environment, and advocating for patient–nurse safety and social changes that impact the public.

As you can see, some of the functions overlap, but the main purpose of each organization is grounded in its social role. These could be conceptualized as protecting the nurse or the individual practitioner (union), protecting the public or society (association or a college), and speaking on behalf of the profession—a service that can be fulfilled either by an organization that exists to protect the nurse or the public or by an association that exists exclusively for this purpose.

Role of Canadian Nursing Organizations

The International Council of Nurses (ICN) is a federation that represents different types of national nursing associations internationally. In 1997, the ICN conducted a survey to identify the nature of its national nursing associations. A total of 62% of national nursing associations identified their major role as representing the profession. They did not have a specific role concerning protection of the public (i.e., regulatory role) or protection of the nurse (i.e., a union role or a socioeconomic mandate). A total of 31% of national nursing associations are unions that negotiate for nurses; only 7% have a regulatory mandate to protect the public (ICN, 2001b).

In Canada, the CNA is a federation of provincial/territorial associations that have the mandate to protect the public and speak on behalf of the profession. The federation includes:

The Association of Registered Nurses of Newfoundland and Labrador
The Association of Nurses of Prince Edward Island
The College of Registered Nurses of Nova Scotia
The Nurses Association of New Brunswick
The Registered Nurses Association of Ontario
The College of Registered Nurses of Manitoba
The Saskatchewan Registered Nurses Association
The Alberta Association of Registered Nurses
The Registered Nursing Association of British Columbia
The Northwest Territories Registered Nurses Association
The Yukon Registered Nurses Association.

The exception among the grouping is the Registered Nurses Association of Ontario (RNAO), which represents the profession in Ontario without a public protection mandate. The protection role is fulfilled by the College of Nurses of Ontario.

BOX 8.1 Membership in the Canadian Nurses Association

What is the Canadian Nurses Association?

The Canadian Nurses Association (CNA) is a federation of 11 provincial and territorial nurses associations representing more than 120,000 Canadian registered nurses. The mission of the organization is to advance the quality of nursing in the interest of the public. To do this, the CNA:

1. Acts in the public interest for Canadian nursing and nurses, to give national and international leadership in nursing and health issues;
2. Promotes high standards for nursing practice, education, research, and administration to achieve quality nursing care in the public interest; and
3. Promotes uniform and high-quality regulatory practices in the public interest, in collaboration with nursing regulatory bodies.

The CNA speaks for Canadian nurses and represents Canadian nursing to other organizations and to government nationally and internationally. It gives registered nurses a strong national association through which Canadian nurses support each other and speak with a powerful, unified voice. It provides registered nurses with a core staff of nursing and health policy consultants and experts in other areas such as communication and testing. The CNA's active role in legislative policy influences the health care decisions that affect nursing professionals every day. It has published a large number of documents, including the *Code of Ethics for Registered Nurses.*

Why should I join CNA?

Individual members of the CNA enjoy many benefits. These benefits include:

1. **National Affiliation**
   Membership connects registered nurses through provincial and territorial associations and national associate and affiliate member groups.
2. **International Affiliation**
   Membership ensures that you can participate in the International Council of Nurses (ICN). The ICN gives Canadian nurses a window on the world and offers nurses the opportunity to assist in achieving the goal of health for all.
3. **Certification Programs**
   The CNA offers national certification programs for nurses working in 14 designated specialties at a reduced rate to CNA members. The certification credential demonstrates knowledge and commitment to nursing and promotes high nursing standards.
4. **Subscription to the *Canadian Nurse***
   Each member of the CNA receives this journal nine times per year. The *Canadian Nurse* updates nurses on advances in practice and provides an opportunity to publish articles about nursing experiences and research. Members also receive *Access,* which keeps them apprised of CNA activities.
5. **Conferences**
   Members obtain discounts to the CNA's biennial conventions. Conventions are held each even-numbered year. They offer dynamic speakers, workshops, and exhibits that bring nurses from across Canada to share and learn together.
6. **Information Resources**
   The CNA is playing a key role in developing a connected network of resources for registered nurses. This network of resources will consist of databases of information and connections to other databases. This network will be your gateway to information necessary for nursing practice.

| BOX 8.1 | Membership in the Canadian Nurses Association (continued) |

7. **Discount on Publications**
   Membership offers you a 20% discount on more than 100 different publications. It offers you free copies of some CNA documents.
8. **Affinity Programs**
   Affinity programs offer registered nurse members discounts on credit cards, insurance, investment plans, and financing.

How do I join CNA?

Nurses automatically become individual members of the Canadian Nurses Association when they belong to one of CNA's provincial or territorial member associations.

Please note that Québec is not a member association of the CNA. Québec nurses who wish to be members of the CNA must hold membership in another province or territory. Both New Brunswick and the Yukon have nonresident categories of membership that are available to Québec nurses.

Source: http://www.cna-nurses.ca

In Canada, the provincial/territorial governments have delegated the right to self-regulation to the nursing profession. These rights have been delegated to many other health professions as well.

The Canadian Federation of Nurses Unions is a national nursing federation that represents provincial nurses unions that have the mandate to protect the nurse and speak on behalf of the profession in the realm of their competencies. Many other national nursing organizations exist that represent nursing's interest in a specific area of competence, in particular, specialty groups, areas of work groups, and the like.

Influence of Professional Organizations

Convergence of action, complementarity of roles, and collaboration among the diverse organizations within a profession increase the power and influence they have to fulfill their social obligations. *Power* is defined as the degree of influence the profession has (Shiflett & McFarland, 1978). Versteeg (1979) identifies five characteristics that affect the power of a group in society:

- Size
- Information of the members
- Expertise
- Available resources
- Personal attributes of the group's spokesperson

In regard to size (of the group that is represented and the percentage it represents of the total group), the CNA speaks for more than 120,000 registered nurses in Canada (CNA, 2005). This number includes almost all nurses in eight provinces and three territories. The exceptions are Ontario and Quebec. In Ontario, the RNAO, which is not a regulatory association, represents more than 20,000 (RNAO, 2005) of 85,187 registered nurses (Canadian Institute of Health Information [CIHI], 2005). In Quebec, the Order des Infirmières et Infirmiers du Québec (OIIQ) withdrew from the CNA in 1985 at the height of the separatism movement. Quebec has 62,494 registered nurses (CIHI, 2005). In 2003, the number of practicing registered nurses in Canada totaled about 241,342 (CIHI, 2005). The CNA has been recognized as the voice of professional nursing in Canada by governments both nationally and provincially as well as by other professional organizations (Box 8.1).

■ THE CANADIAN NURSES ASSOCIATION: NATIONAL VOICE OF NURSING SINCE 1908

In 1908, the first national nurses association was formed so that nurses could exercise their professional responsibilities on behalf of the Canadian public and provide them with a vehicle to join the ICN (CNA, 1968). This first association was known as the Canadian National Association of Trained Nurses (CNATN) before it changed its name to the Canadian Nurses Association in 1924.

Since then, the CNA has been the voice of nursing in Canada, influencing public policies, articulating the viewpoints of nurses on health and nursing issues, and playing a key role in the Canadian political process and in the development of nursing in Canada (CNA, 1958, 1968; MacPhail, 1996; Meilicke & Larsen, 1988). In the past 2 decades, the role of the CNA has expanded considerably in both representative power and self-regulation.

Power of Representation

Since Florence Nightingale's time, nursing leaders have been politically active on behalf of those they represented. Throughout history, many social changes were spearheaded by nursing leaders, although most nurses did not consider their role, either individually or collectively as professionals, to be political activism. One of the first Canadian articles on the topic of grass roots political action by nurses was published in 1974 (RNABC, 1974). The power of representation is exercised most of the time through *political action,* meaning "a systematic series of actions directed toward influencing others into conformity with a pursued goal" (Lemire Rodger, 1999, p. 281). Nationally, since the early 1980s, the CNA has promoted political action by nurses as a means of exercising the power of representation.

Changes in Health Care: Canada Health Act

Nationally, the turning point for representation was in 1985, with the proclamation of the Canada Health Act. Many nurses participated for the first time in political lobbying from coast to coast and influenced changes in national legislation. These changes represented their values and beliefs about the future of the health care system. These beliefs were presented in a brief entitled "Putting 'Health' Back Into Health Care" (CNA, 1980), which has guided pursuant changes by the CNA since its publication.

The advocated changes are based on the principles of primary health care. The principles include health promotion and prevention of disease and injury, accessibility, public participation, multidisciplinary and intersectoral collaboration, and appropriate technology (World Health Organization [WHO], 1978). The changes also incorporate the principles of the Canada Health Act, including universality, portability, accessibility, comprehensiveness, and public administration (Canada Health Act, 1984). These principles are central in the national debate about needed changes in health care.

The CNA's power of representation has had an impact on legislative changes to the Canada Health Act (1984) and has ensured that the national and provincial plans for the future of the health care system are guided by the principles of primary health care and the Canada Health Act (Mhatre & Deber, 1992). The nursing voice was part of the review of the Canadian health care system by the National Health Forum in 1997, when Madeleine Doyon Stout, Margaret Rose McDonald, and Dr. Judith Ritchie, past president of the CNA, participated on behalf of the nursing profession. The nursing voice was also evident in 2001 at the Romanow Commission, the purposes of which are similar to those of the National Health Forum. The commission seeks and entertains close communication with the CNA, including holding private meetings and receiving information before major events as well as invitations to official CNA events.

Research Agenda

Another example of the power of representation can be seen in the overall progress and development of nursing research both nationally and provincially. Nursing has been recognized only recently as a discipline in Canada. In fact, most of the debate about the legitimacy of doctoral programs in nursing related to recognizing nursing as a discipline. Only in the 1980s did the Medical Research Council of Canada and some universities, such as McGill University and the University of Alberta, consider academic approval of doctoral programs in nursing and support for the research infrastructure.

The CNA developed a national plan for the development of nursing research in Canada (CNA, 1984) and has lobbied government, universities, and foundations over the past 2 decades. The power of representation of the CNA was effective even if some of the gains were not sustained (MacPhail, 1996). They include nursing representation at the policy level of the Medical Research Council of Canada in the 1980s and 1990s, and leadership at the National Health Research and Development Program (NHRDP) of the Health Promotion Directorate of Health Welfare Canada (Dr. Mary Ellen Jeans, a nurse, completed her mandate as executive director in 1995).

For the first time, national career awards (three) were instituted for individual nursing researchers at the beginning of the 1990s, and five national nursing research chairs were allocated at the end of the decade (Canadian Health Services Research Foundation [CHSRF], 2001).

The first funded nursing doctoral program at the University of Alberta was approved in 1991 (Lemire Rodger, 1991), and today, nine doctoral programs in nursing are preparing scholars in the discipline. These programs are sponsored by the University of Alberta, the University of British Columbia, the University of Toronto, McGill University, Université de Montréal, the University of Calgary, McMaster University, Université de Sherbrooke, and the University of Victoria by special arrangement (W. McBride, executive director of the Canadian Association of University Schools of Nursing [CAUSN], personal communication, 2002). And, in 1999, for the first time in history, the federal budget included specific funds for nursing research (*CNA Corner,* 1999).

Nursing Workplace and Human Resources

The power of representation was exercised with great determination by the CNA in recent years because issues related to the environment in which nursing is practised have always been part of the CNA mandate under the category of socioeconomic welfare. Issues such as working conditions and contracts negotiated for nurses, human resources statistics, and standards in nursing administration were addressed. The socioeconomic environment of nurses was greatly transformed by the events of the 1990s when major cutbacks in health care funding had a devastating effect on the nursing workforce and the workplace. Thousands of nurses lost their positions when hospital and community services were curtailed by provincial governments across the country. In the workplace, there was a loss of nursing leadership positions, an increase in the number of patients cared for by one nurse, and a loss of support structures for education and research.

In 1997, the CNA commissioned the Ryten Report, which examined the future supply of registered nurses in Canada. The report predicted a serious shortage of nurses by 2011 if no strategic action was undertaken immediately. As a result, the CNA made several presentations to convince federal and provincial governments and associations of employers (CNA, 1998, 1999a, 2000b, 2001c) to act immediately. Further reports (CIHI, 2005) validated the projections, and further attempts were made to convince the governments that the situation was serious and that a lack of action would undermine the sustainability of the Canadian health care system. A concerted effort with the provincial jurisdictions and other nursing and health associations (including the CAUSN, the Canadian Federation of Nursing Unions [CFNU], the Canadian Health Care Association [CHCA], and the Canadian Medical Association [CMA]) was also needed to persuade governments and employers that action was required immediately. The issues of recruitment and retention were addressed in these representations, and the issues of retention and the quality of the professional practice environment became priorities for the CNA (see End 3 in Box 8.2).

The power of representation helped create a national/provincial/territorial agenda on nursing health resources with the reintroduction of nursing advisor positions in many governments, that is, in the federal government and in the following provincial/territorial governments: Nova Scotia, Ontario, Saskatchewan, and British Columbia (Office of Nursing Policy, Health Canada, personal communication, 2002).

BOX 8.2   Canadian Nurses Association Ends

End 1 is the vision, and the missions under End 1 become Ends 2, 3, 4, and 5. In the main document, the ends are not numbered, but they are numbered here for greater clarity.

End 1

The vision of the Canadian Nurses Association is:

Registered nurses collectively contributing to the health of Canadians and the advancement of nursing.

In pursuit of that vision, CNA's mission is that:

- Public policy incorporates the determinants of health and the principles of primary health care and expands the application of the principles of the Canada Health Act across the health care continuum.
- Public trust in nurses is maintained.
- The nursing profession achieves its full potential.
- The Canadian nursing profession contributes to the advancement of global health and equity.

End 2

The end "Public policy incorporates the determinants of health and the principles of primary health care and expands the application of the principles of the Canada Health Act across the health care continuum" is further interpreted to include, but is not limited to:

1. Policymakers are knowledgeable about the relevant issues.
2. Public is supportive of the nursing position on the issues.
3. Nurses are leaders in public policy development.
4. Nurses are an entry point to the health care system.
5. Nurses understand and operationalize primary health care in their day-to-day practices.
6. A national framework for a primary health care-focused system is operationalized.
7. A national nursing strategy exists to discourage the use of publicly funded, private, for-profit delivery of necessary health care.

End 3

The end "Public trust in nurses is maintained" is further interpreted to include, but is not limited to:

1. A coordinated framework for national nursing issues
    1.1 A coordinated regulatory framework.
        1.1.1. A valid and reliable Canadian registered nurse examination that ensures that entry-level registered nurses demonstrate the competencies required to practise safely and effectively in Canada.
        1.1.2. Relevant coordinated regulatory frameworks that support provincial/territorial nursing regulatory bodies in maintaining quality and consistent regulatory practices.
        1.1.3. An assessment instrument to assist and facilitate individual foreign nurses to make informed decisions about their readiness to become registered nurses in Canada.
    1.2 A coordinated national approach to nursing resource planning.
    1.3 An up-to-date, relevant code of ethics for registered nurses that gives guidance for decision making concerning ethical matters.
2. Nurses present an informed view of national nursing and health care issues.

BOX 8.2   Canadian Nurses Association Ends (continued)

3. Nursing self-regulation is maintained or attained.
   3.1 Entry- and advanced-level competencies required for nursing practice are established by nursing regulatory bodies.

End 4

The end "The nursing profession achieves its full potential" is further interpreted to include, but is not limited to:

1. Nursing practice* demonstrates integration of current knowledge.
2. The history of the nursing profession is preserved.
3. Competency and knowledge base for nurses are enhanced.
   3.1. Registered nurses work to their full scopes of practice.
4. Nursing is central to health care delivery.
   4.1. Registered nurses play a leadership role in the identification, development, implementation, and evaluation of best practices and innovations in health care.
   4.2. Practice environments support nurse leadership at all levels.
   4.3. The voice of nursing is influential in health policy and within health services.
   4.4. Adequate numbers of well-prepared nurse leaders are in management roles.
5. Practice environments are conducive to quality nursing care, attracting and retaining registered nurses, and enabling excellence in professional practice.
   5.1. A national nursing strategy exists to direct and support the development of practice environments that enable excellence in professional practice.
6. Canadian standards of excellence in professional practice.

End 5

The end "The Canadian nursing profession contributes to the advancement of global health and equity" is further interpreted to include, but is not limited to:

1. CNA has a leadership role in ICN.
2. CNA has a leadership role in fostering national and international networks for Canadian nurses and international health interest groups.
3. CNA's International Bureau maintains an overseas development program that strengthens nursing's capacity to support nursing excellence globally.

*To include all domains—clinical practice, education, research, administration, and so forth.
Source: Board of Directors, November 2001. Printed with permission from the Canadian Nurses Association.

Representation also helped create a national/provincial/territorial agenda on the development of a nursing strategy for Canada (Advisory Committee on Health Human Resources, 2000) and the creation of a Canadian Nursing Advisory Committee with equivalent committees in provinces and territories to implement the national strategy. Several provincial government plans of action were developed (Newfoundland, Prince Edward Island, Nova Scotia, New Brunswick, Ontario, Manitoba, and Saskatchewan [personal survey, June 2001]). In addition, the topic of nursing recruitment and retention was established as a regular item on the federal/provincial policy agenda for health ministers and even appeared on the First Minister's agenda in 2002. Provincial/territorial premiers meet periodically with or without the prime minister of Canada to discuss issues of importance to them, and nursing is now one of these issues. Thus, the power of representation was effective in creating a national agenda; issues in this area are now addressed.

Self-Regulation

One area that has experienced exponential growth in the past 2 decades is regulation. The CNA always played a supportive role in regulation; for example, the CNA developed a testing service in 1969 to prepare and administer the National Registration Examination. The CNA also played a leadership role in determining the educational requirement for entry into the profession.

Nursing Education

In 1982, CNA members took the position that the entry-level competencies to the profession would be at a baccalaureate level. Today, because of the power of representation of the CNA, provincial and territorial nursing associations—and other partners, such as the CAUSN; the provinces of Newfoundland and Labrador, Prince Edward Island, Nova Scotia, New Brunswick, and Saskatchewan; and the territory of Nunavut—have established baccalaureate education as a requirement for entry to the profession. Manitoba, which had established the same educational entry level, rolled back progress by opening one diploma school of nursing in 2000 as a perceived solution to nursing shortage. As for Alberta and British Columbia, most education is provided in collaborative programs in which graduates can exit after earning a diploma. Most students, however, stay until they earn a baccalaureate degree: In 2000, 131 students graduated with a diploma, whereas 707 students graduated with a baccalaureate degree (RNABC, undated). Lastly, Ontario has identified 2005 as the year a baccalaureate degree will be required for entry into practice.

Educational preparation of registered nurses still encounters opposition from some provincial governments and some nurses; therefore, political action is still needed. The changes in nursing education were also accompanied by major legislative changes. These changes are varied; significant changes relate to the scope of nurses' practice and to the mandate of the association.

Legislative Changes

Most nursing legislation in the provinces and territories has been substantially amended since 1980, as follows: Newfoundland and Labrador, 2001; Prince Edward Island, 1997; Nova Scotia, 2002; New Brunswick, 1984; Ontario, 1997; Manitoba, 2001; Saskatchewan, 1988; and British Columbia, 1988 (personal communication with executive directors of provincial or territorial associations, 2002).

All provincial and territorial nursing associations or colleges regulate the profession and approve the educational program. In Alberta, the approval of educational programs is granted to the University Coordinating Council (UCC). The UCC can delegate this approval to the regulatory bodies, and the Alberta Association of Registered Nurses (AARN) has requested that the delegation be to the Nursing Education Program Approval Board (T. Mark, Nursing Consultant Practice, personal communication, 2002). This is an indication of the importance of legislative reform in health and in the Health Professions Act. In the 1980s, the CNA started developing certification examinations, and, to date, there are 11 nursing specialty certification programs, and more than 10,000 registered nurses are certified (CNA, 2002). The changing legislative environment and the free trade movement within Canada, North America, and the world have increased the need to have a strong national and international voice.

In 1996, the CNA revised its constitution to include a new objective that focuses on supporting nursing regulation (CNA, 2001b) and added this area as one of the goals, or ends, to be pursued more actively by the association (see Box 8.2). In addition, a new Division of Regulation was created within the staff structure to focus on work in this area.

Internationally, a new forum has been created. The forum regroups national nursing associations that are involved in regulation. As a participant, the CNA influences the agenda. To date, an international framework for the development of credentialing (ICN, 2001c) and a registry for credentialing research have been developed to guide the evolution of credentialing in nursing (ICN, 2001d). In 2002, the CNA hosted the third forum that focused on credentialing in clinical practice. Credentialing indicates that an individual, program, institution, or product has met established standards; standards may be minimal and mandatory or above the minimum and voluntary (ICN, 2001c).

■ THE CANADIAN NURSES ASSOCIATION: THE CONTEMPORARY ORGANIZATION

In light of all the social, health, and nursing changes, the CNA reviewed and revised its structure and processes several times over the years.

Structure and Representation

The current structure was adopted by the membership in 1998. Some elements of the previous structure were maintained. For example, each registered nurse continues to be an individual member of the CNA through his or her respective jurisdiction, the jurisdictional members being the nursing body approved in membership (i.e., provincial/territorial associations or colleges and the associate members). Changes to the structure included a smaller board of directors and a different representation on the board. Representation was reduced in the domains of practice (i.e., clinical, management, education, research, and socioeconomic domains), whereas provincial/territorial and public representations were maintained. New areas of representation were created through an associate member's representative and corporate portfolios chosen by the board in line with its priorities. The board is composed of 20 members or directors: a president, a president-elect, 11 provincial/territorial representatives, 4 public representatives, 2 corporate members, and an associate members' representative chosen by associate and affiliate members of the CNA.

The first priorities chosen for the corporate directors were relations with Ontario and Quebec nurses in the hope of finding a way to increase membership in those provinces. This strategy was not successful, and since 2000, the corporate portfolios have focused on workplace quality and primary health care, reflecting current priorities.

The staff structure complements the policy structure and is organized on the same model as the major goals of the board of directors (see Box 8.2). The CNA is represented officially by two spokespersons: the president and the executive director or their delegates (Box 8.3). This representation role calls for attendance at nursing meetings across the country, media relations, governmental relations, and linkage with other strategic organizations. The CNA maintains structures and processes that include a lobbying network to ensure that the CNA is represented at the policy table in health and nursing at the national and

BOX 8.3	Canadian Nurses Association Presidents and Executive Directors, 1980–2006
CNA Presidents	**CNA Executive Directors**
Dr. Shirley Stinson, 1980–1982	Dr. Helen K. Mussallem, 1963–1981
Dr. Helen Glass, 1982–1984	Ginette Lemire Rodger, 1981–1989
Lorrine Bessel, 1984–1986	Judith Oulton, 1989–1995
Helen Evans, 1986–1988	Dr. Mary Ellen Jeans, 1995–2001
Dr. Judith Ritchie, 1988–1990	Lucille Auffrey, 2001–
Dr. Alice Baumgart, 1990–1992	
Fernande Harrison, 1992–1994	
Eleanor Ross, 1994–1996	
Rachel Bard, 1996–1998	
Lynda Kushnir Perkul, 1998–2000	
Dr. Ginette Lemire Rodger, 2000–2002	
Rob Calnan 2002–2004	
Dr. Deborah Tamlyn 2004–2006	

international levels. Regular meetings with the federal health minister and specific meetings with other ministers are part of the structure of representation.

Governance

Once a year, at the general meeting, delegates from each jurisdiction meet to fulfill their fiduciary responsibilities, such as electing a president-elect, choosing an auditor, changing bylaws, and giving guidance to the board of directors through voting on resolutions regarding the policy areas that they believe should be pursued. Although the board of directors is not bound by the resolutions on policy directives, a review of annual reports submitted to membership confirms that almost all resolutions have guided the CNA and have been implemented.

The board of directors is the governing body of the CNA and has provided national and international leadership for nursing in Canada in the areas of standards of practice, educational research, administration, and health issues in the public interest (CNA, 2001a). The board decides on policy options, priorities, and resources, and it also ensures that strategies are implemented satisfactorily by staff. The board appoints an executive director, who has the authority and responsibility to implement the board policies, provide services to members, develop an appropriate network to fulfill the mandate, manage a team of staff members, and ensure linkage with subsidiary (e.g., Assessment Strategies, Inc.) and parallel (e.g., the Canadian Nurses Foundation and the Canadian Nurses Protective Society organizations). The board reports back to the membership at the annual general meeting.

Partnership

Nurses have always worked in partnership, but in recent years, more and larger partnerships have developed to increase the influence of nurses and other health providers. Two large partnerships are the National Nursing Forum (NNF) and the Health Action Lobby (HEAL).

The NNF was initiated in 1996 by the CNA after a review of its strategic directions.

The purpose of the Forum is to provide an opportunity to bring together a broad range of nursing organizations, including the provincial/territorial nursing associations, regulatory bodies, unions, educators, students, and specialty nursing associations. The forum is a venue to discuss issues of concern to the nursing community and to develop strategies to address these issues (CNA, 1999b).

About 50 nursing organizations attend these meetings annually.

HEAL, a coalition of national health and consumer organizations dedicated to protecting and strengthening Canada's health care system, is another successful partnership. The CNA was a founding member in 1991 and cochaired the coalition with the CHCA. HEAL comprises 33 organizations and represents more that 500,000 providers and consumers of health care (HEAL, 1992).

Several multiorganization partnerships have also evolved around specific issues, such as the need to have a strategy focused on health care human resources. In this context, the CNA, the CMA, and the CHCA have met with the federal minister and federal/provincial ministers of health.

Patient safety is another important issue. The representatives of several health professional associations, regulatory bodies, protective societies, legal scholars, and the like are developing a national strategy to reduce errors and omissions in health care. Many other partnerships were developed or reinitiated, such as bilateral executive meetings to discuss issues and plan joint actions with the CFNU, the CMA, the CHCA, and several other organizations.

Internationally, joint meetings with the American Nurses Association are ongoing, as are strategic meetings with some other national nursing associations. Even the ICN changed its structure to encourage national networking and collaboration among the diverse groups of nurses in the country (ICN, 2001b). It is an era in which networking and partnerships are major assets in moving any agenda ahead.

■ CURRENT PRIORITIES AND CHALLENGES FOR CANADIAN NURSING

The national vision for nursing in Canada is that nurses, as a collective, contribute to the health of Canadians and the advancement of nursing. Over the years, the CNA has expressed its commitment to contribute to the health of the public and to the development of the profession, in that order. This vision has been reiterated in corporate objectives and in diverse briefs to governments, health committees, and various commissions. The document on the CNA ends (see Box 8.2) summarizes, in a policy format, the major issues or goals that are current priorities for Canadian nursing.

National Priorities

These goals do not represent all the current issues that a national association has to address, but they help focus the policy work and the resources of the CNA. The CNA board further focuses its work after scanning the environment. The scanning exercise is a survey of national, provincial, and territorial organizations to identify major trends and issues as well as emerging issues that can affect the CNA agenda and is essential for taking advantage of opportunities and for keeping an eye on emerging issues in nursing and health. The board of directors has selected two issues as urgent priorities: primary health care and quality practice and leadership.

Primary Health Care

When the federal government announced that it intended to spend $800 million on primary health care in the 2001 budget, it was an opportunity for the CNA to influence once again national and provincial/territorial policy decisions.

The definition of *primary health care* that was approved at the 1978 WHO conference (WHO, 1978, p. 21) follows:

Primary health care is essential health care based on practical, scientifically sound and socially acceptable methods and technology made universally accessible to individuals and families in the community through their full participation and at a cost that the community and country can afford to maintain at every stage of their development in the spirit of self-reliance and self-determination. It forms an integral part both of the country's health system, of which it is the central function and main focus, and of the overall social and economic development of the community. It is the first level of contact of individuals, the family, and community with the national health system bringing health care as close as possible to where the people live and work, and constitutes the first element of a continuing health care process.

For the past 2 decades, the CNA has been promoting primary health care as a favored strategy to guide reform of the Canadian health care system. In early 1990, when every province/territory assembled advisory committees and commissions to determine the orientation of the health care reform required, they all included the elements of primary health care (Mhatre & Deber, 1992). The CNA influence was evident because it was the only national health association advocating primary health care. Unfortunately, the reform fell short of the direction advocated by the committees and commissions. "Despite the evident political will, the barriers created by the dominant paradigm of the hospital/medical model in most Western industrialized countries, which is antithetical to the principles of a primary health care model, remain a significant challenge for the Canadian nursing profession" (Lemire Rodger & Gallagher, 2000, p. 6).

Today, the dilemma is that the cutbacks in health care funding do not help redirect the system. Community services are as affected as the hospital sector. Funding for primary health care is not integrated in the regular funding but favors a project approach that can be curtailed at will. As a result, the CNA is increasing its efforts to influence future directions. Recently, the CNA developed a primary health care framework that incorporates the principles of primary health care, the determinants of health, and the principles of the Canada Health Act to guide a national strategy. The CNA is also increasing its coordinated lobbying efforts to make a difference in the health of Canadians (CNA, 2001a).

Quality Practice Environment and Leadership

The other priority, quality practice environment and leadership, is also directly related to the effects of the cutbacks in health care funding and the so-called reform that started in some parts of the country, such as Alberta, in the early 1990s, and in other parts of the country, such as Ontario, during the latter part of the 1990s. The infrastructure that supported nursing in the workplace was, in great part, eliminated by the introduction of program management. In program management, generic managers, rather than health professionals, conduct the programs and services. Although the intent of program management was to increase the collaboration of the multidisciplinary team for the benefit of patients, it eliminated direct supports to each discipline, such as mentorship, educational support, research development, and follow-up on standards of practice, to name a few.

Similar changes were implemented in the United States, with nursing leaders becoming generic executives and less visible to their profession. Fagin (1996, p. 30) called the phenomenon a crisis of national discipline leadership in health care and stated, "Our institutions can boast of superb leaders in nursing responding to current political and managerial challenges. However, there seems to be an absence of the visionary, transforming nursing leaders who not only respond to their institutional challenges but also speak for their professions and for the public they serve."

Today, there is evidence that practice environments that do not support nurses have adverse effects on patient outcomes, nurse satisfaction, and organizational impact (Aiken et al., 2001; Baumann et al., 2001). In a time when recruitment and retention of nurses are critical, governments are having difficulty effecting changes in the workplace. The role of the federal government has been mostly through funding while the role of provincial/territorial governments has been mostly through funding and directives, without any accountability mechanism to ensure that required changes are implemented. In response, the CNA has built on previous work and developed a position statement based on the current evidence: "Quality Professional Practice Environments for Registered Nurses" (CNA, 2001a). This position statement will guide a coordinated effort by nurses and other groups to be more effective in bringing about the needed change. The support for further research and the multiple strategies mentioned in the previous section, Nursing Workplace and Human Resources, are part of the national strategy.

National Challenges

Two of the great challenges facing the nursing associations are the complexity of issues and the ability of the profession to be heard.

Complexity of Issues

The transition from the Industrial Age to the Information Age has brought with it an increased visibility of the complexity of issues. The complexity, the speed, and the force of change we are experiencing simultaneously are described by Toffler (1980) in his book *The Third Wave* as a social upheaval. These changes are mirrored not only in society and in a federal and provincial/territorial context but also in health care and nursing; the nursing agenda plays out against this backdrop.

Professional organizations face complexities of their own. An association that is proactive is sensitive to the members it represents and the issues they and the profession are likely to face in the future. The futuristic nature of an effective association is likely to create some tensions within the membership who live in the "here and now." So, some member discontent is a positive indicator of an organization fulfilling its role for the public, the profession, and the members. Too much discontent makes an organization dysfunctional and paralyzes action.

A proactive nursing organization also seeks opportunities in the sociopolitical environment to pursue its objectives and takes advantage of these opportunities to put forth a nursing agenda. The ability to mobilize quickly is very important. At the same time, the finite resources, the challenge of information in a vast country, the membership base represented, and the effectiveness of the spokespersons are part and parcel of this complexity and an association's ability to influence.

Political Voice

The ability to influence and bring about change is one of the powerful tools professional associations like the CNA use. In a complex environment where many agendas compete for attention, this is a very challenging endeavor, and nurses have been preparing themselves for these challenges. Among the most popular themes of conferences and meetings of provincial/territorial, national, and international specialty groups are political action, power and influence, strategies, managing change, and leadership. The topic of political action is also becoming increasingly more visible in the curriculum of many nursing education programs.

The CNA's influence is recognized in changes in the Canada Health Act, the federal budget for nursing research, and entry-level nursing education. As we begin a new century, nursing has never had more attention from governments than it has now. Nursing is explicitly on the political agenda of all provincial/territorial and federal governments. Paradoxically, major issues to be resolved, such as rebuilding professional practice environments, defining workloads for nurses, and increasing enrollment in nursing education programs, are not being addressed adequately. Instead, governments that need a strong nursing profession to ensure sustainability of the Canadian health care system are challenging nursing education, scope of practice, and workloads, among other issues. To have an effective political voice and to manage changes in a very complex environment are major challenges for the CNA.

International Priorities

The national priorities and challenges are reflected at the international level. Among the ICN priorities, the nursing workforce and credentialing are directly related to the CNA's goals.

Nursing Workforce

In the mid-1990s, many countries of the world, in particular the industrialized countries, experienced so-called health care reform or at least cutbacks in health care funding. The impact on the nursing workforce worldwide became evident and of grave concern for the organized profession. In 1996, the ICN developed a forum for discussion around nursing workforce issues facing industrialized countries, including Canada, Denmark, Germany, Iceland, Ireland, Japan, New Zealand, Norway, Sweden, the United Kingdom, and the United States. The CNA has been an active participant in this forum since its inception. Key issues and trends discussed include working conditions, aging workforce, salary, migration of nurses, industrial action, and work hours. The forum also collaborated on joint positions, such as unethical recruiting in developing countries (ICN, 2001a).

Credentialing

Another forum was created in 2000 when the ICN noticed that governments' focus was increasing on professional self-regulation and that free trade discussions would impact regulation of the profession. Internationally, standard setting was also on the increase (e.g., standards for distance learning, international standards for telenursing, and international competencies for generalist nurses).

The forum is composed of countries who are actively involved in credentialing activities or who have well-advanced plans to become involved. They are Canada, Denmark, Ireland, Jamaica, Japan, New Zealand, Spain, Taiwan, the United Kingdom, and the United States. The CNA was again a founding member and contributed to the development of an ICN credentialing framework and an ICN credentialing research registry.

A few of the key issues and trends discussed include terminology, gaining and maintaining competencies, cross-border assessments, and evidence of impact on patient outcomes (ICN, 2001a). These forums are means to leverage international partnerships for the benefit of the profession and the public.

International Challenge

One international challenge that has direct ramifications for the CNA is the need for the ICN to increase its membership and to be more inclusive. With the proliferation of nursing groups representing diverse facets of the profession in most countries, the need to find ways to unite the voice of nurses becomes a serious challenge.

The ICN and its national nursing associations must face the fact that this relationship alone is no longer sufficient to maintain a strong organization. Change is needed—change that will build on diversity and facilitate four outcomes:

- United voice
- Enhanced national and global recognition
- International connection
- Flexibility and choice (ICN, 2001a, p. 8)

The CNA supported the proposal for a new membership model in the ICN and explored for Canada a model of collaboration with other national nursing partners. This new model will increase the power of representation of Canadian nursing on the international scene.

■ THE ROAD AHEAD

The issues are complex, the power of representation is more challenging than ever, and the voice of nursing must be strong and united. Within that context, the representation power of the CNA is important. The road ahead for the CNA will need to include an increased representation base in Quebec and Ontario. It will also need to deal with the issue of leadership. Within the priority of quality practice environments, this issue needs to be addressed very strategically. After the dismantling of the professional infrastructure in health care in the late 1990s, it would be shortsighted to re-create and to count only on positional leadership. The profession needs to move toward a model of leadership and influence by all professionals so nursing values can be present in all disciplinary and multidisciplinary networks in health care. In an ideal model, the following would occur:

- Clinical nurses lead clinical decisions.
- Nurse managers lead decisions about structure, processes, resources, and the environment in which care is provided.
- Nurse educators lead educational decisions.
- Nurse researchers lead knowledge discovery, dissemination, and application decisions.
- Horizontal leadership creates new relationships among nurses for a stronger profession.

The road ahead will also include phenomenal growth in the areas of credentialing and regulation not only at the provincial/territorial level but also at the national level. The ICN framework will guide the need to pursue credentialing of individuals, programs, and products. In Canada, credentialing mechanisms have been developed for individuals in regard to registration for entry to practice and certification in a specialty. We have credentialing for some programs, such as accreditation of a school of nursing or nursing services, but we have not developed credentialing for our products. A lot needs to be done, and the CNA must find

| BOX 8.4 | A Look to the Future by CNA President Dr. Deborah Tamlyn (2004–2006) |

In 2008, we will celebrate our 100-year anniversary. We will celebrate the past and through our strategic planning prepare for a dynamic future. Nursing has not remained static and neither can we. The work of the CNA in an information- and evidence-based society will rely on sharing leadership, embracing change, and preparing ourselves through nursing scholarship. We will need to be visible, vocal, and articulate about what nursing can do for the Canadian health care system.

its role in this new environment. These are a few of the issues Canadian nursing and the CNA will face within the profession on the road ahead (Box 8.4).

■ SUMMARY

This chapter addresses the major roles, priorities, and challenges of the CNA. In Canada, the CNA's role is to protect the public and to speak on behalf of the profession and its professionals.

Some of the characteristics required to increase the influence of a professional association are a specialized body of knowledge and competent application of that knowledge, a code of ethics, standards of practice, autonomy and self-regulation, a tradition of public service, accountability, and professional association.

The CNA is the national voice of nursing. As such, it focuses on the power of representation and self-regulation. The work of the CNA in self-regulation is reflected in the educational field and in the evolution of credentialing in nursing.

Examples of the power of representation include the CNA's influence on the initial Canada Health Act and subsequent legislative changes, nursing research and education, and conditions of nurses' workplaces.

Current national priorities for the CNA are primary health care and quality practice environments and leadership. Current and national challenges for the CNA include the complexity of health care and professional issues and an effective political voice. Future challenges for Canadian nursing are a strong and united voice with increased representation in Quebec and Ontario; development of appropriate leadership models to promote nursing values in all disciplinary and multidisciplinary health care networks; and growth and influence in the areas of credentialing and regulation.

REFLECTIONS on the Chapter . . .

1. Describe a professional association you are familiar with and explain what role it fulfills in society.

2. In the past 20 years, what issues have been affected by the power of representation of the CNA? Select one and describe how the influence of the CNA changed the course of action.

3. Identify the types of members of the CNA and discuss the role each plays in the formulation of policy.

4. What are the two current priorities for the CNA? Discuss one priority and its progress at both the national and international levels.

5. Return to the CNA Web site (www.cna-nurses.ca). Having read the chapter, in what ways is this Web site useful to you as a student and a beginning practitioner? What other suggestions do you have? How would you communicate these suggestions to the national organization?

■ ACKNOWLEDGMENTS

The editors express appreciation to Dr. Deborah Tamlyn for her contributions that assisted in the updating of this chapter.

References

Advisory Committee on Health Human Resources. (2000). *The nursing strategy for Canada.* Ottawa: Author.

Aiken, L., Clarke, S. P., Sloane, D. M., et al. (2001). Nurses report on hospital care in five countries. *Health Affairs, 20*(3), 43–53.

Baumann, A., O'Brien-Pallas, L., Armstrong-Stassen, M., et al. (2001). *Commitment and care: The benefits of a healthy workplace for nurse, the patient and their system.* Ottawa: Canadian Health Services Research Foundation.

Canada Health Act of 1984—Bill C-3. (1984). Ottawa: House of Commons, Government of Canada.

Canadian Health Services Research Foundation. (2001). *CHSRF/CIHR Chair Awards.* [Online]. Available: http://www.chsrf.ca/programs/cadre/chairs/awarded_e.shtml

Canadian Institute of Health Information. (2005). *Registered nurses database.* Retrieved March 2005 from http://www.secure.cihi.ca

Canadian Nurses Association. (1958). *The first fifty years.* Ottawa: Author.

_____. (1968). *The leaf and the lamp.* Ottawa: Author.

_____. (1980). *Putting 'health' back into health care: Submission to the Health Services Review.* Ottawa: Author.

_____. (1984). *The research imperative for nursing in Canada: A 5 year plan towards the year 2000.* Ottawa: Author.

_____. (1998). *The quiet crisis in health care.* Ottawa: Author.

_____. (1999a). *Repair, realign, and resource health care.* Ottawa: Author.

_____. (1999b). *Report on the 3rd National Nursing Forum "Positioning nursing for the next millennium."* Ottawa: Author.

_____. (2000b). *Rebuilding Canada's health system starts with renewing the nursing workforce.* Ottawa: Author.

_____. (2001a). *Board of Directors Minutes, November 2–3, 2001.* Ottawa: Author.

_____. (2001b). *Letters patent bylaws rules and regulation.* Ottawa: Author.

_____. (2001c). *Revitalizing the nursing workforce and strengthening Medicare.* Ottawa: Author.

_____. (2002). Certification. Retrieved September 2002 from http://www.cna-nurses.ca/pages/certification/certification_frame.html

_____. (2005). CNA members retrieved March 2005 from http://www.CNA-Nurses.ca/CNA/about/members

CNA Corner. Nursing research fund created in 1999 federal budget. (1999). *Orthoscope, 5*(2), 6.

Dalton, J., Speakman, H., Duffey, M., et al. (1994). The evolution of a profession. Where do boards of nursing fit in? *Journal of Professional Nursing, 10*(5), 319–325.

Dollinger, M., (2000). Professional associations: Ethics, duty and power. *Journal of the New York State Nurses Association, 31*(2), 28–30.

Fagin, C. M. (1996). Executive leadership: Improving nursing practice, education, and research. *Journal of Nursing Administration, 26*(30), 30–37.

Hawthorne, D., & Yurkovich, N. (1994). Caring: The raison d'être of the professional nurse. *CJNOA, 7*(4), 35–55.

Health Action Lobby. (1992). *Medicare: A value worth keeping.* Ottawa: Author.

International Council of Nurses. (2001a). *Council of National Representatives Meeting, Copenhagen, Denmark, June 2001.* Geneva, Switzerland: Author.

_____. (2001b). *From vision to action: ICN in the 21st century* (revised February 2001). Geneva, Switzerland: Author.

_____. (2001c). *The ICN credentialing framework.* Unpublished manuscript. Geneva, Switzerland: Author.

_____. (2001d). *The ICN credentialing research registry—Draft 1.* Unpublished manuscript. Geneva, Switzerland: Author.

Lemire Rodger, G. (1991). Canadian nurses succeed again! The launch of Canada's first doctoral degree in nursing. *Journal of Advanced Nursing, 16*(12), 1395–1396.

_____. (1999). Intraorganizational politics. In J.M. Hibberd & D.L. Smith (Eds.), *Nursing management in Canada* (2nd ed., pp. 279–295). Toronto: Saunders.

MacPhail, J. (1996). The role of the Canadian Nurses Association in the development of nursing in Canada. In J. Ross Kerr & J. MacPhail (Eds.), *Canadian nursing issues and perspectives* (3rd ed., pp. 31–54). St. Louis: Mosby.

Meilicke, D., & Larsen, J. (1988). Leadership and the leaders of the Canadian Nurses Association. In A. J. Baumgart & J. Larsen (Eds.), *Canadian nursing faces the future* (pp. 421–459). St. Louis: Mosby.

Merton, R. K. (1958). The functions of the professional association. *American Journal of Nursing, 58*(1), 50–54.

Mhatre, S. L., & Deber, R. (1992). From equal access to health care to equitable access to health: Review of Canadian provincial commissions and reports. *International Journal of Health Services, 22*(4), 645–668.

Registered Nurses Association of British Columbia. (1974). Political action influenced health legislation in Quebec. *RNABC News, 6*(1), 11–12.

_____. (1999). *Nursing self-regulation: Nurses govern nursing in the public interest.* Vancouver: Author.

_____. (2005). Membership and services retrieved March 2005 from http://www.rnao.org/membership/index.asp

_____. (undated). *Education requirements for future nurses.* Vancouver: Author.

Ryten, E. (1997). *A statistical picture of the past, present, and future of registered nurses in Canada.* Ottawa: Canadian Nurses Association.

Shiflett, N., & McFarland, D. E. (1978). Power and the nursing administrator. *Journal of Nursing Administration, 7*(3), 19–23.

Styles, M. M. (1983). The anatomy of a profession. *Association of periOperative Registered Nurses, 38*(3), 484–498.

Toffler, A. (1980). *The third wave.* New York: William Morrow.

Versteeg, D. F. (1979). The political process or the power and glory. In D. E. McFarland & N. Shiflett (Eds.), *Nursing Dimensions, 7*(2), 20–27.

World Health Organization. (1978). *Primary health care: Report on the International Conference on Primary Health Care*, Alma Ata, USSR, 6–12 September 1978. Geneva, Switzerland: Author.

Critical Questions

As a way of engaging with the ideas in this chapter, consider the following:

1. Are you aware of which groups of workers in the health care system are regulated and which are not? Who do you imagine is responsible for the regulation of health care workers?

2. In reflecting on what you know about the structure of the Canadian health care system and the tensions between national and provincial political priorities, what would you anticipate as tensions arising in the regulation of registered nurses?

3. Given the mandate of the International Council of Nurses (ICN) and the Canadian Nurses Association (CNA), what role do you imagine they might play in the regulation of registered nurses?

CHAPTER

9

Laurel Brunke

Canadian Provincial and Territorial Professional Associations and Colleges

▶ Registered Nurses Association of British Columbia executive members speak with Canadian Nurses Association Nurse Practitioner Initiative representatives for education at the University of Victoria School of Nursing Summer Institute for Nurse Practitioners.

Chapter Objectives

After completing this chapter, you will be able to:

1. Describe the evolution of nursing regulation in Canada.
2. Recognize how differences in legislation have resulted in different approaches to nursing regulation.
3. Identify differences in the roles and responsibilities of provincial and territorial associations and colleges.
4. Understand issues associated with registration mobility and trends in regulation.
5. Discuss potential implications of current issues facing provincial and territorial colleges and associations.

This chapter will assist the reader in understanding and appreciating the value of nursing self-regulation. To achieve this, the evolution of nursing regulation in Canada is described, as are differences in regulatory approaches across jurisdictions, issues associated with these differences, and considerations for the future of the regulation of nursing by provincial/territorial nursing associations and colleges.

■ REGULATION

The purpose of regulating the nursing profession is straightforward: to protect the public, which makes regulation itself a most complex issue.

The What and Why of Regulation

What is regulation? Simply, regulation is the "forms and processes whereby order, consistency, and control are brought to an occupation and its practices" (International Council of Nurses [ICN], 1985, p. 7). The ICN states the following goals of regulation:

- Define the profession and its members.
- Determine the scope of practice.
- Set standards of education and competent and ethical practice.
- Establish systems of accountability and credentialing processes (Styles & Affara, 1997).

Finocchio and colleagues, with the Taskforce on Health Care Workforce Regulation (1995), take a broader view of regulation. They believe that regulation of the health care workforce best serves the public's interest if it promotes effective health outcomes and protects the public from harm; ensures accountability to the public; respects consumers' rights to choose their health care providers from a range of safe options; encourages a health care system that is flexible, rational, and cost-effective and that facilitates effective working relationships among health care providers; and provides for professional and geographic mobility of competent providers.

Evolution of Regulation

Regulation of professions really began with the formation of crafts and guilds. There was, and always has been, competition among tradespeople in relation to the goods they sold and the services they provided. The crafts and guilds were made up of the people who were known to provide quality products and services, in part because they developed standards for these products and services. Of course, with increased quality came increased costs and, in some circumstances, a monopoly on the products and services the guilds were providing. From these guilds and crafts arose licensing laws intended to protect the public and ensure that only members of the crafts or guilds could provide the specified services and products (Cutshall, 1998).

These traditional licensing laws provided for exclusive scope of practice, or what is sometimes referred to as *turf protection.* Today, there is a shift away from this approach to regulation, a topic discussed later in the chapter.

The nature of regulation has changed in other ways over the years. Historically, professional regulation focused essentially on gatekeeping, that is, setting the requirements for those who can enter the profession and disciplining those who fail to meet the standards of the profession. Finocchio and colleagues (1995, p. vii) have said, in relation to health care workforce regulation in the United States, "Though it has served us well in the past, health care regulation is out of step with today's health care needs and expectations." However, nursing regulatory bodies in Canada have for some time embraced a more contemporary approach to regulation. This approach recognizes that there is more to regulation than gatekeeping.

The Canadian Nurses Association (CNA, 2001a, p. 1) "believes that the public interest is best served when regulatory bodies adopt a framework that strengthens clinical practice and leadership; provides supports to correct and improve practice; and focuses not only on individual nurses, but also on promoting quality practice environments." The Registered Nurses Association of British Columbia (RNABC) and others have adopted a regulatory framework of promoting good practice, preventing poor practice, and intervening when practice is unacceptable. The benefits of promotion and prevention strategies—the quality improvement approach—mean that intervention with unacceptable practice can be kept at a minimum (RNABC, 2000).

■ REGULATION OF NURSING

Many nurses take it for granted that nursing is a profession and that, like other professions, nurses are entitled to collective professional autonomy, that is, the self-regulation of the profession as a whole. Professional autonomy means that, with appropriate public input, professional groups govern themselves. Canada has a tradition that communities of people within society take responsibility for meeting their obligations, both to themselves and the community at large. They do this by managing their affairs in a way that respects and furthers the good of society while recognizing the legitimate interests of their members. This is the essence of self-regulation (RNABC, 2000). However, self-regulation is a privilege of a profession, not a right. In Canada, self-regulation of nursing is less than a century old.

History of Nursing Regulation in Canada

The move to obtain registration for nurses began in 1893 with the formation of the American Society of Superintendents of Training Schools for Nursing of the United States and Canada. This was followed by the development of the Associated Alumnae of the United States and Canada in 1896. Securing legislation to "differentiate the trained from the untrained" (CNA, 1968, p. 35) was the purpose of the Associated Alumnae. When it was recognized that the fight for the nursing legislation had to be fought separately in each country, the Canadian and American groups separated. Consequently, the Canadian Society of Superintendents of Training Schools for Nurses was formed in 1907, with formation of the Provisional Society of the Canadian Nurses Association of Trained Nurses following in 1908 (CNA, 1968).

The development of provincial graduate nurses associations was due in large part to the increase in the number of nursing personnel that occurred at the end of the 19th century. Competition between trained professional nurses and nurses with little or no professional training was evident in the areas of wages and status. Moreover, no mechanisms for ensuring uniformity in nursing service standards were in place (CNA, 1968). Kerr (1996) identified two powerful social forces that affected the pursuit of legislation for the registration of nurses: first, consciousness raising regarding women's rights that was part of the effort to obtain the vote for women; and second, the increased valuing of nurses and nurses' services that occurred during World War I. Kerr speculated that these factors, as well as a general recognition that a mechanism was needed to ensure that nurses were qualified, led to the passage of legislation in all provinces over a 12-year period—a relatively brief time.

In 1910, the nurses of Nova Scotia became the first to have nursing legislation. Registration was voluntary, and nongraduate nurses could still practise. The Registered Nurses Act, which incorporated the Graduate Nurses Association of Nova Scotia, set out, among other things, the powers of the association and the duty of officers, admission of nurses as members, discipline of members, and appointment of examiners. Legislation proclaimed in Manitoba in 1913 was more in keeping with current legislation, as it set out minimum standards for admission, curriculum in schools of nursing, and the registration and discipline of practicing nurses. By 1914, all provinces except Prince Edward Island had a provincial nurses association.

Work to achieve legislation was not easy, as can be seen in the following example from British Columbia, where efforts to achieve legislation began in 1912. In 1914, the government decided that the nurses' bill could not be accepted as a government measure, and the association was advised to have the bill presented as a public measure introduced by a private member.

When the bill was reintroduced in 1916, it was suggested that the president and secretary of the College of Physicians and Surgeons should be members of the council of the nurses association and that the orders, regulations, fees, and bylaws should be subject to the approval of the College of Physicians and Surgeons. The nurses association decided to withdraw the bill rather than include these amendments. A letter was sent to the College of Physicians and Surgeons asking if these amendments met with their approval and if they wished to have graduate nurses under their control. This was unanimously opposed by the college. A revised bill was passed in 1918, and, interestingly enough, the first council was named by the College of Physicians and Surgeons (Kerr, 1944).

Ontario was the last province to achieve legislation for nursing because of objections from nurses who believed they could not meet the qualifications and because some hospital administrators feared that they could not meet education standards. However, by 1922, all nine provinces had some form of nurse registration.

The first act concerning nursing in Newfoundland came into effect in 1931, and the Newfoundland Graduate Nurses' Association was incorporated in 1935. Newfoundland formed as a province in 1949 and enacted legislation for nurses, with mandatory registration, in 1953. Legislation regulating nurses in the Northwest Territories and the Yukon was enacted in 1988 and 1994, respectively. Membership in the Northwest Territories Registered Nurses Association, formed in 1975, was initially voluntary. Before the legislation enacted in 1994 in the Yukon, registered nurses working there had to be registered in another Canadian jurisdiction.

Mandatory Registration

Initial legislation for nursing varied across provinces, and, in some instances, aspects of the legislation were inconsistent with the primary purpose of the regulation of the profession, (i.e., protection of the public). Initially, not all nurses had to be registered to practise nursing. In some jurisdictions, these nonregistered individuals were permitted to use the title "registered nurse" even if they did not meet the requirements for entry to the profession or uphold the profession's standards. In 1922, the Nova Scotia Act was amended to the effect that a register be kept "in which shall be entered the name of every member of the Association" and "only those persons whose names are entered in the register shall be deemed qualified to hold themselves out to the public as registered nurses" (S. Farouse, personal communication, 2002). Although not the same as mandatory registration, it was a first step toward this important mechanism for public protection.

Quebec was the first province to have mandatory licensing with the passing of the Quebec Nurses' Act in 1946 (CNA, 1968). The achievement of mandatory registration took considerably longer in other provinces, with British Columbia and Saskatchewan being the last to make this change to existing legislation. Mandatory registration was a requirement in the first acts for nursing enacted in the Yukon and Northwest Territories.

Authority of Nursing Regulatory Bodies

In Canada, authority to regulate the profession comes from legislation enacted by provincial and territorial governments. The nature of the legislation varies across Canada, although there is an increasing interest from governments in enacting uniform legislation for all professions in a province or territory. Regardless of the form of the legislation, nursing regulatory bodies in Canada generally have authority for the following:

- Standards of education and qualifications for registrants
- Standards of practice and professional ethics
- Use of title
- Scope of practice
- Professional discipline
- Approval of education programs for entry to the profession
- Continuing competence requirements for registrants

With the exception of Ontario, responsibility for regulation of registered nursing rests with the provincial/territorial professional association. In Ontario, this authority rests with the College of Nurses of Ontario (CNO), which also has responsibility for regulating registered practical nurses. In other provinces, this group of professionals, also known as licensed practical nurses or certified nursing assistants, is regulated by separate organizations. Ontario is the only jurisdiction in Canada to have both a regulatory organization and professional association, the Registered Nurses Association of Ontario (RNAO). The RNAO's mission is to pursue healthy public policy and to promote the full participation of registered nurses in shaping and delivering health services now and in the future.

Contrast this with the mission of the CNO to protect the public's right to quality nursing services by providing leadership to the nursing profession in self-regulation. Risk (1992, p. 368) identifies that the uniqueness in Ontario "is based on the philosophical premise that there is an inherent conflict (real or perceived) between professional self-interest and public interest, and that regulatory decisions must be separate from professional advancement." At the heart of this issue is the question of whether an association that has as one of its goals the promotion of the profession can do this in a way that does not interfere with meeting its public interest mandate. There is no evidence to suggest that this combined role has affected the ability of the other Canadian nursing regulatory bodies to meet their public protection mandate. Perhaps that is why the Ontario model is unique, not only in Canada but in many other countries as well.

Other differences between jurisdictional authorities relate to approval of nursing education programs, requirements for continuing competence for registration renewal, requirements for re-entry into practice, language requirements for registration, and approaches to regulation of nurse practitioners.

Approval of Nursing Education Programs

Of particular interest is the authority for approval of nursing education programs for entry to the profession. This authority typically includes establishing the criteria for approval of the nursing education program as well as actually approving the program. Essentially, this gives the profession the authority to establish the education, that is, the competency requirements for entry to the profession. In most instances, approval is limited to education programs for entry to the profession. However, the Association of Registered Nurses of Newfoundland and Labrador has authority to approve the education program for nurse practitioners. Until recently, the responsibility and authority for approving nursing education programs resided with the nursing regulatory body, except in Ontario, Alberta, and Quebec. The 1999 agreement in Alberta to establish the Nursing Education Program Approval Board (NEPAB) transfers the authority from the Universities' Coordinating Council to this board, which is composed of representatives from regional health authorities, educational institutions, the nursing profession, and the public (Way, 2001). Although the Alberta Association of Registered Nurses (AARN) provides funds for the NEPAB support staff, space, and expenses, the AARN has no direct influence on the NEPAB. Until recently in Ontario, authority for approval and monitoring of university programs was vested in the Council of University Programs in Nursing and the university senate or governing council. Recent changes to the regulations under the Ontario Nursing Act provide for baccalaureate programs in nursing to be approved by a body or bodies designated by the council or by the council itself. This is a very significant change because, before this, the CNO had no formal role in the approval of schools. The CNO has selected the Canadian Association of University Schools of Nursing (CAUSN) as the agency to conduct the approval process. In Quebec, the Ministry of Education has responsibility for monitoring diploma programs. In 2002, the Ordre des Infirmieres et Infirmiers du Quebec (OIIQ) was invited to participate in the consultation process for nursing curriculum for the first time.

Regulation of Nurse Practitioners

Another area of notable difference among jurisdictions is in the current or intended approaches to the regulation of nurse practitioners. Registered nurses have been working in extended or expanded roles, predominantly in rural or remote settings, for many years. Although these roles are considered by some to parallel those of the nurse practitioner, authority to carry out functions such as diagnosing, prescribing, and managing labor and delivery comes through delegated medical acts rather than legislation that authorizes registered nurses to carry out these functions autonomously. Pressures related to physician shortages, particularly in underserviced areas, and increasing pressures on health budgets have resulted in renewed interest in implementing the nurse practitioner role. The current status of nurse practitioners across Canada can be seen in Table 9.1, which demonstrates that use of nurse practitioners varies considerably across the country, as does the way in which the role is enacted. In some jurisdictions, collaborative relationships with physicians are mandated; in others, they are not. In some jurisdictions, such as Newfoundland, the title "nurse practitioner" is, or will be, protected; in many others, there are no plans to protect the title. In some provinces, these nurses are identified in different ways; in Ontario, for example, they are registered as RN/Extended Class.

This raises questions as to how the public can be easily informed about which registered nurses have authority for some of the functions commonly associated with the nurse practitioner role. Another significant difference is that, in some jurisdictions, the nurse practitioner has authority for a "package" of functions, such as in Ontario and Newfoundland, whereas in others, such as Manitoba, authority will be given for each individual function.

The evolution of the regulation of nurse practitioners provides a good example of how differences in regulatory approaches can have implications for the consumer of health care. Consider how much easier it would be for consumers and other health care providers to understand the role and the responsibilities of nurse practitioners if the regulatory framework was the same in all jurisdictions. It also provides an example of how differing approaches to regulation can affect the mobility of nurses across the country because the requirements for recognition as a nurse practitioner are beginning to vary across jurisdictions.

■ ISSUES IN REGULATION

As demonstrated in earlier sections of this chapter, there is a need for regulation to evolve to respond to the changing world and the needs of the health care system. Emerging issues in regulation are related to a variety of factors.

Impact of Globalization

Globalization of the economy presents significant challenges to countries to remain competitive in world markets. In this context, policies are being adopted that favor deregulation, decentralization, and, in some instances, a reduced role for government. Advances in technology are already affecting how health care is delivered, with increasing use of video and data communications. At the same time, trade agreements, such as the General Agreement on Trade in Services, the North American Free Trade Agreement (NAFTA), and

TABLE 9.1   Regulation of Nurse Practitioners in Canada

Jurisdiction	Status of Nurse Practitioner Legislation
Alberta	▪ Authority is given under the Public Health Act to provide extended health care services in primary health care settings (the community must be designated by the minister of health and wellness and include some urban settings, such as the inner city in Calgary). In 2002, a regulation was added to include nurse practitioners and to describe what nurse practitioners do. Nurse practitioners are authorized for the following: diagnose and treat; order, perform, and interpret lab and diagnostic tests; prescribe drugs under schedule 1 (all except narcotics); and not be employed unless on the roster. ▪ Nurses are registered on an extended practice register and are authorized to provide the following extended health services: diagnosis and treatment of common disorders affecting the health of adults and children; referral; and emergency services. ▪ Limits on practice, including prescriptive authority, are defined at the regional level.
British Columbia	▪ In 2000, the B.C. government announced its intention to educate, regulate, and deploy nurse practitioners by 2002. ▪ The Health Professions Amendment Act was passed in the fall of 2003 and provides for the regulation of nurse practitioners. ▪ The first students of the two British Columbia nurse practitioner programs will graduate in 2005. Preparation is at the graduate level.
Manitoba	▪ Registered nurses with the required competencies will have the authority to include one or more of the following in their practice: ordering/receiving reports of screening and diagnostic tests designated in regulation; prescribing drugs designated in regulation; and performing minor surgical and invasive procedures designated in regulation. ▪ These nurses will have their names entered on a separate register.
New Brunswick	▪ In 2002, two bills were passed relevant to nurse practitioners. One sets out the nurse practitioner definition and practice; the other provides authority for nurse practitioners to do their work under the authority of other acts (e.g., Pharmacy Act). ▪ A nurse practitioner may: diagnose or assess a disease, disorder, or condition and communicate the diagnosis or assessment to the patient; order and interpret screening and diagnostic tests; select, prescribe, and monitor the effectiveness of drugs; and order the application of forms of energy. Schedules list the x-ray and energy work and lab and other tests that nurse practitioners can order and list formulary drugs they cannot order. ▪ The nurse practitioner title is protected.
Newfoundland and Labrador	▪ The advanced practice nurse practitioner (primary health care) was implemented in 1998, and the advanced practice nurse practitioner (specialty practice) was implemented in 2001.

TABLE 9.1	Regulation of Nurse Practitioners in Canada (continued)
Jurisdiction	**Status of Nurse Practitioner Legislation**
	■ The primary health care nurse practitioner must establish and document a collaborative working relationship with a physician. Regulations outline circumstances in which consultation is required. ■ Regulations set out the diagnostic tests and drugs nurse practitioners can order. ■ The nurse practitioner title is protected.
Northwest Territories/Nunavut	■ The Nursing Profession Act of the Northwest Territories and amendments to the Nunavut Nursing Profession Act were proclaimed in January 2004. Language to include nurse practitioners was established through subsequent amendments to other acts (e.g., Pharmacy Act). ■ The nurse practitioner is entitled to apply advanced nursing knowledge, skills, and judgment to: make a diagnosis identifying a disease, disorder, or condition; communicate a diagnosis to a patient; order and interpret screening and diagnostic tests authorized in guidelines; select, recommend, supply, prescribe, and monitor the effectiveness of drugs authorized in the guideline; and perform other procedures authorized in the guidelines. ■ The nurse practitioner title is protected in both territories.
Nova Scotia	■ The Registered Nurses Act, effective January 2002, gives authority to the College of Registered Nurses of Nova Scotia to regulate nurse practitioners. ■ Nurse practitioners working in collaborative practice arrangements with a physician or group of physicians are authorized to: make diagnoses of diseases, disorders, or conditions and communicate those diagnoses to clients; order and interpret selected screening and diagnostic tests; select, recommend, prescribe, and monitor the effectiveness of certain drugs and treatments; and perform other procedures outlined in collaborative practice. ■ The nurse practitioner title is protected.
Ontario	■ The primary health care nurse practitioner was implemented in 1998. ■ No plans exist at this time to regulate specialty nurse practitioners. ■ Primary health care nurse practitioners can: communicate a diagnosis of a disease or disorder; order a diagnostic ultrasound and some forms of x-rays; and prescribe and administer drugs listed in regulations.
Prince Edward Island	■ There are no provisions for nurse practitioners at this time. Draft legislation is under review by government. ■ It is anticipated that the nurse practitioner title will be protected.
Quebec	■ Legislation was amended in January 2003 to regulate nurse practitioner practice.

(table continues on page 160)

TABLE 9.1   Regulation of Nurse Practitioners in Canada (continued)

Jurisdiction	Status of Nurse Practitioner Legislation
	■ Three specialties have been established: neonatology, cardiology, and nephrology. Primary health care is being considered. ■ Nurse practitioners are authorized to engage in: prescribing diagnostics examinations; using diagnostic techniques that are invasive or entail risks of injury; prescribing medications and other substances; prescribing medical treatments; and using techniques or applying medical techniques that are invasive or entail risks of injury. ■ There are two conditions for nurses to do the above. The nurse must hold a specialist's certificate from OIIQ, and the nurse must be authorized to perform one or more of the acts according to a College of Physicians regulation that defines the specific conditions for the nurse to perform the act. ■ The nurse practitioner title is not protected.
Saskatchewan	■ Amendments to the Registered Nurses Act in 2003 authorize nurse practitioners to: order, perform, receive, and interpret tests; prescribe and dispense drugs; perform minor surgical and invasive procedures; and diagnose and treat common medical disorders. ■ The registered nurse (RN) title is protected.
Yukon	■ In rural communities, 20% of nurses work in nurse practitioner–type roles. ■ Existing legislation governing all registered nurses is broad and provides authority for this practice. ■ Registered nurses will not make full use of their authority to prescribe until related competencies and criteria are established, but legislative changes are not required.

the Treaty on European Union, are facilitating the movement of goods, people, and services across national boundaries. These agreements have significant implications for regulated professions because they promote uniform standards and reduce bureaucratic and regulatory barriers to mobility.

Mobility in Canada

In Canada, the Agreement on Internal Trade (AIT) requires governments to recognize mutually the occupational qualifications of workers who are qualified in any other province or territory and to reconcile differences in occupational standards. Standards, criteria, and indicators to support the registration process are developed by jurisdictions to ensure that practitioners are able to provide safe, competent, ethical nursing care. Registered nurse regulatory bodies are committed to registration processes that are efficient, transparent, and fair and that are guided by the following principles:

1. Public interest.
   Nursing is regulated in the public interest. The purpose of regulation is to protect the public from incompetent or unethical practitioners, to promote efficient and high-quality provision of services, and to strike a balance between the rights and responsibilities of members and those of the public.

2. Flexibility.
   Processes must evolve to allow for growth, change, and innovation.
3. Fairness and equity.
   Demonstration of fairness and equity in all regulatory processes is essential to maintaining the public's trust that the profession should retain the privilege of self-regulation.
4. Administrative efficiency.
   The interests of the public, members, and applicants are best served when regulatory bodies operate in a cost-effective and efficient manner.
5. Mobility.
   Mobility of nurses means that nurses wishing to register in another Canadian jurisdiction encounter only those registration processes necessary to ensure that quality care for the public is not compromised (RNABC, 2001).

Work to achieve registration by endorsement in Canada began in the early 1980s with a series of resolutions passed at the CNA's annual meeting. Initially, discussions centered on developing standards for reciprocity of registration, which implied that a nurse registered in one Canadian jurisdiction could become registered in another jurisdiction simply by showing his or her registration card. Because of concerns that reciprocity, interpreted in this way, did not allow for jurisdictional differences in legislation and might not fully protect the public, it was agreed to work toward endorsement as the mechanism to support mobility.

Endorsement means that once a nurse has established registration in a Canadian province/territory, that nurse should be granted registration on the basis of having been registered in another Canadian province/territory, provided that the nurse's registration is in good standing and that the nurse has met the requirements regarding current practice in the province in which she or he is making application. Standards and criteria, with indicators for each criterion, are used as the basis for endorsement and the identification of differences in requirements between jurisdictions. Four concepts form the basis for the standards: initial competence, continuing competence and capacity to practise, satisfactory professional conduct and character, and confirmed identity (Box 9.1). These standards form the basis of the Mutual Recognition Agreement developed by Canadian registered nurse regulatory bodies in response to the requirements of the Agreement on Internal Trade (AIT). By the fall of 2003, most jurisdictions had signed the agreement. In some jurisdictions, changes in legislation are required before the regulatory body can meet the requirements under AIT. This agreement applies only to registered nurses at this time. Work is beginning to develop a similar agreement for nurse practitioners.

Competencies or Credentials as the Basis for Registration

Because of agreements such as AIT, there is increasing emphasis on competencies rather than credentials as the basis for registration. The challenge is twofold: first, how to achieve consensus across Canada regarding

---

BOX 9.1   Standards for Endorsement of Registration

Standard 1: The applicant has acquired the competencies (knowledge, skills, attitudes, abilities, and judgment) required for entry to practice as a registered nurse in a Canadian jurisdiction.
Standard 2: The applicant has met the continuing competence requirements imposed by the jurisdiction in which the nurse is registered/licensed or was most recently registered to practise.
Standard 3: The applicant demonstrates the capacity to practise as a registered nurse.
Standard 4: The applicant demonstrates the good character and ethical professional conduct necessary to practise as a registered nurse.
Standard 5: The applicant establishes and confirms identity for entry on the register.

the competencies required for registered nurses' practice; second, how to develop an efficient, affordable approach to competence assessment.

Consensus on the competencies required for entry-level practice in 1996 and projected for 2001 for registered nurses, registered psychiatric nurses, and licensed/registered practical nurses was reached in 1997 through the NNCP, the National Nursing Competency Project (CNA, 1997). In addition, the project identified contexts for entry-level practice in 1996 and 2001 for these three nursing groups as well as entry-level competencies that are shared and those that are unique. The competency statements developed were intended to provide information for decision making regarding registration of new graduates, equivalence of out-of-province graduates, requirements for entry examinations, and curricula for basic nursing education programs. It was cautioned that the competency statements would need to be considered in the context of a health care system characterized by constant and rapid change. The report further cautioned that the competency statements are not at a level of specificity that would be required for measurement or assessment, and further work would be required to refine the results (CNA, 1997).

Since the project's completion, several jurisdictional regulatory bodies have engaged in various processes to validate and further refine the competencies for their registrants. Of note is that assessment of the competencies further identified by jurisdictions demonstrates significant consistency between jurisdictions. The competencies for the Canadian Registered Nurse Examination (CRNE) draw on the NNCP competencies and the entry-level competencies used in the provinces and territories. The revised CRNE is one significant means of reducing barriers to mobility of the nursing workforce across Canada as required by AIT. In 2004, a joint project was initiated by several of the regulatory bodies to revise the entry-level competencies. The goal is, over time, to develop one set of competencies that are used at the jurisdictional level.

The 1998 decision by the OIIQ to discontinue using the Canadian Nurses Association's Nurse Registration/ Licensure Examination and develop its own examination has added another dimension to the issue of mobility. At the time the OIIQ examination was implemented in January 2000, no validation and comparison studies had been conducted to compare it and the CRNE. Because successful completion of the CRNE is a requirement for registration in all jurisdictions and for endorsement of registration, OIIQ proposed that for a transition period of at least 2 years, OIIQ would recognize nurses from other jurisdictions who passed the CRNE if those jurisdictions would recognize OIIQ members who passed the OIIQ Professional Examination (H. Rajotte, personal communication, December 23, 1999). Response to this request from jurisdictions has varied, with several not agreeing to this request for accommodation until the validation and comparison studies have been completed. As of the fall of 2004, the validation and comparison studies have not been completed and the situation remains unchanged. This provides another example of how differing approaches to regulation at the jurisdictional level can have a negative impact on the mobility of nurses.

Development of an efficient, affordable approach to competence assessment presents considerable challenge. The reality is that affordable assessment technology is not readily available. If competence assessment is to substitute for credentials as a mechanism for ensuring assessment for practice, the tools must be valid and reliable, and development of these takes both time and money. For example, estimates of the individual cost for assessment of competencies required for certification as a nurse practitioner range as high as $4,000, not including developmental costs for the process. The question is who should pay—the practitioner, the profession through the regulatory body, or the governments driving this change? This is a significant question because competence assessment processes must evolve as practice evolves and therefore do not represent a one-time cost.

Registration Across Borders

As technology increases, the geographic borders of practice begin to disappear. Registered nurses working in call centers, as well as those providing consultation or education services over the Internet, may be providing services to patients in other provinces, territories, or even countries. Canadian nursing regulatory bodies have agreed in principle that, when the nurse and the patient are in two different jurisdictions, the nurse is considered to be practising in the jurisdiction in which he or she is located. As such, the expectation is that registered nurses provide these services in a manner consistent with the code of ethics, standards for nursing practice, practice guidelines, and relevant legal authority of the province or territory in which they are registered and practising. Under this model, registered nurses must ensure that patients are aware of the nurse's name, professional designation, provincial or territorial regulatory body, and place of work to ensure that the patient has the information required to make a complaint regarding the nurse's practice, if needed (CNA, 2001b).

This approach differs from that being implemented in the United States, where the National Council of State Boards of Nursing agreed to establish a model for multistate recognition of the basic entry-level nursing license for registered nurses, licensed practical nurses, and advanced practice nurses. The model, based on the driver's license model, provides for one license only to be issued by the state of the nurse's residence and allows the nurse to practise in other states (remote states) under the authority of the state of residence but the practice requirements of the remote states. Individual states are required to enter into interstate compacts that supersede state laws and may be amended by all party states agreeing and then changing individual state laws. As of the fall of 2004, 17 states had enacted the RN/LPN Licensure Compact with two others pending. Utah is the only state to date to pass the Advanced Practice Compact legislation.

Advantages of the one-license concept include reducing barriers to interstate practice, improving tracking for professional conduct purposes, and facilitating interstate commerce (National Council of State Boards of Nursing, 1996–2001). Nurses will be held accountable to the nursing practice laws and other regulations in the state in which the patient is located at the time care is given.

Remaining to be seen are what differences, if any, emerge in implementing the Canadian versus the U.S. model. Of more relevance is that these models signal that regulation must continue to evolve in response to globalization and increased use of technology in health care. "End Provincial Lock on Professional Licenses" was the title of an editorial printed in a large Canadian newspaper in 2001 (*The Vancouver Sun,* 2001). Its author maintained that national licensing is the only way to ensure that skilled professionals do not have to jump through hoops when they wish to practise their profession in another province or territory. It further suggested that provincial licensing is a waste of time and money. The system of provincial licensing evolved because health, under the Canadian constitution, is a provincial/territorial responsibility, and we continue to see the federal, provincial, and territorial governments struggle with this issue. Is it likely that registered nursing in Canada will move to a national registration system? Perhaps. Is it also likely that the day will come when there will be agreement for nurses to move between countries with licensure or registration only from their home countries? Certainly, there is increasing pressure from the federal government to streamline the process of registration for out-of-country applicants. Significant funds are being directed by the federal government to this issue. If the day does come when nurses move between countries with licensure only from their home countries, care must be taken to ensure that regulatory responsibilities for activities such as monitoring the competence and conduct of members are not diluted.

Changing Approaches to Regulation

Governments across Canada have been exploring and, in some jurisdictions, implementing new approaches to the regulation of health professions. Driving these changes to legislative frameworks are concerns regarding accountability of professions to the public, turf protection, creation of economic monopolies by self-interested occupational groups, and lack of uniformity in legislation regulating health professions causing confusion for consumers.

Scope of Practice Legislation

Traditional licensing laws provide for exclusive scope of practice, or what is sometimes referred to as *turf protection.* As identified earlier in the chapter, governments are beginning to move away from this approach to regulation and toward a model that is the same for all regulated health professions in the jurisdiction. This model includes a broad, nonexclusive scope of practice statement describing what the profession does, the list of reserved acts (also called *controlled acts* or *restricted actions*) that practitioners are authorized to carry out, and protected titles.

Use of broad nonexclusive scope of practice statements is intended to break down unnecessary practice monopolies that limit a consumer's right to choose a health provider, inhibit access to health care through limiting consumer choice, and increase the cost of health care. Although some may consider that this approach serves the interests of powerful groups such as physicians, employers, and government because of the overlapping roles and the potential to use health professionals differently, others argue that this approach will result in new and exciting roles for registered nurses.

An example of a nonexclusive scope statement comes from the Ontario Nursing Act (2004) in which the practice of nursing is established as "the promotion of health and the assessment of, the provision of care for and the treatment of health conditions by supportive, preventive, therapeutic, palliative and rehabilitative means in order to attain or maintain optimal function" (p. 3).

The Ontario Nursing Act does not differentiate the scope of practice of registered nurses and registered licensed practical nurses. Scope of practice statements proposed for registered nurses, registered psychiatric nurses, and licensed practical nurses in British Columbia by the Health Professions Council are virtually identical (Box 9.2). In other jurisdictions, the scope of practice of these three nursing groups differs significantly, which poses the following question: Is there one scope of practice for the profession of nursing, or is the scope different for each of the three nursing groups?

Within the new regulatory framework being implemented, differentiation of practice occurs primarily through the reserved acts that practitioners are authorized to carry out. Reserved acts are tasks or services performed by a health professional that carry such a significant risk for harm to the health, safety, or well-being of the public that they should be reserved to a particular profession or shared among qualified professions (Health Professions Council, 2001). The intended outcome of reserving only those acts that present a significant risk for harm is to ensure that the focus of professional regulation remains public protection and

---

BOX 9.2   Proposed Scope of Practice Statements for Nurses in British Columbia

Licensed Practical Nursing

The practice of nursing by licensed practical nurses is the provision of health care for the promotion, maintenance, and restoration of health and for the prevention, treatment, and palliation of illness and injury, including assessment of health status and implementation of interventions.

Registered Nursing

The practice of nursing by registered nurses is the provision of health care for the promotion, maintenance, and restoration of health; the prevention, treatment, and palliation of illness and injury, primarily by assessment of health status, planning, and implementation of interventions; and coordination of health services.

Registered Psychiatric Nursing

The practice of nursing by registered psychiatric nurses is the provision of health care for the promotion, maintenance, restoration, and palliation, primarily of mental and emotional health and associated physical conditions, by assessment of mental and physical health, planning, and implementation of interventions and coordination of health services.

not the enhancement of professional status or control. The Manitoba Law Reform Commission (1994) identified three factors to evaluate in considering the seriousness of a threatened harm:

- Likelihood of its occurrence
- Significance of its consequences on individual victims
- Number of people it threatens

Examples of controlled acts that registered nurses in Ontario are authorized to carry out include performing a prescribed procedure below the dermis or a mucous membrane; administering a substance by injection or inhalation; and putting an instrument, hand, or finger beyond the external ear canal, beyond the point in the nasal passages where they normally narrow, and beyond the larynx.

Procedures below the dermis include cleansing, soaking, irrigating, probing, débriding, packing, dressing, and performing venipuncture to establish peripheral intravenous access and maintain patency of the vessel using a solution of normal saline (0.9%), in circumstances in which the individual requires medical attention and delaying venipuncture is likely to be harmful to the individual.

Regulations under the Ontario Nursing Act set out the conditions under which registered nurses may initiate and carry out these acts. Legislation in British Columbia and Alberta is similar in its specificity. Important questions for consideration are: What impact will this specificity have on the ability of registered nurses to practise to the full scope of their competence? Can regulations be revised with sufficient frequency to reflect changes in practice? Does legislation such as this reduce nursing to a list of tasks and procedures? Will this approach to regulation ensure public safety while enhancing consumer choice? These questions remain unanswered.

Umbrella Legislation

The changing regulatory approach brings with it a changing legislative framework. Historically, every profession has had its own act that developed over time in response to the needs of the profession and the public it served. The British Columbia Royal Commission on Health Care and Costs (1991) concluded that, in British Columbia, lack of consistency in professional acts contributes to insufficient accountability to the public and that lack of uniformity in the structure, organization, and language of statutes results in confusion for the public. The same conclusions can be drawn from a review of health professions legislation across Canada. For example, in some jurisdictions, some regulatory bodies are called colleges while others are called associations. In Alberta, it is proposed that when the AARN comes under the Health Professions Act that it be called the College and Association of Registered Nurses of Alberta. Processes related to managing complaints from the public vary among professions, as do the legislated responsibilities of regulatory bodies.

Umbrella legislation, seen by some as a mechanism to address these issues, has been implemented in Ontario and British Columbia. In Alberta, the Health Professions Act was passed in the legislature and will come into force as regulations for each profession are developed and approved. Different approaches to umbrella legislation range from one act for all professions to individual acts for each profession with parallel legislative language. The Ontario model relies on the Regulated Health Professions Act to set out the overall guidelines for the health professions, with each profession having its own satellite act. In British Columbia and Alberta, there is no provision for satellite acts. Instead, the requirements unique to each profession are set out in regulations under the act. It remains to be seen what differences in regulatory outcomes, if any, emerge from these differing models. On one hand, there may be more consistency in public policy as it relates to governance of health professions, and the public may be better able to understand how to get assistance with problems. On the other hand, the one-size-fits-all approach may be ineffective in addressing the differing issues of new and established professions and considering how differences in clinical practice should be reflected in regulation of the professions.

Public Participation in Regulation

It should come as no surprise that the public wants to play an increasingly active role in the regulation of health professions. Consumers believe that their complaints about the health care system are not heard, and the

After completing this chapter, you will be able to:

1. Discuss international regulation using the exemplars of Germany and the Netherlands.
2. Explore the effects of regulation or its absence on the advancement of nursing.
3. Describe the influence of government legislation on the regulation of nursing.
4. Account for the evolution of nursing "professionalism."
5. Understand how history, politics, and culture influence the education and regulation of nurses.

This chapter addresses the meaning of nursing regulation internationally and the issues that arise from the way that regulation is influenced by politics and culture. This begins with an understanding of what regulation means, how it is applied in Canada, and how it has been taken up or interpreted in other countries. Specifically, this chapter uses nursing in Germany and the Netherlands as exemplars to illustrate international nursing regulation. These two countries have been chosen to demonstrate the ways in which their political and cultural histories have influenced their regulation of nursing. There are similarities and differences in the histories of these European countries that have resulted in radical differences in the ways in which the nursing profession has evolved in them. To provide an understanding of the context within which nursing in both countries developed, the chapter is structured around common frameworks for analysis, including historical, cultural, and political influences.

■ INTERNATIONAL PERSPECTIVES ON REGULATION

According to the International Council of Nurses (ICN), regulation is the "forms and processes whereby order, consistency and control are brought to an organization and its practices" (Styles & Affara, 1997). The ICN has identified the following goals to address regulation of the nursing profession:

1. Define the profession and its members.
2. Determine the scope of practice.
3. Set standards of education and competent ethical practice.
4. Establish systems of accountability and credentialing processes (Styles & Affara, 1997).

Although the central purpose of regulation has always been the protection of the public, the Taskforce on Health Care Workforce Regulation (1995) has recommended extending this to include the following: the promotion of effective health outcomes, respect for consumer rights to choose among safe options for care, and a flexible, rational, cost-effective system. Regulatory processes can also address effective working conditions and provide professional and geographic mobility for competent members (Finocchio et al., 1995).

Regulation is closely linked to legislation. *Legislation*, as it is used in this chapter, refers to the laws and rules established through the authoritative power of government. In Canada, the authority to regulate the nursing profession comes from legislation enacted by provincial and territorial governments. Nursing regulatory bodies in Canada generally have the authority to determine the following:

- Use of the title
- Scope of practice
- Professional discipline
- Standards of education
- Standards of practice and continuing competence

The goals of the ICN for international regulation and an understanding of the way in which nursing is regulated in Canada form a basis for the discussion of international regulation.

ICN Influences on International Regulations

In a landmark study on the regulation of nursing, the ICN examined the regulatory practices and policies of the nursing discipline worldwide (Styles, 1985). Because the findings of the study indicated a wide variety of definitions of nursing (i.e., basic and specialized nursing education programs) and identified inconsistent regulatory guidelines, the ICN developed practical and concrete guidelines for the development of national nursing regulatory models.

Whereas in the past ICN referred to nurses in terms of *first-* and *second-level nurses*, it later recommended referring to nurses in terms of *nurse* and *nursing auxiliary*. By doing so, the ICN clarified the professional role of the nurse and acknowledged that a broader range of nursing personnel may deliver nursing services.

Specifically, the ICN recommended mandatory licensure for nurses in accordance with each country's regulation of its professions. It was recommended that the entry into professional education and the preparation for nursing practice be comparable to the education and preparation of other professionals. This recommendation indicated that future nurses should meet the same entry criteria into educational institutions as other professionals and stipulated that the academic and clinical preparation of nurses should be firmly grounded in the sciences and humanities to deal with the increasing complexity of nursing practice (Styles, 1985). In addition to providing a clear definition of nursing, the ICN study addressed nursing specialization and recommended a regulatory framework with standards and operational guidelines. This landmark study can be regarded as one of the first efforts to clarify the complex variations of nursing regulation around the world. Styles' study attempts to make clear, through systematization and definitive terminology, what nursing is about and what infrastructure is required to deliver safe practice.

Under the auspices of international trade agreements, European countries formed the European Community in 1957. This group of nations has since become known as the European Union. An international council was formed to identify commonalities in basic nursing curricula and to make recommendations about the instruction and education of nurses throughout the European Union. The advantage of this mandate was that nursing diplomas awarded by European Union member countries would be recognized throughout the European Union. The mandate clarifies the educational terms under which this recognition will be granted (Cutshall, 2000). As a consequence of these directives, the Advisory Committee on Training in Nursing (ACTN) was established in 1977.

In recent years, the ACTN, as well as the ICN and the World Health Organization for Europe (WHO/EURO), have issued reports of recommendations for nursing competency in the European region. In 1998, the ACTN released a report with recommended entry-level competencies, a step toward evidence-based nursing practices. Parallel to this work, the ICN and the WHO/EURO initiated the establishment of expert groups to discuss the functions and roles of the general nurse and the family health nurse (van Maanen, 2001). In the past, qualifications were described in terms of knowledge and experience to be gained during basic nursing education. Today, the scope of education appears to have shifted to clinical judgment and clinical decision-making competencies that enable the nurse to handle complex nursing situations.

It is remarkable that, despite collaboration among the ICN, the WHO, and the WHO/EURO in generating recommendations of the scope of nursing practice, the recommendations of these reports appear to have limited impact. For example, a WHO report in 1986 of regulatory mechanisms for nursing in 25 countries showed that legislation was, in fact, restricting women's access to nursing, midwifery services, and education (WHO, 1986).

A WHO study group that met to examine laws and regulations governing nursing education and practice in Geneva (1983) stated: "Nursing practice and education are governed by legislation that is often archaic, determined by persons from other disciplines, detrimental to the status of the nurse, and not in tune with the needs of society. The primary health strategy involved the re-evaluation of the old policies and this must certainly include nursing legislation" (WHO, 1983 p. 31). These recommendations emphasize that the scope of nursing practice has expanded dramatically in a few countries but is restricted in other countries by legal and social barriers (WHO, 1986). The WHO study group advised initiating a reorientation of basic nursing education and an evaluation of educational programs with respect to the countries' health needs instead of the desires and demands of health care professionals (WHO, 1986).

■ NURSING REGULATION IN GERMANY

German nurses frequently ask why the course of events in nursing developed so differently in their nation than in other industrialized European countries. The cultures of European countries vary from highly industrialized and affluent to predominately rural and less prosperous. Regions may share the same values, but conditions of employment, health, and living differ considerably (Salvage & Heijnen, 1997; WHO/EURO, 1999).

Over and above these cultural and geographic differences, nurses' questions regarding the pace of the advancement of nursing need to be understood as arising in a particular society. It is within this same society that German medical (technical) care has been recognized as one of the leading systems in the world. Barriers to the advancement of nursing in Germany can be understood as issues arising from the societal values with regard to a woman's role and women's work, the history and heritage of the nation with the prominent role of the churches, the (denominational) development of nursing education programs, and the influence of political ideologies on nursing. The term *ideologies* as it is used here refers to a powerful and authoritative voice in society that tells us who we are and how we are to behave (Althusser, 1971).

Culture as a Framework for Analysis

German society is deeply rooted in family values. The family is regarded as the cornerstone of the society. Within the family unit, the mother plays a central role as the facilitator and organizer of family life in the upbringing of the children and the support of the spouse. Outside the family, the mother has social responsibilities within the (church) community. A German statement relates to the role of the woman as determined by "Kinder, Kuche, Kirche," which, translated, means "children, kitchen, church." A mother, *plegt*, is a term synonymous to nursing (Kruse, 1987). Because nursing, by tradition, has been a predominantly female profession, the perception of the nurse tends to be one of a woman who cares for other people in health and sickness. Caring in the sense of *plegt* is traditionally strongly intertwined with the image of *caritas* (a Latin word for charity), in which laypeople as well as professional workers are involved.

History as a Framework for Analysis

German nursing developed along the same trajectory as nursing in other European countries during the early 20th century. The strong commitment to delivering quality patient care and to the proper education of the nurse is reflected in early documentation. This development was interrupted by World War I (1914–1918) and World War II (1940–1945) and by the years preceding World War II, times that affected the nursing discipline in every facet of its practice (Brush et al., 1999). Although the world wars affected the advancement of nursing worldwide, the effects of war on nurses and nursing in Germany are of particular importance. The advancement of nursing was disrupted by both the involvement of Germany in war and by the influence of the political ideologies of the times. One should not underestimate the effects of prewar, wartime, and postwar conditions on the advancement of nursing in Germany.

Only since the late 1980s has there been a systematic recording of advancements in the nursing profession. These advancements have been credited to the financial impetus of grants for advanced nursing education and innovative practice (Stiftung, 1992/1993, 1993b, 1996, 2000). Questions that guide the following discussion of the historical analysis include the following: How have the role of the church, the existence of Red Cross sororities, and the effects of political ideologies influenced nursing history in Germany?

Role of the Churches

The Evangelical and Roman Catholic churches, both state churches, affect the social lives of the German people in many respects. Their influence reaches far beyond religion and church-related activities and embodies many aspects of social life. The churches have strongly influenced the development of nursing in the initiation, implementation, and supervision of nursing education and practice. Nursing was carried out in church-owned facilities, such as hospitals, nursing homes, homes for the aged, and community nursing services. Religious orders were instrumental in framing nursing education within the context of church and society, and Christian values are reflected in basic nursing curricula of hospital schools of nursing. Advanced nursing education is to a large extent organized by church-related institutions. According to both Roman Catholic and Protestant perspectives, nursing is a charitable occupation deeply rooted in the religious tradition of the New Testament, from which the role of the woman is interpreted as enabling, facilitating, and caring (Kruse, 1987). The core of nursing was described as *mein Lohn ist, daf ich darf,* which means "my reward is that I may serve others." This perspective is still reflected in the functions and roles of Protestant deaconesses and Roman Catholic sisters of orders today (Kruse, 1987).

Role of the Red Cross

In the middle of the 19th century, the Red Cross sororities grew out of the women's organizations. Their origins date from the times of war when women took care of wounded soldiers, which required nurses to have formal training. Included in the Geneva Convention in 1864 was support for the idea that capable women, often belonging to the nobility of the country, could be educated as professional nurses (Kruse, 1987). As early as 1902, the Red Cross established an official curriculum for the nurses of their sororities. Within the Red Cross sororities to date, nurses make a voluntary commitment to provide professional nursing services based on the latest developments within the discipline. Although the Red Cross nurse is free to establish a family, she or he, like her or his Salvation Army counterparts, must be prepared to serve the Red Cross sorority in those places where help is required. Today, all the German orders and sororities are integrated into one organization, *Arbeitsgemeinschaft der Deutschen Schwesterngemeinschaften* (ADS), which is the speaking voice of the nominational (or denominational) nursing communities in Germany.

Influences of Political Ideologies on Nursing

German nursing had a rich tradition of community and public health nursing until the early 1930s (Kruse, 1987). However, in the early 1930s, professional nursing began to stagnate in terms of the scholarly advancement of the discipline (Steppe, 1990). This stagnation can be linked, in part, to the emerging political ideologies of the time.

In examining historical documents, one can see how nursing education and practice were gradually incorporated into the ideology of national socialism. Nurses who intended to follow a career path were forced to comply with the national socialist principles of German heritage and racial segregation. Nursing was provided with the "power" to assess the destiny of people with impaired health and handicaps, in particular people who had been identified as having mental and physical disabilities. It is important to note that this so-called power did not emerge from professional advancement of nursing but rather was mandated by law supported by political ideologies. Nursing aims were subordinated to the national socialist system. For example, public health and community nurses in the national socialist system became the uniformed representatives of the political authorities. They were expected to select patients for admission to "special" treatment centers, from which most never returned (Historical museum, Krankenhaus Bremen-Ost; Study trip, Poland, 1997). It is not surprising that the war imposed a severe setback of public health and community nursing and that even today German people are resentful of government interference with their privacy. This resentment raises questions about how this image of nurses interfaces with a cultural ideal of nurses as nurturing and protective (Box 10.1).

BOX 10.1	Nursing Under National Socialism

Nursing under national socialism (NS) in Germany was an occupation that could be characterized as:

- *Diffuse and unclear in its aims*. Nurses worked in dependence of medicine; they indicated that their aims were different but had problems in describing the distinction between nursing and medicine.
- *A woman's occupation*. Nurses were expected to act in an extended role of mothers, caring for and serving others.
- *Determined by law*. Nurses were placed in an assisting role to physicians (*Hilfsberuf*).
- *Unorganized*. The fragmented nursing associations were organized according to religious and social orientation and operated without common goals.
- *Victimized by professional hostility*. The rights and responsibilities of nurses that were granted under the Weimar Republic were not rooted in professional development but were embedded in a political structure that would gradually dictate to nurses what was considered law and order under the system. Nurses were not recognized as professionals but were employed as instruments of war (Steppe, 1990).

Reconstruction of Nursing Education, 1950–2000

Through collaboration with the ICN, German links to the international nursing community that had been disrupted by the war years were re-established in 1949 (Brush et al., 1999; Quinn, 1989). The changing political ideologies and the effects of World War II were to influence significantly the reorganization of nursing in Germany into the present century.

United efforts during the 1950s to reconstruct nursing saw competition among hospitals to provide educational programs. A nursing law passed in 1957 that allowed nursing education programs to be operated under the jurisdiction of labor law prompted criticism from church-related health care institutions. They expressed concern that the control of nursing education and practice would erode as soon as nurses were educated under the jurisdiction of the labor law. Within this restructuring, a controversy was provoked by asking whether educated nurses were really wanted: "German nursing should not be endangered by academically prepared nurses" (Spiegel, 1957, in Steppe, 1990, p. 13). According to Steppe (1990), nursing remained dominated by a moral perspective that focused on women's virtues.

In the 1960s, with the rapid advancement of medical technology, technical specialization in nursing became a trajectory of career planning. Although nurses still emphasized the importance of the person-to-person relationships, medical technology started to prevail over comprehensive nursing care. To solve the acute shortage of nurses, practical nurses were introduced into the health care system. Nursing education, now 3 years in duration, was described in terms of basic nursing (*Grundpflege*) and therapeutic nursing (*Behundlungspflege*). The emphasis was on procedures rather than on processes of nursing intervention.

During these years, the nursing process—the logical analysis of nursing care activities—was introduced, and the recording of patient care was systematized in a patient care record. Through postbasic education, nurses gained the competence to develop innovative strategies and empower themselves as professionals.

In the late 1970s, German nurses became involved in a health-focused perspective on nursing. Health promotion, prevention, and rehabilitation became key concepts to those who supported change and advancement. During this period, Germany hosted several WHO/EURO meetings to facilitate the development and analysis of multicultural action research. An interest in the study and application of foreign nursing theories developed. In the late 1980s, projects were initiated to test and implement these foreign models into some clinical settings.

Professionalization of Nursing

The historical development as described by Steppe (1990, 1996) reflects the highlights of the German nursing scene. In a country with 80 million people and 475,000 nurses, change and development take place gradually. New initiatives may take years before they are regarded as common knowledge, based on professional consensus, and supported by the members of the nursing discipline. An example is the introduction of the nursing process, *Pflegeplanung und Dokumentation,* into nursing practice, which, according to Steppe (1990), started to be systematically introduced as early as the 1970s. However, because nurses in Germany continued to be trained in hospital schools of nursing and were expected to function in rigid health care structures, the real transition toward professional nursing as a collective effort was not substantial until the early 1990s.

According to nurse-educators, the first signs and signals of nursing-focused guidelines for nursing education were reflected when a new 1985 nursing law was passed (Kurtenbach, Golombek, & Siebers, 1994). In this law, the statement that the nursing process is a compulsory component in the education of nurses provided some distancing from medicine (Box 10.2). However, the theoretical education strongly remains a reflection of medical thinking, with emphasis on the preparation for the extended role of nurses within the medical domain. Nursing theory and research are not included in the 1985 nursing law.

Nursing, as a typical women's profession, was not part of the regular educational structure of the German *Bildungssystem* until 1995, and nursing in its professional practice remained vulnerable and outside the mainstream of legislative accreditation and legal protection. However, two decrees (of 1995 and 1997) represent important steps toward change. Through the 1995 decree, nursing education was integrated into the formal German *Bildungssystem,* with all the rights, responsibilities, and perspectives granted to a registered profession. The 1997 decree recommended that, in the future, the education of nurse-educators should be embedded into higher education (Bals et al., 1997; Bundesausschuss, 2000; Sekretariat der Ständigen Konferenz et al., 1995, 1997). These two decrees are significant for the development of nursing education. To prepare German nursing for the 21st century, the next move should be to transfer basic nursing education from hospital schools of nursing into colleges (*Berufsschulen*), the polytechnics' equivalent institutions of higher education.

Legislation and Regulation

Positioned as a typical woman's occupation in Germany, nursing was not registered as a *Beruf* (profession) within the educational structure of the Federal Republic until 1995. This societal position, of course, delayed the educational advances of the discipline (Krüger, 1996; Krüger, Rabe-Kleberg, & Mischo-Kelling, 1993),

---

BOX 10.2　　　The Professional Nurse and the Nursing Process

The responsibilities and expertise of the professional nurse were described in terms of the nursing process approach when a new nursing law was passed. By law, the nurse:

- Can systematically assess and analyze the nursing needs of the patient, group of patients, or patient population
- Can formulate an individual nursing plan or plan nursing interventions, as far as possible, with the agreement of and in collaboration with the patient or group of patients
- Can perform these nursing interventions in a skilled way or delegate the practice and coordination of these interventions
- Is able, when appropriate, to consult with or refer to a colleague
- Reassesses and evaluates the nursing plan and implementation in relationship to assessed needs

From *Nationale Raad voor de Volksgezondheid.* (1988). p. 27; 1992, p. 27, used with permission.

which meant that nursing could be taught and learned by any person with a caring attitude and that the quality of nursing education depended on the vision and competence of the nurses responsible for the nursing curricula and practice.

Whereas the (male) *Berufsbildung* (vocational education) in Germany is embedded in a well-organized, comprehensive educational system and provided by highly qualified teachers and practitioners (*Meister Fachleute*), the traditional women's occupations did not follow this track. Although the nursing discipline undertook several efforts to improve the position of nursing education, changes in the regulation of nursing were required before the discipline could advance as a profession.

The National Nursing Act of 1985 is a federal act that describes nursing as an auxiliary occupation to medicine and regulates nursing education under the jurisdiction of the medical profession (Kruse, 1987; Kurtenbach, Golombek, & Siebers, 1994). This legislative framework has delayed the development of nursing as a discipline. Nursing education and practice have been advanced along the core of medicine, with emphasis on medical technology and the treatment of diseases. This perspective is reflected in the nursing curricula by giving priority to the natural sciences. Nursing students at the University of Bremen (personal communication, 2001) argue that during their nursing training, they have been inadequately prepared in the social sciences and humanities and that such preparation would have enabled them to better deal with the complexity of holistic, comprehensive nursing.

Compared with nursing in other northern and western European countries, German nursing has taken a different trajectory of development. Several initiatives to strengthen the professional role of nurses have been taken over the years. For political reasons, however, these initiatives have had little impact on the anticipated change and development in nursing. As early as 1963, a landmark project in German nursing was the first university-based nurse-teachers program at the Free University of Berlin (Mischo-Kelling & Witneben, 1995). Because of political interventions, this project did not survive; however, the seeds were planted for other initiatives.

In a collaborative effort beginning in the late 1980s, nurse leaders in Germany started to develop educational and research programs aimed at more efficiency and effectiveness in the advancement of nursing. These initiatives were financially supported through grants and bursaries. Experienced, hospital-trained nurses were able to study nursing in other western European countries and gain degrees in nursing sciences. Other nurses took on academic studies in Germany in health-related fields and qualified in the social sciences and humanities. It is through this first generation of academically prepared nurses that the upgrading of nursing management and education into polytechnics and universities has become a reality. To date, 33 programs of nursing, nursing management, and nursing education have been established in German polytechnic institutes, whereas 6 degree programs in nursing science and nursing pedagogies have developed within the universities.

Nurses anticipate that the professional nursing movement will accelerate in the coming years and that, with constructive collaboration among nurse leaders, postbasic nursing programs will increase in quality and depth. With the establishment of programs into the tertiary system, nursing education is, like other practice disciplines, framed within the educational system of the country. Whereas nursing research will primarily be promoted through university departments of nursing science and education, applied nursing studies have become the mandate of polytechnics.

■ NURSING REGULATION IN THE NETHERLANDS

The Netherlands is a small coastal country situated next to Germany, with a high-density population of nearly 16 million people. Nursing in the Netherlands has a long tradition, developing in a way similar to nursing in neighboring western European countries.

In the Netherlands, the Nursing Law of 1921 regulated the education, examination, and registration of nurses. The law protected the diploma and title of the nurse but did not provide substantial direction for the nursing education or nursing practice performed under this jurisdiction (Sindram 1993, 2001; Van der Kooij, 1990). With the advancement of the biomedical sciences, nursing followed in the footpath of medicine and developed an interest in the technical methods underlying the assessment of diagnosis and treatment of patients. The introduction of the human and social sciences in the health care services of the late 1960s and the 1970s forced nursing to re-evaluate its purpose and aims.

The 1970s may be regarded as a phase of professional reflection, an "awakening time" of nursing, characterized by a growing interest in the nature of nursing and its scientific potential. In 1972, the first undergraduate academic program for nurses was established at a polytechnic level, soon followed by an increase of other higher professional education programs for nurses (Nationale Raad voor de Volksgezondheid, 1992).

The 1980s saw rapid development with the establishment of the first university degree program for experienced, postbasic, hospital-trained diploma nurses at the State University of Maastricht. This contributed to a growing cohort of highly qualified nurses. At the same time, the health care institutions became involved in innovations and change, such as team and primary nursing, quality appraisal programs, and nursing audits. The upgrading of nursing education into polytechnics and the state university stimulated interest in the scientific foundation of the discipline.

The 1990s were characterized by a desire to use nursing theory and research as an underpinning for clinical practice. The change of the century sees us focusing on the establishment of clinical nurse specialists, named "nurse practitioners" in the Netherlands. (Grypdonck, 2000; Raatgever, 2000; Roodbol & van de Bunt, 2000; Spijker & Niehuis, 2000). It appears that the nursing profession is restructuring itself, and the legislation of the BIG Law, also known and referred to in this chapter as the Health Professions Act of 1997, provided the impetus for nursing to develop an infrastructure for the licensure and control of professional conduct (NU '91, 2000; Vlaskamp, 2000).

Culture as a Framework for Analysis

The Netherlands is rich in tradition and has strong family values. In the past, the single-family income was seen as the yardstick of socioeconomic well-being. Until the 1960s, the Netherlands had the smallest percentage of working married women in the world (16%). The situation has slowly changed during the past 20 years, with women gradually catching up within the workforce, now representing about 65%. Because most women have part-time jobs, this percentage camouflages the actual employment situation as well as the limited opportunities for career building.

Although the family unit is still regarded as a cornerstone of the society, the Netherlands is among the progressive countries that have accepted alternative ways of partnership and regulated these through legislation. Gradually, the single wage earner (male) employed in the family was replaced by the employment of both partners, leading to a significant change in the traditional family structure. The once-prominent role of the Protestant and Roman Catholic churches, which dominated public life until the second part of the 20th century, gradually eroded, and church-related organizations changed into nondenominational institutions.

Nursing was originally considered to be subservient to medicine. With the changes in societal attitudes toward women and work and the upgrading of nursing education, the discipline has taken on a role more complementary to medicine, a view strongly advocated by the current minister of health, Dr. Els Borst (Koopman, 2000; Van der Pasch, 2000; Van der Veen, 2000).

History as a Framework for Analysis

In reviewing the history of nursing in the Netherlands, one can see that responsibility for caring for the sick, which originally belonged in the family domain, gradually moved into society at large (Van der Kooij, 1990). Many health services emerged from a private initiative and, once well established in the society, were retrospectively brought under the legislation of the Dutch health care system.

In the Netherlands, organized nursing care dates back to 1870. The publication of a nursing journal occurred in 1890, and the first Dutch Society for Nursing (Netherlands Nurses Association, or NNA) was established in 1893. The Netherlands joined the ICN in 1909 and has been an active member of international nursing and health organizations since that time. The first trained nurses received a diploma, awarded by the White Cross, a community-based public health organization in the province of North Holland between 1879 and 1883 (Van der Kooij, 1990). However, the registration of a nursing diploma was not possible until the Nursing Law of 1921 was adopted.

In the Netherlands, as in Germany, the influence of Protestant and Roman Catholic churches significantly influenced the development of nursing as a charitable occupation. Hospital nursing schools with religious affiliation educated deaconesses and religious sisters as well as lay nurses. Since the 1960s, most of these institutions have been integrated with nondenominational, intercultural health services and educational institutions. Although the Red Cross used to possess a few health care institutions with nursing school annexes, its influence was geared primarily toward its international mission in time of war and disaster.

Legislation and Regulation

Nursing regulation in the Netherlands was landmarked by the Nursing Law of 1921 and the Health Professions Law of 1997, under which jurisdiction the nursing profession has been classified. Between 1921 and 1997, several attempts were made to update the legislation to the actual level of nursing practice. The major changes in the intervening decades related to the following:

■ Biomedical advances in health care with immediate repercussions for nursing practice
■ Upward mobility of nursing education from primarily hospital-based training programs to comprehensive, generic nursing education as offered in polytechnic institutions and universities
■ Increased complexity of the nursing process to be managed under frequently restricted resources and time constraints
■ Demand for more in the effectiveness and efficiency of health care delivery

Educational Perspectives

With regard to nursing regulation, a major point of consideration has been the upward mobility of nursing education. In the Netherlands, as in most countries, this upward mobility from vocational training to professional education is planned in various phases. The first phase is to detach the traditional nursing school from the hospital and establish an independent institution for generic professional education, preferably in collaboration with other schools of nursing. Such a program can be offered at a medium or higher level of professional education. Depending on the educational structure within a country, the higher level of education can be identical to the teaching within a polytechnic institution and can lead to a baccalaureate of nursing science degree or diploma. The next step within the tertiary educational system is the university degree program.

International Models of Tertiary Nursing Education

Since the 1960s, the Netherlands and other countries in Europe have been discussing which model of advanced education would serve nursing best in its move toward professionalization. Some suggested selecting experienced clinical nurses to start the process, with or without university entry qualifications, offering them a "bridge" postbasic degree program tailored to the needs of this special cohort. The advantage of this approach would be that these graduates could return to the workplace and be reintegrated in their nursing positions, where they were respected as nurses before attending the university. The disadvantage could be that adult learners with long experience in the workplace would be "set in their ways" and might encounter difficulty with the role transition and academic challenges such as the change from intuitive to problem-oriented reasoning.

The second model suggests encouraging young, qualified high school graduates to enter a nursing degree program at the university and to stimulate a postgraduate degree enrollment soon after graduation to prepare these nurses for academic career paths. This model is similar to the scientific trajectory followed by graduates of the natural, human, and social sciences. The advantage would be academic socialization at a relatively young age and the realistic prospect of a university career. Such a graduate could be disadvantaged, however, upon entering the clinical nursing arena without the expected practical experience. The question arises whether nursing's prime responsibilities as a practice discipline lie in the scientific advancement of nursing, in the clinical conduct of science-based nursing, or in a combination of both.

The preferred model in northern and western Europe has been to educate a selected group of experienced clinical nurses who, after graduation with a postbasic degree, could act as a bridge generation of scholars in preparing the workplace for the changes to come and assisting the next generation of academically prepared nurses to familiarize themselves with the challenges of nursing practice.

Dutch Social Policy Statement on Nursing

Based on the increasing demands for health care of the Dutch population and the trends of nursing developments in other nations, the nursing discipline accepted the mandate to design an educational structure that could meet the expectations for health care of the next century. In 1988, the National Council for Public Health (Nationale Raad voor de Volksgezondheid, 1988) and the Nursing Commission developed a position paper. This paper encompassed an educational structure for nursing and differentiated the various levels of nursing personnel according to the required levels of competencies and accountability. The preparation of vocational auxiliary nurses or short-term trained personnel has never been an option in the Netherlands and, therefore, has not been part of health care personnel planning.

The polytechnic programs that developed between 1972 and 1988 were well established and had demonstrated the usability of professionally educated nurses. University education, started under the jurisdiction of non-nursing disciplines in 1980, was gradually taking shape and gaining definition when the first professor of nursing science was appointed at the state university in 1988. At the start, the university offered an academic program in health sciences with a major in nursing science only, excluding the clinical component that would qualify its graduates as licensed, registered nurses. Therefore, high school graduates who were awarded this degree had difficulty finding employment. This was not the case for registered nurses whose clinical experience was expanded by university study that offered surplus value to their position. To integrate the graduates without nursing background into the health care system, a bridge program was established that enabled them to be clinically prepared as nurses. From a regulation point of view, this was a political move. Because the formal licensure to practise nursing remained at a polytechnic level, the nurse was placed at a different level from other academically prepared health professionals.

To establish clarity at a competency level, the National Council for Public Health and the Nursing Commission designed a structure that was congruent with the decisions about nursing education and service as agreed on by expert panels. This structure accepted the premise that the nurse was expected to possess certain competencies (Box 10.3). In 1992, the council also described the responsibilities of the second-level, or technical, nurse (Box 10.4).

Impact of the Health Professions Act on Registration

Aside from nursing, the Health Professions Act passed in 1997 registered the following health disciplines: medicine, dentistry, pharmacy, clinical psychology, psychotherapy, physiotherapy, and midwifery. In the near future, nurses registered under this health professions law will be subject to a licensure system that articulates the conditions for nurses to practise: It will embody the criteria for safe nursing care. Advanced nursing education will no longer be pursued on a voluntary basis, but it will become mandatory to update nurses' competencies on a continuing basis.

The Health Professions Act expands the accountability of nurses (Table 10.1). The title of nurse remains protected. Further, the nurse becomes subject to disciplinary jurisdiction. By government decree,

BOX 10.3   Nursing Competencies

The structure designed by the National Council for Public Health, the Nursing Commission, expected nurses to exhibit competence in the following:

- Psychosocial aspects of professional practice
- Mastery of instrumental and technical skills for professional practice
- Application of professional knowledge to enable judgment of (complex) nursing situations and to form an independent opinion

Competency requirements were based on the common goals of health care:

- Promotion and maintenance of health
- Prevention and postponement of illness and disability
- Contribution to curing and rehabilitation
- Alleviation of suffering and discomfort (palliative care)

the nurse will be given functional independence with regard to situation-related (authorized) procedures. The register is placed under the jurisdiction of the Inspection for Health Care. Unlike Canada, the Netherlands does not position the register under the authority of the nursing discipline. One reason for this larger jurisdiction is that the Health Professions Act embodies many health disciplines, and its application is to be coordinated by a recognized authority with legislative power. A second reason could be that the nursing profession in transition needs time to prepare for encroaching changes in the organization of its practice. The framework for professional practice is designed, but the consequences of this legislation are in the process of review and development.

The operationalization of the project "renewed registration of nurses" through the Health Professions Act is planned by two leading organizations in nursing: the General Council for Professional and Vocational Nurses and the National Center for Professional and Vocational Nursing. In these two organizations, all the professional nursing associations are integrated, irrespective of nurses' educational backgrounds and nursing specialties. These nursing organizations are important discussion partners of the Ministry of Health and contribute to those health care platforms in which the professional and employment conditions for nursing personnel are discussed (Van der Pasch, 2000). The Health Professions Act has also intensified the dialogue between nursing and medical professions and resulted in several consensual decisions about modes of collaboration in health care delivery (NU '91 and Koninklijke Nederlandsche Maatschappij tot Bevordering der Geneeskunst, 1997).

BOX 10.4   The Technical Nurse

In regard to role and competency, the technical nurse:

- Assists in systematic assessment and analysis of the nursing needs of the patient
- Is able to assist in formulating an individual nursing plan as far as possible with the agreement and collaboration of the patient
- Can perform delegated nursing activities in a skillful way
- Is able to consult with a nursing colleague or members of other disciplines
- Participates in the evaluation and implementation of the nursing plan in relation to the assessed needs

Note: The verbs *assist*, *delegate(d)*, *consult*, and *participate* indicate that the technical nurse is expected to work in close collaboration with the professional nurse.

TABLE 10.1	Health Professions Act (1997) as Applied to Nursing Practice	
Accountabilities	Nurses: Professional	Nurses: Vocational
Title protection	Yes	Yes
Registration leading to... (constitutional registration)	Yes	No
Regulation of specialization	Yes	No
Competence not independent	Yes	Yes
Possibility of providing authority to function independently by government decree	Yes	No
Disciplinary jurisdiction	Yes	No
Measures in case of incompetence	Yes	No
Cause of harm or injury to another person	Not liable to punishment within the domain of professional nursing competence	Not liable to punishment within the domain of vocational nursing competence

Professionalization of Nursing

Implementing the recommendations of the position paper was a first step in developing an educational structure that would ultimately differentiate professional and vocational nursing into five competency levels. In this structure, nurses are educated at three levels (Box 10.5).

Whereas the previous career path of nurses was mainly facilitated through programs of nursing management services and nursing education, nurses in the late 1990s demonstrated a growing interest in the possibility of clinical specialization. This trend was most likely influenced by the career patterns in Canada and the United States. Professionals still propose arguments about which educational program will serve the patient population most effectively. The prime interest of the nursing profession is in the advancement of quality care and the perspective of a career that enables the nurse to pursue her or his interests and enrich both knowledge and experience.

The Ministry of Health has also expressed an interest in the differentiation of nursing positions, but from another perspective. The Ministry of Health would support the position that nurses be authorized to perform routine medical procedures and, by doing so, relieve the burden on medicine. Delegated medical interventions could then be performed at a cost-effective level and help to control the steadily rising costs of health care.

In expressing their concern about the government's perspective, nurses indicate that they are not interested in becoming second-class physicians or physician's assistants. Their response has been that measures should be taken to relieve workloads and improve employment conditions. The attrition rate of nursing

BOX 10.5	Three Levels of Nursing Education

- Nursing colleges that offer generic programs and appear to be the old system enriched with current trends in nursing education
- Polytechnic institutions (HBO-V) regarded as the core preparation for professional nursing
- University level, with emphasis placed on science and research as well as on clinical specialization

personnel is supported by the following data: nurses doing other work (33%), no perspective of personal development (19%), no job satisfaction (19%), the burden of the workload (15%), the family situation (15%), and the financial reward (14%) (Sikking, 2001a).

The waning interest in pursuing a nursing career, combined with the steadily decreasing enrollment in nursing education, is leading to an acute nursing shortage that is not solved by rerouting nurses' responsibilities into medicine. Reports from the higher education programs for nurses relate decreased enrollments of 25% in 2000 and 20% in 2001 (Sikking, 2001b). Nursing vacancies in 2000 were assessed at a 1% to 4% level, particularly in highly specialized nursing areas. In 2001, the shortage of nurses was projected to be at 10% for 2002 (Bruinsma, 2001).

■ SUMMARY

This chapter addresses the progress and challenges of international nursing regulation and legislation, particularly in Germany and the Netherlands, and the roles of various international organizations, such as the ICN, the WHO, and the WHO/EURO, in that regulation and legislation.

The history of German nursing helps explain not only its origin and tradition but also the infrastructure leading to current laws and decrees that regulate nursing.

In Germany, nursing science has accelerated at an advanced pace since the late 1980s. The result is the establishment of nursing management, nursing education, and nursing science programs within polytechnic institutions and universities. A first generation of well-educated nurses is gradually being integrated into the health care system, although it is still too early to evaluate the effect of their contributions.

In the Netherlands, the upgrading of nursing education has had a significant impact on the development of the nursing discipline. A corps of well-educated nurses has been integrated into the health care scene and has started to influence patient care services, nursing management, nursing education, and the scientific advancement of the profession.

The Nursing Law of 1921 was finally replaced by the Health Professions Law of 1997, which included nursing as one of eight health disciplines. The consequences of this law require the nursing profession to register under more stringent conditions for professional practice. The transition process will take a number of years, and regulatory conditions for nursing practice and continuing education are being developed.

The introduction of the Health Professions Act has also revitalized discussions about the nursing specialist, that is, the nurse practitioner with extended accountability. From the perspective of the Ministry of Health, the nurse should be authorized to take over some routine medical procedures. Nurses emphasize that their extended role should focus more strongly on the delivery of comprehensive patient care.

Nursing regulation is the key to the advancement of nursing; it offers the infrastructure for authorized development and change. Nurses in Germany and the Netherlands are actively engaged in building infrastructures that enable them to participate in the establishment of health service delivery, a challenge for which they are prepared.

Online Resources

Add to your knowledge of this issue:

International Council of Nurses (ICN)	**www.icn.ch**
ICN Regulation	**www.icn.ch/regulation.htm**
ICN Regulation Network	**www.icn.ch/regnet.htm**
Nursing Regulation in Europe	**www.clearhq.org/europe.html**
World Health Organization (WHO)	**www.who.int/en**
WHO Nursing and Midwifery Services	**www.who.int/health-services-delivery/nursing**

REFLECTIONS on the Chapter . . .

1. How is regulation talked about in this chapter? How does this compare with the discussion of regulation elsewhere in the text?

2. How does regulation differ in Germany and the Netherlands? In what ways does the interpretation of regulation in these countries resemble or differ from regulation in Canada? What issues do these differences raise for the professional advancement of nursing?

3. How would you account for the differences in the advancement of nursing between Germany and the Netherlands? Are there similarities with the advancement of nursing in Canada?

4. Discuss issues that arise out of the relationship between "women's work" and "nurses' work" in each of these countries. Compare these with issues that Canadian nurses and the profession face in Canada.

5. What stand has the ICN taken on international regulation?

6. What government structures and legislated policies influence regulation in each of these countries: Germany, the Netherlands, and Canada?

7. What issues are raised by the statement "mandatory licensure in accordance with the customs of a country, in the licensure of its professions"?

8. Discuss the difference between "power" gained by nursing through professional advancement and that mandated by law. What issues does this raise for nursing regulation nationally or internationally?

References

Althusser, L. (1971). Ideology and ideological state apparatuses. In B. Brewster (Trans.), L. Althusser (Ed.), *Lenin and philosophy and other essays* (pp. 123–173). London: New Left Books.

Bals, T., Beikirch-Korporal, E., Bischoff-Wanner, C., et al. (1997). *Bundesausschuss der Länderarbeitsgemeinschaften der Lehrerinnen und Lehrer für Pflegeberufe. Bildung und Pflege.* Stuttgart: Thieme Verlag.

Brush, B. L., Lynaugh, J. E., Boschma, G., et al. (1999). Nurses of all nations: A history of the International Council of Nurses 1899–1999. New York: Lippincott Williams & Wilkins.

Bundesausschuss der Lehrerinnen und Lehrer für Pflegeberufe e.V. (2000, May). Structural changes in health- and social care: A challenge for nurse-educators (German text). In *Bildung und Pflege: Die Europäische Dimension* (pp. 62–75). Conference proceedings, Potsdam.

Cutshall, P. (2000). *Understanding cross border professional regulation: What nurses and other professionals need to know.* Geneva: International Council of Nurses.

Deutscher Berufsverband für Krankenpflege (DBfK). (1989). *Nursing research for professional practice.* Workgroup of European Nurse Researchers (WENR). 12th Workgroup Meeting and International Nursing Research Conference. Frankfurt am Main: Verlag "Krankenpflege."

Finocchio, L., Dower, C., McMahon, T., et al. (1995). *Reforming health care work force regulation: Policy considerations for the 21st century.* San Francisco: Pew Health Professions Commission.

Grauhan, A. (1989). Development of nursing research and academic nursing education in W. Germany. In *Nursing research for professional practice* (pp. 12–21). 12th Workgroup Meeting and International Nursing Research Conference. Workgroup of European Nurse Researchers. Frankfurt am Main: Deutscher Berufsverband für Krankenpflege (DBfK).

Grypdonck, M. (2000). De nurse practitioner: Meer dan een nieuwe hype in de Nederlandse verpleegkunde? *Tijdschrift voor Verpleegkundigen TVZ, 110*(10), 299–301.

International Council of Nurses. (1953, 1973, 1997). Code of ethics. In *ICN Statements.* Geneva: Author.

Koopman, P. (2000). De vierde Dinsdag in September: Minister opent bestuurlijk overleg met verpleegkundigen en verzorgenden. *Tijdschrift voor Verpleegkundigen TVZ, 110*(19), 574–575.

Krüger, H. (1996, May). Pflege zwischen besetzten Stühlen? Die Neuordnung der Ausbildung vor dem Hintergrund der Anforderungen neuer pflegerischer Handlungsfelder. In *Bundesausschuss der Länderarbeitsgemeinschaften der Lehrerinnen und Lehrer für Pflegeberufe: Conference Proceedings* (pp. 67–76). Fürth/Bayern.

Krüger, H., Rabe-Kleberg, U., Mischo-Kelling, M. (1993). *Pflegewissenschaft als berufliche Bildung: ein Weg aus der Sackgasse: Entwicklung und Erprobung eines Studiengangs mit berufspädagogischem Fachrichtungsprofil für Lehrkräfte in der Alten—und Kranken/Kinderpflege.* Berufliche Erstausbildung und Lehramtstudium als biografische Bausteine. Werkstattberichte des Forschungsschwerpunktes Arbeit und Bildung der Universität Bremen. Bd. 24. Universität Bremen.

Kruse, A. P. (1987). Berufskunde 11: Die Krankenpflegeausbildung seit der Mitte des 19. Jahrhunderts. Kohlhammer Studienbücher. Berlin: W. Kohlhammer.

Kurtenbach, H., Golombek, G., & Siebers, H. (1994). *Krankenpflegegesetz und Ausbildungs—und Prüfungsverordnung für die Berufe in der Krankenpflege. 4. Auflage.* Krankenhausrecht Köln: Verlag W. Kohlhammer GmbH.

Mischo-Kelling, M., & Witneben, K. (1995). *Pflegebildung und Pflegetheorien.* München: Urban & Schwarzenberg.

Nationale Raad voor de Volksgezondheid. (1988). *Verpleegkundig Beroepsprofiel.* Zoetermeer: Author (National Council for Public Health).

_____. (1992). *Dutch social statement on the nursing profession.* Zoetermeer: Author.

NU '91. (2000). *Evaluatie Wet BIG.* Document National Nurses Association of the Netherlands—Fax of the Ministry of Welfare, Health and Culture 131-71-5253782, Research 17/01/2000.

NU '91 & Koninklijke Nederlandsche Maatschappij tot Bevordering der Geneeskunst. (1997). *Voorbehouden handelingen in de praktijk: Richtlijnen voor de samenwerking tussen artsen, verpleegkundigen en ziekenverzorgenden.* Utrecht: Author.

Quinn, S. (1989). *ICN past and present.* ICN: Scutari Press.

Raatgever, M. (2000). Een nurse-practitioner op de mammapolikliniek. *Tijdschrift voor Verpleegkundigen TVZ, 100*(17), 524–527.

Roodbol, P., & van de Bunt, C. (2000). De "Nurse Practitioner voegt inderdaad iets toe!" Is de kritiek van Professor Grypdonck terecht? *Tijdschrift voor Verpleegkundigen TVZ, 110*(14), 437–438.

Salvage, J., & Heijnen, S. (1997). *Nursing in Europe: A resource for better health.* WHO Regional Publications, European Series, No. 74. Copenhagen: WHO/EURO.

Sekretariat der Ständigen Konferenz der Kultusminister der Länder in der Bundesrepublik Deutschland. (1995). *Rahmenvereinbarung über die Ausbildung und Prüfung für ein Lehramt der Sekundarstufe II (berufliche Fächer) oder für die beruflichen Schulen.* Beschlub der Kultusministerkonferenz vom 12.05.1995. be165bls. Bonn: Author.

_____. (1997). *Bericht der Gemeinsamen Arbeitsgruppe KMK/GMK/ASMK "Studiengänge im Tätigkeitsfeld Gesundheitswesen."* Bonn 24.04.1997 A/Br23-04.Kö. Bonn: Author.

Sikking, I. (2001a). Zorg aan bed komt in gevaar: Drastische afname van aantal studenten verpleegkunde. *Algemeen Dagblad Diagnose, 31*(8), 1.

_____. (2001b). Zorg om de zorg. *Algemeen Dagblad Diagnose, 31*(8), 26. Statistical Data LCVV, research Primant en HBO-raad.

Sindram, I. P. C. (1993). *BIG in zicht: De wet op de beroepen in de individuele gezondheidszorg.* Verplegenden en verzorgenden onder de wet BIG. Utrecht: Nieuwe Unie '91.

Sindram, I. P. C. (2001). *BIG: De wet op de beroepen in de individuale gezondheidszorg—Inzichtelijk.* Verpleegkundigen en verzorgenden IG onder de wet BIG. Uitgave van de Nieuwe Unie '91: Beroepsorganisatie van de verpleging. Venlo: van Grinsven Drukkers.

Spijker, T., & Niehuis, M. (2000). De positionering van de verpleegkundig specialist. *Tijdschrift voor Verpleegkundigen TVZ, 110*(7), 203–204.

Steppe, H. (1990). Krankenpflege im Wandel 1939–1989: von der Berufung zum Beruf–vom Dienen zur Dienstleistung. *Krankenpflege, 1*(90), S.11–15.

_____. (Hrsg.). (1996). *Krankenpflege im Nationalsozialismus. 8. Auflage.* (1. Auflage unter dem Titel: Geschichte der Krankenpflege: Versuch einer kritischen Aufarbeitung, 1984). Frankfurt am Main: Marbuse-Verlag GmbH.

Stiftung, R. B. (Hrsg.). (1992, 1993a). Pflege braucht Eliten. *Denkschrift zur Hochschulausbildung für Lehr—und Leitungskräfte in der Pflege* (3rd ed.). Beiträge zur Gesundheitsökonomie 28. Gesundheitspflege. Gerlinger: Bleicher Verlag.

_____. (Hrsg.). (1993b). *Pflegeförderung: zur Situation in der Bundesrepublik Deutschland.* Materialien und Berichte, Band 39. Gerlingen: Bleicher Verlag.

_____. (Hrsg.) (1996). *Pflegewissenschaft: Grundlegung für Lehre, Forschung Und Praxis.* Denkschrift. Materialien und Berichte 46. Stuttgart: Bleicher Verlag.

_____. (2000). *Pflege neu denken: Zur Zukunft der Pflegeausbildung.* Stuttgart: Schattauer.

Styles, M. (1985). *Report on the regulation of nursing. Report on the present: A position for the future.* International Council of Nurses, Professional Services Committee. Geneva: ICN.

Styles, M., & Affara, A. (1997). *ICN on regulation: Towards a 21st century model.* Geneva: ICN.

Van der Kooij, C. H. (1990). 1980–1990: De vermaatschappelijking van de zorg. In: A. H. M. van den Bergh-Braam, C. H. von der Kooij, & A. E. W. M. van de Pasch (Eds.), *Honderd jaar verplegen* (pp. 13–64). Lochem: Uitgeversmaatschappij De Tijdstroom.

Van der Pasch, T. (2000). "We betrekken verpleegkundigen nog onvoldoende bij de beleidsontwikkeling": Minister Borst over versterking positie verpleegkundigen [Interview]. *Tijdschrift voor Verpleegkundigen TVZ, 110*(14), 434–436.

Van der Veen, A. (2000). Gezondheidszorgberoepen in beweging: Stel een platform in voor beleidsadvisering van de minister. *Tijdschrift voor Verpleegkundigen TVZ, 110*(17), 530–531.

van Maanen, H. (1998, July 5–8). *Two decades WENR: Did history write nursing research or did nursing research write history?* Keynote address, 20th Anniversary Workgroup of European Nurse Researchers (WENR) and 9th Open Conference of the WENR. Helsinki.

_____. (2001, June 10–15). *The family health nurse: An old concept in a renewed appearance. The German experience with community nursing care.* Paper presented at International Council of Nurses (ICN) 22nd Quadrennial Congress, Copenhagen.

Vlaskamp, L. (2000). Verpleegkundige beroepsuitoefening en tuchtrecht. *Tijdschrift voor Verpleegkundigen TVZ, 110*(7), 212–215.

World Health Organization. (1954). *Expert Committee on Nursing: Third report.* World Health Organization Technical Report Series No. 91. Geneva: Author.

_____. (1966). *Expert Committee on Nursing: Fifth report.* World Health Organization Technical Report Series No. 347. Geneva: Author.

_____. (1977). *Criteria for the evaluation of learning objectives in the education of health personnel.* Report of a WHO Study Group. Technical Report Series No. 608. Geneva: Author.

_____. (1983). *New approaches to health education in primary health care.* Report of a WHO Expert Committee. Technical Report Series No. 690. Geneva: Author.

_____. (1984). *Education and training of nurse-teachers and managers with special regard to primary health care.* Report of a WHO Expert Committee. Technical Report Series No. 708. Geneva: Author.

_____. (1986). *Regulatory mechanisms for nursing training and practice: Meeting primary health care needs.* Report of a WHO Study Group. Technical Report Series No. 738. Geneva: Author.

_____. (1988). *From Alma Ata to the year 2000: Reflections at the midpoint.* Geneva: Author.

World Health Organization Regional Office for Europe. (1970). *Trends in European nursing services.* Report on a Working Group, Bern, 1970. Copenhagen: Author.

_____. (1972). *Higher education in nursing.* Report on a Symposium, The Hague, 1972. Copenhagen: Author.

_____. (1984). *Postbasic and graduate education for nurses.* Report on a WHO meeting. EURO Reports and Studies 99. Copenhagen: Author.

_____. (1999). *Health 21: Health for all in the 21st century.* European Publications "Health for All," No. 6. Copenhagen: Author.

NURSING KNOWLEDGE:
How We Come to Know What We Know

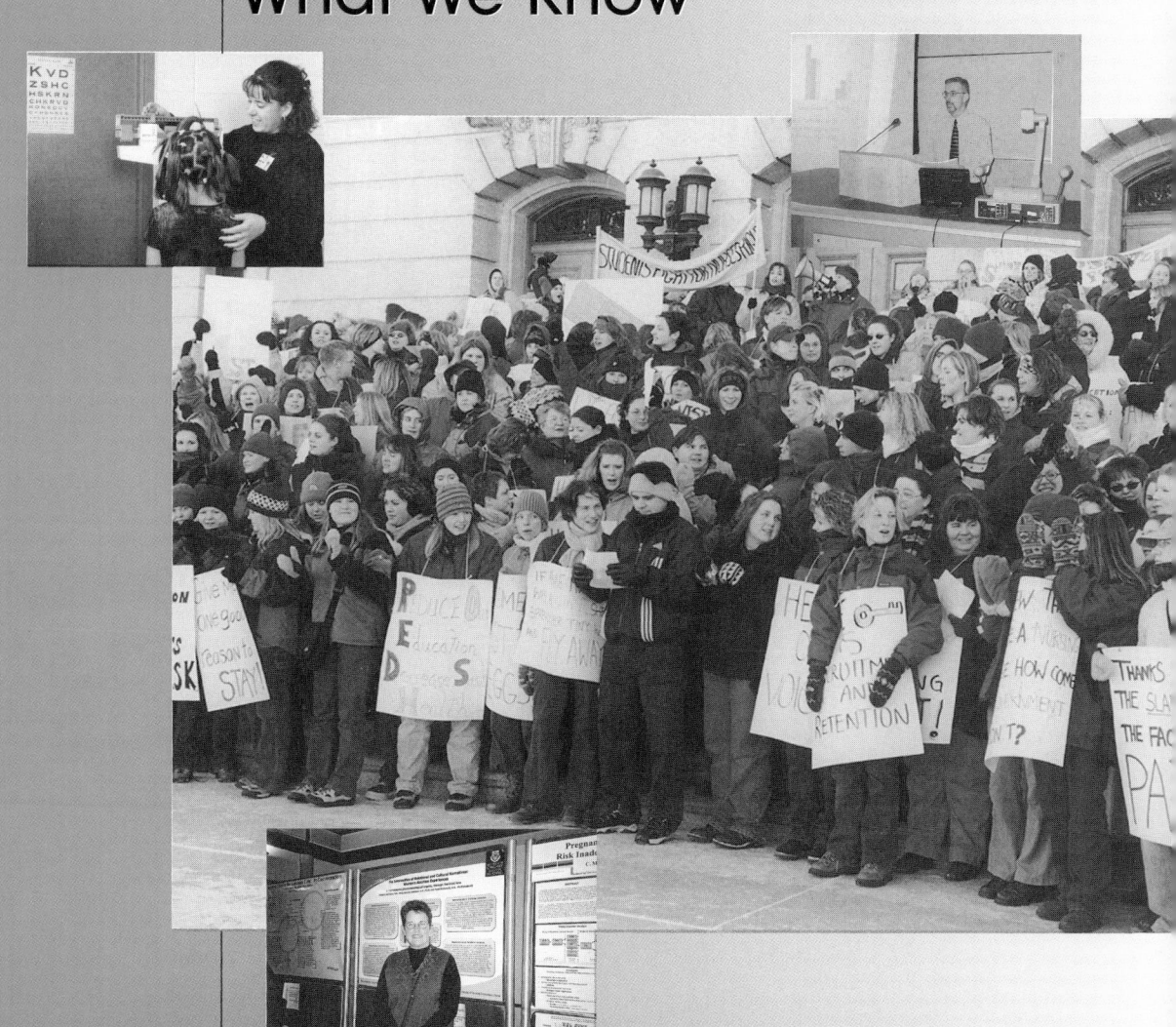

Critical Questions

As a way of engaging with the ideas in this chapter, consider the following:

1. In what ways have you used political processes in your undergraduate nursing education?

2. What would you need to learn to enhance your ability to act politically?

3. What do you imagine might have been the influence of political processes on nurses over time?

CHAPTER
11

Diana Davidson Dick
Betty Cragg

Undergraduate Education: Development and Politics

Undergraduate students on the steps of the Saskatchewan Legislature Building in February 2000, demonstrating in support of the degree as entry to practice. A description of the public debate and the role of students appears in this chapter.

For more than 100 years, undergraduate education has been a major focus of the political and policy initiatives of organized nursing in Canada. The preparation of the next generation of registered nurses (RNs) determines the viability of the profession and its ability to influence the health care system and the health of society. In advocating for changes in undergraduate education, leaders in nursing education and practice have struggled for recognition of their knowledge base and their capacity to determine their own standards. Initiatives to change undergraduate education provide examples of the barriers, innovations, and successes nurses have experienced in their efforts to affect policy and influence legislation to improve the health care of Canadians. Educational changes, such as baccalaureate as entry to practice, also demonstrate how nurses have been able to mobilize the members of their profession, members of the larger society, and governments to contribute to a higher standard of care and to improve patient outcomes through improving undergraduate education.

■ OVERVIEW OF CURRENT ISSUES IN NURSING EDUCATION

This chapter views the contemporary realities and expectations of Canadian undergraduate education not only from a conceptual, informational, and historical perspective but also within the framework of political processes. Two major undergraduate educational issues and concerns are addressed, both of which exemplify the visibility, breadth, and scope of nursing practice and political action:

▨ Achievement of baccalaureate education as the entry standard for practice as an RN
▨ Integration of the political and the nursing processes in educating undergraduate students in a clinical experience

Influence of Nursing and Political Processes

The political process is parallel and integral to the nursing process. Both are problem-solving processes: The nursing process is applied to issues of care and service, and the political process is applied to issues of power and influence. Both include similar key steps, and both are intertwined and nonlinear. Nursing process includes data collection and analysis, diagnosis or problem identification, nursing orders with projected outcomes and dates, implementation, and evaluation. The political process includes data collection and analysis and the identification of issues, goals, or objectives; strategies with projected outcomes; dates and key players; implementation; and evaluation (Box 11.1).

The nursing process and the political process include similar fundamental elements, which are also processes in themselves. These elements include the following:

▨ Developing and maintaining relationships
▨ Identifying and understanding the key players or stakeholders
▨ Planning and organizing
▨ Collecting, analyzing, and disseminating information

BOX 11.1	Comparing the Nursing Process and the Political Process: The Interrelationships

The Nursing Process

Goal: Care and service provision
Steps: Diagnosis/problem identification, expected outcomes/dates, nursing orders, evaluation

The Political Process

Goal: Power and influence
Steps: Issue/goal/objectives identification, desired outcomes/dates, strategies, implementation, evaluation

Common Elements

Opportunity: recognizing or creating it, then seizing it
Relationships: development and maintenance
Identification of key players
Planning and organization
Information and education
Communication
Persistence

■ Educating and communicating
■ Taking advantage of opportunity and acting with persistence

One tends to think of the political process as the application of politics, which has been described as the authoritative allocation of resources—or who gets what, when, and how (Lasswell, 1958). From this definition, one can see that politics is a part of our daily lives. Although the word often has negative connotations, one can also see that "politics" as a concept or an entity is value neutral, neither good nor bad; rather, it exists. How we use politics and the political process determines whether the process is good or bad, just as how we use the communication process determines whether the process is good or bad, effective or ineffective. It is important that we are aware of politics and the political process and, like other processes, that we learn how to use them constructively and effectively (Dick, 1985).

The political process involves the exercise of power that goes on in words—written or spoken (Smith, 1981). Being visible, writing, being read, speaking, being heard, and communicating effectively are requirements for the exercise of power and for the advancement of health and the practice of nursing. Examples of nurses who used the political process to achieve desired education levels and of a clinical group of students and their educator who used political processes to achieve desired results for a patient are presented in this chapter. These examples show that power can be viewed as a health issue. In this context, if you have power, you feel well, or better; if you do not have power, you feel unwell, or less well. The acquisition of power in this context is a worthy goal toward growth, healing, and well-being, and the exercise of power through the political and nursing processes can be seen as an act of caring. It is worthwhile to note that these are principles that a good clinician encourages for his or her patients.

Patricia Benner, nurse leader and researcher, speaks about the "full appreciation for the power that nurses acquire when they articulate the skill and knowledge that is embedded in their practice" (2000, p. ix). Benner (2000, p. ix; bracketed material added) continues:

We have found that discerning and describing the knowledge, competence, and skill that goes into day-to-day nursing work allows nurses themselves to comprehend their work in a more empowering way. It increases nurses' mastery and appreciation of their own work and, by extension, nurses' ability to better care for patients. The articulation of nursing work [or visibility] can not only spur hospital management, politicians and policy makers to value and reward nursing as well as contribute to nurses valuing themselves and each other.

This approach takes the view that nursing is the application of competencies that include a combination of knowledge, judgments, and skills by an individual nurse, or a group of nurses, to make a positive health difference. Competencies are "the knowledge, skills, attitudes and judgment expected of practitioners" (Canadian Nurses Association [CNA], 1997, p. 42). Nursing, which is informed by a large body of theoretical and clinical knowledge, relies on and involves knowledge-based caring and decision making that makes a difference to health.

As well, nursing education, legislation and regulation of nursing practice, social movements, and political processes have a long history of tension and interreliance. This history makes evident the need for Canadian nurses to be involved in the systems, policies, and legislation that have an impact on their capacity to provide safe, effective care and service to the Canadian public. One role of undergraduate education is to convey this background and framework to those who are entering the profession: Canadian undergraduate nursing students.

Key Policy and Political Issues

Policy and political issues about nursing education in the 20th century included the need for registration to recognize nurses who met educational standards, thus protecting the public from those with inadequate nursing preparation. Another issue was which kind of institution (service or educational) should educate undergraduate nurses. A consequential issue is the level at which nurses needed to be educated to meet the competencies required by the bodies that regulate nursing practice and register beginning practitioners.

Since their earliest days, Canadian nursing organizations have made recommendations about undergraduate nursing education designed to ensure that graduates have the competencies to meet the needs of the patient, or population, and to meet the increasingly complex demands of health care systems. Implementation of such recommendations usually depended on legislation and funding. As a result, these organizations have had to influence governments to achieve the most profound and desired changes. Nurses have mobilized and used political processes to create political will. Frequently, in seeking changes for the profession to meet the changing needs of the health care system and the needs of the public, nurses have met opposition from governments, other health professions, other professions, and other nurses.

■ HISTORY OF WOMEN'S PLACE AND NURSING EDUCATION

Formal nursing education in Canada started at a time when women had few rights in Canadian society and were, therefore, disadvantaged politically. Before the 1880s, women could not vote; they could not own property in many places; they were not accepted as full participants in postsecondary education (Errington, 1990). Early in the 20th century, predominantly male professions, such as medicine and law, moved from an apprenticeship model to an educational model and became established in universities. Until the early 21st century, nursing remained a predominantly female occupation, with educational preparation for nursing established mainly in hospitals or at community colleges. As a profession predominantly for women, nursing has reflected many of the problems of women in society. Despite its educational base of science, clinical and professional skills, knowledge, and judgment, the history of nursing education has reflected a social perception that nursing is "women's work," which, therefore, requires little knowledge and preparation, or remuneration (Reverby, 1987).

Nursing has also been seen as a calling, as evidenced by the importance of religious orders of nurses in establishing and providing health care in French Canada. Those with a vocation do the job for love, with little consideration for their own needs or those of the profession. With the influence of Florence Nightingale in the English-speaking world in the last half of the 19th century, nursing became a respectable way for middle-class laywomen to earn a living and display altruism (McPherson, 1996). Nightingale and her followers demonstrated that nurses needed particular skills and knowledge. It was not generally recognized until the second half of the 20th century, however, that nursing comprises a unique body of knowledge and skills (Rogers, 1970, p. xii). The development of nursing theories and research has provided the evidence to justify nursing judgments, decisions, plans, and actions. In some jurisdictions, governments have recently accepted the need, identified by the profession, for specifying competencies nurses must have to function safely and effectively in the current and future health care system. Most regulatory bodies of nursing across the country have concluded that the competencies identified for new RNs require the content of a baccalaureate education program.

Nursing Education in New France

Nursing has a long history in Canada, starting with the founding of hospitals in Quebec City and Montreal in New France by members of religious orders in the 17th century. Jeanne Mance, who founded the Hotel Dieu hospital in Montreal in 1642, has been recognized as the first lay nurse in Canada (The History of Nursing Society, 1929). The Roman Catholic nursing orders sent nuns who had been taught religious observance and care of the sick in their convents in France (Nelson, 1999). Later in the 17th century and in the 18th century, especially after Quebec became a British colony in 1759, which cut off most contacts with France, nursing orders prepared local women to provide care (Gibbon & Mathewson, 1947). A system of hospital-based nursing care developed, and the Grey Nuns under Marguerite d'Youville also started home care in Montreal in 1738. Catholic nursing orders provided early health care to westward-moving pioneers. By the end of the 19th century, these orders had founded hospitals and nursing training schools in various parts of Canada (Ross-Kerr, 1998). Such initiatives reinforced the perception of nursing as a religious vocation and made the provision of nursing care respectable in the cultural context of French Canada. Nuns could exert considerable power and influence within their own settings, controlling the management of hospitals they founded and ensuring that students' educational needs were considered in a way that proved impossible in secular hospitals controlled by boards (Paul, 1998). In a broader social context, religious orders were controlled by the hierarchy of the church and exerted relatively little political influence in secular society.

Nursing Education in English-Speaking Canada

In English-speaking Canada, the religious tradition of nursing was less important. It was not until the influence of Florence Nightingale after the Crimean War in the 1850s that nursing became a respectable occupation for middle-class women and a source of upward mobility for girls from poor homes and farm regions (McPherson, 1996). In the late 19th and early 20th centuries, there was a rapid development of hospitals throughout North America. Nursing schools were founded to train the required nurses and provide staffing for the new hospitals. The founders of new schools of nursing frequently cited Nightingale's principles. However, one of her key principles, the financial autonomy of the nursing school from the hospital, did not occur. Schools in English Canada were usually governed by hospital boards. Therefore, the service needs of the hospital were considered more important than the educational needs of student nurses.

Modern undergraduate nursing education began in Canada in 1874 with the opening of the Mack Training School in St. Catharines, Ontario. The founder was Dr. Theophilis Mack, a physician, who wanted to ensure competent care in hospitals. He believed that middle-class patients would choose modern, scientific hospital treatment if they were assured that they would receive professional nursing care (Gibbon & Mathewson, 1947). Thus began the linkage of nursing education in Canada with the needs of hospitals—and the practice of subservience of nursing to the demands of medicine. It is notable that the motto of the Mack School of Nursing was "I see and am silent" (Coburn, 1981). This contrasts sharply with current professional obligations, responsibility, and accountability to advocate for patients, to question and challenge decisions and approaches to care, and to act and speak to protect patients from harm. From the 1880s to the 1960s, nursing care in Canadian hospitals was provided mostly by nursing students. Graduate nurses worked mainly in homes as private duty nurses or followed the tradition of leaving the workforce after marriage.

Life and Education in Hospital Nursing Schools

In hospital schools, students lived regimented lives, passing uniform inspections, working long hours, and being required to live in residence under strict rules. In the early 20th century, a time of poor working conditions for most workers, students were expected to work 12-hour shifts, with only one-half day off per week (Paul, 1998). In return for their labor, they received free tuition, room, and board. In some cases, they also received a stipend in recognition of the service they provided.

The very restrictive environment of the nursing school perpetuated the notion of the nurse as the physician's handmaiden and discouraged expression of independent thinking or action. Nurses, especially students, were supposed to stand when physicians entered the nursing station, to defer to medical opinions, and to follow doctors' orders for patients. In the hospital schools in the first half of the 20th century, there were few educational or curriculum standards, and the few instructional hours were mainly doctors' lectures, taken by students during off time or in the middle of split shifts (Weir, 1932). Hospitals hired few graduate nurses; therefore, the main practical instruction came from fellow students with only months more experience. As one writer commented, it was an apprenticeship system that had no masters to supervise the apprentices (Paul, 1998). With the exception of a few supervisors who were graduate nurses, hospitals in Canada were staffed and run by student nurses. On evenings and nights, senior students were in charge of wards, supervising the work of their juniors.

Despite the many problems, the hospital training system had advantages for the students as well as the hospitals. It was a source of affordable postsecondary education and an entrance to a respected occupation. Students and graduates felt a strong loyalty to their institution and its patients and often went beyond even the extreme demands of their training for the sake of patient care. For example, student nurses volunteered for literally life-threatening assignments during epidemics of diseases such as smallpox and polio (Garey & Hott, 1988). Living together in residence, students were able to support one another in dealing with the intense demands of life-and-death situations. Much informal debriefing and learning occurred after-hours in the residence. There was no teaching–service dichotomy; therefore, students were integrated into the life of the institution. Even when hospital schools became more educationally focused, the teachers, as employees of the hospital, were an integral part of the unit where they taught. They and their students were not treated as guests but as full participants who were expected to contribute to the quality of the care provided. Boards, administrators, and physicians who wielded power and control within hospitals were motivated to respond to calls for reform within hospital nursing schools because having a nursing school with a good reputation was a source of pride to everyone associated with the institution.

Nursing Programs in the University

The first university nursing program in Canada was founded by Ethel Johns at the University of British Columbia in 1919, providing preparation for nursing in what became known as the "sandwich" model: training in a hospital school sandwiched between first and final years at a university (Mussallem, 1965). After World War I, the need for improved public health and for nurses with university-based public health preparation led the Red Cross to provide seed funding for programs to upgrade diploma-prepared nurses at five additional Canadian universities. The pattern of university education for the next 30 years was created.

Most universities offered post-RN programs that prepared RNs for public health positions or educated those employed in hospitals for leadership positions as nurse educators or administrators. Those who wanted a university degree as their initial preparation for nursing could take the sandwich programs. By incorporating time at the university before and after traditional hospital nursing training, these programs ensured that the students had the general education for which many reformers had called. However, when learning nursing, the students were not required to apply their general education to the situations they were encountering in hospitals. The university had no control over the content or teaching of their nursing courses (King, 1970).

In 1942, Kathleen Russell pioneered an integrated nursing program at the University of Toronto (Carpenter, 1970). A similar program followed shortly thereafter at McMaster University in Hamilton. In integrated programs, the university controlled the nursing as well as the general education portions of the program and, therefore, could ensure that clinical applications and connections were made with the various theory courses the students were taking. The university could also ensure that clinical experiences met students' learning needs and were sequenced in accord with educational principles. Only after Mussallem (1965) studied nursing education in Canada for the 1965 Royal Commission on Health Services were clear recommendations made about the superiority of integrated nursing education. The recommendations led the majority of university schools in the country to move to this model. Entry-level integrated programs began to flourish, but post-RN diploma education also remained a major focus of university education. Many diploma-prepared nurses—who still constituted the majority of the graduates and working nurses—wanted a stronger educational background to satisfy their personal aspirations and increase their career options. Generic baccalaureate education, offered in collaboration with colleges, is becoming the norm. Post-RN diploma baccalaureate degrees will eventually decline, and more emphasis will be placed on graduate education and research within the universities.

■ STRATEGIES TO IMPROVE NURSING EDUCATION

By the middle of the 20th century, educational leaders in nursing were able to persuade their hospital boards that students needed adequate theoretical preparation as well as the practical learning that occurred on the wards. Initial probationary periods with intensive learning of basic sciences and practice laboratories, as well as block scheduling with class times segregated from ward work, represented attempts to ensure more and better-quality nursing education within hospital schools (Paul, 1998). However, projects such as the demonstration school at the Metropolitan Hospital in Windsor in the 1950s (Lord, cited in Mussallem, 1965) and the Nightingale School in Toronto in the 1960s demonstrated that students could reach the same outcomes in 2 years rather than 3, if they were not required to meet the service needs of the hospital.

Concerns about the quality of nursing education led nurses to gather data from external, and therefore presumably more objective, experts to demonstrate that changes were needed. In 1929, the CNA and the Canadian Medical Association commissioned George Weir, a professor of education at the University of British Columbia, to study the current state of nursing education. His report, published in 1932, included scathing indictments of some of the exploitative practices in the hospital nursing system. Among other things, he discovered schools of nursing that accepted students who had grade 7 educations and schools that had hired no instructors to teach students. He identified that a great deal of students' time was spent on what he called "maid's work." Weir (1932, pp. 380–381) commented:

[T]here is abroad in Canada today a certain school of opinion that would single out the nurse from the procession of social progress and ask her to revert to the good old days of apprenticeship and rule-of-thumb standards! A nineteenth century nursing education in a twentieth century world, with its more exacting and specialized demands on intelligence, knowledge, ingenuity, resourcefulness and social adaptability, is sometimes the solution recommended for our nursing problems. Such a strange position is difficult to understand unless it be that these critics believe that nurses should hold membership in a cult of intellectual serfdom....

Weir made many recommendations for improving students' conditions and education. He recognized the need for nurses to have general as well as practical education and recommended that, to meet the needs of the public, universities should, "in the judgment of the Survey, award degrees in Nursing as in Arts, Law, Engineering, Pharmacy, Agriculture, Medicine, or any other field of learning" (Weir, 1932, p. 393). It was almost 60 years before his recommendation was taken seriously outside the nursing profession.

In 1965, the Royal Commission on Health Services provided another case of external recommendations for nursing education that reflected and supported the position of nursing leaders. The commission was influential in the movement of nursing education to postsecondary educational institutions and in the development of integrated generic baccalaureate programs. In the 1990s, the approach used by leaders seeking educational change was to focus on required entry-level competencies. The competencies led, in turn, to identification of the educational level required to meet these standards—a university degree in nursing.

■ CURRENT ISSUES IN UNDERGRADUATE EDUCATION IN CANADA

The considerable changes that have occurred in nursing in the past century often have been led by nurses concerned with educational issues. Among these have been registration, the move to postsecondary educational institutions, and the baccalaureate as the required educational level for entry to the practice of nursing, known as the baccalaureate as entry to practice.

Registration as Recognition of Education

With the establishment of hospital nursing schools at the turn of the 20th century came concerns that nurses who had graduated from formal programs of nursing received no more recognition than women who had picked up whatever skills they might have informally. Therefore, one of the first policy concerns of the nursing organizations in Canada was registration for trained nurses. It is indicative of the importance of entry-level education that one of the first nursing organizations in Canada was the Canadian Society of Superintendents of Training Schools, a precursor, with societies of graduate nurses, of the CNA. As discussed in Chapter 9, they wanted registration as recognition that there should be legislated standards for people who provided nursing care. Registration recognized the value of nursing education from programs that met the standards established by the professional regulatory bodies under provincial legislation and provided the public with an expectation of standards of knowledge, skill, and care from RNs.

Educational Standards

Because the motivation of many hospitals in opening schools of nursing was access to a cheap labor force, another early and continuing concern for nursing organizations was the establishment of educational standards. Could hospitals with fewer than 50 or 75 beds provide enough diversity of experiences to prepare students adequately to provide safe, competent care as graduates? How could specialized hospitals, such as psychiatric institutions, provide students with enough general nursing experience? Did nurses not need more general educational background than could be provided in the limitations of an institution devoted to educating only one type of graduate? Standardized curricula were developed by educators and other nursing leaders in the United States and Canada, but they were not mandatory during this period. However, many schools used these models voluntarily to guide program development.

The Move From Hospitals to Postsecondary Educational Institutions

Those who sought reform and improvement of nursing education advocated transferring nurse education responsibilities from the hospital schools to postsecondary educational institutions (Mussallem, 1965). Moving nursing students from the control of hospital boards would reduce exploitation based on the inherent conflict of interest between the hospitals' need for patient care and the students' need for purely educational classes and clinical experiences. There was also recognition that nurses needed general education in the arts, social sciences, and sciences in addition to the more focused learning related to nursing skills and decision making they received in hospitals. Student nurses should not have watered down summaries of anatomy, psychology, and pharmacology "for nurses." Rather, they need to meet the same standards as other postsecondary students. Change from the hospital sector to the educational sector also required political will because it involved a change in provincial responsibility from ministries of health to the ministries responsible for postsecondary education. It also involved the mechanisms for funding nursing education.

In the 1960s, as community colleges were founded across Canada, several provinces, notably Quebec, Ontario, and Saskatchewan, moved nursing education completely out of hospitals. In Alberta, British Columbia, Manitoba, and Nova Scotia, some hospital schools remained in existence until the mid-1990s, although most schools went to the new colleges.

Hospitals were no longer responsible for the education of nurses. New graduates, many of whom would have clinical experiences in a number of hospitals and community agencies, needed orientation as new employees. This change led to some tensions between educational and service institutions. Employers and others in service agencies have expressed views that nursing graduates are not prepared for the real world; that they are book smart but do not appreciate reality; that they have no loyalty; and that their instructors, whether from the college or university, live in ivory towers and do not appreciate the needs of the workplace.

As Kramer pointed out in the United States in 1974, students graduating from nursing schools suffered "reality shock" in the world of work because the ideals they had been taught in school were not played out in their workplaces. Nearly 30 years later, this phenomenon is still evident in new graduates (Boychuk Duchscher, 2001). Competition for educational clinical placements in health service institutions has become a problem, especially in big cities. Health care agencies, stressed by funding cutbacks and restructuring of the 1990s resulting in nursing position layoffs, the disappearance of senior nursing leadership and management positions, bed closures, shorter lengths of stay, higher patient acuity, and a nursing shortage, are more selective about how many and what level of students they will accept on any given unit and at any time. At the same time, employers and others in the service setting comment that the new graduate has strong skills of problem solving and critical thinking and a strong theoretical base. The recognition that the aim of both education and service is to ensure safe, quality, knowledge-based nursing care for the patient has led to greater dialogue among service agencies and education programs.

Entry to Practice

Educational qualifications for entry level RNs have been a policy issue from the early days of organized nursing. The superintendents of nursing and graduates in the early years of the 20th century wanted to ensure that entry to practice as an RN was restricted to those who had completed approved nursing education programs. In the final years of the century, most nursing organizations in the country were working to achieve the bachelor's degree as the new minimum qualification to become an RN. This policy position became known as "baccalaureate as entry to practice." In 1982, the CNA endorsed a resolution calling for the baccalaureate degree as entry to practice by the year 2000.

By 1989, all provincial professional associations had passed similar resolutions (Bajnok, 1992). However, there was resistance from many provincial governments, from members of other professions, and from a number of nurses. The need for increased education of nurses was questioned on the grounds that existing nurses were adequately prepared, concerns that baccalaureate-prepared nurses would be more expensive to educate and hire, and an implied fear that more educated nurses would be less compliant. Concerns on the part of diploma-prepared nurses that they would lose their jobs if the entry standard were changed were reduced by grandparenting provisions in all provinces and by the realities of a nursing shortage. Leaders were careful to emphasize that diploma graduates should continue their learning in nursing practice as they, like other new graduates, move along the continuum that Benner (1984) identified as being from novice to expert.

Under the authority of legislation, nursing regulatory bodies in each province or territory establish the educational standards and mechanisms to approve curricula, thereby ensuring that graduates will be educationally prepared to meet the minimum competencies required to begin or enter the practice of nursing. Nursing, like law, medicine, and engineering, for example, is a self-regulating profession. For many years, registration as an RN has been based on graduation from an approved school of nursing and success on standardized national registration examinations.

Nursing organizations recognized that nursing competencies for beginning practitioners needed to be clearly identified. The CNA initiated a national initiative to identify entry-level competencies (CNA, 1997). Regulatory bodies are responsible for protecting the public from harm and for the regulation of nursing practice and education. Because nursing is a self-regulating profession, the regulatory bodies determine the minimum educational requirements. Across the country, they have moved to use the competencies as their requirements of entering or beginning RNs to meet standards of nursing practice. To receive provincial approval for their programs from the nursing regulatory body, schools of nursing must prepare graduates who meet these competency requirements. It became evident that the curriculum offered in baccalaureate programs most closely matched the competency and standard requirements. The regulators of nursing concluded, therefore, that to provide nursing care to meet the needs of the Canadian public, educational standards for entry to practice would have to change. In some provinces, no changes in legislation or regulation were required. In others, persuading provincial governments to make the required changes to legislation or regulations, despite the strong evidence for the need for change, has proved to be a major challenge.

Many governments have been slow to support the new entry-level requirement and, some, such as in Saskatchewan and Manitoba, have attempted to move away from baccalaureate as entry to practice after it was established as public policy. A key question to ask is whether these governments would consider reversing support of educational requirements viewed as necessary by the members of the profession for any profession other than nursing. Political action by nurses, nursing students, and other health care providers has been pivotal in persuading provincial governments that nurses do need the content of the baccalaureate curriculum (Buresh & Gordon, 2000).

Canadian Approach to Achieving the Degree for Entry to Practice

The baccalaureate as entry to practice policy position of the profession of RNs has led to cooperation among nursing schools. Now community colleges, institutions, and universities throughout Canada are collaborating to offer nursing degree programs together. Collaboration among colleges and universities in most provinces and territories has been the route chosen to capitalize on the strengths of both types of institutions. This approach maximizes the range of faculty expertise and combines available resources to achieve quality nursing education programs.

Collaboration

Although more complex to administer than stand-alone programs, the commitment of nursing educators to the baccalaureate degree for entry to practice has been reflected in the work of nursing educators to maintain collaborative efforts. Many collaborations were initiated well in advance of the common deadline set by nursing regulatory bodies (in most cases, the year 2000) or before the passage of any legislation. Nurse educators from diploma and baccalaureate programs in several parts of the country got together to create collaborative, joint, or partnership programs that would reflect the best of college and university programs. In some cases, for example in Ontario, these bottom-up collaborative initiatives initially failed because of the reluctance of the provincial government to finance them. However, when the Ontario government adopted the policy of the College of Nurses of Ontario (the regulatory body) that the baccalaureate degree should be the criterion for entry to practice, relationships had been formed and much of the groundwork was in place.

In provinces such as British Columbia and Alberta, collaborative programs were funded but were required to retain a diploma exit after 3 years. The numbers of students who could proceed to the degree were restricted. In other provinces, such as New Brunswick and Nova Scotia, diploma schools have been closed, and the human and physical resources have been allocated to the universities.

Application of Political Processes: Saskatchewan

Policy implementation is well under way across Canada after many decades of lobbying by nurses and nursing organizations through effective, successful use of political processes. For example, in 1984, the Saskatchewan Registered Nurses Association (SRNA), the regulatory and professional association, formally adopted the policy position of the baccalaureate as entry to practice by the year 2000. The Nursing Education Program of Saskatchewan (NEPS), a collaborative program of the Saskatchewan Institute of Applied Science and Technology (SIAST) and the University of Saskatchewan, which accepted its first students in 1996, was set to have the convocation of its first graduates in the spring of 2000.

On January 21, 2000, the minister of health announced that the government did not support the degree as the sole entry to practice but would also recognize a diploma as entry to practice. There were a number of pressures that gave rise to the announcement, one of which was the growing realization of the existing and expected nursing shortage. The SRNA objected to the government's announcement. Its position was that, in keeping with the fact that nursing is a self-regulating profession, the responsibility for regulation of nursing practice and entry-to-practice educational requirements was legitimately that of the SRNA, through legislation and through expertise.

On the day of the announcement, government representatives made presentations to the students and faculty at both collaborative partner program sites in Regina and Saskatoon. With faculty providing powerful models of leadership, nursing students from all 4 years of the program demonstrated their skills in organization, education, information sharing, and communication—and their understanding of the importance of respectful relationships throughout the process. They advanced their strong position in support of their education program and of the degree as the requirement for entry to practice, backed by evidence. Their position, like that of the SRNA, was that nursing students need an undergraduate education that prepares them for an increasingly complex health care system and increasingly complex patient health problems. They advocated for their own education and also for the quality of education of those students who would follow them. They met with politicians, senior public servants, and the media. They planned effective rallies at the legislature in Regina and, during one rally, brought their suitcases as a symbol of their intent to leave the province if they were unable to convince the government of the need for the full content of the nursing degree program.

The SRNA reactivated their previously established political action committee, which had already laid solid groundwork on the issue by having met with all members of the legislative assembly. SRNA officials met with the minister of health, public servants, editorial boards of major media, columnists, and reporters. The deans of nursing at SIAST and the University of Saskatchewan developed two policy option briefing notes for the minister and her staff outlining, first, broad options and, second, educational options to address the nursing shortage. The minister of health met with the deans, faculty, student representatives, and other stakeholders and agreed that there could be a different approach. At a March 13, 2000, meeting, the issue was resolved when the minister, the president of the SRNA, and the deans of nursing signed a Memorandum of Understanding that was based on the policy option briefing notes. The student representatives made a significant contribution to the meeting.

This experience helped students to understand the role of politics and the political process in establishing policy and influencing decisions that directly affected them, their future, their profession, and the public (Box 11.2). This experience was also notable with respect to the actions of the minister of health, who had taken a firm and public policy position on January 21, 2000. In the ensuing days and weeks, the minister was open to reviewing policy options presented by the deans and to hearing the evidence that was presented by many groups and individuals. She is to be commended for having the courage and wisdom to get cabinet support for publicly changing her position, based on sound information; this is a fine example of democracy in action.

Although this situation had a successful outcome, there have been different outcomes in other provinces, such as Manitoba. As of the spring of 2004, the issue of an undergraduate university nursing degree as the educational requirement for beginning RNs had not been consistently resolved across Canada.

BOX 11.2	Reflecting on the Saskatchewan Experience

The processes and outcomes represented in the Saskatchewan experience show how sound policy, leadership, hard work, commitment to an evidence-based position, and collaboration, as well as careful, respectful participation in the political process, can achieve desired results. Identify the elements inherent in the implementation of the political process. Here are some activities to guide your reflection:

■ Identify the policy issue. Comment on the opportunity.
■ Identify the steps of the political process as they were used in this situation.
■ Speculate on the powerful or powerless feeling of the students with respect to the future of the program in which they were enrolled and the future of the profession of nursing from the day of the announcement (January 21, 2000) until receiving news of the signing of the memorandum of understanding (March 13, 2000).
■ Speculate on the range of feelings of the students with respect to esteem, confidence, and health in the time period from the announcement by the minister to the resolution of the policy.
■ Identify the role of visibility and how it was operationalized.
■ Identify the key stakeholders and how they exercised their power and influence.
■ Identify the role of collaboration and innovation.
■ Imagine yourself a student leader in this situation; then develop a political action plan.
■ How would you evaluate the use of the political process and the elements of the process in this situation? What are the ways in which you could define success, had the government not supported the policy?
■ What suggestions would you recommend to acknowledge the minister of health for her leadership and courage in accepting a policy that she did not initially support?

■ ORGANIZATIONS FOCUSING ON UNDERGRADUATE NURSING ISSUES

Although the first university programs began shortly after World War I, it was not until 1942, in the middle of World War II, that the leaders of Canada's university nursing programs got together to form what became the Canadian Association of Schools of Nursing (CASN). The shortage of nurses precipitated by the war created opportunities from which the association could benefit (Kirkwood & Bouchard, 1992). The CNA facilitated the first meeting, and, in the early days, there was much debate about whether this organization should be affiliated with the CNA. Eventually, the deans and directors of the university-based programs decided that they had unique concerns that could best be articulated by a separate organization. With improvements in communications and a clearer vision of the future of undergraduate nursing education, the CASN became one of the first voices encouraging other nursing organizations to endorse baccalaureate preparation as the entry to practice requirement.

The CASN also recognized a need for developing and implementing accreditation of university schools of nursing. Provincial nursing regulatory bodies had standards for schools of nursing that had to be met for students to be eligible for registration. These standards were applied both to diploma and to university schools and were minimum requirements for entry to practice. As a result, the standards did not reflect excellence in academic nursing education. Accreditation was implemented to assess and monitor baccalaureate programs using criteria of excellence in relevance, accountability, relatedness, and uniqueness (CASN, 1995).

In 1985, the first accreditation review was completed (Kirkwood & Bouchard, 1992). Since then, most university schools have undergone the peer-review process that helps schools to recognize their strengths and identify areas for improvement. In Ontario, when the educational standard became baccalaureate as entry to practice by 2005, the College of Nurses of Ontario—the regulatory body in that province—designated the CASN accreditation as the requirement for approval.

With the growth of collaborative programs across the country, community colleges working with universities were admitted to associate membership in the CASN. In 2002, in recognition of the colleges' major contributions to the education of nurses at the baccalaureate level, they were accorded full membership, and the name of the organization was changed to the Canadian Association of Schools of Nursing (CASN).

Students in universities formed their own organization, the Canadian University Nursing Students' Association (CUNSA), in 1971. The CUNSA initially represented only university nursing students. It provided opportunities for exchange of ideas and solidarity among students across the country. The CUNSA regional and national conventions have been sources of inspiration and professional pride for nursing students. The organization decided in 1992 to change its name to the Canadian Nursing Students' Association (CNSA) to be more inclusive and consistent with the partnership innovations in nursing education programs in many parts of Canada. With collaboration among universities and colleges, the concerns of all nursing students could be better served by one organization. Students have taken the lead in recognizing similarities of issues and the strength of one national nursing student organization. The CNSA provides important opportunities for networking, communication, learning, and leadership to its members (Therrien, 1992) and has produced an impressive videotape designed for recruitment to the profession of nursing.

■ FUTURE CHALLENGES IN UNDERGRADUATE EDUCATION

Undergraduate nursing education still faces a number of challenges that must be addressed, including curricula, recruitment, and relationships with clinical agencies.

Curricula

To prepare nurses to meet the requirements of a rapidly changing health care system today and in the future, schools of nursing continually update and modify curricula. The competencies identified by nursing regulatory bodies are the foundation on which curricula are developed and have a fundamental influence on what is taught in nursing education programs. However, programs differed in their approaches to organizing and delivering curricula. For example, the caring curriculum, primary health care and population health, and particular theories have provided the philosophical organizers for different programs.

Research

In recent years, there has been increasing emphasis on research findings to ensure that nursing practice decisions are based on evidence (this is sometimes referred to as research utilization, knowledge transfer, or evidence-based practice). There has also been an increased emphasis on the theoretical underpinnings of nursing practice and decision making.

Most curricula for entry level RNs are designed to educate clinical generalists who can function at a beginning level in a wide variety of health care situations. New graduates need background to function in workplaces ranging from the community to acute care and to demonstrate an understanding of primary health care principles. Most hospital units are highly specialized, with a high level of patient acuity, early discharge, and high patient turnover. Because of these factors, along with a nursing shortage, there is often a tension between employers who would like job-ready employees and educators whose responsibility is to meet the educational needs of students whose future careers are likely to involve work in a variety of settings.

A paradox of employer expectations is that, although there is a desire for nurses who have specialized skills, there is often an assumption in their work assignment patterns that any nurse can work in any setting (i.e., "a nurse is a nurse is a nurse"). The hiring of new graduates in casual positions to float throughout the organization is an example of this approach, which exacerbates the difficulties faced by new graduates adapting to the workplace.

Realizing that health care and the demands for nursing skills are changing and will continue to change rapidly, nursing educators have chosen to concentrate on teaching students skills that will help them to adapt over a working lifetime, with emphasis on critical thinking, attention to process, and decision making based on evidence and analysis. Rapid changes in technology and social expectations mean that specific skills or procedures may not be relevant by the time today's students are established in their careers. Students require basic clinical knowledge and skills, along with skills of analysis and critical thinking, communication and relationships, self-directed learning, problem solving and decision making, and patient teaching. They also need to learn to apply theory and use research-based evidence to inform their care.

Another research issue is the funding of nursing education research. Early research by nurses in Canada focused on nursing education and administration, partly because graduate education in the discipline was not available and nurses had master's degrees and doctorates in education or administration. With the realization that nursing should pursue research in nursing care, the emphasis on education and administration was discouraged by educators and funding agencies. Now there is increased interest in nursing organization and systems research, but there is little emphasis on research into nursing education, especially clinical education. As a result, although nursing educators promote evidence-based practice, they have little evidence on which to base their own practice. With the decrease in clinical placements, the cost of clinical education, and because of the fundamental need for research in teaching effectiveness, this area will need to be embraced and acted on by health care provider education administrators, educators, funding agencies, and policymakers.

Technology

One particular knowledge area for which students must be prepared is the use of technology. As the machinery of acute care and the communications of the Internet and intranets become more sophisticated and are used more broadly in community care, students need the basic skills of informatics to be able to use present technology and adapt to new developments (Hebert, 2000). Students also need the critical skills to assess the benefits and threats that technology may pose to quality of life, collection of data for evidence-based decisions, access to information, and patient confidentiality. They will need the preparation to make informed and ethical decisions about incorporating technologic initiatives into their practice.

Systems and Creating a Culture of Safety

Because nurses need skills to influence their workplaces and to help shape the health care system, there is an ethical and practical imperative to include courses on the political process and systems theory in undergraduate programs. Students need a sound knowledge and understanding about how systems are designed, how they work or fail, and how to influence them. They need this knowledge to function effectively as clinicians for their patients and to survive and thrive as employees and as team members and leaders. Such knowledge can be as important in a nurse's career as the science base and clinical competence; it is enhanced when programs include student representatives in policy development activities.

Of particular importance is the systems approach to patient safety and attention to the reduction of errors and critical incidents that contribute to preventable injuries and deaths in the Canadian health care system. The Canadian Adverse Events Study, reported in the May 2004 *Canadian Medical Association Journal* (*CMAJ*) (Baker et al., 2004), using 2000–2001 Canadian hospital data, reported that 7.5% of patients admitted to Canadian hospitals experienced one or more adverse events. Expert reviewers considered 27% of these to be preventable.

Schools of nursing will increasingly be held accountable for including a systems approach to patient safety in the curricula (Davidson Dick, 2004). One Canadian school of nursing is developing key curricular concepts for integration into courses and curricula. These include the difference in and the complementarity of individual and systems approaches to patient safety; the major components of building a safer system; the concept of root cause analysis; Canadian statistics on errors, preventable injury, and death; systems hazards and defenses; the central role of team coordination and communication; the role of incident reporting and following-up to improve system functioning; and the balance of accountability in the context of shifting from a culture of blame to a culture of safety (Davidson Dick, 2004).

Application of Political and Nursing Processes in Undergraduate Education

The earlier review of how nurses applied the political process to a major public policy issue—the baccalaureate degree as entry to practice—is replicated by the equally important and effective application of the political process integrated with the nursing process in an undergraduate student patient care situation.

A first-year nursing student was one of eight classmates who had an extended clinical experience in a convalescent rehabilitation care setting. Her patient was a young, developmentally delayed woman who required extensive personal care. As a consequence, the nursing student developed an understanding of the character and personality of the patient as well as of her needs and problems. During the course of the clinical experience, the attending physician sought a psychiatric consultation. The student read the consult notes and disagreed with the conclusions the psychiatrist had reached. The adoption of the view of the psychiatrist would have a profound impact on the life of the patient in a particular and limiting direction. The adoption of the view of the nursing student would have an equally profound influence on the life of the patient, but in a more positive and growth-supporting direction that the patient had identified as important to her.

The identification of the issue was based on a clinical assignment. The teacher* had asked each of the students to identify with his or her patient, when possible, one issue that was important to the patient and that would have an impact on the patient's life. The students were to present that issue in the multidisciplinary weekly team conference. The teacher asked the students to use the framework of politics (who gets what, when, and how) and the political process (the problem-solving process applied to issues of power and influence) along with the nursing process (the problem-solving process applied to issues of care and service).

The student discussed the situation with the teacher, and, using the elements of the political process, together they approached the unit manager and then the social worker. In each instance, they presented the findings of the student and her rationale for her position and asked for their support in the weekly rounds, if they agreed with her position. The student was a novice in the situation and was not a confident participant in this new and rather intimidating situation. She practised the presentation of her case in private with classmates, and, when the time came, though very nervous, she presented all of her well-developed case— the analysis and the conclusions—before the large group of professionals. The unit manager spoke up with her support, followed by the social worker, and the student's position was endorsed at the meeting. Her use of politics and the political process were particularly meaningful in this case because the patient could not speak effectively in her own interests.

This was only one of the achievements of the eight students who implemented politics and the political process in representing the interests of their patients at that team conference that day. They each gained an understanding of the relationship of power and health, the interrelatedness of the nursing and political processes, and the key elements of each (Box 11.3).

In contemporary society, nursing students also need an understanding of the social, cultural, economic, and environmental contexts that affect health and the requirements for nursing care. These vary depending on regions, communities, cultures, and the variables that determine health of populations. As graduates, nurses then take these understandings to inform their efforts to influence health and social policy.

---

* NOTE: The teacher was Diana Davidson Dick.

| BOX 11.3 | Reflecting on Nursing Process, Politics, and Education in Action |

Just as the Saskatchewan nurses applied the political process to achieve baccalaureate education for entry to practice, so did a student and her colleagues use the political process to advocate for a patient. Here are some thoughts and exercises to consider in relation to that situation:

■ State the issue that the student identified.
■ Identify the steps of the nursing and political processes as they were used in this situation.
■ Identify the elements inherent in the implementation of the political process.
■ Speculate on the student's feelings of powerfulness or powerlessness.
■ Speculate on the range of feelings of the student with respect to courage, esteem, confidence, and health in the situation.
■ Identify how this student's actions made her role in knowledge-based caring and decision making more visible.
■ Identify the key stakeholders. Identify the role of collaboration and innovation.
■ Imagine yourself the student leader in a similar situation: Develop the nursing process and political process plan.
■ Imagine that the multidisciplinary team had not supported the perspective of the student. What process would the student need to use to achieve the best result for the patient?

Recruitment and Retention

With an aging population that will require more health care, the impending nursing shortage, and the aging of qualified faculty to teach in nursing programs (Canadian Institute for Health Information [CIHI], 2001), recruiting qualified students, faculty, and academic leaders is a pressing concern for nursing educators. There is a global skills shortage, and nowhere is it more pronounced than in nursing and nursing education.

Sufficient Students, Educators, and Administrators—and the Transition of New Graduates to the Workplace

During the 1990s, as part of dramatic downsizing and restructuring of the health care system across Canada, thousands of RNs lost jobs, and nursing positions at all levels of service organizations were eliminated. Although other groups of employees were affected, nursing was by far the hardest hit. The federal government's financial transfers to provinces for health care and education were decreased from $18.5 billion to $12.5 billion between 1996 and 1999 alone (CNA, 1998). At the same time, some provincial governments decreased funding for nursing education seats. These events had a domino effect, creating a shortage of nurses in practice and education. In some jurisdictions, there has been a shortage of qualified applicants to nursing schools because people made career plans based on the reality of news stories about nursing position cuts and lack of availability of jobs in the health care workplace. Equally serious and significant was the deletion of senior nursing leadership and management positions. This was an international phenomenon and one of the most stunning examples of policy decisions being made and implemented without adequate research or evidence.

There has been a pattern since the 1960s of nursing shortages followed by oversupply. Governments, administrators, and educators have made decisions that have long-term consequences without adequate data for human resource forecasting. In some cases, these decisions reflect a lack of vision about the future of health care or a lack of agreement on the vision. Because there is a lag time of about 5 years between application and graduation from a baccalaureate nursing program, the education system has often been out of step with the numbers of employees needed by the workplace. Reactive rather than proactive planning for future needs has meant that undergraduate nursing programs have been unable to satisfy demands even when they have been able to predict trends. Policies producing cutbacks, followed by reinstatement of nursing positions, have had impacts throughout the system, including reduction in applications to nursing programs in some geographic areas. The number of new graduates is thus reduced, and the long-term impact on health care will be felt for many years. Bed closures and budget cuts in community health and home care and throughout the system have meant that there are fewer clinical placements available for student learning, increased workloads, and stressful work environments along with fewer nurses to serve as mentors to novice nurses.

The transition of the new graduate to the workplace is one area that needs attention and cooperation between education and service. Initially described as "reality shock" (Kramer, 1974), this phenomenon continues and has been exacerbated by today's intense clinical environment. This area is being explored, with new strategies proposed (Duchscher, 2004).

Nurses in all areas are aging. The Nursing Strategy for Canada (Advisory Committee on Health Human Resources, 2000) recommended that governments increase student enrollment by 10% to allow for replacement of the nurses older than 40 years of age who can be anticipated to retire as the baby-boom generation reaches senior citizen status. The mean age of faculty is about 6 years older than the mean age of staff nurses (43.3 years and 48.8 years, respectively; CIHI, 2001). There will be a crisis in the capacity to prepare new nurses unless effective strategies to ensure replacement of nursing educators are implemented immediately. Both the Kirby report to the Senate (2002) and Romanow's Royal Commission Report (2002) recommended strategies to improve the tracking, recruitment, and retention of health human resources, including nurses.

Diversity

As well as ensuring adequate numbers of new nurses and the faculty to teach them, it is important that the nurses and those who educate them reflect the diversity of Canada's population. Cultural issues are included in curricula of schools of nursing largely because Canadian RNs can expect to care for and provide service to an increasingly culturally diverse patient base—individuals, families, groups, and communities (CNA, 2000). Although the principles of cultural diversity theory provide the framework for this area of competence, examples and application differ according to regional differences across the country. For example, in Saskatchewan and northern British Columbia, where there is a high aboriginal population, emphasis would be on understanding the culture and health practices of native peoples, whereas the focus in Vancouver or Toronto would reflect the cultural diversity of immigrant populations in those locations.

In contrast to the past when Weir (1932) reported that 84% of the Anglophone student nurses who responded to his questionnaires gave their ethnic origin as English, Scottish, or Irish, the RN student population has become increasingly diverse. There was a time when the great majority of students entered nursing schools directly from high school and nursing studies were their major responsibility. Although students continue to come from high school, large numbers enter programs with degrees, diplomas, or other credentials in other disciplines, from other occupations and careers. Many have many roles and responsibilities in addition to those of student; they may be parents, be caregivers for elderly relatives, and have full- or part-time jobs.

Despite this diversity, most nursing students in many schools of nursing continue to be white and female. Faculty who teach, coach, and guide, and administrators and managers of nursing programs (deans, directors, program heads), are even less culturally diverse. This is a concern on a number of levels. Women of color, men, men of color, and those whose culture and race are not reflected in their school or profession lack role models. They rarely see themselves and their particular concerns reflected in their peers, faculty, and nursing education administration or in the practice settings. As well, there are many options available to white women, the predominant group in the majority of Canadian schools of nursing. As a matter of policy and practicality, there is a need to develop strategies to replenish, recruit, and support students from a much more diverse pool than has been the practice (Sullivan, 2000). The Canadian government developed and has proudly championed cultural diversity through promoting public policy and celebrating multiculturalism, and Canada's population has become increasingly culturally diverse.

In light of these factors, it is increasingly important that the population of working nurses and, hence, the nursing student population, should be proportionally culturally representative of the general population of a province, territory, or region. For example, a number of initiatives are under way to recruit and retain aboriginal nursing students (see Chapter 24). There are solid examples of this in nursing education programs across the country.

Changing Relationships Among Educational and Service Agencies and With Other Health Care Disciplines

As they face the challenges of dealing with recruitment issues and shortages of nurses, nurses working in educational and service institutions are developing new relationships and new models for educating nurses. Demonstration projects where educators, unit nurses, and students work together to break down some of the barriers within health care (Horsburgh et al., 1998) are being proposed and tested, as are new ways of preceptoring, mentoring, and supervising student practice. The pressing need for research in this area as indicated above cannot be overemphasized.

Trends in health care that emphasize interdisciplinary teams working collaboratively have implications for the education of nurses and all other providers of health care. Romanow (2002, p. 109), in his Royal Commission Report, *Building on Values: The Future of Health Care in Canada*, stated, "in view of . . . changing trends, corresponding changes must be made in the way health care providers are educated and trained. If health care providers are expected to work together and share expertise in a team environment, it makes sense that their education and training should prepare them for this type of working arrangement." In response to this recommendation, the federal government is providing funding for projects to improve interdisciplinary education of health care professionals.

In the next few years will come challenging and demanding new initiatives that will continue to change the face of undergraduate nursing education to meet rapid changes in health care and an increasing demand for new approaches to the provision of nursing care and services with stronger links among education, practice, research, and administration. As the move to reverse some of the negative outcomes of restructuring and program management continues, one result is likely to be that nursing leaders in management positions in education and service come together to support an environment for evidence-based or research-based nursing practice and the conduct of applied research in the clinical or service setting.

■ SUMMARY

Since the first modern nursing schools opened more than 100 years ago, undergraduate nursing education in Canada has been influenced by policies of nursing organizations, health service agencies, educational institutions, and governments. The health care system throughout Canada is highly political, and it is one of the most highly valued publicly funded social programs. Its maintenance is a profound concern of the Canadian public and a number of stakeholders. It is a system with many subsystems, such as rural, remote, northern, community, acute, and home care, with a range of disease-based specialties and approaches to health such as population health and primary health care. An understanding of the intertwining of relationships, systems, and nursing and political processes is needed by students and graduates if they are to be effective clinicians and participants in decision making. This understanding is needed to achieve positive outcomes for patients and the effective functioning at many levels of the systems in which patients receive care and service. All of these factors have current and future implications for the curriculum and for student learning, and they play a role in job satisfaction.

Nursing educators have a responsibility to be proactive in identifying and researching improvements in curricula and teaching–learning strategies and also to be open to responding to initiatives and recommendations of others. Research is one of the mandates of university faculty. With the establishment of educational programs based on partnerships of colleges and universities, coupled with a pressing need to make the most efficient use of resources, there will be increased emphasis on collaborative research among university and college faculty and students. One of the challenges facing nursing education is the need for increased emphasis on asking the questions and collecting the evidence on which sound educational policies can be based and for developing a stronger research base in the area of effective teaching–learning strategies in undergraduate education.

Nursing has identified four domains: practice, education, research, and administration. There is an urgent need to increase the domains to six, with the addition of leadership and policy, both of which need to be integrated into the curricula of undergraduate nursing education.

REFLECTIONS on the Chapter . . .

1. What strategies would you use to attract into nursing men and members of other underrepresented groups?

2. How could educational and service organizations work together to improve the clinical education of undergraduate students? What policies would need to be in place for students and for faculty? Would there be an effect on patients?

3. What is the regulatory body in your province or territory? Has the policy of the baccalaureate as the minimum educational requirement for entry to practice been implemented?

4. Discuss the established domains of nursing (practice, education, research, and administration). What would the likely impact be of adding leadership and policy as two additional domains of nursing?

References

Advisory Committee on Health Human Resources. (2000). *The nursing strategy for Canada* [Online]. Ottawa: Health Canada. Available: http://www.hc-sc.gc.ca/english/pdf/media/nursing_strategy.pdf

Bajnok, I. (1992). Entry-level educational preparation for nursing. In A. J. Baumgart & J. Larsen, (Eds.), *Canadian nursing faces the future* (2nd ed., pp. 401–419). Toronto: Mosby Year Book.

Baker, G., Norton, P., Flintoft, V., et al. (2004). The Canadian Adverse Events Study: The Incidence of Adverse Events Among Hospital Patients in Canada. *Canadian Medical Association Journal, 170* (11), 1678–1686.

Benner, P. (1984). *From novice to expert: Excellence and power in clinical nursing practice.* Menlo Park, CA: Addison-Wesley.

_____. (2000). Forward. In B. Buresh & S. Gordon. *From silence to voice* (p. ix). Ottawa: Canadian Nurses Association.

Boychuk Duchscher, J. E. (2001). Out in the real world: Newly graduated nurses in acute-care speak out. *Journal of Nursing Administration, 31*(9), 426–438.

Buresh, B., & Gordon, S. (2000). *From silence to voice: What nurses know and must communicate to the public.* Ottawa: Canadian Nurses Association.

Canadian Association of University Schools of Nursing. (1995). *Accreditation guidelines.* Ottawa: Author.

Canadian Institute for Health Information. (2001). *Canadian Institute for Health Information reports moderate rise in registered nurses workforce, fewer RNs working on casual basis, more working full-time* [Executive Summary, Online]. Available: http://secure.cihi.ca/ cihiweb/dispPage.jsp?cw_page=media_23may2001_e

Canadian Nurses Association. (1997). *National nursing competency project final report.* Ottawa: Author.

_____. (1998). The quiet crisis in health care: A proposal for a federal government investment in quality health care [Brief, Online]. Retrieved 2002 from http://www.cna-nurses.ca/pages/qcrisis/frames/qcframe.htm

_____. (2000). Cultural diversity: Changes and challenges. *Nursing Now, 7,* 1–4.

Carpenter, H. M. (1970). The University of Toronto School of Nursing: An agent of change. In M.Q. Innis (Ed.), *Nursing education in a changing society* (pp. 86–108). Toronto: University of Toronto Press.

Coburn, J. (1981). "I see and am silent": A short history of nursing in Ontario. In D. Coburn, C. D'Arcy, P. New, et al. (Eds.), *Health and Canadian society* (pp. 182–201). Toronto: Fitzhenry & Whiteside.

Davidson Dick, D. (2004, March). Designing a safer health care system: What it means for nursing education (excerpt, Message from the dean, SIAST Nursing Division News). *Canadian Nurse, 100*(3), 32–33.

Davidson Dick, D., and Hoffman, C. (2004, October). *Designing a safer system: Nursing education embraces partnerships.* Paper presented at the meeting of the Registered Nurses Association of Ontario, International Nursing Education Conference, Toronto.

Dick, D. D. (1985). *Politics, power and the political process.* Tel Aviv, Israel: ICN Quadrennial Congress.

Duchscher. J. E. B. (2004). Transition to professional nursing practice: Emerging issues and initiatives. In M. H. Oermann & K. T. Heinrich, *Annual Review of Nursing Education* (Vol. 2, pp. 283–303). New York: Springer.

Errington, J. (1990). Pioneers and suffragists. In S. Burt, L. Code, & L. Dorey (Eds.), *Changing patterns: Women in Canada* (pp. 51–78). Toronto: McClelland & Stewart.

Garey, D., & Hott, L. R. (Producers). (1988). Sentimental women need not apply: A history of the American nurse [videorecording by Florentine Films]. Willowdale, ON: McNabb & Connolly.

Gibbon, J. M., & Mathewson, M. S. (1947). *Three centuries of Canadian nursing.* Toronto: MacMillan.

Government of Canada. (1964–1965). Royal commission on health services [E. Hall, Chairman]. Ottawa: Queen's Printer.

Hebert, M. (2000). A national education strategy to develop nursing informatics competencies. *Canadian Journal of Nursing Leadership, 13*(2), 11–14.

The History of Nursing Society, School for Graduate Nurses, McGill University. (1929). *Pioneers of nursing in Canada.* Montreal: Canadian Nurses Association.

Horsburgh, M. E., Stamler, L. L., Snowdon, A. W., et al. (1998, July). The role of the professional nurse mentor and staff nurse outcomes in the clinical education unit. In *Proceedings of the Workgroup of European Nurse Researchers, 9th Biennial Conference* (Vol. 1, pp. 342–348). Helsinki, Finland: International Council of Nurses.

King, M. K. (1970). The development of university nursing education. In M. Q. Innis (Ed.), *Nursing education in a changing society* (pp. 67–85). Toronto: University of Toronto Press.

Kirby, M. J. L. (2002). *The health of Canadians—The federal role.* Ottawa: The Standing Senate Committee on Social Affairs, Science and Technology, Government of Canada. Available: http://www.hc-sc.gc.ca/english/hhr/1

Kirkwood, R. A., & Bouchard, J. L. (1992). *Take counsel with one another: A beginning history of the Canadian Association of University Schools of Nursing, 1942–1992.* Ottawa: Canadian Association of University Schools of Nursing.

Kramer, M. (1974). *Reality shock: Why nurses leave nursing.* St. Louis: Mosby.

Lasswell, H. D. (1958). *Politics: Who gets what, when, how.* New York: World Publishing.

McPherson, K. (1996). *Bedside matters: The transformation of Canadian nursing 1900–1990.* Toronto: Oxford University Press.

Mussallem, H. K. (1965). *Nursing education in Canada* [submission to Royal Commission on Health Services]. Ottawa: Queen's Printer.

Nelson, S. (1999). Entering the professional domain: The making of the modern nurse in 17th century France. *Nursing History Review, 7,* 171–187.

Paul, P. (1998). Nursing education becomes synonymous with nursing service. In J. C. Ross-Kerr (Ed.), *Prepared to care: Nurses and nursing in Alberta 1859–1996* (pp. 129–153). Edmonton: University of Alberta Press.

Reverby, S. (1987). A caring dilemma: Womanhood and nursing in historical perspective. *Nursing Research, 36,* 5–11.

Rogers, M. E. (1970). *An introduction to the theoretical basis of nursing.* Philadelphia: F. A. Davis.

Romanow, R. J. (2002). *Building on values: The future of health care in Canada—Final report.* Ottawa: Government of Canada. Retrieved September 27, 2004, from http://www.hc-sc.gc.ca/english/pdf/care/romanow_e.pdf

Ross-Kerr, J. C. (1998). *Prepared to care: Nurses and nursing in Alberta, 1859 to 1996.* Edmonton: University of Alberta Press.

Sullivan, B. (2000, September/October). Gender diversity vs cultural diversity. *Journal of Professional Nursing, 6*(5), 253–254.

Therrien, L. (1992). *CUNSA & CNSA: A beginning history* [Online]. Available: http://www.cnsa.ca/publications/history/

Weir, G. M. (1932). *Survey of nursing education in Canada.* Toronto: University of Toronto Press.

As a way of engaging with the ideas in this chapter, consider the following:

1. Have you ever considered graduate education in nursing as a possibility for yourself?

2. What would it be important for you to consider in making a decision to pursue graduate education in nursing?

3. What difference might nurses prepared at the graduate level make to the study and practice of nursing?

4. What do you imagine is influencing the current proliferation of Canadian graduate programs in nursing?

CHAPTER
12

Sally Thorne

Graduate Education

University of Victoria School of Nursing faculty and graduate students. ▶

After completing this chapter, you will be able to:

1. Understand the implications of the historical context associated with graduate nursing education in Canada.

2. Identify specific challenges faced in Canada by nurses with graduate preparation at various levels.

3. Recognize the impact of various social, historical, economic, and political forces on the practice realities of Canadian nurses who have graduate degrees.

4. Interpret major issues and controversies associated with graduate nursing education in Canada.

5. Examine current social, political, and economic trends as they shape current graduate nursing education.

6. Identify opportunities by which the profession of nursing in Canada can direct its future through strategic advancement of graduate education.

This chapter focuses on the contributions made to the health care system by nurses educated at the graduate level. A special emphasis is placed on the contributions of nurses prepared at the master's level, whose focus is advanced practice, and those prepared at the doctoral and postdoctoral levels, whose focus is research.

Building on a historical overview of the evolution within graduate education in Canada, this chapter examines the impact of graduate education in general as well as some of the specific contributions made by Canadian nurses with graduate level educations. Within this discussion, the reader will find a further exploration of some of the realities of graduate-prepared nurses in their places of work, the issues that arise for these nurses in practice, and the barriers that need to be addressed if the full potential of these nurses is to be realized.

■ HISTORY OF GRADUATE NURSING EDUCATION IN CANADA

The second half of the 20th century brought graduate nursing education into the mainstream for the profession in Canada. In 1959, the first master's program in the country was launched at the University of Western Ontario, followed quickly by the inauguration of three more within the next decade, at McGill, Montréal, and the University of British Columbia (UBC). With a handful of new programs becoming available each decade, 22 universities were offering master's degrees in nursing by 2004 (Association of Universities and Colleges in Canada [AUCC], 2003). The first doctoral program in the country, at the University of Alberta, admitted students in 1991, and, within the next 12 years, the country boasted nine established doctoral programs in nursing (AUCC, 2003; Canadian Association of Schools of Nursing, 2004). The history of the evolution of graduate programs in Canada explains something of the shape that graduate nursing education has taken in comparison to that of other jurisdictions and provides a foundation for understanding some of the issues that face nurses with graduate preparation in the current academic, scientific, and social context.

Evolution of Master's Degree Programs

Although graduate degrees in other disciplines have been available to nurses for a much longer time, the history of master's programming in the country is one of only 40 years. As can be seen in Table 12.1, there has been a relatively stable proliferation of new master's degree programs in nursing every decade throughout

TABLE 12.1	Proliferation of Graduate Nursing Programs in Canada	
University	**Master's Program**	**Doctoral Program**
Athabasca University	2003	
Dalhousie University	1975	2003
Laurentian University	2004	
L'université de Laval	1991	
L'université de Moncton	1997	
L'université de Montréal	1965	1993
McGill University	1961	1993
McMaster University	1994	1994
Memorial University	1982	
Queens University	1994	
Université du Québec	2001	
University of Alberta	1975	1991
University of British Columbia	1968	1991
University of Calgary	1981	1999
University of Manitoba	1979	
University of New Brunswick	1995	
University of Ottawa	1993	2004
University of Saskatchewan	1986	
University of Toronto	1970	1993
University of Victoria	2003	
University of Western Ontario	1959	2003
University of Windsor	1994	

Note: Data compiled from most recent Canadian statistics AUCC (2003) and CASN (2004). Not listed above are graduate programs leading to a degree other than nursing (such as the Master of Health Sciences, Master of Science in Community Health, Maîtrise en sciences cliniques, interdisciplinary PhD, Doctorat en sciences cliniques) or graduate nursing degrees occurring outside of an approved program, such as doctoral degrees by special arrangement.

the latter part of the 20th century. However, graduate programs designated as *nursing* degree programs still compete with a range of other options open to nurses in Canada, and nursing programs remain only one of several routes by which Canadian nurses obtain graduate education.

Before the local availability of master's nursing programs in Canada, many nurses obtained their graduate preparation in other countries, particularly in the United States. Others undertook graduate work at Canadian universities in such fields as public health, education, medical science, social science, or business administration (Field, Stinson, & Thibaudeau, 1992). Although some of these degree programs drew nurses away from the main focus of their discipline for much of their academic development, others were quite sensitive to the special needs of nurse leaders and produced graduates with specialization in the study of problems directly relevant to their profession. In some instances, nursing faculty members with cross-appointments augmented the learning opportunities for nurses in those disciplines. In other instances, some nurses managed to retain their disciplinary focus within academic environments that were not entirely supportive.

For reasons of proximity and preference, many Canadian nurses continue to obtain graduate education outside of the discipline, and, for the most part, the profession has enjoyed the healthy skill-set mix that can derive from an interdisciplinary perspective. In the early years, however, nurses tended to be less confident that their discipline would produce the highest-quality graduate level preparation for their advancement within such fields as nursing education and health administration (Beaton, 1990; Field et al., 1992); hence, consciousness raising about the relevance of graduate preparation within nursing has been an ongoing challenge.

A continuing complication has been the availability of graduate programs designed specifically with nurses in mind but located somewhat outside of the disciplinary core, such as Master of Health Science programs. In some universities, these programs have evolved collaboratively with the involvement of other disciplines as an evolutionary step toward more comprehensive nursing master's degree offerings (McBride, 1995).

In recognition of the urgent need for augmented graduate educational opportunities for nurses to advance the general academic level of professional nursing in Canada (Mussalem, 1965), nursing leaders creatively pursued a variety of strategies and mechanisms in developing master's programs. Among the strongest supporters of this initiative was the Kellogg Foundation. This foundation was a major presence in Canadian nursing education from 1949 through 1981 (Wood & Ross-Kerr, 2002). The foundation's fellowships to individual nurses helped Canadians obtain graduate degrees elsewhere, and its development grants helped many Canadian universities to support initial programs in their early phases. Approvals to deliver graduate programs were accomplished individually by each university's senate and, in most instances, were explicitly built on a foundational history of high-quality undergraduate programming (McBride, 1995).

Within the Canadian nursing master's programs, the initial focus was primarily on filling the articulated needs within nursing education or nursing administration (McBride, 1995). Since the mid-1970s, that focus has shifted from these functional areas toward clinical specialization and leadership (Allen, 1986; McBride, 1995). Although nursing theory and science are still integral to the curriculum, the primary role of master's degree programs in preparing nurse researchers has gradually shifted since the 1980s as more Canadian nurses have had access to doctoral programs. Although rigorous research preparation was the standard within Canadian nursing master's programs until the advent of doctoral programs in 1991 (Kerr & McPhail, 1996), the master's thesis has become increasingly controversial since then. Some master's programs in nursing continue to require a research-based thesis or include a thesis option; others no longer provide direct research training at this level (Gein, 1994; Kerr & McPhail, 1996; McBride, 1995).

Over its 40-year history, master's education in Canadian nursing has also experienced the effects of other trends and innovations. The rate of admission into graduate programs has not yet attained a sufficient level to meet the profession's projected need to fill senior practice, education, and administrative positions (Kerr & McPhail, 1996). Because Canada's geography makes proximity to learning experiences a significant barrier for many nurses, and because the dominantly female constitution of the profession implies multiple demands upon learners, accessibility and flexibility of graduate education have been important aspects of the ongoing discussion (Broughton & Hoot, 1995; Kerr, 1988). Over the years, a number of innovations in distance learning have been noted (Kerr, 1988), and some components of many of the existing programs are available by distance delivery or Web-based format. Beyond those now delivered entirely by distance format, alternative format master's programs are likely to proliferate across the country as the technology becomes available to ensure high-quality interactive learning experiences (Canadian Nurses Association [CNA], 2004). Two early innovations in the formatting of master's degree programs were the clinical training master's program available at the Family Nursing Unit in Calgary (Wright, Watson, & Duhamel, 1985) and the generic master's program at McGill (Ezer, MacDonald, & Gros, 1991). Although the dominant language of master's instruction in the country has remained English (with 15 English language and 3 French language programs currently available), the University of Ottawa was the first to offer a bilingual program, in 1993 (Kerr & McPhail, 1996).

Although master's programs have rapidly proliferated and produced a generation of leaders for nursing practice, administration, education, and research, this evolution has not resolved the leadership shortage, let alone addressed the projected future demand at this point in our history (Kerr & McPhail, 1996). It is well recognized that, in the early 21st century, Canada has insufficient numbers of adequately prepared nurse educators (Beaton, 1990; Ford & Wertenberger, 1993) and that a significant percentage of the current cadre of nurse educators is within sight of retirement age (May, 2000; Nursing Education Council of British Columbia, 2001). In addition, consensus remains elusive as to what constitutes graduate education in nursing, how it ought to be funded and delivered, and whether academic or professional jurisdictions ought to take the lead in shaping the direction of future developments in master's preparation for Canadian nurses (Beaton, 1990).

Evolution of Doctoral Degree Programs

The evolutionary process for doctoral nursing education in Canada has been much more recent and strategic than the development of master's degree programs. In 1978, the CNA sponsored a national seminar in which nursing leaders endorsed the value of working toward making doctoral nursing education possible in Canada (Zilm, Larose, & Stinson, 1979). From that, the Canadian Nurses Foundation (CNF) and the Canadian Association of University Schools of Nursing (CAUSN) developed a proposal dubbed Operation Bootstrap to obtain funding for the infrastructure on which doctoral programs in nursing might be established (Kerr & McPhail, 1996). Although that proposal was never funded, the cooperative efforts involved in its development stimulated nursing educational leaders across the country to engage in sufficient strategic dialogue to create the basis on which explicit program proposals became successful a decade later. Through this process, Canadian nursing leaders developed a consensus with regard to the general conditions under which doctoral programs ought to be established, including the following:

- Universities with a successful track record in undergraduate and master's programming in nursing
- Close proximity to a full range of interdisciplinary doctoral/medical degree programs
- Sufficient number of doctorally prepared faculty members
- Explicit research development resources (such as programs of research or research units)
- Sufficient levels of research funding and a high degree of scholarly productivity shared among a range of faculty members (Field et al., 1992)

Although the first Canadian nurse to obtain a doctoral degree was Sister Denise Lefebre, SQM, PhD (Docteur de Pédagogie) from l'université de Montréal in 1955, the first to graduate with a doctoral degree in nursing on a special-case basis was Francine Ducharme from McGill in 1990 (Banning, 1990). Such special-case arrangement programs, allowing nurses to obtain doctoral degrees with a substantial nursing component, developed in a number of universities before the launching of actual nursing doctoral programs (Field et al., 1992; Wood & Ross-Kerr, 2002) and have continued in some universities to the present. They differ from interdisciplinary doctoral degrees or degrees taken in another discipline in their explicitly nursing focus but lack the programmatic core disciplinary component that the established nursing programs offer (Kerr & McPhail, 1996).

In 1991, the University of Alberta was the first in the country to launch a fully funded doctoral program in nursing, and its first graduate was Joan Bottorff in 1992, having begun her studies as a special-case student. The political negotiating involved in obtaining funding for that program and admitting the first group of students attracted considerable excitement across the country and was recognized as a landmark achievement (Brink, 1991; Field et al., 1992; Godkin & Bottorff, 1991; Rodger, 1991; Trojan et al., 1996). A second program, at UBC, admitted its first students later that same year (1991), and, in rapid succession, programs were launched at the University of Toronto and by collaborative arrangement at McGill and Montréal in 1993, and at McMaster a year later (Kerr & McPhail, 1996).

Because of the commitment to dialogue and strategic planning throughout the developmental phase of advancing graduate education for the country, the character and shape of the Canadian doctoral nursing programs evolved in a somewhat distinct manner from those in other parts of the globe. A forum on doctoral education in Canada, which was held in late 1990 in Edmonton just before the country launched its first programs, compared the history of doctoral nursing education in the United Kingdom, the United States, and Europe and took advice from such international leaders as Rozella Schlotfeldt and Lisbeth Hocky. By unanimous agreement, the Canadian leaders who were present concluded that doctoral preparation in Canada should lead to a doctorate of philosophy in nursing, and not to a professional doctorate (Jeans, 1990).

A second invitational conference, held in Toronto in April 1995, brought together student and faculty representatives from the five doctoral programs in existence at that time, as well as from universities in which special-case opportunities were available for doctoral degrees in nursing, to examine the substantive context of Canadian PhD nursing programs as they were evolving and developing (Wood, 1997). It was noted that the Canadian programs all had a rather similar structure, requiring an average of four or five courses in core disciplinary knowledge. On that foundation, both coursework and research training were individualized in conjunction with a carefully matched faculty supervisor for each student. Led by Ada Sue Hinshaw, who drew on American examples to point out the quality and resource challenges that a rapid proliferation of doctoral programs could create, participants at that meeting also grappled with such challenging questions as how many doctoral programs Canada should support.

As doctoral programs took hold within the profession's national consciousness, it became apparent that they provide nursing not only with high-quality research training but also, and perhaps more importantly, with the following:

■ The capacity to study the clinical phenomena pertinent to the discipline
■ The conceptual leadership to direct the development of scholarly practice
■ The grounded analytic skills to design systems of nursing practice and health care delivery (Field et al., 1992)

In so doing, these programs create a cadre of future leaders with expertise in both the art and science of nursing.

However, the development of doctoral nursing education in Canada is not without its ongoing challenges. Among the most pressing has been the difficulty in obtaining funding to support nurses pursuing doctoral education. In contrast to the more traditional academic model in which doctoral degrees are pursued before the establishment of family and professional responsibilities, most Canadian nursing doctoral students to date have been mid-career professional women, for whom full-time study is often problematic and expensive. Financial support exclusive to nursing has been scarce, with the CNF able to provide only small numbers of graduate fellowships (Wood & Ross-Kerr, 2002). Further, the kinds of substantive problems relative to nursing care delivery and its outcomes that nurses want to investigate have seldom been viewed competitively within the clinical (medical) and social science funding arenas (Field et al., 1992). The CNA has called on partners within government, health care agencies, universities, and nursing associations to plan cooperatively and share resources to support doctoral education for nurses (CNA, 2003).

With the advent of the Canadian Institutes of Health Research in 2000, many nursing leaders became actively involved in trying to shift the traditionally narrow direction of research support beyond basic and clinical (biomedical) science to include such concerns as the social determinants of health, the psychosocial experience of illness, and the impact of the caring sciences. On the basis of this effort, there is considerable optimism that the profession will continue to make progress in the funding of doctoral nursing education (Wood & Ross-Kerr, 2002). Without doubt, the exceptional quality and productivity of Canada's early nursing doctoral program graduates bode well for the profession's continuing success in this regard.

■ PRACTICE REALITIES AND CHALLENGES FOR GRADUATE-PREPARED NURSES

In the early years of graduate nursing education in Canada, advanced preparation was generally understood to be a route away from the bedside and into teaching or administration. However, as the percentage of Canadian nurses prepared at the master's level has risen, it has become increasingly apparent that a significant proportion of nursing's professional leadership and scholarship ought to be in the clinical practice arena. Although all aspects of nursing scholarship play a significant role in advancing nursing knowledge and influence, the unique contribution of the discipline to the Canadian health care system inherently depends on the application of knowledge in the practice arena.

Thus, since the early 1980s, a number of master's programs have explicitly shifted their emphasis to professional and clinical leadership as a primary objective. Moreover, they have expanded the opportunities for a range of clinical leadership learning options. Similarly, when doctoral programs came on board in the 1990s, most nurses assumed that their primary goal would be to produce the next generation of academic nurse researchers. Although many graduates have gone on to faculty positions, the potential for developing clinical scholarship leaders at that level has also been recognized. Thus, the practice reality for nurses with graduate preparation in the discipline is a moving target, in keeping with the rapid changes in the population, the health care system, and knowledge proliferation within society.

Among the more subtle but challenging practice realities for nurses at the graduate level has been the general level of skepticism and distrust within the mainstream nursing population for the value that advanced education brings to the profession. In preparing this chapter, a wide range of students and recent graduates were interviewed for the purpose of clarifying the issues that might be included in the discussion. Many of them pointed out that, although attitudes are slowly shifting, it is not uncommon for nurses "coming back to do their master's work" to report the absence of endorsement or support from their colleagues. Even those who remain active in their clinical roles for the duration of their studies may find it an ongoing challenge to convince their colleagues that the university has anything relevant to provide to the practice setting.

Where expertise and professional leadership are clearly evident within the practice setting, it is often attributed to the special qualities of an individual nurse rather than to knowledge and skills that graduate education can bring to the effectiveness of nursing practice.*

Perhaps because nurses have had long-standing debates about entry-to-practice levels and scope of responsibility, some remain reluctant to recognize the value of diversifying to achieve collective aims. Pressures from union ideologies, an inherent democratizing ideal, and a reluctance for self-promotion have made nurses more comfortable with the general notion that "a nurse is a nurse is a nurse" than with the ramifications of leveling and specializing nursing contributions. By packing extreme amounts of content and experience into tightly crafted curricula, and by sending new graduates out into a health care system that is exceedingly complex and strained, nurses sometimes feel that their educational programs have set them up for failure (Griffiths, 2000). This pressure may be felt particularly strongly by diploma-level graduates in the context of the current climate of health reform and instability.

Sadly, however, nurses have not always provided one another with a mechanism for understanding how their practice reality is shaped by the prominent forces of the day. Many simply fail to appreciate that the profession is advantaged, not disadvantaged, by an increasingly educated majority. Thus, nurses as a group have not always been supportive of the continuing educational advancement of their peers and may interpret "going back to school" as abandonment rather than as adding ammunition for the collective battles. Certainly, an emphasis on increasing social awareness and political analysis among the mainstream of practicing nurses will continue to be an important element in the general experience of graduate education and the practice reality of nurses prepared with graduate degrees.

A somewhat similar climate of misunderstanding can occur for doctorally prepared nurses with primary appointments in a clinical practice setting. Although the profession has had a generally high level of collective comfort with the traditional model of the academic researcher-educator, it seems much less comfortable with how to apply the skills of doctorally prepared nurses into the clinical context. Nurses in clinical leadership and scholar positions may find, for example, that the research component of their role is less valued than is the administrative aspect. As a result, although nursing has made great strides in

---

*As a teacher of a core master's level class that students often take early in their programs, I have been fascinated over the years by how prominent these rather negative attitudes are within the profession and how resistant they are to change. I do know that graduate students are increasingly recognizing the "ambassador" role that they can play to help their colleagues appreciate the value of the new learning they obtain from their graduate degree programs and to recognize that the confidence, critical thinking skills, and "big-picture" thinking that they begin to apply to their practice are not simply coincident with their going back to school. –Author

cultivating a generation of accomplished researchers, this may have been at the expense of other critically important leadership roles. For example, many of the recent dean and director searches for Canadian nursing schools have been long and protracted, and it is generally understood that the available applicant pool has been diminished by other opportunities in research and scholarship as well as by an extended period of time in which nursing administrative scholarship was relatively unsupported. Thus, in contrast to the situation that faces the master's prepared nurse attempting to re-enter the practice domain, doctorally prepared nurses graduate into a professional culture characterized by an inordinate valuing of specialized research training and acquiring protected time away from distractions to attain the highest level of research funding possible. In its own way, this attitudinal climate is as problematic and counterproductive as that of the academically resistant mainstream.

■ ISSUES AND CONTROVERSIES IN GRADUATE EDUCATION

In contrast to the career paths typical of many professions, nurses still perceive the option to take their graduate education in nursing or consider advanced study in other disciplines. Although the proliferation of programs at the graduate level across the country and the increased availability of distance offerings have made higher degrees in nursing a viable option for all Canadian nurses, many decide to look elsewhere for their academic advancement. Certainly, the history of the nursing profession in Canada has been well served by many noted leaders who returned to the fold after completing their master's or doctoral degrees in such fields as education, psychology, business administration, public health, anthropology, medical sciences, or sociology. From those disciplines, we have derived benefits in theoretical diversity, methodology, and analytic processes. We also recognize that the world in which nursing is practised is inherently interdisciplinary and, therefore, that nurses have a natural affinity for the models, methods, and substantive knowledge of a range of disciplines.

At the same time, despite individual exceptions, leaders who lack an in-depth understanding of the complex theoretical, historical, and philosophical grounding of the nursing discipline can be considerably disadvantaged when they attempt to articulate a nursing perspective. Even more problematic may be that they do not even know they lack this understanding. Because nursing is and remains difficult to describe, delineate, and encapsulate in language, because of its ineffable nature and complexity, Canada needs a cadre of leaders who are adept at conceptualizing the discipline and its contributions in a changing context. Because of this, although graduate preparation in nursing will remain a high priority for the discipline's development in this country, there are many opinions on how best to achieve it.

Theoretical Debates

An explicit concern for issues of a theoretical nature evolved in the second half of the 20th century in response to the explosion of new knowledge in the physical and social sciences and the availability of new theoretical challenges arising from the core projects of a variety of academic disciplines. Nursing theory emerged as a mechanism for organizing and making sense of "this infinitely dynamic and complex body of information" so that nurses could use knowledge in a "professional, accountable, and defensible manner" (Beckstrand, 1978).

As the influence of physicians and the medical model on health care delivery systems expanded, new species of health care professionals and technicians proliferated and nursing curricula evolved away from the more traditional medical science and apprenticeship structure. As such, nurses began to recognize an urgent need to articulate the uniqueness and distinctiveness of their profession among others in the health care system (Chinn & Kramer, 1999; Engebretson, 1997). To do this, they began to create conceptual maps that would depict the manner in which nursing informational and decisional processes might relate to a theoretically infinite range of clinical situations (Ellis, 1968; Johnson, 1974; McKay, 1969; Wald & Leonard, 1964). In calling such conceptual frameworks "nursing theory," they located nursing thought within the rather rigid academic and scientific community of the era and thereby created a context within which nursing science could be legitimized and acknowledged (Cull-Wilby & Peppin, 1987; Jones, 1997).

The conceptual model–building era that lasted from the mid-1960s through the mid-1980s was remarkable in its optimism and enthusiasm for extending the boundaries of existing scientific and philosophical thinking. In a context in which theory development in science was understood to follow linear causation and reductionistic models, the nursing theorists were essentially attempting to capture complexity and infinite variation within a rigorous and systematic scientific matrix.

Considering some of the philosophical and scientific innovations with which we can now reflect on the project, some aspects of their efforts may seem naïve in retrospect. However, it can also be said that their efforts to develop a science accounting for both the generalities of substantive knowledge and theory as well as the particularities of an infinite range of new applications was impressive in its capacity to recognize the complexities inherent in excellent clinical nursing reasoning and to respect the diversities of expanding knowledge within which nursing operates (Barnum, 1994; Benner, Tanner, & Chesla, 1996; Meleis, 1987; Raudonis & Acton, 1997; Thorne & Perry, 2001).

However, the model-building enterprise was not well understood within the dominant mainstream of nursing and, for the most part, remained a distinct enterprise from the research scholarship that developed through the latter decades of the century. As the theorists themselves became embroiled in debates about whose conceptual structure should dominate the discipline, much of academic nursing tired of the discourse and began to consider the theoretical debates a minor embarrassment in nursing's history (Engebretson, 1997). Indeed, where comparative analysis of the theoretical models had been a prominent aspect of graduate education in nursing, many programs eliminated the issue from their curricula in favor of a shift toward what Meleis (1987) termed the *substance* of nursing theory.

Because it is arguable that mainstream nursing theorizing was evolving toward embracing aspects of those directions anyway, the "revolution" in nursing thinking became something of a turf war in which ideologic claims about the inherent intentionality of theoretical positions took the form of abject generalizations about the beliefs and motives of those who did and did not sit on the same side of the paradigm fence (Thorne, Reimer Kirkham, & Henderson, 1999). Further, instead of welcoming debate, some proponents of simultaneity theory have elected to interpret challenges to the inherent value of simultaneity theories within the discipline as nothing more substantive than a "vicious diatribe" (Cody, 2000) or an intentional "mis-take"(Pilkington & Mitchell, 2003) and have even suggested that criticism from outside of that paradigm cannot be taken seriously because it is inherently misguided (Parse, 1998). Perhaps one advantage of this unfortunate turn of theorizing is that it brought the relevance of theoretical thinking back into the forefront of academic nursing and stimulated many nurse scholars to pay attention to the debates. Because of this, critical analysis of the implications of theoretical positioning has come back into favor in graduate nursing education as a relevant and entirely necessary body of scholarship. Further, the explosion of misunderstanding and accusation among the discipline's theorists has forced academic nursing to recognize the imperative of understanding more fully its philosophical underpinnings.

Philosophical Challenges

Among the most overt and easily recognized philosophical challenges facing nursing scholarship from the 1980s to the present has been the qualitative–quantitative methodologic debate. Although research methodology has technical aspects, much of this debate underscores a number of much deeper and more complex philosophical schisms within the scientific and academic communities of which nursing is a member. Overt attention to the philosophy of science was at one time rare in nursing curricula at any level, but it is now well recognized as a hallmark of a credible graduate program in the discipline and has crept downward into undergraduate curricula as well. Thus, an appreciation for the philosophical positioning of the ideas of the discipline has emerged as a critically important element in professional leadership.

As a result of the popularization of Kuhn's (1962) treatise on scientific revolution, academic discourse is no longer characterized by indisputable facts and truths, but rather by claims and positions. In a climate in which postmodern thinking permeates society, knowledge previously considered immutable by virtue of its scientific grounding has become fodder for deconstruction and revisioning (Haack, 1998; Hacking, 1999). The evolution of scientific knowledge is no longer understood as linear and rational, but rather as an entirely human enterprise, subject to ideational and political pressures over time (Van Doren, 1991). What we knew to be true yesterday is entirely disputable today and may be considered reactionary tomorrow. For a discipline such as nursing, the dramatic shift from a realistic ontologic orientation, in which factual truths exist, toward consideration of knowledge as social construction, in which there may be different ways of understanding truth, has had tremendous appeal. For example, nurses know that every practice principle must have its legitimate variations and that every theoretical claim one might make about human health and illness experience will break down in the face of individual human uniqueness. To some degree, one might argue that theoretical relativism has always been philosophically consistent with the kind of flexibility and adaptability that is the hallmark of excellent nursing practice. Because of this, nursing scholarship has enthusiastically embraced qualitative methods, subjective knowledge, and critical-emancipatory inquiry as consistent with its general moral underpinnings.

In a climate in which theoretical truths are no longer as comfortable as they once were, however, many nurse scholars now find themselves struggling to find purchase on an increasingly slippery platform of disciplinary knowledge. For the profession to have a social mandate, certain basic philosophic truths or positions seem to be prerequisites. For example, although it might be interesting to philosophize about whether human pain and suffering exist apart from our ability to apprehend them subjectively, nursing is solidly morally bound to an assumption that they do and that nurses have an obligation to ameliorate them when possible, despite the individual variations they might manifest and the possibilities that they might simply be profound subjective constructions within the minds of those afflicted. Thus, in reaction to the notion that qualitative methods were more true to human subjective experience and, therefore, more relevant to the knowledge required for nursing practice, many scholars now recognize the inherent limits of any methodologic approach for generating knowledge suitable to a practice science. To develop useful knowledge in relation to a substantive field, for example, nursing might require population-based surveys, linear regression modelling, phenomenologic interpretation, and emancipatory action research. Thus, the members of the academy are scrambling to expand beyond their traditional methodologic expertise and develop the more rounded philosophical and methodologic buttressing that scholars of the future will require. For doctoral programs in nursing, this means that skill within a range of inquiry methods, including qualitative research, quantitative research, and philosophical analysis, will be foundational to producing a new generation of excellent scholars.

Although traditional doctoral training has relied heavily on mentorship models, the scholarship of the future will inevitably require a shift in student and supervisor relationships. The postmodern challenge within academia has raised awareness that traditional science re-creates itself, such that genuine innovation must inevitably resist and react against the dictates of older models and authorities. Of course, in the extreme version, the notion of expertise is rejected entirely (Thorne, 1999). However, although that extreme version clearly exists within the academic community in Canada (Good, 2001), nursing's professional practice mandates seem to have kept it somewhat more grounded in a perspective in which the ideas one holds have meaningful implications for the society we live in and the individuals who constitute it. However, it also seems quite common for Canadian nursing graduate students, especially those at the doctoral level, to view the scholarship forms of their mentors with a critical lens, to envision combinations of methodologic and philosophical approaches that extend beyond the specific expertise of their supervisors, and to chafe under academic regulations that create barriers to building their own programs of scholarship in a less rigid and bounded science than did their predecessors.

Practical Challenges

Although many of these debates underscore the challenge of understanding the theoretical and philosophical nature of the discipline, there are also a number of somewhat technical and practical issues that relate centrally to the question of core disciplinary knowledge. Historically and currently, Canada has almost no dedicated source of funding for the development of nursing knowledge (the relatively minor amounts available from the CNF notwithstanding). The issue of a separate nursing fund was hotly debated during the developmental phase of transforming Canada's research infrastructure from the Medical Research Council and the National Health Research Development Program into the Canadian Institutes for Health Research. Although many nurses felt confident in their ability to compete for dollars with other disciplines in the context of the mandates of specific institutes, others recognized that an opportunity might be lost to sustain inquiry pertaining to the core of nursing. In other words, although new knowledge considered part of the national health agenda might be supported, that which would be considered specific to the discipline would be much more difficult to accomplish.

In many instances, this insight may have been elusive for those whose graduate preparation was outside the discipline, for whom the problems of core nursing knowledge seemed tangential to the larger enterprise. Given the contentious nature of the nursing theoretical debates, their reluctance to engage in these issues seems understandable. However, this tension between allegiance to "substantive" knowledge (such as children's health or family health) and "disciplinary" knowledge (such as the nature of nursing or the dynamics of clinical nursing reasoning) has played itself out in graduate nursing curriculum and program development as well, with some nursing scholars advocating immersion in the substance and others pressing for the disciplinary competence within which to ground it. Ongoing debates with regard to the relative importance of such topics as the philosophy of nursing science in comparison to the interdisciplinary knowledge associated with distinct fields of nursing specialization are likely to continue and to complicate curricular planning for the foreseeable future.

A related practical challenge derives from the applied and practical nature of the science of nursing. Although graduate education has not always been understood as an inherent adjunct to the practice of nursing, increasing numbers of master's and doctoral students seek advanced degrees for the explicit purpose of enhancing and strengthening their practice effectiveness. Although it has been natural for the discipline to consider the conduct and dissemination of research as a scholarly enterprise, the notion of practice scholarship has been much more difficult to articulate. Although many Canadian universities continue to support and encourage advancement of practice knowledge using a variety of strategies, the continuous pressure to evaluate the quality of academic units on the basis of the research dollars they attract and the publications they produce is unavoidable. Thus, particularly at the doctoral level, there has generally been less overt support for scholarship in the practice tradition than for more conventional health research scholarship, and students seeking to create practice scholar careers may find themselves seduced by the apparent credibility afforded the more usual career track strategies.

As graduate education continues to proliferate in this country, nursing will confront many permutations of the theoretical, philosophical, and practical challenges that have been mentioned. As graduate education becomes the norm rather than the exception, increasing pressure toward flexibility and access will inevitably occur, and smaller academic nursing units will start to feel left behind if they are not offering graduate degree programs.

■ CHALLENGES FOR GRADUATE-PREPARED NURSES

Nurses prepared at the graduate level are the current and future leaders of the profession in Canada. In that capacity, they are vulnerable to the effects of the current health care climate. Various health reforms in Canada since the 1990s have reflected attempts to control health spending by shifting resources from the acute care to the community sector, mechanisms to rationalize resource allocation decision making, and efforts to bring health care system decision making closer to home within national regions (CNA, 2000). The strongly held principles articulated in the Canada Health Act, and traditionally embraced by nurses, have been challenged as never before in the context of this conflictual health reform climate (May & Ferguson-Pare, 1997). Nursing shortages and the "graying" of the profession (Bradley, 1999) occur in a climate in which nursing leadership is increasingly scarce (King, 2000).

The weight of navigating the discipline's journey through the health reform process over the next several decades will undoubtedly sit squarely on the shoulders of practice leaders, many of them prepared at the master's level. Clearly, their capacity to make nimble adjustments in health human resource planning, economic accountability, health policy processes, and professional practice leadership will determine the shape of professional nursing for the next generation. Because these fields of inquiry have not been dominant within nursing's disciplinary scholarship over the most recent decades, there is a recognized shortage in scholarship related to nursing work, nursing service, and the delivery of nursing care. Because formal research scholarship has eclipsed academic and administrative leadership as a priority since the 1980s, it will take some time before graduate nursing programs can take a sufficient shift in course to cultivate a new generation of professional leaders. In the meanwhile, collaborative partnerships between practice settings and universities will be essential to resolve the challenges inherent in the shortage of nursing personnel at all levels and in the conditions of nursing work. Thus, we can expect issues of the workplace to take an increasingly prominent position among the scholarship arenas of graduate education, such that issues traditionally considered the domain of the functional specialization of nursing administration will become mainstream and foundational expectations of nursing in any leadership role.

Although the number of nurses entering graduate programs continues to increase at all levels, the pressures on nurses to extend their academic commitment have also exponentially increased. First-rate graduates of master's programs are quickly seduced into doctoral programs, doctoral graduates are encouraged to shift immediately into postdoctoral training, and postdocs are expected to seek career award funding to protect their research investment. Although each of these progressions is laudable and necessary, it is also important for the profession to remain vigilant to the continuing need for nursing scholarship and leadership throughout the system. University (and college) programs will increasingly be hungry for new faculty members to teach the next generation of nursing students, and clinical agencies will be desperate for nurses capable of combining practice knowledge with policy work, administrative strength, evidence-based practice development, and corporate leadership. As the current generation of faculty and administrators retires from the active roster, the demand for the next generation to fill the gaps will clearly exceed the current capacity of the profession to train and groom appropriate numbers. Thus, we can anticipate that the global effects of Canada's nursing shortage have only just begun (Canadian Institute for Health Information, 2003).

In the current climate, the health care community will more urgently demand that the university play a strong role in resolving the critical human and material resource challenges that Canada will face in its development and delivery of health services to an increasingly diverse and complex population. Pressure to meet the emergent needs of the system will take the form of new professional practice roles, increasingly specialized training expectations, and greater numbers of excellently prepared graduates. Without dialogue and debate to create a national consensus on our shared beliefs, role definitions, and disciplinary core values, nursing may well experience discord and organizational disarray. And with the urgent demands on the system insinuating themselves on our education and practice contexts as well as on our research, it may be difficult in the next few decades to take the time we require to reflect on our past and direct our future.

■ STRATEGIES FOR ADVANCING GRADUATE EDUCATION

Canadian nurses have been strong advocates for the principles embedded in the Canada Health Act, and they have also been consistently proud of a national tradition of high-quality professional education and service delivery. As the pressures to increase the number of graduates inevitably lead to more programs and more diverse program delivery modes, it will be important for Canadian nursing to attend to the quality of the educational opportunities on which its leaders build their professional careers.

Nursing has no quality-monitoring mechanism at the graduate level. Programs preparatory to professional licensure are all regulated by provincial statute and professional organizations, and there is a voluntary accreditation system by which the quality of baccalaureate nursing programs is well supported. Although the Canadian Association of Schools of Nursing (CASN) has created position statements on master's and doctoral level education (Box 12.1), graduate program approval is entirely within the authority of the individual university senate. The approval is typically based on the market demands of the specific institution as well as on the degree to which it considers conventional academic quality criteria in its program decisions.

A number of additional universities are preparing proposals to deliver doctoral programs in nursing. Because doctoral students bring in fellowship dollars, increase the rate of faculty publication, and expand the research capacity of the organizational unit, many university administrators may not be all that concerned that there is insufficient support within the nursing department for core disciplinary knowledge, research training, or scholarly mentorship.

Similarly, there is continuing pressure to expand the flexibility and accessibility of master's programs (CNA, 2004). A review of the CNA's current program listings suggests that most Canadian nursing master's programs have some courses available by distance delivery mode or are working toward complete program delivery online or using modern information technology. Although there is no doubt that these fulfill an identified need, the implications of responding to the pressure *en masse* should be an important agenda for national discussion and deliberation. Some of the less objective attributes of a high-quality master's program, such as developing the skills of collegial networking, challenging one's own concepts and core values, and being mentored by knowledge brokers and generators within the discipline, all become experiences of a different nature when conducted in intellectual isolation. Thus, it seems more important than ever for Canadian nurses to remain vigilant to the question of quality monitoring of graduate education and to take ownership of the standards by which excellence (and mediocrity) can be judged.

Because the financial imperatives of universities will undoubtedly continue to create the conditions under which scholarship is evaluated in the external academic community, nursing academics and their leaders will have to find strategies by which a balance between lucrative and meaningful inquiry can be supported. At present in Canada, there is an influx of opportunity for funding research projects, programs, and training centers within the national agenda of health system and health service demands. To the extent that nurses can align their scholarship with those national agendas as they unfold, they will be increasingly successful in attracting additional resources to their academic units. Unfettered adherence to these agendas, however, would have predictable and unacceptable effects on the culture and nature of nursing academic departments. Within any department offering graduate degree programs, it will remain important to have faculty who teach as well as do research, who engage in practice scholarship as well as traditional research, and who examine the philosophical and theoretical problems of the discipline as well as respond to the immediate expressed needs of the society around them.

Indeed, one of the most complex challenges for academic nursing will be to enact strategies and processes that reward a range of professional leadership and scholarship (Boyer, 1990; Glassick, Huber, & Maeroff, 1997) and to create the kinds of learning environments that are grounded strongly within the discipline and are active and credible in the larger arena. In support of this endeavor, a number of national initiatives are under way. CNA and CASN have been working together to enact a number of the recommendations arising from the recent Canadian Nursing Advisory Committee workforce study (CNAC, 2002). CASN's Education Committee is in the process of revamping and updating its position statements on master's and doctoral education in nursing (CASN, 1998), and CASN has established a task force on doctoral education, which is working with Health Canada's Office for Nursing Policy to create recommendations for a national policy on the proliferation of doctoral programs in nursing. The task force will grapple with the complex issues associated with such challenges as ensuring the quality of research-intensive training programs in an era of rapid proliferation, considering the potential value of professional nursing doctorates in Canada, and maintaining the integrity of doctoral education within the context of increasing pressure within the discipline for flexibility and accessibility.

BOX 12.1   CASN Position Statements on Graduate Education (2004)

On Master's Level of Nursing

At the Master's level, students build upon the knowledge and skills acquired at the baccalaureate level. Emphasis is placed on developing ability to analyze, critique, and use research and theory to further nursing practice. Provision should also be made for examination of current issues in health care and the ethical values that influence decision making. The Master's curriculum should include a definitive component designed to enable students to synthesize research, theory and practice at an advanced level. The focus of Master's study may include the preparation of nurses with advanced skills in the practice of nursing (e.g., nurse practitioner). Master's programs encompass a *program continuum* that includes programs that require a master's thesis, programs that require a major project or practicum, and programs that are course based. Individual Master's programs may include both required and elective courses designed to prepare graduates to assume positions in advanced nursing practice, teaching, administration, policy development and/or to provide a foundation for PhD study.

The purposes and nature of Master's education are based on the following assumptions:

■ Nursing practice is an inclusive term that incorporates care of individuals, families and communities as well as involvement in nursing education, administration, research, and policy development.
■ Many nursing practices are founded on rationales that have not been critically validated or critically examined.
■ Nursing practice is enhanced by nursing-related research/scholarship and theory.
■ The Canadian health care system needs advanced practice nurses with knowledge and skills necessary for appraising the "state of nursing science" in areas relevant to nursing practice, and transferring this to the practice setting.
■ Master's level education is the minimum requirement for advanced nursing practice, leadership positions, and faculty positions in nursing education programs.

On Doctoral Education in Nursing in Canada

Canada will require significant increases in the number of nurses with doctoral preparation in order to:

■ build the faculty base necessary to educate sufficient numbers of new graduates to meet the health care system workforce needs,
■ generate the evidence required to address the health problems of Canadians, and
■ advance the knowledge base within which the practice of nursing is grounded.

Recommendations:

1. That innovative and creative delivery models for PhD training be explored to improve access to formal research training to qualified potential students.
2. That Canadian doctoral programs in nursing be held to explicitly articulated quality criteria, including:

■ Research-intensive academic nursing units, housed within universities with well established graduate program infrastructure and access to high quality interdisciplinary interactions.
■ A critical mass of active faculty researchers capable of supporting the mentorship, research training and socialization required to engage in the full complement of roles associated with success in the competitive Canadian health research context.
■ Learning experiences related to at least three core components: 1) research training, 2) core disciplinary knowledge related to the history, context, and theoretical underpinnings

BOX 12.1   CASN Position Statements on Graduate Education (2004) (continued)

of nursing, and 3) knowledge of the current state of science and scholarship within a substantive field within the discipline.

■ A combination of a modest amount of coursework, comprehensive examinations, and completion of a dissertation.

■ Opportunities for active engagement in a scholarly learning environment.

■ Evidence of a rigorous external evaluation benchmarking research effectiveness and productivity, infrastructure and resources, and outcomes.

3. That the critical attributes of graduates of Canadian programs include

■ Obtaining competitive research funding.

■ Conducting research that is both rigorous and original to address a problem of concern to the discipline.

■ Articulating and establishing a program of research.

■ Communicating effectively through peer-reviewed journal publication, presentation at scholarly meetings, and in professional and scientific interactions.

4. That CASN/ACESI undertake further work to more fully articulate necessary and expected attributes of PhD in Nursing programs in Canada and implement processes whereby high level quality standards can be assured.

5. That the PhD in Nursing in Canada remain a research-focused degree program.

6. That the Professional or Practice doctorate not be focused on as a direction for Canadian universities at this time.

7. That we work to develop strategies to reduce geographic and demographic barriers to access, including creative and collaborative mechanisms to accommodate nurses through such means as interdisciplinary doctoral programs, special case doctoral initiatives or collaborative distance delivery approaches.

8. That we establish a clear and coherent communication mechanism whereby the explicit outcome criteria associated with the PhD in Nursing are distinguished from other doctoral preparation options and interpreted to potential students, potential employers and others.

9. That we create strategies to actively target potential students at earlier points in their academic programs and in their career and actively support their continuing development through to senior research and academic leadership roles.

10. That we establish explicit predictions of the number of doctorally prepared nurses that will be required and develop coherent strategies to meet those targets.

11. That we seek significant increases in funding for doctoral students, for nursing research infrastructure, and for the infrastructures for graduate programs within Schools of Nursing.

12. That we work with other nursing organizations to develop and implement a unified nursing voice to address the funding challenge at a national level.

Approved November 16, 2004. Canadian Association of Schools of Nursing. (2005). Retrieved from http://www.causn.org/Education/Position_Statements/DOC_Pos_Statement.pdf

Nurses in Canada have made great strides toward developing professional scholarship and academic credibility during an era in which the pressing problems of society have demanded unprecedented attention. They have attempted to stay true to a vision of professional integrity as they flow with the changing tides of acceptable inquiry methods and theoretical locations. In an increasingly interdisciplinary world in which truth is never static and credibility is always open for discussion, nurses have collectively assumed

After completing this chapter, you will be able to:

1. Understand the historical and political evolution of nursing competencies.
2. Describe the mechanisms by which competencies become "facts" within nursing.
3. Articulate the relationships between competencies, accreditation, and auditing practices.
4. Trace the relationship between a competency framework and self-regulation.
5. Account for differences in competency development in Canada and elsewhere.
6. Discuss individual and organizational differences in responsibilities for nurses' competence.

Competencies are ubiquitous. Internationally, competency statements underpin curricula, define and maintain professional standards, delineate specialist practice, and perform a multitude of functions related to the accreditation and regulation of practice. A concise definition of competency according to the Alberta Association of Registered Nurses (AARN, 2000, p. 20) states that "competence is the ability of the nurse to integrate and apply the knowledge, skills, judgement, and personal attributes required to practise safely and ethically in a designated role and setting."

A fairly recent occurrence in nursing's professional history, competency-based practice has transformed the Canadian nurse's manner of conceptualizing and ordering practice. This chapter examines not only the success of the competency movement in Canada and abroad but also the possibility that the movement as conceived weakens nursing's influence in holding governments accountable for the resources that enable competence in practice.

This chapter also explores the competency phenomenon by examining the genesis of competencies, considering the reasons for their success, and comparing Canadian competency models with others, such as those in Australia and the United States, where the competency movement in nursing has a slightly longer history. The range of competencies, the kind of nurse produced by competency-based formulations, and the applications of these competencies are discussed in relation to what they reveal about the nursing profession and its changing place in the health care system.

■ HISTORICAL UNDERSTANDINGS OF COMPETENCY STANDARDS

The Canadian competency movement is a fairly recent innovation adopted by nursing professional associations across the country to assist the process of determining whether educational programs are preparing nursing students for entry into the profession of nursing. A national consensus process was engaged in by nurses across the country for a 2-year period (1995 to 1997), during which time the National Nursing Competencies Project (NNCP) was undertaken. At the culmination of this project, entry level nursing competencies for licensed practical nurses, registered nurses, and registered psychiatric nurses were established. Each provincial association then went through a more local process of validating the relevance of the competencies within the context of local nursing practice settings.

This Canadian process was predated by processes in other countries that also culminated in the production of competency statements, and, in each case, quite different processes developed. To illustrate this, the next sections review processes for the development of practice competency statements in Australia and in the United States.

Australian Approach

During the 1980s, the Australian federal government moved to reform and revitalize the economy and the workplace. Each profession was expected to develop competency-based standards. The goal was standardization of education and portability of qualifications, which would thereby produce a more efficient workforce.

As part of this innovative and world-leading program of initiatives, the National Training Reform Agenda and then the National Training Board (Gonzi, Hager, & Oliver, 1990) were established to review vocational education and training programs across the country. The timing of these national initiatives was significant; the Australasian Nurse Registering Authorities Conference (ANRAC) had begun the process in 1986. After a period of vigorous debate within the profession, Australian nurses took the lead in this movement and became the first profession or industry to develop national competency standards as part of the structural reform of the Australian workplace in its drive for market efficiency (Gonzi, 1993).

Nurses' enthusiasm for competencies has not been confined to Australia. From Benner's work in the 1980s in the United States, which had international impact (Borbasi, 1999; Gallaher, 1999; Hegedus & Pearson, 2000; Krugman, Smith, & Goode, 2000; Sarvimaki & Stenbock-Hult, 1996; Thompson, 1999), to the formal requirements for continuing license to practise in Canada, competencies have been seized by nurses, employers, registration authorities, and educators as the scaffold upon which to design curricula, develop legislation, and assess continuing safety to practise.

American Approach

A major impetus for introducing competencies in the United States came from the Pew Health Professions Commission Taskforce on Health Care Workforce Regulation (Pew Commission), released in December 1995 (Lassiter, 1997; Sharp, 1998).

Aimed at reforming the health workforce regulation system, the Pew Commission disbursed grants totalling $300,000 to stimulate the health professions to restructure the health system in ways that focused attention away from profit making and toward effective, competent practice.

In the manner of all successful innovations, competencies take the appearance of logical, even inevitable, developments (Lassiter, 1997). Their unproblematic and almost universal adoption by the profession internationally, however, merits reflection. How was it that competencies were so enthusiastically endorsed and adopted by nursing? How has the adoption of competencies as a framework for training, assessments, and professional development changed the way nursing understands itself? How have competencies changed the nurse? By what mechanisms have competencies become facts within nursing?

■ INVENTION OF COMPETENCIES

To explore these questions, one may follow an intellectual path developed by British sociologists Thomas Osborne and Nikolas Rose (1999) in their analysis of the creation of new phenomena. In examining the mechanisms by which competencies have become facts, the concern is in determining what facts have become *true* in our world (i.e., competencies), how they have become true, and with what consequences. It may be helpful to think along the following lines: This is a matter of the emergence of certain descriptions *rather than others;* some descriptions will survive *if it is possible to do things with them* and use them *to produce effects.* So, how did competence emerge as a favored way of making determinations about the ability of nurses to fulfill a particular role within society? What sorts of things become possible once a nursing association identifies particular competencies as being necessary attributes for nurses to demonstrate—and to demonstrate in particular ways? What are the effects produced in the world through these processes, which are mandated by professional associations that demand competence from nurse members?

To the extent that these questions can be answered, one can say that the conditions underlying the creation of a phenomenon as set out by Osborne and Rose (1999, p. 373) are met. And, as a result, one may say that a particular knowledge practice has created a phenomenon. The significance of engaging in this analytic process is that it illustrates the socially constructed basis of the competency movement as it is currently being implemented within the Canadian context. As such, nurses are invited to examine for themselves a range of purposes the competency statements serve.

Osborne and Rose (1999) used the example of public opinion in their study of the way in which social sciences create phenomena. They argued that "new ways of describing and acting have been used to create all sorts of effects" (1999, p. 377). In the case of competency development, the manner in which this formulation of practice has "entered into the true" (Osborne & Rose, 1999, p. 367) can be productively analyzed by considering the mechanisms that generate them and the conditions of their acceptance by the nursing profession worldwide.

For Osborne and Rose (1999), the target was the history and philosophy of science literature and what they consider its failure to engage with the process through which the social sciences *actively create truths*. For nurses, these processes, rather than the epistemologic concerns of Osborne and Rose, are of primary concern. Namely, by what mechanisms have competencies become facts within nursing? Or, to paraphrase historian Peter Brown (1967, p. 393), what is the choice of problems that nursing regards as important? And why have these particular approaches been designed to particularize and solve those problems?

Evolution of the Canadian Competency Movement

The competency movement of the 1980s and 1990s has a particular genealogy. Fundamental to the successful application of a competency model are corresponding systems of accreditation and standardization. Competencies can operate only within a framework that sets up standards for practice that arise from the quality assurance movement with its accreditation and auditing processes. After decades of refinement, the quality assurance movement achieved the extension of these accreditation and auditing technologies to the professions.

To implement the auditing of personnel within the total framework of industry accreditation, training and skill reviews became implicit components. It was the skill base of professionals, who ostensibly satisfied the training and educational preparation requirements for any audit procedures, that was targeted. Historically, the professions had been immune to ongoing review of their skill base (Angus, 1959). Therefore, it is significant that the competency movement breached the defenses of the professions and demanded they introduce processes to standardize curricula, implement skill audits for registration, and set in place processes to monitor lifelong learning compliance (Figure 13.1).

What is significant about these imperatives is that they have been facilitated not by draconian measures but by self-regulation. The success of the competency movement has been in its general acceptance as a framework that enables the more effective self-regulation at all levels: professional, organizational, and

FIGURE 13.1 Used with permission, Faculty of Nursing, University of Calgary.

individual. These are not processes that individuals are forced to undertake but rather are engaged by individuals through self-review.

Early Frameworks of the Competency Movement

Australia provides us with an example of this. For Australian nurses, the competency movement had three main stages:

1. Development of standards for entry to practice level
2. Development of standards for advanced practice
3. Development of standards for specialty practice

Each stage involved different actors, served different objectives, and achieved distinct outcomes.

Entry Level Competencies

Entry level competencies grew out of the 1984 in-principle decision of the Australian federal government that nursing education be moved from a hospital-based education system into the university sector, thereby setting a bachelor's degree as the entry to practice qualification for Australian nurses. Executing this momentous shift in the provision of nursing education involved a major reworking within the postsecondary education sector and the development of new curriculum standards. It also involved a period of intense collaboration among clinical leaders, registration authorities, professional and industrial associations, and the universities over curriculum, standards of practice, and registration (Australian Nursing Council, Inc. [ANCI], 1993).

The competency framework mandated by the federal government provided a timely mechanism for reconstituting nursing education and professional preparation. It was not uniformly welcomed by Australian nurses, however. Kim Walker (1995, p. 97), an Australian nurse-educator, assessed the competency movement as demonstrating rampant positivism that places nursing at the mercy of macro-political concerns. Less sophisticated was the commonly held concern that nursing's professional aspirations may be damaged by the embrace of the competency movement. After all, the Australian competency framework had emerged from the vocational education sector wherein skilled workers rather than professionals were prepared according to competency principles. For nurses who had finally achieved their goal of a university qualification for entry to practice, there was widespread concern that nursing curricula based on competencies reinforced the perception of nursing as a *skilled* rather than a *professional* pursuit (Pincombe, 1993; While, 1994). Despite these misgivings and strongly voiced opposition, government imperatives and the obvious benefits to industry prevailed. As sociologists Osborne and Rose (1999) argue, with the development of all phenomena constituted by the social sciences, "At a certain point, the controversy is settled. The phenomenon exists: now it is time for it to be investigated, explained. . . . It becomes a *usable* kind of thing" (p. 372, emphasis added).

In fact, it is this very utility of competencies that is so important. The process of developing competencies reveals this to be one of the most critical aspects of their success—*competencies are generated through consensus*. This has certainly been the case with nursing competency standards. "In fact the process actually reinforces consensus and the sense of objectivity of what has been discovered" (Osborne & Rose, 1999, p. 368).

In the case of undergraduate nursing, the universities, the profession, the unions, the regulators, and industry engaged in a process of structured consultations to agree on a set of competencies for entry level practice. As Osborne and Rose (1999, p. 390) noted: "One then observes a rather complex work of alliance between academic researchers and professionals and practitioners, in which the practitioners call upon the academics to boost their credentials, and the academics draw upon the pragmatic credit of their appeal to a professional audience to increase their likelihood of research funding and the like."

The process outlined here resonates with contemporary experiences of seeking research funding. Research grant-writers have developed strategies that capitalize on an "appeal to a professional audience"—at the same time, those same researchers experience the constraints such associations bring to the research endeavor.

Advanced Level Competencies

For the advanced level practitioner, all the nursing organizations in the country engaged in a protracted series of consultations. An action research project was undertaken, leading to the development of consensus statements as to what constituted a generic set of competencies for advanced practice (Australian Nursing Federation [ANF], 1997). Action research was both a method to achieve the research aim of the production of advanced level competencies and a process to develop participants' and the profession's thinking forward through the creation of such competencies. The collaborative philosophy of action research, where researchers and participants move together toward a shared change agenda, proved a useful approach to the development of competencies.

Specialist Competencies

Finally, in the case of specialist nursing, such as that engendered by the Australian Confederation of Operating Room Nurses (ACORN), the creation of competencies served extremely useful functions. It, too, generated consensus among practitioners about the scope of specialty practice and engaged them in defining and delineating practice boundaries. Again, the favored model was an action research design of multiple methods and a high level of participant engagement (ACORN, 1999). Action research provided the overall methodologic and theoretical framework for a project that involved a combination of qualitative and quantitative methods. Thus, at the end of the competency process, areas of specialty practice could be said to exist legitimately; a set of truths about that specialty were now written into the professional literature. The active constitution of the area was dynamically achieved through the enactment and reenactment of these competencies as the basis for recognition as a specialist practitioner. Through these processes, competencies can be said to exist as real things. And, by means of the creation of such realities, practices that may be as archaic as nursing itself can now be described in new and accountable ways.

These new realities are created in a systematic way that draws into play relations between state authorities, professional organizations, and individual nurses. Under *advanced liberalism,* which can be understood as a stance held in relation to questions of the governing of conduct of citizens, certain self-evaluative techniques related to competent practice, which are discussed later, provide the mechanism through which compliance with workplace reforms and improved efficiencies is achieved.

Compliance Initiatives

In the case of Australia, the federal government demanded compliance of all professional regulatory authorities. In the United States, nongovernmental but highly influential organizations (such as the Pew Commission) led the charge with funded programs that set the agenda for workplace reforms through a competency framework.

In Canada, partnerships between the state (i.e., regionalized health authorities), professional associations, and other regulatory authorities and educators reframed both the expectations and the responsibilities of the profession and the individual practitioner. Regulatory authorities take responsibility to ask whether the practitioner remains competent to practise, but the practitioner is now expected to complete an official document and make an honest assessment of his or her competence. Self-declarations of competence need to be supported with a portfolio of evidence. The characteristics of this evidence are highly questionable when considered in relation to the stated goals of competency projects.

■ COMPETENCY MODELS AND IMPLICATIONS FOR NURSING

Since early in the year 2000, individual nurses across Canada have been receiving brightly colored print materials from their professional associations. These materials offer directions for nurses in each provincial jurisdiction on how to engage with a set of complex legal requirements in demonstrating their "continuing competence." The requirements for such demonstration have been established through provincial legislation and require that health care professionals forward documentary evidence of their alignment, as individual practitioners, with statements established by regulatory bodies to support their claims to competence in nursing practice. How are these textual materials being taken up by these regulatory bodies to become usable in ways anticipated by Osborne and Rose's argument about how phenomena are created?

"A key aspect of the creativity of phenomena in the social sciences pertains to the subjective attributes of the persons themselves: the kinds of persons they take themselves to be and the *forms of life they inhabit and construct*" (Osborne & Rose, 1999, p. 392, emphasis added). Of particular interest here is how the process of demonstrating competence has "produced a version of the world that [has] entered into the true" (Osborne & Rose, 1999, p. 367)—that is, a process that is generally unquestioned by nurses who engage enthusiastically in the construction of themselves as particular sorts of competent practitioners. Significantly, nurses will practise their competence within everyday circumstances that render invisible the responsibilities of the wider sociopolitical system for offering financial and material resources necessary to support competent practice.

A comparison of target audiences embedded in competency documents produced by professional organizations in Canada and Australia offers a starting point to question the emphasis on competence within these two particular jurisdictions. Evident in even an initial comparison of Canadian and Australian competencies is that the focus on the individual nurse in Canadian documents is largely missing from Australian documents.

Alberta Association of Registered Nurses' Model

The AARN defines *competence* as "the ability of the nurse to integrate and apply the knowledge, skills, judgement and personal attributes required to practise safely and ethically in a designated role and setting" (AARN, 2000, p. 20). Other associations emphasize similar aspects of competence.

The AARN definition goes on to suggest to nurses that, "Just as nursing is more than a set of procedures or tasks, competence is *more than just a set of skills which must be performed safely and efficiently.* It is the integrating of knowledge with skills and applying it to the practice of nursing in a *safe, ethical* manner, based on the standards of the profession" (AARN, 2000, p. 20, emphasis added).

Safe practice is the central issue, and the individuated nurse is the target of the message. That is, competence is defined against "the ability of the nurse" to enact specified knowledge functions, such as applying relevant knowledge to particular circumstances, practising in a skilled manner, making relevant and appropriate judgments about the ever-changing condition of the patient, and so on. In this definition, there is no indication that the *context* within which opportunities to know particular things are embedded would have any influence on the nurse's ability to fulfill the required knowledge functions. The individuated focus is reinforced in additional ways: first, in the reference to "personal attributes" and, with this, the association of safety with ethics.

Safety is used in two different ways in this definition. Initially, nurses are informed that they are "required to practice safely and ethically in a designated role and setting." Next, they are advised that competence is "more than" safely and efficiently performed skills. An intellectual process of "integration and application" is signaled here, although the actual set of knowledge, skills, judgments, and personal attributes that constitute "safe and ethical" practice are left unspecified. (In a footnote, readers are advised that these attributes "include but are not limited to attitudes, values, and beliefs.")

Authors of the AARN definition of competency-based practice and the accompanying workbook containing explanatory notes provide some historical and political context for the focus on safe and ethical practice. Indeed, many regulatory bodies offer similar rationale for developing procedures to measure and monitor competence. That is, they establish a link between the requirements for demonstrating competence with legislative reviews of acts pertaining to health care professionals. Authors of the AARN document offer the following explanation for why the AARN asks members to submit themselves to the competency review process (note the primary reference to the impact of health service restructure):

Over the past ten years, the health care system has undergone massive changes, and the public has asked for reassurance that health professionals have maintained and upgraded their knowledge and skills for the role and setting in which they practise. The government has placed the responsibility for protection of the public on registering bodies, such as the AARN, and has responded to this public request by requiring that the AARN and other regulatory bodies develop continuing competence programs for their members. In 1999, the Alberta government passed the Health Professions Act *(HPA). It requires that all health professions develop a continuing competence program and that all health professionals demonstrate that they are maintaining their competence throughout their careers. This means that the AARN is required to develop a continuing competence program, and that, "regardless of the role or setting in which you work, you will need to fulfill the program requirements and demonstrate that you are continuing to be competent in your practice" (AARN, 2000, pp. 2–3).*

The issue, as we see it being formed through a series of consensus-making opportunities involving professional associations, governments, and health care employers, is that "competence" emerges as a personal attribute, completely within the control of the individuated nurse. In the foregoing quotation, the Alberta Association of Registered Nurses acknowledges the extent of change that health care services have been exposed to over the preceding decade and that the public demands assurance that nurses continue to be as competent now as they were before the changes started. Notwithstanding that acknowledgment, we argue that the consensus-making project of nationally agreed competency standards has produced the competent practitioner of nursing as a decontextualized individual.

It is our assessment that this has been the overall effect of the competency movement—certainly in Canada. We recognize this to be a contentious assessment: It may be read as positioning nurses to speak against competence—something that would be very difficult for a well-socialized nurse to do. So, to foster an understanding of our position, we want to draw to readers' attention what is *not* happening because of this particular formation of competency in relation to professional nursing.

One of the disturbing consequences of the decontextualized and idealized basis of competency assessment for practicing nurses is that they are forced to participate in the fabrication of themselves as individually competent actors. Moreover, this individual actor either bears the full load of responsibility for a failing health care system or colludes in the pretense that good nursing care rests on the individual—not the system. In framing competence as resulting through personal effort to enact particular attributes such as selflessness, conceiving of all errors as resulting from personal failings and deference to all authority, nurses are left in a position of having to lie when they complete their continued competency workbooks. Nurses are positioned to lie about experiences of refusing mandatory overtime. They have to lie when negative patient outcomes arise out of situations where appropriate material resources are not available to support high-quality practice. Nurses have to lie when they are bullied into maintaining poor practice through a lack of organizational support for necessary and critical engagement in collective discussions about what it would take to achieve high-quality patient outcomes.

These represent serious consequences of the current focus of competence as resting entirely with the nurse. Alberta is not alone in this focus. Other Canadian jurisdictions also focus attention on nurses as individually responsible to enact themselves as competent practitioners. Perhaps in recognition of the rather vulnerable position this leaves nurses in, some regulators seek to ameliorate the message—adding further confusion to the issue rather than clarifying it.

Registered Nurses Association of British Columbia's Focus

The Registered Nurses Association of British Columbia (RNABC) is quite explicit that specification of the *content* of safe and ethical practice is expressly *not* the point of the exercise of reporting on practice competencies by individual nurses. Instead, the exercise of competency review is designed to explicate a process that RNABC claims all nurses already engage in:

RNABC's personal practice review requirements provide a framework for nurses to identify and address their learning needs. It offers a systematic approach for nurses to maintain their competence to practice and demonstrate accountability to the public. The requirements are not designed to assess competence. *An underlying belief of the personal practice review requirements is that nurses are competent professionals. The additional continuing competence requirements provide an opportunity to formalize the process that registered nurses already use to maintain their competence to practice" (Retrieved April 2, 2005, from http://www.rnabc. bc.ca/pdf/340.pdf; emphasis added).*

The RNABC offers the following rationale for establishing safe practice standards to its members:

The Nurses (Registered) Act requires RNABC to establish and maintain a continuing competence program. This is a legislated mandate required of all health regulatory bodies in B.C. RNABC's personal practice review requirements provide a framework for nurses to identify and address their learning needs. It offers a systematic approach for nurses to maintain their competence to practice and demonstrate accountability to the public" (Retrieved April 2, 2005, from http://www.rnabc.bc.ca/pdf/340.pdf).

As in the AARN statement, members of the RNABC are advised that the continuing competence program is a "requirement" that the association is mandated by provincial legislation to undertake. Also evident in this explanation are references to the fact that such programs are not required only of nurses but that "all health regulatory bodies" in the province are required to address this mandate.

This might be interpreted as an attempt by RNABC to resist any breaching of its authority as a professional and autonomous body. But such an interpretation denies the extent to which such regulatory bodies are networked and, thus, discipline one another into forms of consensus and compliance. In claiming that the process merely formalizes practices already engaged in by individual nurses, this statement, too, has an individuating effect: It pulls the individual nurse out of widely diverse practice settings and locates her or him in a space of accountability that is somehow supracontextual, that of individual accountability.

The authors of these definitions intend for the processes of integration and application to move nurses to engage in practices that are both safe and ethical. However, references to efficiency denote an organizational influence on nursing practice. In contrast to this, the reference to ethics denotes the centrality of the individual, professional nurse as holding primary responsibility for the conduct of safe and competent practice.

College of Registered Nurses of Manitoba's Position

Emphasizing the point about "an increased awareness of health care issues [and] the changing roles of health care providers" in a way echoed in the AARN publication, the College of Registered Nurses of Manitoba (CRNM) offers the following rationale for its introduction of competency procedures to its members:

There is an increasing emphasis on and interest in the continuing competence of registered nurses and other health care professionals. This is due in part to an increased awareness of health care issues, the changing roles of health care providers, and the recognition that there is a link between quality care and the practitioner's competence to provide it (http://www.crnm.mb.ca/competence.php.htm; Finocchio et al., 1998).

The rationale for this explanation links it to the work of the Pew Commission. Mentioned earlier in the chapter, this commission's role was to develop standard competencies for a broad audience of health professionals. The report by Finocchio, cited in the CRNM rationale for the need to engage in a review of competence in practice (Finocchio et al., 1998), refers to a report focusing on strengthening health

---

BOX 13.1　　　　**Twenty-One Competencies for the 21st Century**

1. Embrace a personal ethic of social responsibility and service.
2. Exhibit ethical behavior in all professional activities.
3. Provide evidence-based, clinically competent care.
4. Incorporate the multiple determinants of health in clinical care.
5. Apply knowledge of the new sciences.
6. Demonstrate critical thinking, reflection, and problem-solving skills.
7. Understand the role of primary care.
8. Rigorously practise preventive health care.
9. Integrate population-based care and services into practice.
10. Improve access to health care for those with unmet health needs.
11. Practise relationship-centered care with individuals and families.
12. Provide culturally sensitive care to a diverse society.
13. Partner with communities in health care decisions.
14. Use communication and information technology effectively and appropriately.
15. Work in interdisciplinary teams.
16. Ensure care that balances individual professional system and society needs.
17. Practise leadership.
18. Take responsibility for quality of care and health outcomes at all levels.
19. Contribute to continuous improvement of the health care system.
20. Advocate for public policy that promotes and protects the health of the public.
21. Continue to learn and help others learn.

From the Pew Commission (1998).

---

care consumer protection within the United States. One of the major contributions of the commission was the development of "Twenty-One Competencies for the 21st Century." The list of these 21 competencies appears in Box 13.1.

■ IMPACT OF CANADIAN COMPETENCY REQUIREMENTS ON NURSING

Two points stand out regarding the genesis of a rationale supporting the introduction of the continuing competence movement within the Canadian nursing professional body context:

- First, the competency requirement is directed at individual nurses—their knowledge, skills, and personal attributes. Nurses are targeted as responsible for the conduct of safe and ethical care—in the absence of any acknowledgment that the organizational context shapes possibilities and opportunities for engaging in ethical conduct (Latimer, 1998; Varcoe & Rodney, 2001).
- Second, the work of explicating nurses' competence in this highly individualized manner represents a significant departure from the way in which competencies were conceived of by those contributing to the Pew Commission's report, which is cited as a central, founding document supporting the development of nurse competencies in Canada.

As the list of 21 competencies indicates, those working within the context of the Pew Commission were setting forth an agenda designed to link consumers and providers. Such an agenda has a particular meaning within the largely for-profit health care industry of the United States. Consider the following data: The U.S. Census Bureau reports that for the year 2003, 45 million people lacked health insurance, or 15.6% of the population. That represents an increase on 2002 from 43.5 million (http://www.census.gov/ hhes/hlthins/hlthin03/hlth03asc.html). In light of what have become annual increases in both levels of poverty as well as levels of American citizens who are uninsured for health care coverage, the Pew Commission's competency statements for the 21st century can be read as a national agenda for health care provision within the context of inequitable access to basic health care services.

In contrast to the situation in the United States, universal access to health care in Canada is mandated by federal statute in the form of the 1984 Canada Health Act (Government of Canada, 2001). The act mandates that health care be delivered through a funding structure whereby federal and provincial levels of government share costs through public, not-for-profit insurance providers. The key point here is that the relationship among governments, health care providers, and citizens seeking access to health care is vastly different between these neighboring countries. The competencies set out by the Pew Commission reflect an interest in positioning health care delivery as a form of social responsibility. Ethical practice within this context reflects an interest in attending to the myriad ways in which people seeking health care might be discriminated against within the American context (Allen, 1996). That is, the competencies set out by the Pew Commission must be interpreted, in the American context, as politically motivated.

One may argue that the Pew agenda for social responsibility already underpins the Canadian system of publicly funded, universally accessible health care. And so the reference to this commission's work prompts many questions about how Canadian nursing regulatory bodies are defining ethical practice and how they intend that definition to be taken up by Canadian nurses. Before exploring this perplexing question, let's first examine the target of competencies in the Australian context. As suggested earlier, the competency agenda has developed quite differently within different national contexts, and the Australian case illustrates this difference quite clearly.

Contrasts in Competencies

In stark contrast to the tone of the competencies developed in Canada are the competencies set out by the ANCI (2001) for beginning practice and the Advanced Nursing Competencies (ANF, 1997). In the ANCI's competency standards, one can see that organizations employing nurses and other health care workers are responsible for enabling competent practice.

Competency units (CUs) for registered nurses are established in four domains: professional and ethical practice, critical thinking and analysis, management of care, and enabling (Box 13.2). Even from these titles, it is possible to see some linkage to the competencies set out by Canadian professional bodies, particularly in regard to professional and ethical practice. However, the target for responsibility around the achievement of competent practice in this domain is rendered in quite different language within the detailed description offered. For instance, within this domain of professional and ethical practice, the first competency unit (CU 1) relates to "functions in accordance with legislation and common law affecting nursing practice." The specific competencies set out within this unit relate to a specific knowledge base: common law regulating safe practice. Nurses are responsible for knowing about this law, how it affects their actions, and what the reporting requirements are should they witness a breach of the law. This statement is quite different from the lack of specificity related to knowledge requirements established for Canadian nurses.

Similarly, CU 2 demands that nurses conduct nursing practice "in a way that can be ethically justified," again in relation to a specified document: Element 2.1 of the professions' code of ethics.

The 14 ANCI competencies are targeted at entry to practice level nurses. Consequently, they focus on the responsibilities that the new nurse must be ready to shoulder as a registered professional. They incorporate expectations regarding the nurse's approach to nursing work by specifying the issues of research (CU 6), assessment (CU 7), planning (CU 8), and evaluation (CU 10). The competencies also place the

BOX 13.2   Practice Domains and Units of Competency for Australian Nurses

Domain: Professional and Ethical Practice

Competency Unit 1: Functions in accordance with legislation and common law affecting nursing practice.
Competency Unit 2: Conducts practice in a way that can be ethically justified (in relation to the professions' code of ethics [Element 2.1]).
Competency Unit 3: Protects the rights of individuals and groups in relation to health care.
Competency Unit 4: Accepts accountability and responsibility for own actions within nursing practice.

Domain: Critical Thinking and Analysis

Competency Unit 5: Acts to enhance the professional development of self and others.
Competency Unit 6: Values research in contributing to developments in nursing and improved standards of care.

Domain: Management of Care

Competency Unit 7: Carries out a comprehensive and accurate nursing assessment of individuals and groups in a variety of settings.
Competency Unit 8: Formulates a plan of care in collaboration with individuals and groups.
Competency Unit 9: Implements planned nursing care to achieve identified outcomes within scope of competency.
Competency Unit 10: Evaluates progress toward expected outcomes and reviews and revises plans in accordance with evaluation data.

Domain: Enabling

Competency Unit 11: Contributes to the maintenance of an environment that promotes safety, security, and personal integrity of individuals and groups.
Competency Unit 12: Communicates effectively with individuals and groups.
Competency Unit 13: Manages effectively the nursing care of individuals and groups.
Competency Unit 14: Collaborates with other members of the health care team.

Source: http://www.anci.org.au/competencystandards.htm

nurse's role within the context of multidisciplinary teams and heterogenous service structures, emphasizing the collaborative and collegial demands of nursing (CUs 8, 12, and 14).

Likewise, the competencies developed by the National Nursing Organisations (NNOs) with the ANF set the basis for advanced practice in the work of the nurse as opposed to the ethical or personal attributes of the nurse (Box 13.3).

As with the entry to practice level competencies, the function of the ANF's advanced nursing standards was consensus building. The advanced standards project set out to reflect current practice and to acknowledge the evolving framework of national standards. Another goal was to put in place standards that reflect the practice of nurses beyond the minimum level reflected in the ANCI competency standards. Additional objectives included informing ongoing professional education, contributing to ongoing development of specialty competency standards, and achieving endorsement by nurses across Australia (ANF, 1997, p. 6).

BOX 13.3 Competency for Advanced Practice Nursing in Australia

The advanced practice competencies advanced by the Australian Nursing Federation (ANF) evince a pragmatic and contextualized view of nursing performance. These competencies set out 12 standards that provide a broad framework for advanced nursing practice. Essentially, they state that the advanced practice nurse:

■ Uses multiple approaches to decision making
■ Manages the care of individuals and groups
■ Engages in collaborative practice to achieve patient outcomes
■ Provides a supportive environment for colleagues
■ Manages staff and physical resources
■ Engages in ethically justifiable nursing practice
■ Protects the rights of individuals and/or groups
■ Engages in activities to improve nursing practice
■ Develops therapeutic and caring relationships
■ Fulfills the conduct requirement of the profession
■ Acts to enhance the professional development of self
■ Functions in accordance with the legislation and common law affecting nursing practice

From Australian Nursing Federation. (1997). *Competency standards for the advanced nurse*. Melbourne: ANF Federal Office.

Thus, in the ANCI's minimum standards for practice, the ANF's advanced standards, and the separate specialty standards (such as those advanced by ACORN), the emphasis is on consensus building in a fractured educational and regulatory framework. Scope of practice, curriculum framework, and ethical and legal issues dominate, and the standards provide an ordered and coherent path around which these diverse practice and educational and regional interests can successfully cohere. As previously mentioned, the competencies also fill a void of public and professional confidence in consistency in the standard of nurse education, a void which has existed since the abolition of state registering examinations in favor of moving Australian nursing into the postsecondary education sector in the 1980s.

Australian Concerns: Corporate-Shared Responsibility

The focus of these standards appears to be on the scope of practice and the educational and professional preparation required of nurses rather than on the individual nurse's ability to meet the values set out in the formulated competencies. The *choice of problem* addressed by the Australian competencies was the development of national curricula and clinical experience requirements within the tertiary sector for new graduates and advanced practice in the clinical specialties.

Canadian Concerns: Individual Responsibility

These concerns appear largely absent from the Canadian competency material. One indication of the "choice of problem" Canadian competencies are trying to address can be found in Appendix 11 of the National Nursing Competency Project Final Report, which was published in 1997 (pp. 138–172). This section is entirely devoted to the complex task of discrimination between shared and unique competencies for the licensed practice and registered nurses. It even tabulates then current (1996) and future (2001) competencies between the two levels of nurses. As such, the competencies attempt to clarify the muddy waters of multiple entry to professional practice.

In contrast, Australia's competency document is only directed at a specific level of professional nurse designation: the registered nurse. The problem of multiple levels of nursing practitioners in Australia, then, was not one requiring solution through the competency process. Instead, the competencies solved a problem of irregular educational standards across the country. In the shift of nursing education from hospitals to universities, the process of national examination was lost. In this case, the competencies provided an informal framework for the evolution of a national curriculum, with recent calls for a national nursing curriculum based on competencies seeking to formalize this process (National Review of Nursing Education Committee, 2001).

The most radical example of departure from the pragmatic and context-based competency model of Australia comes from Alberta, where the focus is solely on the individual nurse and the nurse's capacity to determine continuing education needs and attend to them. The AARN triple component, "We Trust You, Tell Us, Show Us," asks reregistering nurses to assess their own practice according to the set standard (on a scale of 1 to 5), to collect feedback from colleagues and patients, and to develop an appropriate learning plan that will be evaluated. Set forth in writing, the AARN documents present a professional climate of not only self-surveillance but also cosurveillance, with substantiation of the individual nurse's claims to have achieved and maintained critical competencies required from those around him or her.

Written in the first person, the AARN continuing competence handbook leaves no doubt as to who is fully responsible for continuing competence in the nursing profession—the individual. Moreover, the confessional tone of the document is further heightened by requiring the nurse to identify limitations and define how to redress them. Given that the exercise is entirely subjective and that the document is unable to be verified, the document radically fails as a conventional audit of continuing competency.

But perhaps this is not its purpose. That these competencies institute mandatory reflective practice is illuminating, particularly because these reflective techniques are a means to reconstitute subjective attributes, performing a "specialized form of self-culture" (Nelson, 2000, p. 88). As the tool of choice by regulatory authorities, reflective practice provides the mechanism whereby nurses internalize the new professional ethos. Clearly, one can see that nurses are under surveillance by the registration authorities to make sure this reconstitution of the nurse is achieved.

■ FUTURE IMPLICATIONS: NURSING'S CHANGING PLACE

One thing that is clearly articulated and "enters the true" is a changing relationship between the public and those professionals who have undertaken advanced education to learn practices designated as effective in providing health care services. What the development of competencies signals is that an initial preparation as a nurse is no longer sufficient guarantee of the competence of that practitioner to deliver appropriate care. Instead, elaborate processes (which, as we have argued, fail on any conventional measure of competency audit) have been designed apparently to assuage the fears of the public that health care practitioners might somehow be "out of practice." Yet no strong evidence exists that the public has expressed these fears. Instead, the competency movement seems to have emerged out of a much longer-term interest (of governments and, more locally and by implication, health service managers) in breaching the immunity held by professional groups to any sort of external reviews of their skill bases' effectiveness.

■ SUMMARY

The analysis of the competency movement in several jurisdictions establishes an argument that, particularly in the Canadian case, review processes fail to provide the very guarantee of effectiveness that the competency movement seeks. This does not mean, however, that the competency movement has failed. Instead, it has been spectacularly successful in producing a range of consensus statements that serve as powerful narratives of consistency.

Competencies fill a void of public and professional confidence in consistency in standards of nurse education. In Canada, registering examinations are devised at the national level. As such, diversity in the capacity to deliver on a range of health care services resulting from regional economic disparity can be masked by federal and provincial legislators through demands for professionals to create narratives of consistency. In contrast, the registration examination did not survive the shift from hospital schools to university-based education in Australia. In that context, competencies provided a surrogate framework for an evolving national curriculum.

Professional bodies such as the ANF and the AARN share an interest in demonstrating guarantees of competence to the public by responding to government demands. In so doing, however, they undermine their capacity to hold governments accountable for providing resources that make such competent practice much more likely.

The success of the competency movement within nursing deserves careful and cautious attention by the profession. Far from fulfilling the promise of detailing an evidential basis for professional practice, alignment with the competency movement alienates nurses as individuals and as members of a professional body from holding managers and governments accountable for the provision of resources, such as staff-to-patient ratios that enable nurses to work collaboratively with patients to deliver care that acknowledges and respects their goals for health. It is our belief that it is this sort of condition that underpins safe and effective care. Instead, by drawing on highly suspect strategies of self-surveillance and cosurveillance, the blame for poor practice outcomes can be placed on individual nurses. Where nurses are naïve enough to believe that quality improvement is the aim of the competency exercise and who, on that basis, willingly report their failings, these nurses will only prove themselves to be trustworthy and, for their truth-telling efforts, will have their registrations revoked. Such responses to truth telling will only encourage others to tell complex lies that create an illusion of competence within working conditions where such promise of competence cannot possibly be fulfilled.

Online Resources

Add to your knowledge of this issue:

The Canadian Nurses Association	www.cna-nurses.ca
Provincial and Territorial Organizations	
Alberta Association of Registered Nurses	www.nurses.ab.ca
Association of Nurses of Prince Edward Island	www.anpei.ca
Association of Registered Nurses of Newfoundland and Labrador	www.arnn.nf.ca
College of Nurses of Ontario	www.cno.org
College of Registered Nurses of Manitoba	www.crnm.mb.ca
College of Registered Nurses of Nova Scotia	www.crnns.ca
Nurses Association of New Brunswick	www.nanb.nb.ca
Ordre des Infirmieres et Infirmies du Quebec	www.oiiq.org
Registered Nurses Association of British Columbia	www.rnabc.bc.ca
Registered Nurses Association of the Northwest Territories and Nunavut	www.rnantnu.ca
Registered Nurses Association of Ontario	www.rnao.org
Saskatchewan Registered Nurses' Association	www.srna.org
Yukon Registered Nurses Association	www.yrna.ca

REFLECTIONS on the Chapter . . .

1. The authors of this chapter claim that, despite the spectacular success of the competency movement in Canada, it undermines a nurse's capacity to hold governments accountable for providing resources that would make such competency possible. Do you agree with this argument? Support your position.

2. Go to your province's Web site (listed in Online Resources) and download the most recent document related to competencies for practice. Review this document and discuss how this fits or does not fit with this chapter.

3. Discuss with colleagues or classmates what they see as the purpose of the competencies for practice documents. How does your view fit with those of your colleagues or with those expressed in this chapter?

4. Demonstrated evidence of competence is required by law in some provinces. What is the intended purpose of such legislation? What are the effects of such legislation for nurses? For health care organizations? For health care practices?

5. Discuss the implications of competencies for nursing curricula generally and for continuing education of nurses in particular.

6. What are your thoughts about the notion that nurses are targeted as responsible for providing safe and ethical care in the absence of any acknowledgment that the organizational context shapes possibilities and opportunities of engaging in ethical conduct? Review existing documents on competencies for your province to see if and how this might be true. Take a stance that supports or challenges this claim.

7. In considering the chapter, your province's documents, and your own thoughts on this matter, what issues can you identify for nurses, nursing practice, and the health of Canadians? What frameworks can you identify that help you to articulate these issues? What barriers to resolving these issues can you identify? What strategies for resolving these issues can you suggest?

References

Alberta Association of Registered Nurses (AARN). (2000). *AARN continuing competence handbook.* Edmonton: Author. Available: http://www.nurses.ab.ca/contcomp/docs/Core%20Information.pdf

Allen, D. G. (1996). Knowledge, politics, culture, and gender: A discourse perspective. *Canadian Journal of Nursing Research, 28,* 95–102.

Angus, N. C. (Ed.). (1959). *The expert and administration in New Zealand.* London: Oxford University Press.

Australian Confederation of Operating Room Nurses (ACORN). (1999). *Validation of ACORN Competency Research Project Report.* Adelaide: Author.

Australian Nursing Council, Inc. (1994). National validation of ANCI competencies for beginning level enrolled nurses across all areas of nursing practice: Report to ANCI Competencies Committee 1993. Canberra: Author.

_____. (2001, August 1). *ANCI national competency standards for the registered nurse and the enrolled nurse* [Online]. Available: http://www.nursesreg.nsw.gov.au/RNcomp_b.htm

Australian Nursing Federation (ANF). (1997). *Competency standards for the advanced nurse.* Melbourne: ANF Federal Office: Author.

Borbasi, S. A. (1999). Advanced practice/expert nurses: Hospitals can't live without them. *Australian Journal of Advanced Nursing, 16*(3), 21–29.

Brown, P. (1967). *Augustine of Hippo.* New York: Dorset.

Commonwealth of Australia. (1990). *The identification and assessment of competencies: The Nursing Project and its implications.* Department of Employment, Education and Training, Research paper No. 4. Canberra: Australian Government Publishing Service.

Finocchio, L. J., Dower, C. M., Blick, N. T., et al. (1998). *Strengthening consumer protection: Priorities for health care workforce regulation.* San Francisco: Pew Health Professions Commission.

Gallaher, L. (1999). Expert public health nursing practice: A complex tapestry. *Nursing Praxis in New Zealand, 14*(3), 16–27.

Gonzi, A. (1993, December). *Competence and competencies: A global perspective.* Paper presented at the First National Conference on Competencies in Nursing, Adelaide.

Gonzi, A., Hager, P., & Oliver, L. (1990). *Establishing competency-based standards in the professions.* Department of Employment, Education and Training Research paper No. 1. Canberra: Australian Government Publishing Service.

Government of Canada. (2001, August 1). *Canada Health Act overview* [Online]. Available: http://www.hc-sc.gc.ca/main/hc/web/datapcb/datahins/chaover.htm

Hegedus, K. S., & Pearson, G. S. (2000). Articulating professional nursing practice in Hungary: Ripples that extend to waves. *National Academies of Practice Forum: Issues in Interdisciplinary Care, 2,* 187–190.

Krugman, M., Smith, K., & Goode, C. J. (2000). A clinical advancement program: Evaluating 10 years of progressive change. *Journal of Nursing Administration, 30,* 215–225.

Lassiter, F. (1997). Pew Commission's state initiatives program to Reform Health Care Work-force. Regulation grant activity update [Health Policy Issues]. *AORN Journal, 6*(5), 923–926.

Latimer, J. (1998). Organizing context: Nurses' assessments of older people in an acute medical unit. *Nursing Inquiry, 5,* 43–57.

Masters, G., & McCurry, D. (1992). *Competency-based assessment in the professions.* Department of Employment, Education and Training Research paper No. 2. Canberra: Australian Government Publishing Service.

National Review of Nursing Education Committee. (2001). *National review of nursing education.* Discussion paper. Canberra: AusInfo.

Nelson, S. (2000). *A genealogy of care of the sick: Nursing holism and pious practice.* Southsea, Hants: Nursing Praxis Press.

Osborne, T., & Rose, N. (1999). Do the social sciences create phenomena? The example of public opinion research. *British Journal of Sociology, 50*(3), 367–396.

Pincombe, J. (1993, December). *Competencies: Do we need them?* Paper presented at the First National Conference on Competencies in Nursing, Adelaide.

Sarvimaki, A., & Stenbock-Hult, B. (1996). Intuition: A problematic form of knowledge in nursing. *Scandinavian Journal of Caring Sciences, 10,* 234–241.

Sharp, N. (1998). October 1998 Pew Report: Supportive of NP goals. *Nurse Practitioner, 23*(12), 72.

Thompson, C. (1999). A conceptual treadmill: The need for "middle ground" in clinical decision making theory in nursing. *Journal of Advanced Nursing, 30,* 1222–1229.

United States Census Bureau. [Online]. Available: http://www.census.gov/hhes/hlthins/hlthin03/hlth03asc.html

Varcoe, C., & Rodney, P. (2001). Constrained agency: The social structure of nurses' work. In S. Bolaria & H. Dickinson (Eds.), *Health, illness and health care in Canada* (3rd ed., pp. 108–128). Toronto: Harcourt Brace.

Walker, K. (1995). Courting competency: Nursing and the politics of performance in practice. *Nursing Inquiry, 2,* 90–99.

While, A. E. (1994). Competence versus performance: Which is more important? *Journal of Advanced Nursing, 20,* 525–531.

Critical Questions

As a way of engaging with the ideas in this chapter, consider the following:

1. What are your assumptions about the usefulness of technology in nursing education and professional nursing practice?

2. How do you think that nursing compares with other professional practice disciplines in regard to the use of technology in practice and in education?

CHAPTER

14

W. Dean Care
David Gregory
Christina Whittaker
Wanda Chernomas

Nursing Technology and Informatics: An Easy or Uneasy Alliance?

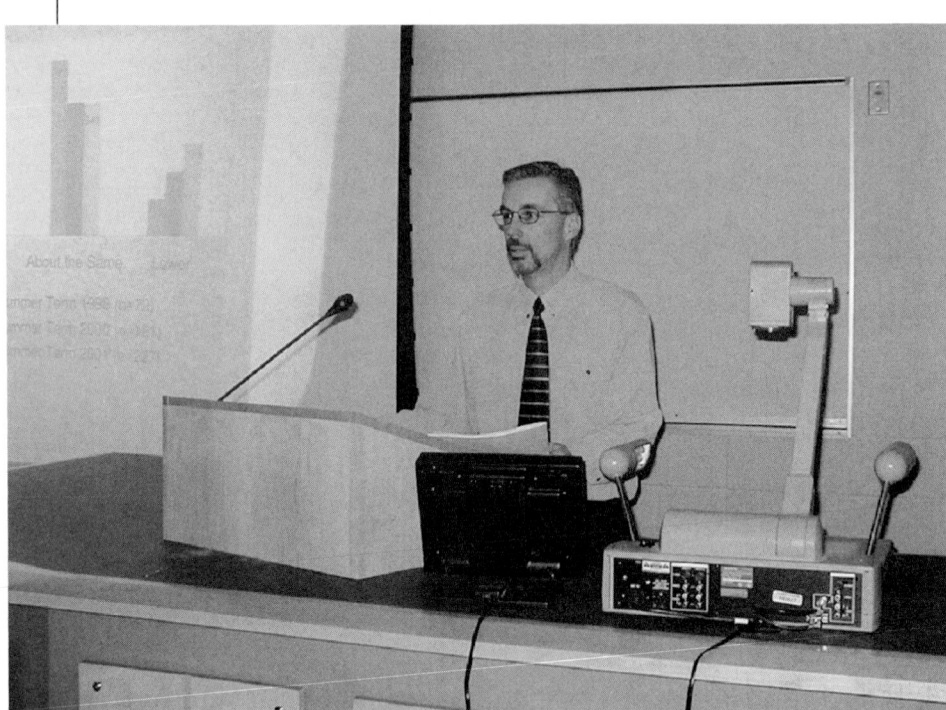

Teaching by videoconference to northern Manitoba. Used with permission, University of Manitoba, Faculty of Nursing.

After completing this chapter, you will be able to:

1. Discuss the relationship between nursing and technology.
2. Describe the role of technology and informatics in nursing practice.
3. Explore the possibilities of the use of technology and informatics in nursing practice.
4. Discuss the issues related to applying technology and informatics in practice.
5. Identify the barriers to resolving these issues in practice.
6. Formulate strategies for resolving these issues in practice.

It is the year 2007. You are a public health nurse with the newly reorganized regional health authority. Your primary responsibilities include following up on clients who have been discharged from the cardiac surgery program at the local tertiary care hospital. Clients are now being discharged 3 to 4 days after surgery. The care you provide includes teaching, wound care, symptom management, assessing and monitoring health status, and coordinating the interdisciplinary team. Most (80%) of the clients you serve have access to the Internet and personal computers (PCs) in their homes.

A typical day for you looks something like this: You arrive at work and log on to your desktop PC. You receive notice of the cardiac clients who were discharged yesterday. You call or e-mail five of these clients and set up appointments for the day. Having downloaded their electronic medical records onto your desktop computer, you review the files in preparation for the home visits. You then transmit these files onto a wireless, hand-held, personal digital assistant (PDA), which accompanies you on all home visits. It provides access to your e-mail messages and Internet databases, and it has an intranet feature that allows instant access to the other members of the team. This tool is also a cell phone, and it contains your appointment schedule, word processing documents, and address book; it is your personal organizer. It has 512 MB of memory and contains a voice recognition system that allows you to verbally record and store your "Nurse's Notes," which will be digitalized and downloaded to appropriate permanent record when you get back to your office.

Most of your clients wear electrocardiogram (ECG) leads. You are able to monitor their cardiac rhythms and vital signs from both your desktop and PDA. Each client has an e-mail account from which they can send you messages and ask you questions. Before you leave the office, you receive a call from a 10-day postop client who is experiencing chest discomfort. You ask him to turn on his video Web-cam, a piece of equipment provided to each client upon discharge. It is mounted on top of his desktop PC and provides you with a visual image of his appearance and allows you to assess his medical condition and speak with him "face to face." He attaches a Dynamap to his arm, and you receive instant blood pressure and pulse readings; an oxygen saturation reading is transmitted from the finger probe he is wearing. Using your desktop computer, you upload his ECG to get a "real-time" image of the client's cardiac rhythm. Next, you upload a visual image of his normal cardiac rhythm and compare it to his current ECG. You decide to make a home visit to assess this client's situation more thoroughly.

This brief vignette sets the stage for a discussion of the issues and trends arising from technology and informatics as they apply to nursing. Like this vignette, the chapter focuses on common uses and applications of technology in nursing practice and education. It also identifies issues arising from this technology and broaches the future of technology in nursing and health care. Relevant historical events are introduced, particularly as they relate to the significant shift in Western society from an industrial focus to an information ethos. Both rely heavily on technology, but in vastly different ways.

The Industrial Age was characterized by an emphasis on productivity, efficiency, division of labor, and hierarchical organizations. In contrast, the Information Age is distinguished by a heavy dependence on telecommunications, knowledge and information explosion, global operations, decentralized organizations, and networked employees. The Information Age provides society with rapid access to information. In the area of health care, the Information Age fosters advances in health and telecommunications technology, which has had, and will continue to have, a profound effect on nurses and the organizations for which they work.

The relationship between technology and nursing has traditionally been marked by tension and unrest. Until recently, nursing and technology have been framed as a dichotomy—nursing at one end and technology at the other—polar opposites, in a sense. Technology has been viewed as masculine, scientific, mechanistic, and reductionistic. In contrast, nursing in this dichotomous thinking has been conceptualized as feminine, nurturing, a soft science, humanistic, and holistic. Thus, technology has been identified as innately negative and dehumanizing to nursing—potentially obstructing or impeding nursing care (Erlen, 1994; Gadow, 1988).

Understanding technology simply as "scientific care" and nursing as "sympathetic care" does great injustice to the science of nursing care (Sandelowski, 1999). Like technologic advancements, nursing care is based on science and empirical evidence. Technology and its relationship with nursing are being considered in more sophisticated and complex terms. For example, nurses can use technology as an intentional way of expressing caring (Schoenhofer & Boykin, 1998). Expert nurses can and do use technologies as part of their holistic care (Sandelowski, 1998). In this way, nurses can potentially render technology as unobtrusive as possible while achieving maximum therapeutic benefit for the whole person (Purnell, 1998). With technology, nurses look beyond the technical to "touch" patients (Ray, 1987, as cited in Sandelowski, 1998). Touch includes physical, psychological, emotional, and spiritual aspects of care.

Nurses serve as "cultural brokers" between technology and patients. In this role, nurses translate technology for patients and provide explanations about the technology. Bridging the worlds of technology and nursing care, however, is not without a host of challenges. Despite expert nurse clinicians and their brokering activities, these challenges do have the potential to undermine the relationship between nursing and technology.

■ RELATIONSHIP BETWEEN NURSING AND TECHNOLOGY

What exactly is the relationship between nursing and technology? Nurses are rarely "at the table" in regard to developing technology that affects their practice. As a profession, nursing most often inherits or receives technology developed by other disciplines. Medical technology is not nursing technology, and yet this technology is most often imposed on nursing (Purnell, 1998). This has, in great measure, contributed to the strained relationship between technology and nursing. Because of this, *technology inheritance*—an understanding of technology's impact on the illness experience, or how a disease or condition is experienced by a patient and integrated into her or his life, remains mostly unknown.

Additionally, the relationships among technology, patients, and nursing care are of great concern to nursing. Assessing the impact of technology entails considerations of efficacy, safety, cost, legal ramifications, and social and ethical impact on the lives of patients and their families (Purnell, 1998). This is supported by the Canadian Nurses Association (CNA, 1992) in the following statement:

While technology has the potential to improve health care, science has advanced so quickly that some technologies have been put into use with little understanding of the possible impact on clients, families, health care professionals and the health delivery system. Nurses are often called upon to use technologies with limited training, and with little technical or administrative support. The introduction of new technologies can lead to higher overall costs, particularly if the technologies are not planned and managed properly.

The adoption of new technology also has an impact on the nature of nurses' work. Nurses incorporate technology into their work on a regular and ongoing basis, and they must learn how the new technology works, consider its demands for nursing time and knowledge, and decide how best to blend it into nursing care. One of the challenges of technology is that time previously dedicated to patient care may be short-shifted as a consequence of the technologic demands. Nurses use technology and the data it produces in clinical assessments, decision making, and nursing interventions. However, accompanying the technology are time demands and an impact on independent nursing interventions. With the introduction of new technology comes a litany of tasks. For example, in combination chemotherapy, oncology nurses engage in the following activities: checking dosages, starting intravenous therapy, mixing and administering premedications, obtaining blood specimens, and giving antiemetic medications (Brown, 1992). These tasks draw on the limited time available to oncology nurses as they provide supportive patient care.

Nurses, as patient advocates, are concerned about the illness experience. Nurses attend to how new technologies impinge on patients and their families. As Sandelowski (1998, p. 8) observed, "Nurses have a special 'angle of vision' by virtue of their distinctive epistemologic, social, and moral position on the front lines and at the point of impact of technologies on patient care." It is incumbent upon nurses to conduct research on the impact of technology on their work. This will provide valuable information to refine how and why technology is used in practice.

■ NURSING INFORMATICS

According to Simpson (1998, p. 22), "Part of the reason nursing informatics is so hard to define is because it's a moving target." A workable definition of nursing informatics, however, is essential for understanding its role in practice. It will ensure that nurses are taught "not just how to use computers, but how to collect and use information to truly further care delivery" (Simpson, 1998, p. 24). Graves and Corcoran-Perry (1996, p.15) state that informatics is "an application of computer science and information science to the management and processing of data, information and knowledge in the named discipline." Simpson (1999, p. 91) further expands this idea to include in a definition, "all the activities involved in managing and processing nursing data for use in care delivery. It also includes conceptual frameworks and such theories as information processing and decision theory and language development and human-computer interfaces, among others."

Today's nurse is affected by an ever-changing health care system dominated by a focus on outcomes, evidence, performance measurement, and the use of technology to provide and support care delivery. In their evolving role as "knowledge workers," nurses are increasingly being called on to access information systems to facilitate evidence-based practice. The evolution of this role can be hampered if nurse educators lack the necessary knowledge and competence in information technology. In addition, as more patients become comfortable with information technology, expectations will be placed on nurses to have similar skills. "In fact, nurses may find that their patient education encounters will increasingly occur through distance technology" (Gassert, 1998, p. 266).

The rapid explosion of both computer technology and telecommunications makes it essential that faculty clearly articulate the need for information technology in nursing curricula. According to Gassert (1998), all nurses will need core informatics skills to practise effectively. These skills include word processing, use of electronic mail, familiarity with a variety of spreadsheets, ability to search and access databases, bibliographic retrieval, and ability to develop graphic presentations and to access and critique Web-based information.

■ APPLICATIONS OF NURSING INFORMATICS AND TECHNOLOGY IN PRACTICE

The application of nursing informatics as an umbrella concept takes various forms in practice. At this time, the most common form is telehealth, with the telephone, electronic mail, and Web-based information as the vehicles for knowledge dissemination. Electronic health records are also discussed in this section.

Telehealth

The term *telehealth* encompasses a broad range of health care and service delivery systems provided through distance or electronic technology (Gassert, 2000). *Telehealth* can be defined as "the use of advanced telecommunications technologies to exchange health information and provide health care services across the geographic, time, social, and cultural barriers" (Reid, 1996).

The geographically dispersed population of Canada provides an ideal opportunity for the application of telehealth to reduce barriers related to health care access. Telehealth has the potential to provide borderless, seamless, and accessible health care in all reaches of the country, delivering fast, accurate diagnoses and treatments in situations where face-to-face visits may not be possible.

The proliferation of terms relating to care practices using distance technology has created confusion and difficulty when exploring related issues. Terms such as *telemedicine*, *nursing telepractice*, and *tele-education* are used in the literature. Collectively, they refer to different components of health care delivery through technology and, in certain instances, as subsets of telehealth. A national working group chaired by the CNA has defined *nursing telepractice* as patient-centered forms of nursing practice that occur through, or are facilitated by, the use of telecommunications or electronic means. Nursing telepractice uses the nursing process, which encompasses patient assessment, planning, and implementation through the provision of information, referral, education and support, evaluation, and documentation (CNA, 2000).

An example of nursing telepractice, Tele-HomeCare is the provision of a range of services to patients in their own homes through an integrated approach to service delivery by home and hospital care providers, a hospital-based monitoring center, the use of videoconferencing equipment, and remote vital signs monitoring (Hospital for Sick Children, 2001). Through 24-hour interactive video systems, a patient can contact the nurse specialist any time for consultation on a wide range of issues that would previously require visits to emergency facilities either at great distance or considerable difficulty.

In real time, nurses can perform a wide variety of assessment, education, and intervention skills at varying frequencies. They can listen to heart and chest sounds, read and interpret ECG results, assess wound status, review downloaded blood glucose information, and observe and educate the patient's self-care (Russo, 2001). The opportunities for nursing within this area may be limited only by the technologic resources available and the knowledge and ability of nursing to advocate for our expanded role in implementation, care, and evaluation.

Within telehealth, the need remains for nurses to practise according to the established standards of practice, codes of ethics, legislation, and competencies of their provincial regulatory bodies. Several related issues and challenges are apparent within the telehealth environment. There are standards of telephone practice in some jurisdictions, but not all provinces have such policies for their practitioners. These telephone standards of practice do not address the range of practice now possible within a telehealth environment. Policies on the provision of telehealth across provincial registering bodies have yet to be developed through coordinated efforts. In addition, educational standards or credentials have not been established for this area of practice nor have issues related to maintenance of privacy and confidentiality been adequately addressed. Without a comprehensive consideration of the aforementioned issues, liability issues and employer responsibilities become unclear.

Some questions needing clarification include:

1. What is the nurse's liability in regard to nursing care provided to patients who reside in a province where the nurse is not licensed to practise?
2. How do professional nursing organizations and regulatory bodies promote safe and competent practice, prevent substandard nursing practice, and intervene or investigate complaints as necessary when the registered nurse and patient may be thousands of miles apart and their interactions are electronic?
3. How are provincial associations addressing these developing issues?

Care Delivery by Telephone

The earliest use of the telephone as a tool for providing public health or private duty nursing occurred in the early 1920s (Sandelowski, 2000). Only recently, however, has consultation with patients over the telephone become a distinct nursing intervention, with specialized protocols for practice.

Many of the current telephone health care delivery programs evolved from the emergency room. However, telephone practice is no longer just an extension of emergency health service. Standards of practice have been developed for nursing care offered by telephone. Two examples of provincial standards from regulatory bodies include (1) the College of Nurses of Ontario: Telephone Nursing Practice Standards and (2) the College of Registered Nurses of Manitoba: Telephone Nursing Standards. A wide range of protocols also exists to guide nurses' decision making and judgment. Questions and issues remain regarding the frequency of review of protocols, the qualifications and education required of the practitioner, and nurses' involvement in developing these standards.

Manitoba's Health Links is an example of telephone technology that provides 24-hour provincewide nursing access for health information and advice. Experienced registered nurses with a broad range of expertise and skills usually provide this service. Another example is British Columbia's HealthGuide NurseLine, which makes 24-hour, toll-free, provincewide nursing access available. Nurses use software to assist in guiding patients' health care decision making. NurseLine is part of an expanded program endorsed by the Registered Nurses Association of British Columbia. The program consists of a printed HealthGuide handbook and an online health database. Commercially available software can be customized, at a cost, to meet needs for evaluation and monitoring of calls, including the number and type of calls and users, automated evaluation of disposition or outcome, patient satisfaction, and patient knowledge of services.

Whether the protocols are available online or on paper, telephone nursing can be contrasted to the more traditional triage. Telephone nursing uses nursing assessment to guide or coach the decision making of the patient concurrently with an empowerment approach rather than directed decisions. The inability for nurses to incorporate nonverbal patient behaviors can be viewed as a limitation, or as a challenge, to their assessment skills. However, the advent of visual images may address this limitation.

The Aboriginal Nurses Association of Canada (ANAC) supports the use of telehealth practices to improve the health of First Nations and Inuit communities. According to a recent discussion paper, "inequities exist in the health and the health care services of Aboriginal people compared to the general population of Canada" (ANAC, 2001, p. 9). The introduction of telehealth services into aboriginal communities has the potential to address these inequities. However, patients from these communities or others without phones, computers, or computer skills are at a disadvantage. The introduction of advanced technology may create a two-tiered system: those people with financial and technical resources will have access to health services; those who do not will be at a disadvantage.

Electronic Mail and the Internet

Electronic mail (e-mail) and the Internet are means of providing telehealth services. As more patients become comfortable with and gain access to e-mail, this form of communication will be used increasingly as a means of contact and consultation with health care providers. Some patients may experience greater comfort using e-mail as a form of communicating, especially if their concerns are of a personal or sensitive nature. With e-mail, patients and nurses have some flexibility in regard to the timing of consultations, inquiries, and responses. However, the issues of privacy and confidentiality remain unresolved. Additionally, it may not be possible to verify that the individual initiating communication is indeed the patient, nor that the question and the nurse's response will not be read by others. The nurse's e-mail response could also be circulated to other care providers, with the nurse's response misinterpreted out of context to that particular patient or prior communication. The lack of live communication may belie the complexity of the patient's situation, leading to tendencies for both the patient and provider to simplify or exaggerate inadvertently their concerns, assessments, and responses. Liability for care practices and potential misdiagnoses or care provided through distance or electronic technology are issues warranting careful exploration.

Health-Seeking Behaviors

Similarly, the Internet has provided the opportunity for health-seeking behavior by patients, often before contact with a health professional. Potentially, the Internet offers privacy, immediacy, breadth of information, different perspectives, and infinite repetition of information (Bischoff & Kelley, 1999). Conversely, the potential for greater patient involvement in health choices can be overwhelming because of the variety and often-conflicting health information.

An uneasy alliance with this information technology can result as patients and care providers may be unaware of how to evaluate the accuracy and credibility of Web-based information. Provider resources for such evaluation are growing, as exemplified by the inclusion of guidelines and standards for Web-based publishing on many Web sites. The nurse may find her or his practice extending into patient education about how to evaluate Internet sites, just as various local public and academic libraries are beginning to provide information on how to do just that. An example of such a service is the Consumer and Patient Health Information Service at the University of Manitoba.

An example of an interactive Internet service that promotes health-seeking behaviors with palliative care patients is the Canadian Virtual Hospice. This represents a network of information and support for people dealing with life-threatening illness and loss. After registration, people can access this Web site as a patient, friend/family member, health care provider, or volunteer. This is a credible and well-recognized health service offered by health care professionals. This is in contrast to the myriad unregulated Internet sites that have been established and maintained by nonprofessional "experts" in various areas of health care. Consumers of health and those seeking health care information need to be aware of the potential for information that is not validated or credible being posted to authentic-looking Web sites.

Online Support Groups

In addition to its use for patient self-education, the Internet is used for support groups through online synchronous chat rooms (real-time discussion) and asynchronous interaction (any-time discussion), which provide patients with the opportunity to seek support and to consult with others independently. The content of online health care and related discussions may vary according to the nature of the disorder and the composition of the group (White & Dorman, 2000). Topics may revolve around general themes, such as personal experience and opinion, encouragement and support, treatment, symptoms, alternative therapies, caregiver concerns, and coping strategies. As with electronic mail, using technology may ease communication for those who feel inhibited by face-to-face support groups, who seek the company of those who are similarly affected, or who are geographically isolated. Future research will need to explore the role that nurses play in such online support groups, how effective groups are conducted, and the role of such groups in health promotion. Active participation or "listening" to online support groups also helps the nurse to understand patients' concerns. Nurses need to be familiar with the opportunities that online support groups provide.

Despite the challenges of this technology, e-mail, the Internet, and telehealth practices have the potential to decrease substantially the indirect and social costs of health care. Costs associated with travel to health care facilities and absenteeism from family, school, or work may be reduced. This is particularly relevant to patients and families isolated by geography or care needs.

Electronic Health Records

The definition that best summarizes the intent of *electronic health records* (EHRs) is the health record of a person that is accessible online from many separate, interoperable automated systems within an electronic network (Office of Health and the Information Highway [OHIH], 2001). This definition infers the complexity of the issues involving EHRs, such as the additional resources, infrastructure, and economic challenges related to access to an integrated electronic network, including the various regional, provincial, and federal approaches to health care delivery.

The move to EHRs has been stimulated by technologic development, increased social mobility, public and government demand for accountability, and care by a wider range of health care professionals—all of whom will require information (OHIH, 2001). Health care decision makers and policy analysts increasingly require access to data for the evaluation and support of appropriate health care programming. The availability of a patient's record electronically promotes accessibility of the information by a variety of health care providers who are involved in the patient's care and who are linked to the network. EHRs could eliminate duplication of services, improve efficiency of the system, and provide accurate documentation over time.

Patient access to health records also becomes a possibility with EHRs. Such access may support enhanced personal decision making in health behaviors. Potentially, patients can be more informed about their health status, which may facilitate discussions with health care providers. However, patient access may inhibit professionals from freely recording data on sensitive issues or from offering potentially controversial assessments, such as "patient is malingering." Patient access may also pose legal ramifications in certain circumstances, such as those involving illicit drug use. Additionally, patients could misread or misinterpret findings in the health record, causing distress pending clarification.

As Nahm and Poston (2000) report, nurse and patient satisfaction with EHRs is mixed. Nurses identified a number of considerations in adjusting to EHRs, such as time required for charting; time for acquiring appropriate skills and knowledge; quality of documentation; change in care, charting, and privacy related to using wireless terminals; technologic difficulties, including "viruses" and "worms"; and potential changes in quality of patient care.

The benefit of wide and simultaneous availability of EHRs also raises concerns related to the potential threat to privacy of health records. Challenging questions include the following:

■ Who decides which health care providers have access to information about patients?
■ Should the patient have a role in determining which health care providers are entitled to access?
■ Should there be a mechanism to ensure informed consent around access?
■ What mechanisms should be designed for the detection and sanction of access violations, and who should perform such monitoring?

Answers to these questions have ethical and legal implications and, as such, should be addressed before the health care system adopts EHRs as a primary means of record keeping.

■ ISSUES IN THE APPLICATION OF TECHNOLOGY IN NURSING PRACTICE

A study by Cooper and Powell (1998) revealed how technology created extreme uncertainty and profound physical, emotional, psychological, and spiritual vulnerability among patients undergoing bone marrow transplantation. It was, however, nurses who attended to these vulnerabilities. The researchers observed the following about how nurses incorporated technology as part of their nursing care:

It is no exaggeration to suggest that these nurses created a sacred space in this highly technologic enterprise for patients to do the work of making meaning of the experience.... One extraordinary feature of this [nursing] care resides in the fact that it occurred in the context of a highly technical endeavor. Capturing the essence of this feat, one patient insightfully asked, "How can the nurses be at the end of technology [in a spectrum of technology and care] and thank goodness they are because I'm here today because of it—and then how can they be at this touch-feel end at the same time?" (p. 65).

Ethical Dilemmas

The nurse experiences firsthand the ethical dilemmas associated with new technology. Ethical and moral knowledge moves nurses to action in relation to technology. Reproductive technologies, for example, are a special concern of women, their families, and practitioners, and within nursing, there is a substantial body of work related to the ethics of reproductive technology. Availability of genetic testing requires women to examine their personal situations and beliefs to determine whether they wish to access the technology. Nurses may need to provide counselling as a woman sorts through the best decision for her. Additionally, society at large varies in its perception of the right or the need of government, resource availability, funding, and community values to influence the utilization and distribution of technologies.

Decision Making

Decision making regarding access to available technology has further ethical implications when technology is costly or in limited supply. Who should have access? What criteria should be used? Who should develop the criteria for access? These are some issues that emerge in the face of new technology. For example, at this time, not all people who need dialysis have locally available access to this technology. One mechanism to address determination of access under high-demand, limited-availability situations is to refer decision making to review boards. Such boards establish criteria in reviewing candidates for access to the technology. Nurses may be members of such boards, or they may be called on to assess a patient's suitability for access to the technology. Then, too, nurses are in positions to provide information, advocacy, and emotional support to patients and families denied access to these services.

Decision-making criteria to purchase technology or make it accessible to units are also limited (Purnell, 1998). In most instances, incorporation of technology onto nursing units occurs as a consequence of criteria established by medical and, increasingly, non-nursing administrators. As nurses are left out of technology development, they are similarly distanced from decision making related to technology application in their workplaces.

■ ISSUES IN THE ALLOCATION OF TECHNOLOGY IN EDUCATION

Timothy, a nursing student, is about to graduate and thinks he is well prepared to face a workplace filled with technology. Computers were commonplace in his life as a student. Nursing Informatics was a required course that he took at the beginning of his program. He used a word processing program to construct and format papers. He found that electronic mail and Internet access were helpful to search Web sites, stay in touch with classmates, keep informed about university and faculty information, and take courses offered by WebCT. He became adept at locating electronic information and was skilled at critiquing the quality of the information. Timothy's program offered him a number of options in course delivery. His favorite course offered by WebCT was Leadership in Nursing Practice, in which he applied course concepts in an assignment that had him plan how he would introduce practitioners not knowledgeable about computers to their use in patient education. He participated in courses that were videoconferenced to other sites. It was enlightening to hear the perspectives of students from the north because this was one of the places Timothy was considering for his senior practicum experience.

The computer is a significant tool for education and practice. Brown (1992, p. 9) states, "To become appropriate role models for students regarding the use of computers, faculty must integrate computers into the curriculum and demonstrate comfort and lack of fear in using them." It is important to define what knowledge and skills in relation to computers will be required of students in nursing programs. It is evident that if nurse educators want students to be able to use computers in their practice, students must become proficient and comfortable with computers in their own basic programs. Saranto and Leino-Kilpi (1997) identified the following content areas for teaching information and communication technologies: introduction to computers, skills in software application, system security, data transfer, skills in computerized patient monitoring, how to teach about hospital information systems, how to teach nursing informatics, and the educator's role.

Extent of Computer Literacy

Computers are available in most schools of nursing, but their use is neither systematically nor routinely included in programming, unlike the situation described in the previous vignette. Until recently, no program in Canada had a required nursing informatics course. Postsecondary institutions may believe that incoming students possess the necessary computer skills because of their experience with computers in primary and secondary schools. However, empirical evidence shows that although nursing students had access to computers in primary and secondary schools, they had limited opportunity to use them for tasks other than word processing (Gassert, 1998).

The life experiences of today's students are vastly different from previous generations'. The new generation of student, often called "millennials," represent those students born after 1980. This cohort exhibits unique learning characteristics and needs (Zemke, 2003). These young learners function better in learning activities that are structured, involve teamwork and experiential activities, and include the use of technology (Collins & Tilson, 2001). Millennials want quick access to information, have little tolerance for delays, and prefer interactive learning styles. They represent a challenge for traditional instructors who rely on a teacher-centered lecture style of course delivery.

Many institutions of higher learning are increasing their use of computers and other technologic innovations. In some cases, technology is being used to address the issue of increasing student numbers, multiple-site campuses, declining numbers of faculty, and limited financial resources. The potential then exists that technology will become a means to address these complex administrative problems without due consideration for maintaining educational standards and quality programming. Educational facilities need to guard against the temptation of substituting quality of instruction for increased student access and financial gain.

Options for Distance Learning

Nursing education is experiencing unprecedented changes in student characteristics. The student of the 21st century is more likely to be older, in pursuit of a second degree or career, closely linked to a community, and working to balance career and home responsibilities (Bates, 2000). These demographics are fueling the need for educational facilities to consider distance-learning options. The same can be said for providing opportunities for practicing nurses who require enhanced job skills, such as physical assessment or leadership abilities.

Technology-based pedagogy enables us to conceive of education without the restrictions of the classroom; hence, the usual mechanisms and parameters around course delivery need to be rethought. For example, traditional lectures, which often are the foundation of content delivery in higher education, become nonexistent in a learner-centered, Web-based environment. In this scenario, a faculty member and student may never see each other despite having lengthy "discussions" that have the potential to shape a student's thinking for life. At the same time, nursing education values strategies that facilitate the learning of a wide range of skills. Nursing education also values knowledge that includes assessment skills, promotion of health in families, adoption of the ethical values of the profession, and communications skills.

The use of technology in nursing education is not a recent phenomenon. Advances in technology have affected the way nurses have been educated since the late 19th century (Sandelowski, 1999). Instructional technology has evolved from the use of a chalkboard and overhead projector to innovations such as computer-assisted instruction, interactive television, presentation media, electronic mail, and virtual classrooms.

Learning Distribution Systems

Four general categories of distributed learning systems in use today support instructional delivery and communication. These include (1) print, (2) audioconferencing, (3) videoconferencing, and (4) computer technology (Billings & Bachmeier, 1994).

Print-Based Delivery

Print-based and correspondence courses employ prepackaged courses and self-contained learning modules. Faculty–student interaction is limited to occasional telephone contact and written feedback on submitted assignments. In recent years, distance education providers have incorporated technologic advancements such as facsimile machines, electronic mail, and assignment submissions through the Internet to supplement print-based courses. This mode of course delivery requires maintaining an expensive and extensive infrastructure. A team of instructional designers, administrators, and support staff are needed to design, manage, plan, and implement the course beyond the work of the faculty member in teaching the course.

Audioconference Delivery

Instructional delivery has been enhanced by advancements in digitalized audio capabilities. This medium includes two-way telephone interaction between the faculty member and groups of students gathered at remote sites. Courses can be offered anywhere in the world that has telephone lines. Audioconferencing provides for real-time delivery at a fairly reasonable cost. It is ideally suited to students who cannot attend courses offered on campus or who do not have easy access to computer technology. One drawback of this method is the lack of visual stimuli to enhance the teaching–learning experience. This is especially evident for students who have been exposed to video games, television, virtual learning experiences, and other hi-tech classes with slide presentations and graphic illustrations of course materials.

Videoconference Delivery

Interactive video networks use compressed digital video technology to deliver two-way audio signals and visual images to distant sites. Although the initial investment in videoconferencing requires an expensive technologic infrastructure, ongoing costs are usually limited to long-distance telephone charges and technical support. Student participation is encouraged through the use of multimedia presentations and interactive capabilities. Recent innovations in technology include the development of desktop video applications and simulations.

This form of delivery best approximates a face-to-face learning experience. It also permits students in remote locations to have access to faculty expertise that they may not have available in their locale. However, the expectations of this technology are often exceeded by the realities of the technical difficulties that can occur. The more complex the technology is, the more complex the problems; this is one reason that more technical support is needed before and during course delivery. Preparing for a videoconference course requires considerable preliminary planning, knowledge of the technology, and the ability to solve problems and use the available technology to its fullest. Another drawback is that students on the receiving end tend to feel isolated from the faculty member, which may result in a perception of substandard and unequal treatment. Extensive faculty development is needed to assist educators to use this method of teaching.

Web-Based Delivery

To participate fully in a Web-based course, students must have regular access to a computer with Internet capacity. Web-based delivery allows students to engage in online interaction with the teacher and other students in a virtual learning environment. The instructional medium is through such software programs as WebCT and Blackboard. Interaction occurs through bulletin boards, chat rooms, and e-mail. New hybrid learning technologies combine the use of audio, video, and/or computer applications, creating multidimensional course delivery options. Courses can be structured as synchronous (real time) or asynchronous (any time) offerings. This delivery method virtually eliminates geographic and access barriers to education. As a result of this fairly recent movement to Web-based instructional technology, the issues associated with this delivery system are emphasized in the following discussion.

■ ISSUES IN ADOPTING TECHNOLOGY IN NURSING EDUCATION

The adoption of advanced instructional technology, like Web-based delivery, has become commonplace in continuing and higher education. It has been viewed as both an educational boon and a technologic "money pit." Using advanced instructional technology in higher education also challenges educators to rethink the teaching and learning enterprise.

Changing Models

In the traditional paradigm of education, the educator is the "sage on the stage," with lectures being the dominant teaching practice. Students are expected to listen passively and absorb large quantities of content in a single serving. This "tell 'em and test 'em" approach sees the teacher as the expert and provider of information. In a learner-centered paradigm, the principles of constructivism, that is, "a learning philosophy that focuses on the ways in which individuals come to know or understand..." (Wambach et al., 1999, p. 268), can be applied in a Web-based course. In this constructivist paradigm, teachers facilitate the learning process and, as such, become "guides on the side" for students.

Changing Roles

The adoption of technology in education requires a paradigm shift that has a dramatic impact on the roles of faculty and students. The role of facilitator has been commonly used to characterize how an educator functions in the technology-based pedagogy (Billings, 1997). In relation to Web-based instruction, specific aspects of the faculty role have been defined as assisting with access and navigation, explaining expectations for students, clarifying the faculty role, stimulating critical thinking, sharing professional expertise, and providing encouragement to online students (VandeVusse & Hanson, 2000). This shift points to the potential discrepancies between necessary computer skills for future nurses and the skills possessed by faculty (Austin, 1999; Carty & Rosenfeld, 1998). How will teachers be able to assist students to develop such skills without developing the computer knowledge and skills themselves?

Carryover to Curricula

Rapid advances in the use of technology in practice have put pressure on faculty to integrate the types of technology used in health care and nursing into already "packed" undergraduate curricula. Educational programs need to make decisions about the extent of use of technology in the delivery of program. Will all educators be expected to adapt their courses or teaching strategies to include advanced instructional technologies?

Demands on Time and Career Activities

A troublesome area for faculty in regard to adopting technology into their teaching is time. The use of technology may actually increase the amount of time needed for teaching. This takes faculty away from other aspects of their academic roles and responsibilities, such as scholarly and research activities. VandeVusse and Hanson (2000) found online courses increased faculty workload, at least in the course development phase. Link and Scholtz (2000) support the premise of allocating preparation time to allow faculty to develop and deliver online courses.

One of the greatest barriers to implementing Web-based instruction in higher education is the lack of recognition it affords faculty. University environments, in particular, place a high value on research and scholarly achievements in the criteria for tenure and promotion. Faculty members who persist in incorporating advanced instructional technologies in their courses serve the curriculum in significant ways, but the time spent on this activity may be perceived by them as detracting from their other academic roles. If so, faculty may be reluctant to take on this type of instruction. Faculties and schools of nursing need to make important decisions about the value placed on using advanced technologies in their programs. Sufficient resources and faculty development activities will help to reduce this significant barrier.

Gains and Losses

One of the benefits of Web-based, online instruction is increased access by students who live in remote locations. For example, education becomes a reality for underrepresented populations like the aboriginal community. A concern with this instructional medium is the loss of face-to-face contact between teachers and students and among students themselves. What becomes of the high value placed on socialization, role modeling, and development of the student–teacher relationship? Can a chat session replace the level of dialogue and discourse that exists in a traditional classroom? It is only after these issues are resolved that faculty will feel comfortable adopting this approach on a large scale.

Isolation

The inherent nature of distance education includes the geographic separation of students from faculty and from other learners. This can often contribute to feelings of social and psychological isolation. Moore and Kearsley (1996) coined the phrase "transactional distance" to describe the psychological distance that occurs in learners. This transactional distance is often caused by miscommunication and psychological gaps occurring between learners and instructors. In a traditional classroom, students are in touch with the nuances of nonverbal communication. Their presence in class contributes to a sense of community with other students and the instructor. In a virtual classroom, the instructor must make a conscious effort to bridge the psychological distance experienced by learners. This can be achieved by promoting the establishment of a community of learners among students.

Effect of Advanced Instructional Technology on Career Choices

There is a call for a critical examination of the use of and growing reliance on technology in education. Mallow and Gilje (1999) caution faculty about the rapidity of adopting technology in nursing education without careful thought about its impact. They note that research to date supports the effectiveness of technology in conveying factual information, and they report student satisfaction. However, little evidence exists regarding "student progress in affective domain criteria such as outcomes related to humanism, moral knowledge development, ethical development, interdisciplinary communication, or caring attributes." Mallow and Gilje recommend that educators consider the core values and social processes of the profession before using technology in the curriculum. Faculty often struggle to balance the use of technology with the need to develop valuable working relationships with students.

In Canada, it is becoming clear that certain areas within nursing practice are "passed over" by students in favor of more technologically challenging environments. Nursing students are drawn to the "power and prestige" of technology. This was substantiated in a longitudinal study by Australian researchers (Stevens & Crouch, 1998). Of note was how nurse educators and nurses in clinical settings championed high-technology areas of nursing practice (e.g., emergency room, intensive care nursing) and created favorable technologic bias in students. The 156 students who were studied responded accordingly and, after graduation, gravitated toward these high-technology nursing practice domains. Because of this socialization by educators and clinicians, students valued specialized training experiences (e.g., intensive care, spinal trauma, pediatric/neonatal intensive care) over basic nursing. Students and graduate nurses in the Australian study perceived that high-technology activities attracted power, prestige, and the nod from the elite of the profession, whereas basic nursing had low status and no power and was marginalized from the profession (Stevens & Crouch, 1998, p. 14). At issue then, is how will the new generation of computer-literate, technologically savvy nurses be attracted to and retained in low-technology practice areas, such as long-term care, or in practice agencies that do not have the financial means to support the newest technologies?

Information and instructional technologies can enhance the quality of the educational experience if used for the right purpose. The adoption of advanced technology in education does not in and of itself guarantee a positive outcome. How can this technology contribute to the overall effectiveness of the educational process in a way that maximizes student learning? Until this question is adequately addressed, educators must be cautious of wading into the technologic sea.

■ FUTURE OF TECHNOLOGY IN EDUCATION AND PRACTICE

Although the future is unclear, one thing is certain: Technology will continue to evolve and advance. The computer has become to the Information Age what the automobile was to the Industrial Age. The Internet is accessed by millions of people daily. The explosion of a digital society has brought about significant transformations in the way people interact, access and process information, and solve problems. Health care professionals are only beginning to appreciate the impact this revolution will have on the ability to deliver comprehensive and safe care. These challenging times call for health care professionals who can think critically and adapt to change quickly.

Impact of Nursing Science on Practice Technology

The development of nursing science, that is, knowledge relevant for nursing practice, will have an impact on the development and use of technology in nursing practice. Clinical nursing information systems, for data categorization and storage, depend on the taxonomic structures developed to reflect the phenomena of the discipline (Graves & Corcoran-Perry, 1996). If nursing science continues to be reflected in numerous classification systems, those that are selected to frame data management programs will have their presence more strongly embedded in the discipline.

Extent of Informatics in Curricula

At this point in nursing's history, it is not surprising that there is a need for more education, support, and research for optimal utilization of computer technology and information systems for practicing nurses, educators, and undergraduate and graduate students (Link & Scholtz, 2000; Smith, Young-Cureton, Hooper, et al., 1998). As the next decades unfold, improved understanding and skills among all these groups are likely, as is concurrent acceptance of advanced information technology as part of nursing.

The Canadian Nursing Informatics Association recently completed a national research study of undergraduate nursing education informatics in Canada (Clarke & Nagle, 2003). Among its recommendations, the study suggested a holistic approach to nursing informatics and that the use of information and communication technology be required in education, health care, research, and policy development. Schools of nursing should also plan and implement a strategy for faculty development in the area of nursing informatics.

As a result, the extent of inclusion of nursing informatics within nursing undergraduate curricula is now being discussed in faculties across the country. New curricula that emerge in the coming years will incorporate decisions about this vital issue. Research into the effectiveness of advanced technology in nursing education will provide valuable information in refining how we incorporate technology into delivering nursing knowledge in undergraduate programs.

Potential for Greater Learning Access

Technology has the potential to improve availability of basic and continuing nursing education for those for whom geography or other barriers have prevented access. This is a particularly significant issue in Canada for nurses and students who live great distances from major cities where higher education or facility-based continuing education is more likely to be located. Today's public demands education that is convenient and flexible. Moreover, in the face of busy lives, the ability to access education from home is appealing. Developments in the kind of available distance education modalities have expanded the options available and increased the quality of communication that is now possible with students who prefer to obtain degrees from their living rooms.

Faculty and student roles will change as the means of communication between faculty and students takes different forms. This can also be said about nursing practice as technology is further incorporated into the health care system. Although computer skills and knowledge will be important in the 21st century, interpersonal relations that rely on basic language and communication skills will remain significant in the provision of nursing care. Being with patients and their families can be facilitated through technologic advances, because it is the way nurses enact their knowing with patients that defines the practice. Technology facilitates and alters this but does not replace nursing knowledge about the work with patients.

Whatever technologic innovations emerge in the future, nursing must remember that technology offers the profession tools to use in its mandate to provide care to individuals and their families in illness and in health promotion. Technology is a means toward the goal of health and quality patient care. Thoughtful development and use can serve nursing and recipients of care well.

■ SUMMARY

Nursing informatics—the application of computer and information science to managing, processing, and documenting nursing data—has a profound effect on nurses and the organizations where they work. The relationship between technology and nursing is marked by tension, with technology viewed as scientific, mechanistic, and reductionistic and nursing viewed as sympathetic, humanistic, and holistic.

The advent of nursing informatics presents challenges and opportunities. The Canadian Nurses Association recognizes that technology can improve health care, but technology without training and support may also impact clients, families, health care professionals, and the health system in untoward ways.

Some applications of nursing informatics are telehealth (the use of advanced telecommunications technologies to exchange health information and provide health care from vast distances), videoconferencing, remote monitoring, and electronic health records.

Challenges associated with technology include "short-shifting," as real-time demands replace patient care with a litany of technical tasks and a focus on outcomes (evidence), performance measurement, and technical expertise that calls for acquiring related knowledge and competence in information technology.

Applied informatics will require nurses to adhere to standards of practice, codes of ethics, provincial legislation, and competencies established by regulatory bodies. To this end, nurses will need to develop or follow telephone standards of practice, policies on providing telehealth across provinces, educational standards and credentials, provisions for maintaining privacy and confidentiality, protocols to guide decision making and judgment, and advice on professional liability issues and employer responsibilities.

Additional challenges to nursing practice are the geographic invisibility of the client and liability for care practices—potential malpractice or misdiagnoses—delivered by distance or electronic technology. On the other hand, changes influenced by informatics will be incorporated into the health care system, offering nurses tools to use in promoting health and caring for the sick.

Benefits to practice include greater client involvement in health-seeking behaviors and health choices, possibly because electronic communication is perceived to offer privacy, immediacy, breadth of information, and different perspectives.

Additional benefits apply particularly to education. One of the benefits of Web-based, online instruction is increased access by students who live in remote locations. Information previously disseminated in classrooms and in textbooks and other print media is now available to students and faculty in remote locations at nontraditional times. Examples include audioconferencing, videoconferencing, and Web-based information delivery. The benefits are obvious, as are the challenges prompted by change. Faculty must clearly articulate the need for information technology in nursing curricula to ensure that all nurses have the skills needed to practise effectively. Faculty must acquire technical skills and adjust to altered roles as collaborators, facilitators, and guides.

Online Resources

Add to your knowledge of this issue:

Aboriginal Nurses Association of Canada: Technology Information	anac.on.ca/web/techinfo.html
Breakthru Counseling Care	www.therapyexpress.com
British Columbia Health Guide, B.C. Ministry of Health	www.bchealthguide.org/kbaltindex.asp
British Computer Society Nursing Specialist Group	www.bcsnsg.org.uk
Canadian Association for Distance Education	www.cade-aced.ca
Canadian Coordinating Office for Health Technology Assessment	www.ccohta.ca
Canadian Nursing Informatics Association	www.cnia.ca
Canadian Society of Telehealth	www.cst-sct.org
COACH–Canada's Health Information Informatics Association	www.coachorg.com
Cochrane Collaboration	www.cochrane.org/index0.htm
Hospital for Sick Children Telehealth Program	www.sickkids.on.ca/telehealth
Nursing Informatics	www.allhealthnet.com/Nursing/Informatics
Office of Health and the Information Highway (OHIH)	www.hc-sc.gc.ca/ohih-bsi/menu_e.html
Telehealth Association of Ontario	www.rohcg.on.ca
Telemedicine Research Center	trc.telemed.org/telemedicine/education.asp

REFLECTIONS on the Chapter . . .

1. From your experience, consider the application of technology and informatics in your practice.

2. How would you describe the relationships among technology, informatics, and nursing practice in these examples?

3. Identify issues related to the use of technology in your practice or in practice situations you have observed.

4. What strategies have you used or observed being used to overcome barriers to the use of technology and informatics in practice?

5. What barriers have you experienced in using technology in your nursing studies?

6. What strategies have you used or could you use to overcome these barriers?

References

Aboriginal Nurses Association of Canada. (2001). *Impact of technology on Aboriginal nursing: A discussion paper.* Ottawa: Author.

Austin, S. I. (1999). Baccalaureate nursing faculty performance of nursing computer literacy skills and curriculum integration of these skills through teaching practice. *Journal of Nursing Education, 38*(6), 260–266.

Bates, A. W. (2000). *Managing technological change: Strategies for college and university leaders.* San Francisco: Jossey-Bass.

Billings, D. M. (1997). Issues in teaching and learning at a distance: Changing roles and responsibilities of administrators, faculty and students. *Computers in Nursing, 15*(2), 69–70.

Billings, D. M., & Bachmeier, B. (1994). Teaching and learning at a distance: A review of the nursing literature. In L. R. Allen (Ed.), *Review of research in nursing education* (Vol. 6, pp. 1–32). Indianapolis: Indiana University School of Nursing.

Bischoff, W. R., & Kelley, S. J. (1999). 21st century house call: The Internet and the World Wide Web. *Holistic Nursing Practice, 13*(4), 42–50.

Brown, J. (1992). Nurses or technicians? The impact of technology on oncology nursing. *Canadian Oncology Nursing Journal, 2*(1), 12–17.

Canadian Nurses Association. (1992). *The role of the nurse in the use of health care technology.* Ottawa: Author. Available: http://www.cna-nurses.ca/sections/cna_issues/ps_html/role_healthtech.html

_____. (2000). Telehealth: Great potential or risky terrain? *Nursing Now: Issues and Trends in Canadian Nursing, 9.*

Carty, B., & Rosenfeld, P. (1998). From computer technology to information technology: Findings from a national study of nursing education. *Computers in Nursing, 16*(5), 259–265.

Clarke, H., & Nagle, L. (2003). OHIH research project: 2002–2003—Final report. Available: http://www.cnia.ca/OHIHfinaltoc.htm

Collins, D. E., & Tilson, E. R. (2001). A new generation on the horizon. *Radiological Technology, 73,* 172–177.

Cooper, M. C., & Powell, E. (1998). Technology and care in a bone marrow transplant unit: Creating and assuaging vulnerability. *Holistic Nursing Practice, 12*(4), 57–68.

Erlen, J. (1994). Technology's seductive power. *Orthopedic Nursing 13,* 50–52, 56.

Gadow, S. (1988). Covenant without cure: Letting go and holding on in chronic illness. In J. Watson & M. Ray (Eds.), *The ethics of care and the ethics of cure.* New York: National League for Nursing.

Gassert, C. A. (1998). The challenge of meeting patients' needs with a national nursing informatics agenda. *Journal of American Medical Informatics Association, 5*(3), 263–268.

_____. (2000). Telehealth and nursing. In B. Carty (Ed.), *Nursing informatics: Education for practice.* New York: Springer.

Graves, J. R., & Corcoran-Perry, S. (1996). The study of nursing informatics. *Holistic Nursing Practice, 11*(1), 15–24.

Hospital for Sick Children. (2001). *What is tele-homecare?* [Online]. Available: http://www.sickkids.ca/telehomecare/program.asp#whatis

Link, D. G., & Scholtz, S. M. (2000). Educational technology and the faculty role: What you don't know can hurt you. *Nurse Educator, 25*(6), 274–276.

Mallow, G. E., & Gilje, F. (1999). Technology-based nursing education: Overview and call for further dialogue. *Journal of Nursing Education, 38*(6), 248–251.

Moore, M.G., & Kearsley, G. (1996). *Distance education: A systems view.* Belmont, CA: Wadsworth.

Nahm, R., & Poston, I. (2000). Measurement of the effects of an integrated, point-of-care computer system on quality of nursing documentation and patient satisfaction. *Computers in Nursing, 18*(5), 220–229.

Office of Health and the Information Highway, Health Canada. (2001). *Toward electronic health records* [Online]. Available: http://www.hc-sc.gc.ca/ohih-bsi/ehr/ehr_dse/ehr_dse_e.html#Overview

Purnell, M. (1998). Who really makes the bed? Uncovering technologic dissonance in nursing. *Holistic Nursing Practice, 12*(4), 12–22.

Ray, M. (1987). Technological caring: A new model in critical care. *Dimensions in Critical Care Nursing, 6,* 166–173.

Reid, J. (1996). *A telemedicine primer: Understanding the issues.* Billings, MT: Art Craft Printers.

Russo, H. (2001). Window of opportunity for home care nurses: Telehealth technologies. *Online Journal of Issues in Nursing, 6*(3). Available: http://www.nursingworld.org/ojin/topic16/tpc16_4.htm

Sandelowski, M. (1998). Looking to care or caring to look? Technology and the rise of spectacular nursing. *Holistic Nursing Practice, 12*(4), 1–11.

_____. (1999). Troubling distinctions: A semiotics of the nursing/technology relationship. *Nursing Inquiry, 6*(3), 198–207.

_____. (2000). Thermometers and telephones: A century of nursing and technology. *American Journal of Nursing, 100*(10), 82–85.

Saranto, K., & Leino-Kilpi, H. (1997). Computer literacy in nursing: Developing the information technology syllabus in nursing education. *Journal of Advanced Nursing, 25*(2), 377–385.

Schoenhofer, S., & Boykin, A. (1998). Discovering the value of nursing in high-technology environments: Outcomes revisited. *Holistic Nursing Practice, 12*(4), 31–39.

Simpson, R. L. (1998). A few points about point-of-care technology. *Nursing Management, 29*(11), 19–22.

_____. (1999). The state of nursing informatics. *Nursing Administration Quarterly, 23*(3), 90–92.

Smith, C. E., Young-Cureton, V., Hooper, C., et al. (1998). A survey of computer technology utilization in school nursing. *Journal of School Nursing, 14*(2), 27–34.

Stevens, J., & Crouch, M. (1998). Frankenstein's nurse! What are schools of nursing creating? *Collegian, 5*(1), 10–15.

VandeVusse, L., & Hanson, L. (2000). Evaluation of online course discussions: Faculty facilitation of active student learning. *Computers in Nursing, 18*(4), 181–188.

Wambach, K., Boyle, D., Hagemaster, J., et al. (1999). Beyond correspondence, video conferencing, and voice mail: Internet-based master's degree courses in nursing. *Journal of Nursing Education, 38*(6), 267–271.

White, M. H., & Dorman, S. M. (2000). Online support for caregivers: Analysis of an Internet Alzheimer mailgroup. *Computers in Nursing, 18*(4), 168–179.

Zemke, R. (2003). Here come the millennials. *Training, 38*(7), 44–49.

Critical Questions

As a way of engaging with the ideas in this chapter, consider the following:

1. How do you understand the claim that research conducted by nurses is not necessarily "nursing research"?

2. What areas of research, apart from nursing research, do you imagine that nurses draw on in practice?

3. In your practice so far, what questions have come up for you that might benefit from research or inquiry?

CHAPTER
15

Dorothy Pringle

The Realities of Canadian Nursing Research

Publications, professional conferences, poster sessions, and scholarship exchanges are key ways to disseminate the nursing research findings that are central to determining what constitutes "best practice." Photography by Beverly Anderson. Used with permission.

Chapter Objectives

After completing this chapter, you will be able to:

1. Appreciate the history of nursing research in Canada.

2. Identify significant milestones in the evolution of nursing research in Canada.

3. Describe obstacles nurses and nursing have had to overcome to develop research.

4. Describe how nurses can use research in their practice.

5. Identify challenges confronting the continued development of nursing research.

6. Discuss ways in which these challenges can be overcome.

esearch has become an important force in Canadian nursing. This has not happened quickly, and, whereas the ultimate impact of research is still not clear, it has the potential to revolutionize nursing. To illuminate the impact of research in nursing, this chapter traces the evolution of nursing research in Canada, examines the influence it currently has on nursing practice and education and how it exercises that influence, and speculates on the potential influence of nursing research. This chapter also explores the contribution nursing research has made to the health of Canadians. Finally, this chapter discusses issues regarding getting nurses to become involved in the utilization of research and the future of nursing research in Canadian health care.

■ THE EVOLUTION OF NURSING RESEARCH IN CANADA

This section could easily have been called "The Revolution in Nursing Research in Canada" because the last 4 decades of the 20th century represent no less than a revolution. Revolutions are not one-battle affairs. They are fought over time and include many skirmishes as well as a few large-scale battles. Usually, only the battles make their way into the history books. Although there were no declarations of war and no lives lost, nurse researchers in Canada struggled to establish nursing research firmly during the second half of the century and finally achieved that status in the 1990s.

The evolution of Canadian nursing research can best be appreciated against the landscape of its counterpart in the United States. Canada followed the American model of nursing education rather than the British model in that it identified nursing education as appropriately located in universities. This does not mean that all or even most nursing education occurred there, but in Canada, from 1919 onward when the University of British Columbia commenced a program to prepare nurses for public health, nursing was associated with universities. This was very important in the evolution of nursing research because universities are where the vast majority of health-related research occurs. Furthermore, the usual academic progression of baccalaureate to master's to doctoral education was adopted in Canadian nursing (as it was in the United States), and this set the pattern for the preparation of nurse researchers in the same mould as other academic disciplines.

In Britain, the voyage has been more difficult than in North America because of early decisions that nursing education should occur in hospitals and that specialization should be through hospital-based certification programs rather than through the pursuit of master's degrees. Nursing education essentially did not move to universities until the 1990s. There were exceptions, such as the University of Edinburgh, which has had a nursing program since the 1940s, but few nurses pursued their initial nursing education through university programs.

Publishing Nursing Research

Nursing research began in Canada in the 1920s with a focus on nursing education. However, over the next half century, only occasional studies were conducted by the few people prepared to undertake research

(Ritchie, 1992). This contrasts with the United States, where nursing research began developing momentum in the 1940s and 1950s. *Nursing Research*, the first research journal in nursing, was initially published in the United States in 1952. The first nursing research text, *Better Patient Care Through Nursing Research* (Abdellah & Levine), appeared in 1965. The impetus for much early nursing research came from McGill University and the leadership of Dr. Moyra Allen. Dr. Allen completed her PhD at Stanford University and returned to Canada and to McGill. She saw the need for a nursing research journal to serve Canadian researchers, and *Nursing Papers* was launched in 1969 with just two editions per year. In 1975, *Nursing Papers* became bilingual, publishing both French and English articles and providing abstracts of the articles in the other language. The French language name, *Perspectives en Nursing*, was added (Gottlieb, 1999) at that time. It was renamed the *Canadian Journal of Nursing Research/Revue Canadienne de Recherche en Sciences Infirmiéres* in 1988. Gottlieb traced the history of this journal in the editorial that introduced the 30-year anniversary edition published in 1999. Maintaining this journal represents one of the struggles in the development of nursing research in Canada. There was never enough money, manuscripts—particularly in the early days—were hard to come by, and circulation was low. However, it was crucial and remains so for Canadian nurse researchers to have a vehicle in which to publish their works, some of which address topics of particular interest to the Canadian scene. For example, in 2002, Butler and colleagues produced a report on a workshop that was held to develop a national strategy for integrating supportive care in research, practice, and policy. In addition, the editorials reflected issues in Canadian health care and nursing education and what research had to bring to these issues (Gagnon, 1999). The journal remains at McGill and issues four editions a year.

Many other journals have been established in Canada since 1969, including journals that support specialty fields, for example, the *Canadian Journal of Cardiovascular Nursing,* the *Canadian Journal of Nursing Leadership and Perspectives,* and the *Canadian Gerontological Nurse*, the journal of the Canadian Gerontological Nurses Association. Several of these journals began by publishing articles about clinical practice with very little research reflected in them. This has changed over the years. They all now publish reports of research on topics relevant to practitioners in their specialty areas. Most have introduced peer review, which means that the reports submitted by the researchers are reviewed by people with research expertise in that field to determine whether the research is sufficiently sound to warrant publication. The reviewers are not informed who the authors are; hence, the peer review is called a "blind" review. This prevents the reviewers from bringing positive or negative biases colored by any relationships they might have with the authors of the research.

Canadian researchers publish well beyond journals based in Canada and well beyond nursing journals. Many excellent nursing research journals are now available, including *Research in Nursing & Health*, the *Journal of Nursing Scholarship* (formerly *Image*), *Qualitative Nursing Research,* and the *Western Journal of Nursing Research*. Despite the excellence of many journals and the filter of the peer-review process, the caveat "reader beware" still holds true. Consumers of research must bring a critical perspective to reading all published research to determine whether the findings of the study can or should be generalized to their own practice.

Funding of Nursing Research

Until the mid-1990s, being a nurse researcher in Canada was challenging because of the lack of resources available. The conduct of research takes funds, and funds were scarce to support the kinds of research that nurses undertook. The Medical Research Council (MRC) of Canada was launched in 1960 with a mandate to "promote, assist and undertake basic, applied and clinical research in Canada in the health sciences" (MRC Act), but because of the meager funding available, MRC decided to limit its support to biomedical research. This did not change in any fundamental way until the mid-1990s and, as such, did not support research by nurses.

The alternative major national source of funding available to nurses (and other non-biomedical researchers) was the National Health Research and Development Program (NHRDP) of Health Canada (previously Health and Welfare Canada). Unlike the MRC, which operated in an arm's-length relationship with the government and could develop its own research priorities, the NHRDP was a department of the government and was expected to support research that assisted the government to meet its objectives. The size of their budgets differed enormously: Although the MRC had a budget of about $150 million in 1990, the budget for the NHRDP was about one tenth of that and fluctuated every year depending on the government's largesse. Because the NHRDP was the major general research fund (i.e., not limited to a specialty area) available to nurses at the national level, the competition was fierce and the size of the available grants was limited. Grants could be as large as $300,000 for a 2-year project, but most were less than $100,000 annually.

Despite the constraints of both a limited budget and government-directed focus, the NHRDP proved to be a great benefactor of nurses. Many nurses who pursued doctoral education from 1975 until 2000 received fellowships from the NHRDP that supported them during their studies. Nurses won these fellowships in national interdisciplinary competitions that demonstrated their ability to compete head-on with the best candidates from other health disciplines. The scientists who gained this training went on to become some of the best researchers in the country. Academically able, they were admitted to excellent research training programs in nursing and other disciplines in Canada and elsewhere and worked with some of the best supervisors available.

The NHRDP was also a source of grants needed by nurses for the actual conduct of research. Charitable organizations with special interests in particular diseases, for example, the Heart and Stroke Foundation, the Diabetes Association, and the Cancer Society, raise money to support research into those diseases. Many tended to favor biomedical research because of its orientation to seek cures rather than to focus research on caring for individuals with the disease. However, some nurses were successful in receiving grants from competitions held by these organizations and built important research programs based on this funding. Fortunately, the policies of many of these foundations evolved over the years, and nursing research is now part of the range of studies they fund.

Because of the very limited funding available at the national level, the Canadian Nurses Foundation (CNF) was established by the Canadian Nurses Association (CNA) in 1962 initially to provide support for nurses studying at the master's and doctoral levels. (See Ritchie [1992] for a description of the development of the CNF.) In 1984, small grants for the conduct of research were added. As with many nursing-based endeavors, the CNF has struggled since its inception to secure sufficient funds to keep itself in business. Much of its support has come from donations from nurse researchers themselves. In the days before NHRDP and MRC funding, the CNF was frequently the sole resource nurses could turn to. Even today, the CNF will fund studies that address topics unique to nursing that would not likely be successful in interdisciplinary competitions. The investigation of nursing-specific themes, such as the nature of the nurse–patient relationship, is appreciated as vital to understanding nursing as a discipline in peer-review committees dominated by nurses. This is not necessarily true of interdisciplinary committees unless a strong nursing research advocate is a member of the committee. In 2002, the CNF entered into a partnership with the Canadian Health Services Research Foundation (described later) to increase their resources substantially. For the first time in its history, the funding future looks secure, and the CNF will be able to support substantially more graduate fellowships at higher dollar levels and provide larger grants to support research projects.

The Social Sciences and Humanities Research Council of Canada (SSHRC) has been and continues to be an important source of funding for many nurse researchers. The SSHRC is a national foundation established in 1977 on the same basis as the MRC, that is, arm's length from government. (The third national body in Canada that makes up the research funding triumvirate is the Natural Sciences and Engineering Research Council, or NSERC.) The SSHRC also derives its funding from the federal government but always has had a substantially smaller budget than the MRC. In 2001–2002, its budget was $156.5 million. In contrast, the successor to the MRC, the Canadian Institutes of Health Research (CIHR), had a budget of $560 million for that same year. As its name suggests, the SSHRC funds research that examines questions relevant to the social, cultural, and economic dimensions of life. For many qualitative nurse researchers and those interested in ethical, historical, and psychosocial dimensions of nursing, the SSHRC is a major source of funding. The peer-review committees understand and value qualitative methods to address questions and have expertise in content areas relevant to nursing. Nurses also have received doctoral fellowship support from the SSHRC. However, the size of the overall budget dictates that most SSHRC grants are relatively modest in comparison to those available from the MRC and the CIHR.

Some provincial granting bodies have had a tradition of providing funds to nursing research, for example, the Fonds de Researche Scientifique du Québec (FRSQ), the British Columbia Health Research Foundation, and the Ministry of Health of Ontario. Unfortunately, the Ontario program, which was an enormous contributor to nursing research in the 1980s and early 1990s (O'Connor & Bouchard, 1991), is no longer in operation, but the British Columbia Foundation was replaced by the Michael Smith Foundation for Health Research (MSFHR) in 2001 to honor British Columbia's first Nobel Prize winner. The MSFHR has developed a variety of innovative ways to support research in British Columbia, and nurses have successfully capitalized on these opportunities.

In 1980, Alberta was enjoying a booming economy, and the government decided to invest some of the money not needed for current provincial needs into the Alberta Heritage Foundation for Medical Research (AHFMR). A $300 million endowment was created to fund basic biomedical and medical research. New research positions were created, and new competitions for doctoral and postdoctoral training were initiated. Nurses in the province objected, and, after a major initiative led by Dr. Shirley Stinson of the University of Alberta, the Alberta Nursing Research Foundation (ANRF) was established in 1982 and provided with an expendable $1 million yearly budget. This contrasted with the large endowment provided for biomedical research but nevertheless was a breakthrough for nursing research in Canada.

The ANRF was certainly welcomed by nurse researchers in the province, but the fund was too limited to award large grants, for example, more than $100,000 per year for several years. Furthermore, it separated nursing from the more intense interdisciplinary competitions that one finds at the national level. However, provincial competitions are good training grounds for learning to write strong, coherent grant applications that will survive and be successful at the national level. The ANRF was terminated in 1994, but Alberta nurses once again successfully mounted a campaign, and the AHFMR expanded its mandate to include nursing research and nurse researchers among those eligible to compete for their funds. Since then, nurses have successfully competed for grants, doctoral and postdoctoral training awards, and research scholar awards to support young investigators. In fact, the AHFMR has become a major source of support for nurse researchers in Alberta and a model of an innovative granting body for the rest of the country.

At the national level, a lot happened in the 1990s. The Canadian Health Services Research Foundation (CHSRF) was established in 1997 with an initial endowment of $66.5 million that was increased by an additional $60 million in 1999. Its mandate is to fund research on health services management and policy. In 1999, as a result of successful lobbying of Health Canada by the CNA, $25 million was allocated to the CHSRF for the funding of nursing research over a 10-year period. The CHSRF was the recipient of the funds because the CNA argued that workplace difficulties and workforce shortages were at crisis levels in Canada and required serious research attention. The agreement between Health Canada and the CHSRF specified that $500,000 per year was to be spent on clinical research; the rest was to go to health services and policy research relevant to nursing. The CHSRF and the CNF have developed the Nursing Care Partnership Fund for the administration of the clinical research dollars.

Almost simultaneously with the CHSRF developments, the MRC—led by Dr. Henry Friesen—undertook a national study that resulted in a reinterpretation of its mandate to embrace all types of research. New peer-review committees were developed, and nurses and researchers from other disciplines, such as occupational and physical therapy, epidemiology, and family medicine, were able to compete. This was followed quickly by a redevelopment of the entire health research enterprise. The CIHR was approved by the government of Canada in June 2000. The MRC and the NHRDP, as such, ceased to exist, and the CIHR became the depository for the bulk of national health research funding.

Thirteen "virtual" interdisciplinary institutes were created to represent such diverse areas of science as genetics, aging, cancer, aboriginal health, and gender and health. Each institute reflects four pillars or types of research: basic biomedical, clinical, health services, and population health. A scientific director heads each institute and is assisted by an advisory board. The CIHR started with a budget of $339 million, which increased to slightly more than $600 million by 2004. A target was set to try to achieve $1 billion in funding annually by 2006. As this date approaches, the likelihood of reaching that target becomes less. This is a problem for all health researchers and speaks to the limited commitment of the federal government to research relative to other countries' such as the United States' and Britain's.

Nurses are an integral part of the CIHR. Dr. Nancy Edwards, an outstanding nurse researcher who holds a CHSRF nursing research chair in the School of Nursing at the University of Ottawa, is a member of the council, which is the policymaking body of the CIHR. A nurse scientist, Dr. Miriam Stewart, is the scientific director of the Institute of Gender and Health, and another nurse, Earl Nowgesic, is the assistant director of the Institute of Aboriginal Health. There are nurses on most institute advisory boards, and nurses sit on all the appropriate peer-review committees. They chair some committees and serve as scientific officers on others. Nurse researchers now compete for much larger grants available through the CIHR and take their place alongside scientists from all other disciplines.

The structure of the CIHR was not what nursing had hoped for. Given the frustration created by the MRC's exclusion of nursing research for so many years and the very tentative steps to include an applied research agenda in the 1990s, nursing had hoped that the new approach to research funding would include an institute for nursing research. However, very early in its development, the CIHR embraced a strictly interdisciplinary agenda and declared that no institute would be disciplinary based. Despite this assertion, the Canadian Association of University Schools of Nursing (CAUSN) and the Canadian Association of Nurse Researchers (CANR) mounted a campaign for a nursing-specific institute. The two organizations successfully competed for funds from the SSHRC and the CHSRF to undertake a planning exercise for a new institute. Representatives met and debated the relative advantages of advocating for a nursing research institute versus a nursing and caregiving research institute. The latter was seen to accommodate an interdisciplinary thrust while acknowledging nursing as the lead discipline. The decision was made to go with the latter, and a proposal for such an institute was developed and submitted to the CIHR interim council, which acted as a planning committee. The application was not successful.

In the United States, nursing research has had a different history. After many years of concerted and well-coordinated lobbying by nurses, a National Center for Nursing Research was created in 1985 as part of the National Institutes of Health (NIH). The center was elevated to the status of a National Institute of Nursing Research (NINR) in 1992. The American National Institutes of Health are organized very differently than their Canadian counterparts in that they have dedicated buildings, they conduct research within the institutes (intramural research), and they mount competitions for researchers to apply for funds (extramural research). Also in comparison to their Canadian counterparts, they have relatively large budgets, many in the billions of dollars. The NINR's autonomy and resources (a budget of $134,579 million in the United States in 2004) mean that American nurses are able to identify areas of particular interest to nursing or areas that require special attention and establish special competitions (in addition to their regular competitions) to drive research into them. For example, they have identified five themes that require specific nursing research attention, including changing lifestyle behaviors for better health and enhancing the end-of-life experience for patients and their families.

Canadian nursing cannot do this under the CIHR structure and must seek other routes to gain attention for special needs areas. This battle for the recognition of nursing research is not over. Nurses are well positioned within the CIHR, and there is no reason to believe that individual nurse researchers will not do well in competitions for grant support. However, the discipline has yet to develop strategies for working with the various institutes so that nursing is heard when new initiatives are required to understand issues and problems that either are unique to nursing or are those in which nurses play a major role.

Preparation of Nurse Researchers

The conduct of nursing research depends on having well-prepared researchers. This requires programs of study and funds for students while they study. Preparation at the doctoral level is seen as necessary for most people to undertake the role of principal investigator, the person who takes major responsibility for designing and managing research studies. Canada was late to develop doctoral programs in nursing relative to other countries. Our first programs occurred in the early 1990s, whereas the United States already had four doctoral programs by 1975. By 1990, the United States had 45 programs, and Finland, Japan, Korea, and Thailand all had doctoral programs in nursing.

In the mid-1980s, McGill University, followed closely by the University of Alberta, began to plan in earnest for doctoral programs in nursing. In the case of McGill, the governing body of the faculty of medicine—of which the School of Nursing was a department—challenged the plan. The faculty of medicine did not think that nursing had demonstrated sufficient resources or a sufficient body of knowledge to justify a PhD degree in the discipline. The faculty of nursing at the University of Alberta saw their program approved at the university level, but the government was not prepared to provide funding for it. The faculty decided that it should not try to mount the program in the absence of funds; essentially, they determined that if the doctoral program could be mounted without additional government funding, even if it were difficult, the government would never provide the funds.

Both programs went on hold while these internal and external political situations were resolved. However, both McGill and the University of Alberta had provisions within the universities that made it possible to admit individual students to studies in areas in which doctoral programs were planned. Both nursing schools used these provisions to admit nurses to *ad hoc* studies, and several nurses were able to complete the requirements for a PhD in nursing before formal programs were established. One of these nurses was Dr. Francine Ducharme, the first person to complete a PhD in nursing in Canada. Dr. Ducharme completed her doctoral program at McGill University.

Although it took a long time to initiate doctoral education in Canada, once started, 5 programs began within a 3-year period. After intensely lobbying the government, the University of Alberta received funding to begin a doctoral program in nursing in January 1991, and the University of British Columbia followed with a program later that same year. The University of Toronto opened a program in 1993, and a joint bilingual program between McGill University and the University of Montreal opened that same year. McMaster University completed this quintet with a program in 1994. Additional nursing PhD programs have been added at the Universities of Calgary, Ottawa, Victoria, and Western Ontario and at Dalhousie University and Laval University. Individual students can study with specific supervisors at the Universities of Saskatchewan and Manitoba and receive PhD degrees, but these universities do not have programs per se. These programs started with small enrollments of between 3 and 5 students, but, by the year 2002, a total of 271 students were enrolled in these doctoral programs. Between 10 and 20 students graduated each year from 2000 to 2002 (Canadian Nurses Association/Canadian Association of Schools of Nursing [CNA/CASN], 2004).

The graduates of these early programs are becoming the major Canadian nurse researchers of the early 21st century. Dr. Ducharme holds the endowed chair in gerontological nursing research at the University of Montreal. Dr. Bonnie Stevens, another graduate of the *ad hoc* doctoral program at McGill, holds the Signy Hildur Eaton Chair in pediatric nursing research at the Hospital for Sick Children at the University of Toronto. Dr. Joan Bottorff, a graduate of the University of Alberta *ad hoc* program, held an NHRDP research scholar award, and Dr. Carole Estabrooks, another Alberta graduate, is a CIHR/MRC health scholar and an AHFMR population health investigator, and she directs the Centre for Knowledge Transfer at the same university.

Like everything else in the establishment of the nursing research enterprise in Canada, the mounting of doctoral programs did not come easily. Nursing had to prove itself once again as a legitimate academic field of study in several of the universities. Only a few faculties and schools actually received additional funding to support these programs, and the rest stretched their budgets to include this new resource-intensive activity. Now this most important battle may be declared won.

These programs provide the infrastructure for the continued production of researchers without which all the other elements of the conduct of research could not proceed. Furthermore, after 10 years of experience, a clearly Canadian model of the PhD degree in nursing has emerged. Canadian programs require only a few courses, four to five on average, including a course on the philosophic underpinning of science (in general) and nursing science (in particular), one or two research design and statistics courses, and one or two courses on theories and content specific to the students' research. The dissertations are a very large component of the programs and are begun immediately upon entering the program. These dissertations are substantial in scope, and the supervisory committee is usually interdisciplinary in composition.

This model contrasts markedly with the design of doctoral programs in the United States, which include a large number of courses, usually around 20, a smaller dissertation which the doctoral candidate does not begin until completing much of the course work, and a supervisory committee composed largely of nurse scientists. In Britain, there is usually no required course work, and the entire focus of the PhD degree program is on the conduct of the research, which is supervised by one individual.

All of these models are consistent with the approach to doctoral work in general in their host countries. One design is not superior to another, but they do tend to produce researchers with somewhat different strengths. Graduates of Canadian programs have strong research design skills and an appreciation of what other disciplines bring to the conduct of research even when that research is focused on answering questions relevant to nursing. This is an important orientation given the strong interdisciplinary bent of the national funding agencies.

Funding to support nursing doctoral students has not proved as buoyant as the programs themselves. The absence of a specific source of funds for nurses is felt every time the CIHR releases the list of successful candidates for doctoral fellowships. There is an enormous demand for doctoral support, and the CIHR funds fewer than 20% of the applications it receives. The limited access to funds means that many doctoral students work full- or part-time throughout their programs. This tends to slow their progress and creates a great burden on the individual who may be raising a family at the same time. This is a continuing struggle and one that requires creative solutions by nursing agencies.

Although completion of a doctoral program was sufficient to commence a research career until recently, it is increasingly common for graduates to undertake 2 to 3 years of postdoctoral studies before accepting an academic or research position. The graduates of Canadian nursing PhD programs have achieved a high level of success in national and provincial competitions for funding to support their postdoctoral work. Most Canadian funding sources require candidates to change their locations and their supervisors to get the maximum benefit from further studies. Postdoctoral work is intended to turn young researchers into independent researchers and render them competitive for grants, which PhD studies alone sometimes cannot or do not do.

Research takes time: time to undertake the review of the current state of knowledge in the area of interest; time to assemble a research team and to meet with them; time to determine the most appropriate design, data gathering approach, and measurement instruments; time to figure out the data analysis strategies; and time to write the grant and get ethics approval. Because it is so time intensive, research frequently is relegated to second or third place behind other responsibilities. Nurses in academic settings find themselves with heavy teaching loads, a situation which requires them to fit research into weekends and evenings. Similar dilemmas are faced by administrators and clinical nurse specialists, who have heavy demands on their time but are expected and encouraged to do research. One way of managing this is for the researcher to apply for a "personnel award." These awards have a number of different titles depending on the granting agency and the stage of the individual's career: research scholar, career scientist, scientist, and national scientist, among others. Personnel awards provide a researcher's employer with at least half of the researcher's salary, with an expectation that 75% of the person's time can be spent on research.

These awards are very important, particularly to young scientists who are just launching their independent research careers. As noted earlier, because the MRC and most disease-related funding charities did not support nurses, young scientists depended on the NHRDP and a few provincial funding agencies for personnel awards. In the 1970s, Dr. Moyra Allen at McGill won an NHRDP National Health Scientist award to study the health-promoting activities nurses undertook at the nursing-run health station in Montreal. A few other nurses were awarded the NHRDP research scholar funding. In the 1970s, awards were granted to Dr. Shirley Stinson of the University of Alberta and Dr. Jacqueline Chapman at the University of Toronto; in the 1980s, awards went to Dr. Sharon Ogden Burke at Queen's University, Dr. Gina Browne at McMaster University, Dr. Joan Anderson at the University of British Columbia, and Dr. Janice Morse at the University of Alberta. These were important breakthroughs for nursing as a discipline, but they were too few to move the development of nursing science ahead at a pace that reflected the size of the profession. Much more was needed, particularly to assist young investigators to launch their research careers.

Dr. Ginette Rodger was executive director of the CNA in the 1980s, and, in 1986, she was appointed to the MRC council. Only one nurse before her, Dr. Dorothy Kergin, then the director of the McMaster University School of Nursing, had ever sat on the decision-making body of the MRC. Dr. Rodger used this opportunity to encourage the MRC to work with the NHRDP to create a new set of research scholar awards for nurses only. After huge initial resistance, the agencies capitulated, and the Joint MRC/NHRDP Research Scholar awards were launched in 1988. Schools of nursing had to compete for these awards on behalf of their best young researchers. The program got off to a rather slow start, but, over the subsequent 7 years of its existence, 17 nurse researchers from 8 universities received 5-year awards. (The 17 included Drs. Hilary Llewellyn-Thomas and Diane Irvine, University of Toronto; Annette O'Connor, University of Ottawa; Celeste Johnston, McGill University; Louise Levesque, Francine Ducharme, Lise Talbot, and Sylvie Robichaud, University of Montreal; Lesley Degner and Linda Kristjanson, University of Manitoba; Sharon Ogden Burke and Carol Roberts, Queen's University; Marilyn Ford-Gilboe and Helene Berman, University of Western Ontario; and Janice Morse, Jane Drummond, and Beverley O'Brien, University of Alberta.) Building on their earlier successes, some went on to compete for and receive the NHRDP research scholar awards for another 5 years. These awardees, with few exceptions, have become leaders in nursing research in Canada.

Nurse researchers now compete for the CIHR personnel awards along with all the best scientists from other health disciplines and are enjoying a reasonable level of success. Is this another battle won in the road to research respectability and achievement or one that is still in progress? The CIHR is still too new to be able to draw any definitive conclusions about whether nurses can continue to rely on it as a major source of support for funding that will allow them to devote a significant portion of their time to research. Although the absence of the NHRDP as a consistent funding source is felt, several provincial governments (Ontario, Alberta, Quebec) offer competitions for these types of awards, and nurse researchers have done well in them.

Research chairs are now a major resource on the national scene. There have been research chairs for many years, but the 1990s saw an avalanche of new chairs become available. The creation of named chairs became a popular fundraising target for universities and hospitals. Dr. Ellen Hodnett assumed the first endowed research chair in nursing in Canada, the Heather M. Reisman Chair in Perinatal Nursing Research, a joint chair between Mt. Sinai Hospital and the University of Toronto. The CHSRF added five more nursing chairs in 2000. These chairs are not endowed but will support the incumbents for 10 years. Research chairs are filled by researchers who have international reputations for their work and who have made outstanding contributions to specific fields of knowledge. At the beginning of the 21st century, the number of newly endowed chairs is outstripping the number of senior nurse researchers available to fill them. The University of Toronto and its teaching hospitals alone have five endowed nursing research chairs they have been unable to fill. This is a new phenomenon for nursing (i.e., to have more resources than it is able to absorb), and it puts pressure on the discipline to continue to support young investigators, protect their time, and assist them to develop the reputations that will make them eligible to assume chairs in the future.

A final indicator of the maturing of nursing research in Canada is reflected in the amount of funding nurses are receiving to conduct their research. The CAUSN compiled the research funding received by nurses as principal or coinvestigators on grants throughout the 1980s, and O'Connor and Bouchard (1991) published the CAUSN results for the 1988–1989 academic year. In total, nurses had received $4,491,000. Close to $3 million of these funds were received by universities in Ontario. Ten years later, in 1998, the total amount of grant money for research on which nurses were either principal or coinvestigators essentially doubled to $8,584,611 (Table 15.1).

What followed over the next 3 years was an almost exponential growth in funding: $14,390,303 in 1999, $19,323,971 in 2000, and an all-time high of $27,528,277 in 2001 (CASN, 2002). This escalating growth is attributable to both an increased number of nurses conducting research and an increase in the amount of funding available to do the work. By 1998, the first graduates of the Canadian doctoral programs in nursing were applying for grants. The beginning productivity of this new stream of researchers bodes well for the future of research. Nurses are now successfully competing for funds provincially, nationally,

TABLE 15.1	Summary of Research Funding by Region in Canada, 1998–2001			
Amount of Research Funding ($)				
Region	1998	1999	2000	2001
Western Canada	2,041,378	4,127,076	5,585,288	11,433,161
Ontario	5,225,348	8,441,655	10,969,440	13,537,441
Quebec	203,454	172,245	467,328	721,818
Atlantic Canada	1,114,432	1,649,327	2,301,915	1,835,857
Total Canada	8,584,612	14,390,303	19,323,971	27,528,277

Source: Canadian Association of Schools of Nursing, as of March 9, 2002.

and internationally. Several Canadian nurses (Dr. Janice Morse from the University of Alberta, and Drs. Bonnie Stevens, Ellen Hodnett, and Souraya Sidani from the University of Toronto) hold, or have held, NINR grants worth millions of dollars because they have been able to demonstrate that there is no one in the United States who can mount the same research as they are proposing.

■ INFLUENCE OF RESEARCH ON NURSING PRACTICE AND EDUCATION

After touring the status of historical and current nursing research in Canada, one is likely to ask what nursing research is and where it fits into the spectrum of human sciences research.

Research, and especially research in a profession like nursing, is a service to the people who require the assistance of nurses and to the health care providers, especially nurses, who provide that assistance. Some disciplines can investigate phenomena simply to satisfy the curiosity of the investigators. Nurses do not enjoy that luxury. It should always be possible to explain the relevance of each research study that is undertaken.

Defining nursing research rather precisely occupied nurse researchers for several decades in the last century, but this question receives little attention now, and there is little angst about the answers. Bloch (1981) developed a model of nursing research and nursing science that nicely locates these within the larger landscape of science. She describes a communal pool of what she calls "fundamental research" to which researchers of all disciplines contribute. This pool includes knowledge about life, health, and disease. Before this knowledge can be applied directly in practice, it must first be translated into a series of interventions. Nursing develops its interventions based on this fundamental knowledge, as do all other applied disciplines, such as psychology and medicine. An important message in Bloch's perspective is that nursing must draw on knowledge developed by many other disciplines to develop interventions that are unique to its practice. These interventions are tested, and their results, taken together, form nursing science or the science of nursing practice. Nurse researchers have a responsibility to contribute to the pool of fundamental knowledge as well as to address questions that affect nursing practice. This perspective does not preclude researchers from other disciplines undertaking research on nursing practice problems.

The reality is that in addition to research that is of particular interest to nurses, nurse researchers work on many studies that do not directly impinge on nursing practice but to which they bring expertise that benefits the study. A good example of this is found in the work of Dr. Ellen Hodnett. The focus of her research is care of mothers and families during labor and delivery, particularly the benefits of one-to-one supportive care by nurses. However, Dr. Hodnett is part of a team of researchers that includes obstetricians, pediatricians, epidemiologists, and statisticians who study a whole range of issues related to perinatal care of women.

Among many others, she was a coinvestigator on a large international trial that investigated breech positions of babies and whether allowing breech deliveries or intervening with cesarean sections was more beneficial to the mothers and babies (Hannah et al., 2000). Clearly, nurses do not make decisions about cesarean sections, but they are parts of teams that make those decisions, and they need to understand the nature of the issues that drive decisions one way or the other. Furthermore, the care of women during the long difficult labor when a breech presentation is involved is of significant importance to nurses. Dr. Hodnett brought her deep understanding of perinatal care and her skill in designing multisite, international, randomized clinical trials to the team. The outcome of this particular study was interesting: The trial was terminated early because the evidence for both mothers and babies was overwhelmingly in favor of intervening and delivering the babies by cesarean section rather than letting the labor proceed to a vaginal delivery. This was not an outcome that the investigator team had predicted (Hannah et al., 2000).

Influence on Practice

Throughout the 1970s and part of the 1980s, much was made of nurses delivering theory-based practice. This referred most frequently to the grand theories that a number of nurses had developed to understand and explain patient behaviors and the relationships between what nurses did and patients' responses to these interventions. Among these were King's Interacting Systems Framework, Rogers' Science of Unitary Human Beings, and Neuman's Systems Model (Fawcett, 1989). The term *theory-based practice* is rarely heard now because the era of evidence-based practice has replaced it.

Evidence-based practice, which is sometimes referred to as *best practice,* means that the type of care delivered (or in health-promotion arenas, the health-promotion strategy used) is based on the best research evidence about that practice integrated with knowledge about the patient's preferences, culture, emotional status, information needs, and unique physiologic responses, among other things.

Research is now regarded as central to the determination of what constitutes best practice. Basing care on research evidence was not possible until recently because there was simply not enough research available in most areas of nursing practice to influence the decision. This is still the case in some areas of nursing practice, such as the care of patients with dementia or chronic psychiatric disorders. Nevertheless, the evidence is mounting, and increasingly nurses can turn to research studies to help them determine what is best for individual patients or classes of patients, for example, patients being supported by mechanical ventilation or recovering from coronary artery bypass surgery. This represents a significant change in how nurses approach patient care and will change the view that nurses turn to each other rather than to research literature to answer questions about what is the most current thinking on the care of patients with specific problems.

One research study in an area tells us something about that area but is rarely sufficient in scope or size to support a change in practice. An exception might be a large, multisite, randomized controlled trial with thousands of patients enrolled, such as the study on breech births referred to earlier. Clinicians seek out a series of studies that focus on a specific type of practice, but this requires a method for integrating the findings from across the studies so a determination can be made of what the true conclusion is. Two approaches are used: systematic reviews and meta-analysis. In systematic reviews (sometimes called *integrated reviews*), all the studies that relate to a topic are retrieved from published and unpublished sources, the individual studies are assessed for their methodologic quality, and then the findings from all the studies, taking into account the quality of the research, are examined to reach a decision on what is the state of knowledge on that topic (Mulrow & Cook, 1998). If possible, a recommendation is made to change practice. However, if the evidence is conflicted or the quality of the studies is poor, then a recommendation for further research is made specifying the questions it must address and the designs needed before a conclusion can be reached.

A meta-analysis takes the systematic review a step further and integrates the actual data from all the studies to reach a statistical decision about whether a particular intervention improves outcomes. This is reported in the form of an odds ratio or an effect size, depending on whether the data are continuous or dichotomous (Lau, Ioannidis, & Schmid, 1998). This latter technique is applied mainly to analysis of findings from randomized controlled trials. Systematic reviews and meta-analyses are now commonly found in journals, and the Cochrane Library provides meta-analyses on a wide range of topics, including many that are relevant to nursing. These analyses are updated regularly as new research is published.

It is a common misconception that systematic reviews can be undertaken only on experimental research and that the randomized controlled analysis is the gold standard for all research (Jennings, 2000; Petticrew, 2001). Nursing research includes an increasing number of randomized controlled trials, but much of nursing practice does not lend itself to experimental treatment. Nursing relies heavily on qualitative research to help understand phenomena from the perspective of the patient; furthermore, interventions that include a strong interpersonal component are difficult to subject to the methodology of randomized controlled analysis. Nevertheless, nurses need to know what the state of knowledge is in the range of patient care issues that confront them. Systematic reviews provide a method for summarizing the state of knowledge across the range of research methods used to address nursing research questions (Petticrew, 2001).

Conclusions from systematic reviews and meta-analyses frequently are integrated into clinical practice guidelines or care maps for patients who share a common diagnosis or clinical condition. Most of these guidelines are interdisciplinary in nature and provide the type and timing of tests, interventions, and medications across all the disciplines providing patient care.

The development of electronic databases has made the search for and location of research studies and systematic reviews immensely easier. Access to these databases in all hospital libraries and frequently through computers located on hospital patient care units or public health units has provided nurses with findings from research never before possible. As well, there are Internet Web sites that house clinical practice guidelines that teams of practitioners can access rather than having to start from scratch every time to develop their own. In practice, however, most teams find it difficult to incorporate other teams' guidelines without studying the issues, reading the original research or at least the systematic reviews, and finally adapting the guidelines to their own environments and patient populations.

As difficult as it is to believe, doing the research and accessing the research reports, the systematic reviews, the meta-analyses, and the clinical practice guidelines on patient care units are the easy parts of evidence-based practice. The difficult part is getting the individual practitioner—whether that person is a nurse, physician, or physical therapist—actually to change her or his practice to conform to the evidence. There is a huge gap between what is known as a result of research and its application in patient care. Research utilization is a developing area of science, and Canadian nurse researchers, in particular Dr. Carole Estabrooks (1998) of the University of Alberta Faculty of Nursing, are taking a lead in explicating the factors that influence health professionals to use or ignore research findings in their practice. It seems that simply knowing what works best does not necessarily lead to practising on the basis of that knowledge. The issue is change and the difficulty in getting individual nurses and teams of nurses to become informed about research, to give up their usual practice, and to adopt new methods.

Several theories have been developed to try to guide research utilization. The difficulty with many of them is their linearity (Kitson, Harvey, & McCormack, 1998); that is, there are a series of steps that, if followed in a simple straightforward manner, will result in practice changes. The reality is quite different. Kitson and coworkers have proposed a conceptual framework that acknowledges how messy and complex the process is. Their framework for implementing research in practice explicates the formula:

$$SI = f (E,C,F)$$

that is, **S**uccessful **I**mplementation is a **f**unction of **E**vidence, **C**ontext, and **F**acilitation. Rather than treating this as a linear formula, the elements of evidence, the environment, and the presence of a facilitator whose role it is to make things easier for those being asked to change are considered simultaneously. Each of these components has several dimensions:

- Evidence includes research, clinical expertise, and patient choice.
- Environment incorporates an understanding of the culture, of human relationships as explicated in leadership roles, and of how the organization measures its system and service performance.
- Facilitation involves determining how the facilitator uses interpersonal and group skills to influence change.

In this framework, each of the elements is assessed along a continuum (high to low). Depending on how the three elements are assessed, the facilitation approach changes (Kitson et al., 1998).

None of the research utilization theories guarantees successful change to best practice; however, the theories represent the state of the art of our understanding about how to bring about practice changes early in our experience. Clearly, this is an area of great potential for future development, but the patients and the practitioners cannot wait until the "right" theory comes along that will guide change with more predictable results. The facilitators, nurse educators, and clinical leaders must use the theories and frameworks available now to approach research utilization in as systematic a way as the theories allow.

A second force for research on the horizon is an increasingly better-educated nursing workforce. Research will increasingly influence the way nurses practice as more nurses are educated to read research with authority, to conduct systematic reviews, and to seek out research as their first resource when trying to answer practice questions.

So far, this discussion on evidence-based practice has skirted the question of how much research actually influences current practice because the question cannot be answered definitively. In some settings, most frequently the highly specialized areas of practice like intensive care units, coronary care units, and transplantation units, clinical practice guidelines that incorporate best practices are widely used. Nurses in these units are challenging long-standing practices, such as the routine introduction of saline solution into artificial airways to facilitate suctioning of mucus. A number of well-designed studies demonstrate that saline solution does not necessarily improve suctioning and may harm the patient (Druding, 1997). In other units, the concept of best practice has not yet been discovered let alone incorporated into daily life. This will not continue for long. Nursing in Canada is in the very early days of research production and utilization. Nursing practice will be influenced and changed as more nurses are educated to use research and as more nurses attend conferences in their specialty areas and hear presentations on research on common practices. Nursing practice will be influenced and changed as more nurses read their specialty journals and encounter not let-me-tell-you-how-we-do-it-on-our-unit articles but articles describing why questions were raised about a nursing practice and how research was conducted to answer those questions. Nursing practice will be influenced and changed as nurses change employment and move from units or organizations that operate on best-practice principles to ones that do not. It is possible to predict that, by the end of the first decade of the 21st century, nursing practice will be greatly influenced by research. The term *best practice* may not be heard very commonly then because it will be so embedded in the daily lives of nurses as not to require comment or attention.

Influence on Education

Nursing education has been profoundly affected by the development of research in terms of what is taught and who teaches it. Forty years ago, faculty members in university programs were educated at the baccalaureate or master's levels, and teachers in diploma programs themselves had only diplomas or baccalaureate degrees. Research had little presence in the programs by virtue of the fact that little existed. Textbooks were the cornerstone of course work. In the 21st century, this has changed dramatically. Most university professors of nursing now hold a PhD, and the minimum preparation found throughout nursing education programs is the master's degree. These are not just paper qualifications. They mean that the faculty in nursing programs are both educators and researchers. This profoundly changes teaching.

The journal replaces the textbook as the source of knowledge. Students are guided to use the journal collection as their major resource. Increasingly, the assigned readings for courses are collections of research articles assembled and printed, in accord with Canadian copyright laws, and sold to students. Course content focuses on findings from research on the topic. Faculty members bring their own research into the classrooms to teach the content students are to acquire. If courses in the 21st century are taught the same way as they were even 10 years earlier, they are not reflecting the changes in knowledge nor the source of knowledge.

In larger research-intensive university programs, opportunities are available to undergraduate students to work as research assistants on research projects throughout their education. This frequently serves as an incentive for these students to pursue graduate education immediately to acquire the research skills that will allow them to become principal investigators. They get bitten by the research bug, and they want to do it all.

Nursing is still struggling with how to make research an attractive and attainable career goal for an increased number of students entering the profession. Most students enter nursing to realize their desire to care for people who are ill. In the course of their studies, they find that many different career paths are available to them. If they are exposed to research and have the opportunity to participate actively in it, they might come to see research as a possible future.

In schools of nursing with master's and doctoral programs, undergraduate nursing students are exposed to graduate-level students in those programs. The students interact in their roles as teaching assistants or in social encounters. This makes graduate education very real and attainable. If undergraduate students are not in a research-intensive environment, then faculty members have to use imaginative ways of making research live for the students. It may mean attending research days at other universities, days when faculty and graduate student research is presented, or having researchers or doctoral students come and meet with students, present their work in interactive seminars, and discuss the realities of research careers. Students need encouragement to see graduate school as a logical step in their career plans. They also need tangible financial support to be able to pursue their education. Students who are excited by the possibilities of research, who in the course of their studies raise questions that have been investigated or can be investigated using research methods, and who challenge current practice are excellent candidates for future research careers in nursing.

■ CONTRIBUTION OF NURSING RESEARCH TO THE HEALTH AND HEALTH CARE OF CANADIANS

It would be very nice if the contributions of nursing research to Canadians' health could be numbered and neatly listed. It is not that simple. Nursing research has contributed in many different ways to Canadians' health and health care, but the nature of the research undertaken by nurses does not usually result in products like the identification of the gene for muscular dystrophy, the discovery of insulin, or the development of pablum—all the outcomes of medical research by Canadian scientists. Instead, nursing research has helped us to understand how parents manage multiple encounters with the health care system when they have a chronically ill child (Burke et al., 1991), how pain is experienced by premature infants in pediatric intensive care units (Stevens & Johnston, 1994; Stevens, Johnston, & Horton, 1994), how chronic illness is experienced and how people change their lives to cope with it (Paterson, 2001; Thorne & Paterson, 2001), how patients are comforted during painful treatments in the emergency rooms (Morse & Proctor, 1998), and how patients with cancer want to have control over the type and amount of their treatments (Degner, 1992). Much of what nursing research has done to date is inform clinicians (nurses and all health care professionals) of what patients are experiencing and what they prefer in the way of treatment, information, and approach. This positions the clinicians to work in more sensitive, helpful, and therapeutic ways with patients. Nurses increasingly are undertaking experimental research, whether it be randomized controlled trials or theory-based experimental studies advocated by Sidani as more appropriate for many of nursing's questions (Sidani & Braden, 1998). Randomized controlled trials have demonstrated how to control pain in babies undergoing such procedures as heel sticks (Stevens et al., 1999), how to help family caregivers of older people with dementia adjust to the institutionalization of their relatives (Ducharme et al., 2001), and how to use exercise to manage fatigue in patients with cancer (Graydon et al., 1998). These few examples all focus on what research by Canadian nurse researchers has contributed to our understanding of how to care for people having a variety of illnesses or undergoing medical treatments. Clearly there is much more; the journals are replete with reports of studies.

Nurses have also contributed research that has increased the health of Canadians. They have explored how to assist pregnant women and new mothers to stop smoking or to extend periods of nonsmoking (Johnson et al., 2000), and they have studied how to help mothers protect their infants from environmental smoke (Ratner, Johnson, & Bottoroff, 2001). Much work has been done on how to reduce falls among individuals living in the community and in institutions because falls are a major contributor to morbidity, reduced quality of life, and premature death (Edwards, Cere, & Leblond, 1993; Gallagher & Scott, 1997; Morse, 2001). An inventory has been compiled of interventions carried out by public health nurses and other community health workers that are effective in improving health and preventing morbidity and mortality (Ciliska et al., 1996; Ploeg et al., 1996).

An area to which nurse researchers, and Canadian nurse researchers in particular, are making impressive contributions is in our understanding of how to staff and manage the health care system. Doran and McGillis Hall at the University of Toronto have undertaken a series of studies on the impact of staffing ratios and nursing skill mix (the proportion of registered nurses, licensed practical nurses, and nonprofessional workers) on a variety of patient outcomes and several aspects of nurses' work (Doran et al., 2002; McGillis Hall et al., 2001). Tourangeau and colleagues (2002) at the University of Alberta have demonstrated that better nurse–patient ratios reduce the death rate among patients with cardiovascular disease and shorten their hospital stays. An interdisciplinary team of researchers with nursing leadership (O'Brien-Pallas et al., 2002) found that nurses with baccalaureate degrees working in home care reduced the number of visits patients required to achieve the desired outcomes. O'Brien-Pallas (2002) has launched a program of research to develop a model for explicating the complex phenomenon of determining the size and nature of the nursing workforce required to meet Canadian's health care needs in the future.

This type of research, which relies heavily on databases that house information about patient case mix, lengths of stay, and mortality, rather than on the collection of primary data, is increasingly important to our understanding of how to staff the health care system to achieve maximum efficiency and maximum patient outcomes. It is relatively new to nursing and requires that nurse researchers have the expertise to use, link, and extract data from these types of databases, which are a national resource. The Canadian health care system makes it possible to establish national databases drawn from the systems in each of the provinces that house information about patients, their diagnoses, treatments, lengths of stay, use of medications, and outcomes in terms of morbidity. Ontario is planning to establish databases that include patient outcomes reflective of nursing's input. These databases will allow questions to be answered regarding the relationship between nursing inputs, such as skill mix, the number of nursing hours per patient days, or the educational level and experience of nurses, and patient outcomes such as self-care ability and functional status (Pringle & White, 2002).

■ ISSUES FACING NURSING RESEARCH

A number of issues have been identified throughout this chapter, but the following three, in particular, deserve special attention:

■ The need to produce sufficient researchers for the future
■ The need to use the CIHR's structure and resources to serve nursing research and the role of interdisciplinary research in nursing's future
■ The need to increase research utilization in practice

Shortage of Nurse Researchers

Canada entered the 21st century in the throes of a nursing shortage and with the probability that this shortage would intensify over the next decade. The shortage is distributed across all dimensions of the profession. There are insufficient staff nurses, too few nurse educators, not enough senior researchers to fill the chairs available, and not enough junior researchers to replace the cohort of researchers who will retire during the next 10 to 15 years.

Canada needs more nurse researchers, not fewer. Medical science is making enormous progress in addressing the treatment of disease. For every development in medical care, nursing must respond by determining patients' responses and needs and by developing interventions that complement the medical treatment. Furthermore, there is much catching up to do. Because the undertaking of nursing research is so recent, most of what nurses do and most of what patients experience and need to understand about their health situations has not been studied.

In an overall nursing shortage, every dimension of nursing competes with every other to attract nurses. When there are lots of well-paying positions, it can be very difficult to convince undergraduate students to forego immediate employment and stay in school to pursue research training or to leave well-remunerated positions and return to school. This difficulty is compounded in situations of insufficient funding to allow students to remain in school. The increasing cost of nursing education has resulted in more students graduating with debt. Most find it untenable to take on more debt in the course of acquiring graduate degrees.

Because nurse researchers compose the majority of nurse educators, unless incentives are put in place to make it possible for nurses to undertake graduate work, there will be not only insufficient researchers but also insufficient educators to prepare the nurses to staff the health system. In the United States in the 1960s, the federal government put in place "nurse traineeships" so all students undertaking graduate degrees in accredited nursing programs received a tuition waiver and a monthly stipend. Over the years, this program allowed the federal government to manage shortages in selective areas, such as psychiatric nursing, by offering more traineeships in these areas and fewer in areas where numbers were greater.

There are alternative strategies that serve as incentives for nurses to seek advanced preparation:

- Academic debt-forgiveness programs if students pursue research training
- Tuition reimbursement programs
- Special graduate scholarships
- Awards available to schools with graduate programs

With the exception of the small MRC/NHRDP research scholar program of the early 1990s, Canadian nursing has not been the beneficiary of incentive programs designed specifically to support nurses to achieve or accelerate research careers. And they are needed more now than ever before. However, they will not be successful unless young nurses see research or academic careers as attractive, achievable, and rewarding. Interested students need to be exposed to successful nurse researchers who are enthusiastic about their career choice and can serve as role models and mentors to less experienced nurses. Developing opportunities for young nurses or nursing students to work as research assistants to successful and positive researchers is an important recruitment device.

Creating incentive programs to support nurses while they pursue graduate education and developing creative and stimulating opportunities to help undergraduate and graduate students see research as a viable and desirable career choice are desperately needed to ensure the future of nursing research.

Canadian Institutes of Health Research Structure

As noted earlier, Canadian nursing does not have its own institute within the CIHR structure and must seek other routes to attract attention for special needs areas. Furthermore, the CIHR emphasizes interdisciplinary research. Nurses are well positioned within the CIHR institutes, but the discipline has yet to develop strategies for working with the various institutes so nursing is heard when new initiatives are required to better understand issues that are either unique to nursing or in which nurses play a major role.

The peer-review committees that review applications and make recommendations for grants to support research projects and personnel awards are separate from the CIHR institutes. Many of these peer-review committees include nurses but usually not more than 1 or 2 in a total membership of 12 to 15. When applications from nurses reach these committees, the nurse members may find themselves having to interpret the relevance of the project and to argue for its worth. Nursing must find a way to ensure that there are nurses on all peer-review committees to which nursing proposals might be assigned so proposals are reviewed by knowledgeable researchers who respect the nature of the work.

Additionally, nursing needs to develop ways of connecting with the CIHR institutes that have special-relevance nursing, such as cancer research, aging, circulatory and respiratory health, human development, and child and youth health. These connections might be made through nursing's specialty organizations, such as the cancer nurses association, the cardiovascular nurses group, and the gerontologic nursing societies. These specialty organizations could develop special relationships with their institute counterparts to design special initiatives that would serve nursing. Keeping in mind that the institutes must be interdisciplinary in their orientations, the initiatives would have to be of interest to other disciplines and incur their support. *Interdisciplinarity* in research has become the watchword of the CIHR. As an organization, the CIHR is convinced that better research results from investigators from a variety of relevant disciplines working together and merging their expertise. This may be true. However, interdisciplinarity results from individuals well prepared in their own disciplines coming together. Interdisciplinarity depends first on disciplinarity. Preparing experts in their own disciplines in an environment that rewards interdisciplinary teams who write grants and conduct research is a real challenge and, in Canada, one that nursing must address.

Nurses will have to be creative to work with the CIHR to ensure that nursing's unique needs and orientation are addressed. It will take imagination and relationship building different than the routes available to American nurses, who have their own NINR; however, it is not impossible, and nurses' presence in important positions throughout the institutes and on the CIHR council is a good starting place.

Research Utilization

A third critical issue facing nursing research is the need to accelerate the transfer of research into practice. As discussed earlier, the uptake of research into best practice is at an early stage of development in nursing and in all the health disciplines. The rate of research production in nursing, however, means that if the transfer process does not accelerate, research knowledge will languish in journals years before it is used in patient care. This is wasteful and unfair to the public that has funded the research in the first place. Nursing needs an understanding by and commitment from all practicing nurses to attend to research findings and to seek opportunities to use the results of research in their practice. This means that nurses must be prepared in their initial education or through continuing education opportunities to read, comprehend, and critique research. It puts a special demand on nursing practice leaders, such as nurse managers, clinical nurse specialists, and nurse educators, to assist nurses to appreciate the value of research and to find creative ways of bringing research into practice. Organizations that employ nurses have a special responsibility to provide the resources and the infrastructure supports that make it possible for nurses to access research, to have time to read it, and to have individuals available to them to assist them in using it.

■ THE FUTURE OF NURSING RESEARCH

Notwithstanding the challenges confronting nursing and nurses in the creation of nursing research, the future has never been more encouraging, more robust, or more exciting. Nursing internationally, and particularly in Canada, has never before in its history had so many well-prepared and productive researchers. They are increasingly successful in funding competitions; they see their research published in the best nursing journals and highly regarded interdisciplinary and medical journals; they are sought out to participate in research studies examining a wide range of health issues; and they are well placed in the new structures that support Canadian health research. The doctoral programs that were created in the 1990s have proved to be solid and sustainable. Their products are credible and successful. The research conducted by the students is sound and relevant.

Canadians have every reason to be confident that the money they are investing in nursing research is paying off in better understanding of what matters to them about their health, how they can sustain their health, how their health care and nursing care can be better designed and delivered, and how they can achieve their objectives through the health care system. It is a good time to be a nurse researcher.

■ SUMMARY

Nursing research has been developing since the 1960s in Canada, and enormous strides were made in the 1990s. Doctoral programs in nursing were launched, and more nurses than ever before achieved doctoral preparation. The funding environment changed, new sources of funds became available to support nursing research, and a number of opportunities developed to allow nurses to devote more of their time to the actual conduct of research. Nursing research achieved an increasing share of the research dollars that are distributed annually. These changes did not come easily. Opposition both inside and outside universities had to be overcome before the PhD programs became established, and nurses had to work very strategically to ensure that they gained access to the new sources of funding.

Research is now regarded as central to determining what constitutes best practice, that is, care delivered based on the best research evidence available combined with knowledge about the patient's unique circumstances. An understanding of how to bring about best practice and research utilization more broadly is in its infancy, but new theories and robust programs of research are slowly contributing to knowledge in this area.

Nursing education has been profoundly influenced by research. Nurse educators are better prepared and bring knowledge about research into their teaching. Increasingly, students are assigned journals rather than textbooks as their first source of information about patient care.

Despite its relative youth, nursing research has made major contributions to our understanding of what patients are experiencing and what they prefer in the way of treatment, information, or approach to their care; how to better care for patients experiencing a variety of health conditions; how to run the health care system more effectively and efficiently; and how to help people to live healthier lives. The potential for even more substantive contributions is immense, particularly because more research funding is available, and more nurse researchers are in positions to design, develop, and conduct programs of studies.

Of the many issues facing nurses, three stand out: the challenge to prepare sufficient researchers to replace those who will retire over the next 10 to 15 years and to meet future demands; the challenge of using the structure and resources of the new CIHR to meet the needs of nursing research; and the challenge of dramatically increasing research utilization in practice.

Future nursing research will help Canadians better understand how to sustain their health and how health care and nursing care can be better designed and delivered. Nurses have never before been as well prepared or had the amount of support available to them to meet these expectations.

Online Resources

Add to your knowledge of this issue:

Alberta Heritage Foundation for Medical Research	**www.ahfmr.ab.ca**
Canada Association for Nursing Research (CANR)	**www.canr.ca**
Canadian Association of Schools of Nursing (CASN)	**www.causn.org**
Canadian Health Services Research Foundation (CHSRF)	**www.chsrf.ca**
Canadian Institutes of Health Research (CIHR)	**www.cihr-irsc.gc.ca**
Canadian Nurses Association (CNA)	**www.cna-nurses.ca**
Canadian Nurses Foundation (CNF)	**www.canadiannursesfoundation.com**
Fonds de Researche Scientifique du Québec (FRSQ)	**www.frsq.gouv.qc.ca**

Michael Smith Foundation for Health Research (MSFHR)	**www.msfhr.org**
Natural Sciences and Engineering Research Council of Canada (NSERC)	**www.nserc-crsng.gc.ca**
Social Sciences and Humanities Research Council of Canada (SSHRC)	**www.sshrc.ca**

REFLECTIONS on the Chapter . . .

1. Identify one or two nurse researchers whose work interests you. Trace their publications through electronic databases such as CINAHL and MEDLINE. What journals are they publishing in? Are they working alone or with a consistent team of collaborators? How would you summarize their contributions?

2. Think about an area of practice that interests you, for example, managing the symptoms of children being treated for cancer or helping mothers maintain a sense of control during labor, and then develop a nursing practice question. Go to the electronic databases and search for research that addresses that question. Has research been done on it? If there is research, who has done it, and how much of it has been done by nurses? If there is no research, are there opinion pieces, editorials, or descriptions of how various places manage? Describe the state of knowledge at this time on the practice. Would you recommend research or more research on the question?

3. Think of one practice setting you have been in. What strategies are in place to apply research findings to practice? How successful are they? If there are no obvious strategies, describe what could be done to bring research to practice.

4. Go to the CIHR Web site, http://www.cihr-irsc.gc.ca/. Visit the Web pages of the 13 institutes. Review their mission statements and the types of research they are interested in. How many are focused on research that is relevant to nursing? Look at their staffing and the members of their advisory boards. How many have nurses on their boards? Is there a relationship between mission and research focus and the membership of their boards?

References

Abdellah, F. G., & Levine, E. (1965). *Better patient care through nursing research.* New York: Macmillan.

Bloch, D. A. (1981). Conceptualization of nursing research and nursing science. In J. McCloskey & H. Grace (Eds.), *Current issues in nursing* (pp. 81–93). Oxford, UK: Blackwell.

Burke, S. O., Kauffmann, E., Costello, E., et al. (1991). Hazardous secrets and reluctantly taking charge: Parenting a child with repeated hospitalizations. *Image: The Journal of Nursing Scholarship, 23,* 39–45.

Canadian Association of Schools of Nursing (CASN). (2002). Nursing research funding database. Retrieved from http://www.causn.org/Databases/nursing_research_database.htm

Canadian Nurses Association/Canadian Association of Schools of Nursing (CNA/CASN). (2004). The national student and faculty survey of Canadian schools of nursing 2002–2003. Retrieved from www.cna-nurses.ca/_frames/resources/statsframe.htm

Ciliska, D., Hayward, S., Thomas, H., et al. (1996). A systematic overview of the effectiveness of home visiting as a delivery strategy for public health nursing interventions. *Canadian Journal of Public Health, 87*(3), 193–198.

Degner, L. (1992). Patient participation in treatment decision making. *AXON, 14,* 13–14.

Doran, D. I., Sidani, S., Keatings, M., et al. (2002). An empirical test of the nursing role effectiveness model. *Journal of Advanced Nursing, 38*(1), 29–39.

Druding, M. C. (1997). Re-examining the practice of normal saline instillation prior to suctioning. *MEDSURG Nursing, 6,* 209–212.

Ducharme. F., Levesque, L., Gendron, M., et al. (2001). Development process and qualitative evaluation of a program to promote the mental health of family caregivers. *Clinical Nursing Research, 10*(2), 182–201.

Edwards, N., Cere, M., & Leblond, D. (1993). A community-based intervention to prevent falls among seniors. *Family & Community Health, 15*(4), 57–65.

Estabrooks, C. A. (1998). Will evidence-based nursing practice make practice perfect? *Canadian Journal of Nursing Research, 30(*1), 15–36.

Fawcett, J. (1989). *Analysis and evaluation of conceptual models of nursing* (2nd ed.). Philadelphia: F. A. Davis.

Gagnon, A. J. (1999). Do editors have anything to teach us? A review of 30 years of journal editorials. *Canadian Journal of Nursing Research, 30(*4), 23–26.

Gallagher, E. M., & Scott, V. J. (1997). The STEPS project: Participatory action research to reduce falls in public places among seniors and persons with disabilities. *Canadian Journal of Public Health, 88*(2), 129–133.

Gottlieb, L. N. (1999). From nursing papers to research journal: A 30-year odyssey [Editorial]. *Canadian Journal of Nursing Research, 30(*4), 9–14.

Graydon, J., Sidani, S., Irvine, D., et al. (1998). Literature review of cancer-related fatigue. *Canadian Oncology Nursing Journal, 8*(Suppl 1), S5.

Hannah, M. E., Hannah, W. J., Hewson, S. A., et al., for the Breech Trial Collaborative Group. (2000). Planned caesarian section versus planned vaginal birth for breech presentation at term: A randomized multicentre trial. *Lancet, 356,* 1375–1383.

Jennings, B. M. (2000). Evidence-based practice: The road best traveled? [Editorial]. *Research in Nursing & Health, 23,* 343–345.

Johnson, J. L., Ratner, P. A., Bottoroff, J. L., et al. (2000). Preventing smoking relapse in postpartum women. *Nursing Research, 49,* 44–52.

Kitson, A., Harvey, G., & McCormack, B. (1998). Enabling the implementation of evidence-based practice: A conceptual framework. *Quality in Health Care, 7,* 149–158.

Lau, J., Ioannidis, J. P., & Schmid, C. H. (1998). Quantitative synthesis in systematic reviews. In C. Mulrow & D. Cook (Eds.), *Systematic reviews.* Philadelphia: American College of Physicians.

McGillis Hall, L., Doran, D. I., Baker, G. R., et al. (2001). *The impact of nursing staff mix models and organizational strategies on patient, system and nurse outcomes. Final report.* Toronto: University of Toronto.

Medical Reesearch Council of Canada. [Online]. Retrieved April 2, 2005, from http://strategis.ic.gc.ca/epic/internet/inrti-rti .nsf/en/te01458e.html

Morse, J. M. (2001). Preventing falls in the elderly. *Reflections on Nursing Leadership, 27*(1), 26–27.

Morse, J. M., & Proctor, A. (1998). Maintaining patient endurance...the comfort work of trauma nurses. *Clinical Nursing Research, 7*(3), 250–274.

Mulrow, C., & Cook, D. (1998). *Systematic reviews.* Philadelphia: American College of Physicians.

O'Brien-Pallas, L. (2002). Where to from here? *Canadian Journal of Nursing Research, 33*(4), 3–14.

O'Brien-Pallas, L. L., Doran, D. I., Murray, M., et al. (2002). Evaluation of a client care delivery model, Part 2: Variability in client outcomes in community home nursing. *Nursing Economics, 20*(1), 13–21.

O'Connor, A. M., & Bouchard, J. L. (1991). Research activities in Canadian university schools and faculties of nursing for 1988–1989. *Canadian Journal of Nursing Research, 23*(1), 57–65.

Paterson, B. (2001). The shifting perspective model of chronic illness. *Journal of Nursing Scholarship, 33*(1), 21–26.

Petticrew, M. (2001). Systematic reviews from astronomy to zoology. *British Medical Journal, 322,* 98–101

Ploeg, J., Ciliska, D., Dobbins, M., et al. (1996). A systematic review of adolescent suicide prevention programs. *Canadian Journal of Public Health, 87*(5), 319–324.

Pringle, D. M., & White, P. (2002). Nursing matters: The Nursing and Health Outcomes Project of the Ontario Ministry of Health and Long Term Care. *Canadian Journal of Nursing Research, 33*(4), 115–121.

Ratner, P. A., Johnson, J. L., & Bottoroff, J. L. (2001). Mothers' efforts to protect their infants from environmental tobacco smoke. *Canadian Journal of Public Health, 92,* 46–47.

Ritchie, J. A. (1992). Research issues. In A. J. Baumgart & J. Larsen (Eds.), *Canadian nursing faces the future.* St. Louis: Mosby.

Sidani, S., & Braden, C. J. (1998). *Evaluating nursing interventions: A theory-driven approach.* Thousand Oaks, CA: Sage.

Stevens, B. J., & Johnston, C. C. (1994). Physiologic responses of premature infants to a painful stimulus. *Nursing Research, 43,* 226–231.

Stevens, B., Johnston, C., Franck, L., et al. (1999). The efficacy of developmentally sensitive interventions and sucrose for relieving procedural pain in very low birth weight neonates. *Nursing Research, 48,* 35–43.

Stevens, B. J., Johnston, C. C., & Horton, L. (1994). Factors that influence the behavioural pain responses of premature infants. *Pain, 59,* 101–109.

Thorne, S., & Paterson, B. (2001). Health care professional support for self care in chronic illness: Insights from diabetes research. *Patient Education and Counseling, 42,* 81–90.

WORKPLACE REALITIES

Carol McDonald
Marjorie McIntyre

Issues Arising From the Nature of Nurses' Work and Workplaces

Nurses work in many environments and adapt to many conditions. The setting for these nurses is the inner city. Photography by Chuck Russell. Used with permission from *Canadian Nurse*.

1. Understand the nature of nurses' work.

2. Discuss the significance of nurses' work issues.

3. Articulate issues arising from the nature of nurses' work and their workplaces.

4. Frame and analyze issues arising from the nature of nurses' work and the places in which that work is carried out.

5. Identify barriers to resolving issues arising in nurses' work and workplaces.

6. Formulate strategies for resolving issues arising in nurses' work and workplaces.

7. Trace the links between nurses' work, nurses' health, and the health of Canadians.

8. Recognize the conflicting loyalties between the goals of organizations and nurses' professional goals.

This chapter highlights relevant issues arising from the nature of nurses' work and the significance of these issues for the health of nurses and the health of Canadians who need nursing care. Issues arising from the nature of nurses' work are closely related to and sometimes overlap the issues arising within the environments in which nurses' work takes place. However, there is increasing Canadian and international research substantiating the importance of understanding the nature of nurses' work as distinct from nurses' work environments. Therefore, this chapter highlights some of the distinctions between the issues arising from the work that nurses do and the places in which this work takes place.

■ THE NATURE OF NURSES' WORK

Themes throughout the literature on the changing nature of nurses' work include confusion about what constitutes nurses' work, the increasing demands of nurses' work, the lack of control that nurses have over the work they do, and the incongruity between what nurses are prepared as professionals to do and what they are expected to do in practice.

The lack of clarity in defining nurses' work is due in part to the lack of clear boundaries between nurses' work and non-nurses' work and the increasing expectation that nurses perform work other than nursing care. Changes in administrative structures and in the way auxiliary workers are utilized means nurses take on work that has been traditionally performed by others. In other situations, nursing practices have been relinquished to auxiliary workers. In addition to the increasing demand to do more work, nurses are also faced with the increasing demands of the work itself. Patients in care are more acutely ill, and the care nurses provide is increasingly complex. There are demands on nurses for increasing technical competence.

In practice, nurses are often faced with a lack of control over the work they do. Decisions about what care will be provided, who will provide that care, and in what setting the care will be provided are made by someone other than the nurses expected to provide the care. Nurses' work often occurs in a climate of diminished resources without support to meet the demands of their work with competence and confidence. The increased demands of nurses' work and the lack of support provided to sustain the work may contribute to the disturbing reality that nurses are unable to nurse in the ways that they have come to expect they should. Nurses increasingly experience incongruities between the work that they are prepared to do, both educationally and philosophically, and the expectations that they encounter in practice.

■ THE NATURE OF NURSES' WORKPLACES

The nature of nurses' work and the workplaces themselves are interrelated; both contribute to nurses' experiences of job satisfaction, recruitment and retention, and well-being. For example, many writers and researchers have linked Canada's current nursing shortage to inadequate and inferior work environments (Ceci & McIntyre, 2001). Baumann and others (2001, p. iii) claim, "Canada's nursing shortage is at least in part due to a work environment that burns out the experienced and discourages new recruits. But that environment can be changed." Despite the seriousness of the real and potential shortcomings of nurses' work environments, there is evidence that governments, employers, and nurses are taking action to improve the situation. Further, there is an acknowledgment on the part of these groups that they must work together to create and maintain healthy nurse workplaces. Research suggests that recruitment and retention strategies will be successful only if this action is implemented on a large scale (Sochalski, 2001).

Understanding what constitutes a healthy work environment and selecting those environments in which to work will positively affect not only the individual's work–life experience but also the quality of care that individual is able to deliver. As more desirable work environments are created, nurses already in practice will undoubtedly be attracted to those employment situations, promoting the continued production of healthy work environments. Many employers are beginning to offer to nurses and other employees onsite services that have been identified as indicative of a quality work environment (Box 16.1).

■ THE SIGNIFICANCE OF NURSES' WORK ISSUES

Issues arising from the nature of nurses' work relate directly to the recruitment and retention of nurses, the health of the nursing workforce, and the quality of care that nurses are able to deliver. The belief that all we need to do to address the recurrent shortages of nurses is to produce more nurses overlooks the point

BOX 16.1

Research (Baumann et al., 2001) shows that the workplace for professional practicing nurses would be improved through the integration of these initiatives:

- Support for new nurses through mentoring programs
- Support for continuing and advanced education
- Nurses' participation in policy and governance
- Clear distinction between nurses' and non-nurses' work
- Provision of adequate resources, including human and material resources

Indicators of a quality workplace include (Baumann et al., 2001):

- Provision for onsite child care
- Safe, accessible, and affordable parking
- Nutritious and hot food services 24 hours a day
- Onsite fitness centers and classes
- Wellness programs, such as those for smoking cessation, back care, and stress management
- Counseling for mental health issues and substance use and misuse
- Programs for workplace safety
- Programs to reduce workplace violence

TABLE 16.1 Employment Predictions for Nurses in 2011			
Between 1993 and 2011 Number of Nurses Must Increase	Low Growth: 23%	Medium Growth: 34.5%	High Growth: 46%
Number of RNs employed, 1993	235,630	235,630	235,630
Number of RNs employed, 1996	227,830	227,830	227,830
Projected number of RNs required, 2011	290,000	317,000	344,000
Additional RNs required, 2011	62,000	89,000	116,000
Projected number of RNs available, 2011	231,000	231,000	231,000
Projected shortage of RNs	**59,000**	**86,000**	**113,000**

Source: Compiled from data collected by the Canadian Nurses Association. Used with permission.

that it is the issues arising from the nature of nurses' work that sustain and perpetuate nursing shortages. Unless these issues are addressed, it is unlikely that existing vacancies will be filled, that student enrollments will increase, or that nurses, given other opportunities, will stay in nursing. This chapter challenges the inevitability of health care systems doing more with less in the short term when downsizing and restructuring occur at the expense of nurses' health and well-being (Table 16.1).

For the most part, nurses' work environments are and always have been complex, and barriers to providing quality professional practice environments are considerable. However, given the authority, adequate resources, and support of colleagues, it is assumed at the outset of writing this chapter that nurses can provide such quality practice environments as those envisioned by the Canadian Nurses Association (CNA).

According to the CNA position statement (2001, p. 1) on nurses' work environments, nurses have an obligation to their patients to "demand practice environments that have the organizational and human support allocations necessary for safe, competent and ethical nursing care." The CNA position states that a quality nursing practice environment for professional nurses is one in which "the needs and goals of the individual nurse are met at the same time the patient or client is assisted to reach his or her individual health goals, within the costs and quality framework mandated by the organization where the care is provided" (p. 1). The CNA holds that the development and support of quality practice environments for professional nurses are responsibilities shared by practitioners, employers, regulatory bodies, professional associations, educational institutions, unions, and the public.

■ ISSUES ARISING IN NURSES' WORK AND WORKPLACES

In the face of indisputable evidence that there are too few nurses to fill current positions and predictions that the shortage will worsen, there is only beginning recognition that issues related to the nature of nurses' work can and must change. In any discussion of nurses' work, one cannot overlook the nature of the work itself and the availability of nurses to do this work.

Despite the positive initiatives of select groups of employers, for many Canadian nurses the realities of the workplace continue to be reflected in themes of professional and social isolation; disrupted workplaces, resulting in alienation from nurse leaders, peers, and other professionals; inadequate educational, mentorship, and orientation programs; decreased levels of support for professional development; and the failure of governments and the public to recognize and support the need for change in nurses' workplaces. Despite the well-documented lack of control over their work and work environments, nurses continue to be held accountable for, and in some cases hold themselves accountable for, providing quality practice environments and safe, competent, ethical care. The following sections contain an expanded discussion of each of these issues.

Increasing Demands of Nurses' Work

Although one can cite many examples of the increasing volume of nurses' work, it is important not to overlook the demands of increasing acuity and complexity of patient care. Baumann and coauthors (2001, p. 4) conclude that the discrepancy between the work demanded of nurses and what nurses can reasonably give because of increased patient acuity and complexity of care creates an imbalance that threatens the health of nurses and "puts patients throughout Canada at risk."

The care provided by nurses is thought to be more complex than ever before. O'Brien-Pallas and associates (2001) reported that the acuity of patients has increased steadily since 1994. Nurses have the added responsibility of providing care not only to individual patients but also to families and communities; this suggests that nurses' work is increasingly physically, intellectually, and emotionally demanding (Baumann et al., 2001). Studies also show that, in addition to the increased demands brought on by patient acuity and complexity of care, the effects of hospital downsizing and restructuring have intensified nurses' work. The result is obvious: Nurses work harder (Burke & Greenglass, 2000).

Other research highlights the "load" that nurses' work puts on nurses (Gaudine, 2000). In a descriptive study in which 31 nurses were interviewed, Gaudine offers compelling narration of the experiences of workload—and work overload—from the accounts of these nurses. Although nurses' descriptions of what constituted work overload varied significantly, a brief glimpse of the richness of these accounts is offered in the following examples.

Simultaneous demands were apparent in situations in which study subjects talked about being expected to do more than one thing at a time and to be in more that one place at a time:

A doctor is asking me questions. . . . Meanwhile a patient's relative is standing beside me and wants something, and the phone is ringing. I have to get a patient ready to go to X-ray. Then the doctor wants a dressing changed and I know the vitals need taking on my patient receiving blood (Gaudine, 2000, p. 24).

In a second example of work overload, Gaudine (2000, p. 25) describes "qualitative work overload," in which the nurses' experiences of work overload are attributed by the nurses to the unfamiliar nature of the work. The following example richly illuminates one nurse's experience with this:

It was the night shift, and I had never done TPN before. I had eight charts to look over. The TPN lines hadn't been changed on days and had to be done for around 8 PM. I spent a half hour with the procedure manual, which for me is useless. I want to see it, not just read it. The dressing set didn't have what the procedure book said it would. It was 9:30 PM by the time I finished it, and I hadn't even looked at the other patients' charts.

"Heavy load" is another dimension of the work that Gaudine (2000, p. 25) describes. Heavy load involves situations in which there is just too much work to do and is exemplified by this nurse's response:

I can't believe we have to be here for twelve hours and often have to miss our breaks. And I just get the expectations of nurses is really, like super nurse, to do an incredible amount, and I think it is just too much. To work twelve hours, and I can't even go out to lunch, like at any other job.

The final example of work overload is illustrated by a situation in which nurses are, by virtue of their competence and experience, responsible directly for the care of the patients assigned to them and also responsible indirectly for the patients assigned to other nurses on their unit. One of the nurses in Gaudine's (2000, p. 25) study talks about this dilemma in a way that resonates with other accounts throughout the literature:

Most [nurses] are more junior than me and may have trouble doing new things. . . . Just to be cautious, I stayed on the unit at break today, because there was a very sick child and so many new nurses.

Many researchers and practicing nurses identify workload as the most significant issue for nurses directly and indirectly because of links between nurses' work, nurses' health, and the health of patients in their care (Baumann et al., 2001; Burke & Greenglass, 2000; Cockerill & O'Brien-Pallas, 1990; O'Brien-Pallas et al., 1997; Shullanberger, 2000; White, 1997).

Incongruities Between Nurses' Work as Taught and Practised

The lack of clarity about what constitutes nurses' work and the increasing demands of nurses' work life have hindered the development of a professional role for nurses. The professional role of nurses is further hindered by incongruities that exist between "nursing as taught and nursing as practiced, between nursing as experienced by nurses and nursing as perceived by others" (Ceci & McIntyre, 2001, p. 123). The incongruities that are raised "when nurses find themselves unable to nurse as they had envisioned, as they can or believe they should" (p. 123), undermine the meaning that nurses find in their work. Researchers who interviewed practicing nurses claim "nurses find meaning in their work when they are able to care for patients performing in a way that conforms to the philosophy of care held by the nursing profession" (Baumann et al., 2001, p. 8).

In considering the meaning that nurses find in their work, it is important to recognize that nurses have a different experience than other members of the health care system. And this difference, rather than being trivial or blatantly obvious, "holds ethical and political meanings and implications for nurses and for our practices" (Ceci & McIntyre, 2001, p. 127). The professional role for nurses (i.e., their understanding of their scope of practice) develops through both education and practice experiences. For many nurses, this scope of practice makes central a holistic approach to the care of patients and their families. However, in contemporary practice, a "treatment-oriented medical model" often overrides the nurse's scope of practice (Baumann et al., 2001, p. 9). When faced with demanding workloads and the dissonance of conflicting approaches to care, nurses' work becomes reconfigured as tasks. In addition, when nurses' interpretations of what is occurring in practice are excluded from policy discussions, "a sense of being incorrect, in some essential sense, in their understanding of themselves and their work comes into play" (Ceci & McIntyre, 2001, p. 123).

Lack of Control Over Nurses' Work

Commitment and Care: The Benefits of Healthy Workplaces for Nurses, Their Patients and the System, by Baumann and others (2001), makes an important contribution to our understanding of issues arising from the nature of nurses' work in Canada. Drawing on the earlier work of Kristensen (1999), Baumann identified six principles that constitute an optimal work environment for nurses' social and psychological well-being. Baumann's work incorporates a review of current literature, including relevant policy documents on the topic as well as the findings of focus group discussions with nurses in practice across Canada.

This chapter draws on the findings of Baumann's work to support discussions of issues of control and support in nurses' work. The term *control* as it is used here can be understood as both control over the work that nurses do and control over the ways in which that work is organized in practice. Baumann and colleagues introduce the finding that "establishing a professional role is a prerequisite for establishing control over practice" (2001, p. 9). They further link control over practice to job satisfaction and greater latitude in decision making to decreased turnover of nurses in practice.

Baumann and others reported that focus group participants strongly supported the need for nurses to have input into the "patient-care decisions related to their practice" (2001, p. 9). Nurses stressed the importance of having their say in "all aspects of care within their scope of practice, including serving as patient advocates" (p. 9). Nurses in this study experienced difficulty in playing "significant roles in policy-making" or in communicating "effectively with decision makers" because of being "under-represented in institutional hierarchies" (p. 10).

For nurses to experience control over their work, they must be central in the policy decisions that direct work–life issues, such as scheduling, full-time to part-time staff ratios, casual nurses, and auxiliary workers. Although nurses are often left with the responsibility of calling in relief staff and implementing mandatory overtime, there are still too few instances in which nurses have meaningful input into the policies that determine these arrangements. The failure to gain control over and have meaningful input into one's practice, generated by the demands of mandatory overtime and the high rates of relief staff, influences nurses' commitment to their practice and the decisions they make about remaining in practice. Nurses who are satisfied with their work and the organization of their work schedules show a higher commitment to their practice. Research shows that the job satisfaction level of the nursing staff strongly determines the satisfaction level of the patients in their care (Baumann et al., 2001).

Lack of Support for Nurses' Work

Central to the discussion of nurses' work is the decline of emotional and cognitive support available to nurses in their workplaces (Baumann et al., 2001). In place of full-time positions, in which nurses knew the people they worked with and were familiar with their places of work, many working nurses have "moved away from the traditional workplace to a world where employers may offer part-time or casual work and employees have several jobs" (Baumann et al., 2001, p. 7). In full-time, long-term work situations, nurses' social support for dealing with professional and personal issues came from managers, supervisors, and colleagues. Cognitive support came from preceptors, mentors, and organizational policies that provided the needed in-service and continuing education for professional and career development.

In the absence of leaders to protect them from overwork, some nurses have turned to absenteeism as a way to deal with feelings of diminished competence, work overload, and mandatory overtime (White, 1997). Research shows a relationship between nurses' satisfaction with support in their work and absenteeism (Blythe, Baumann, & Giovannetti, 2001). It is significant that nurses have lower rates of absenteeism in part-time than in full-time work, suggesting that absenteeism may be related to the strain of working longer hours (Burke & Greenglass, 2000).

During the restructuring of health care services, as nurses face increasing demands in their workloads, the cognitive or educational support that could once be counted on has been withdrawn. The financial and professional support for ongoing education and in-servicing has diminished at a time when there is an increasing pressure for nurses to account for their continued competency. Despite the profession's commitment to advanced education among its members, employers provide little support or remuneration for the pursuit and attainment of advanced degrees (Table 16.2).

Workplace Isolation

A review of literature on social support in the workplace and an examination of employer practices suggest that nurses' commitment to their employing organizations has decreased (Baumann et al., 2001). This diminished commitment is due, at least in part, to a belief that employers no longer support them. The

TABLE 16.2 Levels of Education Among Canadian Nurses	
Education in Nursing in 2003	**Education in Nursing in 1999**
69.1% (166,824) diploma	76.2% (174,085) diploma
28.6% (69,093) baccalaureate	22.2% (50,664) baccalaureate
2.1% (5,150) master's	1.6% (3,591) master's
0.1% (275) doctoral	0.1% (194) doctoral

Source: Canadian Nurses Association: Highlights of 2003 nursing statistics.

TABLE 16.3   Where Do Nurses Work?

Location	Percentage of Canadian RNs (%)	Number of Canadian RNs
Hospital	59.9	144,675
Nursing home/home for the aged	10.5	25,292
Community health center/agency	9.7	23,290
Home care agency	2.9	7,026
Educational institution	2.7	6,512
Physician's office/family practice	2.1	5,071
Other	10.8	26,117
Not stated	1.4	3,359

Source: Canadian Nurses Association: Highlights of 2003 nursing statistics.

dismissal of chief nursing officers, head nurses, and middle managers during restructuring has meant that nurses receive less professional support on the job. Unit nurses do not have the opportunity to build relationships with their managers, an important source of professional and social support in the past. The nurse working in the practice environment has no one to turn to for professional support, such as advice on patient- or unit-related problems.

Nursing teams that take time and commitment to build have been decimated by the redeployment of nurses from their usual practice environments. This redeployment of nursing teams has also reduced the collaboration in patient care and relationships with other health care professionals because of the uncertainty of professional practice environments.

One example of organizational initiatives to create healthy workplaces is the Victoria Order of Nurses in the Ottawa region. In this setting, nursing teams have been established to support nurses working with specialized groups of patients. In these teams, where nurses are able to develop and use their expertise, nurses not only nurse better but also derive more satisfaction from their work (Baumann et al., 2001).

Although many, if not all, nurses experience some degree of professional and social isolation in their workplaces, rural nurses, community health nurses, and new graduates are nurses whose sense of isolation can be linked clearly to the workplace. The following sections discuss these select groups of nurses (Table 16.3).

The Experiences of Rural Nurses

Whereas nurses working in rural locations have more independence in their practice than other nurses have, they have other workplace issues to contend with. Rural nursing environments often include both inpatient and outpatient practice areas, and rural nurses attend to medical, surgical, obstetric, pediatric, and emergency room patients, possibly on the "same shift and frequently alone" (Winters & Mayer, 2002, p. 79). Scharff (1998, p. 20) describes experienced rural nurses as "expert generalists" because they must know a great deal about a "variety of practise areas," possess a "high level of flexibility, work independently, transition smoothly from one task to another and one patient to another" in constantly changing environments. However, not all nurses working in rural settings have the experience and education needed to provide care in such varied situations. Nurses working in isolated communities seldom have opportunities to update their knowledge and skills that nurses working in major centers have. Additionally, rural nurses face professional isolation in that there are not always other nurses to draw on.

These nurses may find themselves alone with professional care and decision making while being highly visible to the community. "Nurses working in sparsely populated areas lack anonymity, which means they are visible and identifiable within their communities and experience diminished personal and professional boundaries" (Winters & Mayer, 2002, p. 79). An example of the conflict that can arise from high visibility or lack of anonymity for nurses in small communities is demonstrated by nurses' privileged access to confidential information about community members. Unlike nurses in larger centers, rural nurses cannot avoid social interaction with patients and their families. In instances in which a patient's circumstance has social consequences, such as alcohol or substance abuse, the nurse can be placed in an uncomfortable or conflictual situation.

Community as Workplace

Although much of the distance nurses experience from leaders, peers, and other professionals can be attributed to restructuring and the deployment of nurses, in some cases, the particular workplace undermines the relationship of nurses and the leaders who work there. Home care nurses practise in isolation and frequently provide nursing care that remains invisible to administrators of home care services and to the decision makers who fund these programs. Nurses who work in home care settings may be asked to exclude from their caseloads patients to whom they have been providing nursing care. These excluding practices are based on criteria set by administrators rather than on what the home care nurses know from providing care. Purkis (2001) describes how home care nurses find themselves caught in the tension between what they know particular patients need and what administrators and government agencies expect nurses to provide.

Nurse administrators who supervise home care nurses are also caught in a tension, but their conflicts are different. Nurse administrators are situated between the home care nurses' desire to base their decisions for excluding patients from services on their professional assessments and the pressure they face as administrators "to reduce the deficits in the face of major cuts in federal health and social spending" (Purkis, 2001, p. 142).

Mentorship and Orientation Programs for New Graduates

Another group of nurses for whom the professional practice environment is an issue is new graduates whose precarious job situations as occasional "on-call" nurses have become a way of life (Viens, 1996). To understand better what it means for new graduates to fit into current practice environments and to understand the rate at which new graduates leave the profession, Viens explored the experiences of 31 new graduates over 18 months from 5 different Quebec hospitals. In this study, new graduates discovered very early on that "they have entered a brave new world where the work situation proves to be very different from what they have been taught" (p. 44). In the absence of the stability that a consistent environment might bring, new graduates struggle for "professional survival." Adapting to a constantly changing environment produces what Viens (1996, p. 44) dubbed the "functional nurse"—the nurse who learns to be "available at all times, to provide care with no continuity and without any hope of ever belonging to a unit." Is it any wonder these new graduates question the quality of care they give or their future as nurses? How is it that new graduates are expected to take their places in this constantly changing practice environment?

In an initiative to support new graduates, the Calgary Health Region has hired nursing instructors to orientate and mentor new staff. Numerous innovative programs across the country support new graduates and their mentors through the provision of release time and reduced responsibilities for both participants. Examples of these programs are in St. Michael's Hospital in Toronto, in the Winnipeg Health Authority, and through British Columbia's Health Action Plan (Baumann et al., 2001).

Disrupted Workplaces

During restructuring, health care organizations decreased their level of support for professional development. The shift to program management meant that mentoring and evaluating junior nurses became less common and resources for continuing education were often eliminated. Today, staff shortages make attendance at educational courses difficult even when they are available. In 1988, the CNA developed a position statement on nurse administrators that emphasized the role of the nurse administrator in providing an environment conducive to quality patient care and nurses' well-being. In 1993, the CNA developed a position statement on the role of chief nursing officers, and, in 1996, it developed a position paper on nursing leadership. These statements have been repeatedly updated and offer clear direction for change (CNA, 1996a, 1996b).

However, hospital downsizing and restructuring have undermined existing leadership structures and the vision the CNA documents provide for nursing. Significantly, positions such as the chief nursing officer are being eroded. In some instances, they have disappeared altogether. Changes in the role of nurse managers have led to these roles becoming more diffuse with "a broader scope of services to administer and more managerial tasks to accomplish" (McGirr & Bakker, 2000, p. 7). These changes tend to distance managers from practice and give added professional practice and coordination responsibilities to staff nurses at a time when fewer nurses are available.

Framing and Analyzing Issues Arising From the Nature and Conditions of Nurses' Work

Issues arising from the nature of nurses' work and the conditions within and under which this work is performed are not new. Although the rationale for making nurses' work-related issues a priority has varied across time, overall, governments, employers, and even nurse leaders have failed to address these issues in a way that resulted in lasting effects.

Clearly, more than the temporary provision of resources or superficial changes in nurses' working conditions is at stake in this issue. Each of these elements—numbers, working conditions, and work satisfaction—incorporates underlying and unexamined assumptions about the nature of nurses' work, nursing knowledge, and the relationship of each to power structures in health care and society. What follows is a discussion of different frameworks for analysis and the possibilities they generate for understanding issues arising from the nature and conditions of nurses' work.

Historical Understandings of Nurses' Work

In reviewing historical literature, one gets a sense that the nature of nurses' work has always been idealized—and less than ideal (Gibbon & Mathewson, 1947). What we can learn from historical analysis is how the issues have been sustained over time and the implications that this has for the current situation and for long-term planning of health care provision.

Despite the evidence of declining enrollments and an inadequate supply of nurses to fill current positions, many employers continue to assume that one can still "recruit women interested in self-denial, servitude and the expression of their natural qualities as women . . . the workplace still operates to some extent on that basis—expecting nurses to work harder than ever for less and less" (Stuart, 1993, p. 22). Although many nurses in the past expressed a deep dissatisfaction with nurses' work, what has changed is that, today, nurses are more likely to view themselves as professional and their work as a career rather than to understand nursing as a calling to servitude. With this view of professional work, nurses who stay in the profession do so knowing they have choices. Nurses have many more opportunities to leave the profession and work elsewhere than in the past.

Social and Cultural Analysis

Priorities placed on nurses' work and the value attributed by society and by nurses to this work have often been linked to economic rather than social realities (Donner, Semogas, & Blythe, 1994). The issues arising from the nature of nurses' work would benefit from a social and cultural analysis that considers the social realities of nurses' lives, nurses' health, and the quality of patient care.

A social and cultural analysis reminds us that considering the realities of nurses' lives must include consideration of the realities of the lives of women in our society. Nurses facing issues of increasing demands and lack of support for their work simultaneously experience the demands of the multiple roles in their nonworking lives as women. Prevailing attitudes in society suggest that work and personal lives are separate domains. This attitude privileges particular members of society and fails to take into account the realities of the lives of women as mothers, care providers, community supporters, and volunteers juggled alongside their paid work as nurses. Issues that arise from mandatory callback, overtime, and the increased workload demands of nursing compromise the quality of nurses' lives, their well-being, and their energy to participate fully in both their personal and professional lives.

Professional organizations and individual nurses have lobbied, and continue to lobby, government representatives for changes that would empower nurses to control their workplaces and that would provide the resources needed for safe, competent, and ethical nursing care. Yet as our history unfolds, it is the values and priorities of the dominant culture rather than those that are representative of nursing or the recipients of nursing care that continue to influence this issue.

Despite a growing awareness of how professions whose members are predominantly women are disadvantaged, decisions about nurses' work and their workplaces continue to be made by non-nurses. Decisions about nurses' work and nurses' work environments are increasingly based on criteria derived from business, management, and economic models rather than on the needs of the populations nurses serve (Taft & Steward, 2000; White, 1997).

Nurses and their managers continue to hear explanations of budget cuts that have forced them to reconceptualize services without the opportunity for nurses or their leaders to provide input about what patients need in terms of care. Moreover, nurses have insufficiently understood and critiqued the ways in which these values and priorities put the needs of the dominant culture over other members of society (Davies, 1995).

The aging of the nursing workforce is well documented in the literature (Table 16.4). Dominant views of society regarding the devaluing and dispensability of older workers threaten to undermine the contribution that nurses continue to make to the profession as they age. Operating on a framework that views all nurses as the same, with expectations that each nurse will perform the same work in a given setting, erases the realities of the differences among nurses, including the differences that may be associated with aging. A British Columbia setting provides a useful model that recognizes both the realities of nurses' lives and the contribution that is fluid throughout nurses' careers. This program enables senior nurses to be relieved of up to 30% of their patient assignment in return for mentoring new nurses (Baumann et al., 2001).

TABLE 16.4   Age of RNs Employed in Nursing in Canada in 2003

Age	Number	Percentage (%)
<25	4,681	1.9
25–29	17,413	7.2
30–34	24,115	10.0
35–39	31,672	13.1
40–44	36,973	15.3
45–49	42,339	17.5
50–54	41,476	17.2
55+	42,650	17.6
Not stated	23	10.0

Average age of RN employed in nursing in 2003 was 44.5; average age in 1999 was 42.8.

Source: Canadian Nurses Association: Highlights of 2003 nursing statistics.

Political Analysis

Typically, issues arising from the nature of nurses' work come to the foreground when recruitment and retention issues arise, but these issues tend to fade from public awareness and concern once the numbers (shortages) problem is averted. Significantly, once vacant positions are filled, concern about nurses' work tends to be put aside as a topic for serious debate. The failure of governments, employers, professional organizations, and nurses to address adequately the issues arising from the nature of nurses' work is linked to the failure to understand the implications of such conditions and their significance for the health of Canadians.

A political analysis asks who benefits from this issue being resolved and who benefits from things staying the same. Nurses and the patients they care for stand to benefit from the resolution of issues arising from the nature of nurses' work. Employers, however, may benefit from some of these issues remaining as they are. For example, the lack of clarity between nursing and non-nursing work allows employers to exploit nurses in assigning multiple roles to them. This exploitation serves managers well as nurses take on the work of other professionals and clerical staff when needed, but it undermines the control that nurses have over what constitutes nurses' work. When nurses are engaged in non-nursing work in addition to their patient care, it is the patient care, the real work of nurses, that is compromised.

Critical Feminist Analysis

A critical feminist analysis directs us toward the consideration of power structures and ideologies and to the question of what it means to be a subject of one's own life. This analysis highlights how realities such as other people defining and controlling nurses' work influence how nurses see themselves. As the subject of their own work life, nurses would retain control of their work and work arrangements rather than be objects that are manipulated and controlled by structures of power.

Nurses are complicit in the maintenance of power structures when they fail to make central their own beliefs and ideas or the ideas of nurse leaders. *Complicity* as it is used here refers to nurses perpetuating power structures and unexamined ideologies that work against them.

Although the nursing literature and other human care literature highlight the importance of relationships accompanied by an ethic of care in the work of nursing, there is still an unquestioned assumption that implicitly or explicitly nursing is an expression of women's natural capacities, a view that effectively erases the knowledge required by nurses to comprehend and respond to the needs of another (Ceci & McIntyre, 2001, p. 128). Still "other discourses obscure or slide over the emotional labor and stress involved in nurses' work and instead emphasize the instrumentality [of nurses' work], the tasks that need to be done and [the] pairs of hands" (p. 128) needed to perform them. It is not difficult to see how "these ideas about women, about women's work and how it does or does not require significant knowledge, responsibility and skill are embedded in nursing and become part of nursing's taken for granted reality" (p. 128).

Ethical Analysis

Professional codes, such as the CNA *Code of Ethics* and the provincial and territorial scope of practice guidelines, direct nurses to advocate for patients in the provision of health care. Legislative acts, such as the Canada Health Act and the Health Professions Act, mandate nurses as professionals to provide competent, ethical care. Collective bargaining and labor laws are in place to protect nurses from the demands of overwork, to control the hours of work, and to ensure safe practice standards. Despite these multiple levels of regulation of nurses' work, governmental agencies and employers continue, uninterrupted, to demand work of nurses that erodes these guidelines.

Ethical questions are raised about the health of nurses and the subsequent health care provided to patients. These quandaries include the risks to patients when a nurse who has worked many shifts without a leave or entire shifts without a break becomes vulnerable to fatigue and to a subsequent increased risk for making errors. Ethical questions may also evolve from the added responsibility felt by nurses when they are working with other nurses whose competence is compromised by unfamiliarity with the work demanded of them or with the fatigue of overwork.

Economic Analysis

An economic analysis highlights how the forces of supply and demand work in a particular issue. For issues related to nurses' workplaces, one may explore the influence nurse leaders have in challenging purely cost-containment strategies when the health of Canadians is thought to be at risk. A purely economic analysis of these issues could lead, and has led, to nurses being asked to do more with less. Sochalski (2001, p. 15) reminds us that "economics provides the framework for the allocation of resources," and the economics question facing nursing is not what the value of nursing care is but rather "how to allocate this valuable resource to best meet the health care needs of our patients and our population."

The difficulty with talking about health care and nursing care in purely economic terms is that it overlooks other costs. What needs to be made more transparent to the public is the high cost and incredible waste of resources resulting from the short-term slashing of funds, closure of needed health facilities, and withdrawal of life-sustaining services. A point to consider here is that the position statement obligating nurses to demand quality practice environments includes a phrase suggesting that this be done "within the costs and quality framework mandated by the organization where the care is provided" (CNA, 2001, p. 1). The concern is that such wording supports the claim that governments would provide differently if they could, a point that, in many cases, has been accepted without question.

■ BARRIERS TO RESOLVING WORK AND WORKPLACE ISSUES

One of the largest barriers to making decisions about the amount and nature of work one nurse can be expected to do is that there is little, if any, consensus on what nurses' work is and what it is not. For example, many systems designed to measure nurses' workload measure only a portion of the work done (O'Brien-Pallas et al., 1997). Typically, the focus of such systems is tasks performed without taking into account the complexity of the patient assignment, the nurses' knowledge and skill to provide the required care, and the context in which the care is to be provided. Incomplete assessment of what nurses know and do in their practice results in nursing effort and expertise being inadequately recognized or compensated (Baumann et al., 2001, p. 5).

"Nurses' views of the world are both overshadowed and undermined" by the views of others who "define what nurses are and what nurses are for" (Ceci & McIntyre, 2001, p. 126). This places nurses in the "uncomfortable position of trying to render their perspectives believable or credible using terms of reference which are not necessarily their own" (p. 126). Many employers think of nurses as versatile. In addition to the care their education and experience have prepared them to give, they are known to be able to provide "services for which the hospital sometimes employ nurses' aides, secretarial and clerical personnel, lab technicians, pharmacists, physical therapists and social workers. They commonly assume hospital management roles after hours and (under certain circumstances) substitute for physicians in the community" (Stuart, 1993, p. 22).

A second major barrier to changing the issues arising from the nature of nurses' work is the failure of Canadians generally and governments and employers specifically to acknowledge the impact of the nature of nurses' work on nurses' health and on the health of patients. Nurses' work, in particular adequate staffing levels, has been linked through research to improved patient outcomes (Aiken, Sloane, & Sochalski, 1998) and to the health of nurses (O'Brien-Pallas et al., 2001).

The reality that staffing decisions are based on funding rather than on the level of nurse preparation or the number of nurses needed to achieve the desired outcomes is the third barrier to resolving these issues. Despite the tools and systems available to help with making staffing decisions, the literature reviewed expresses skepticism about these tools and the need for senior nursing positions whereby those with the expertise would make these decisions. The staffing of patient care units must be based on the needs of the patients and the corresponding "staffing required to achieve desired outcomes" (Blegen, Goode, & Reed, 1998, p. 49).

A fourth barrier that undermines the control that nurses have over their work and that interfaces with the lack of clarity about what constitutes nurses' work is the balancing of the ratio of registered nurses to auxiliary workers. It is not always easy or even possible to assess accurately how many registered nurses are needed to achieve desired outcomes of care. As discussed earlier, difficulty in assessing nurses' work is compounded by difficulties distinguishing nurses' work from other work that nurses do. Although existing tools for determining a good skill mix have been judged inadequate, there is support among nurses for refining these tools. In addition to the limitations of existing tools, however, the literature is very clear that much more important than the tools are the relationships among nurse managers, nurses, and other team members involved in and influenced by the staffing decisions made (Gaudine, 2000).

A fifth barrier to resolving issues of nurses' work conditions is a failure to see the link between job security and nurses' absenteeism from work, nurses' organizational commitment, and nurses' satisfaction or dissatisfaction with work. Similar to other workers involved in research studies, nurses reported that job security (i.e., being able to count on full-time work despite changes and restructuring) was associated with less absenteeism from work, more commitment to employers, and better physical and emotional health (Blythe et al., 2001).

■ STRATEGIES FOR RESOLVING WORK AND WORKPLACE ISSUES

Recent research studies provide compelling evidence that the issues arising from the nature of nurses' work can and must change (Baumann et al., 2001). They challenge the notion that these issues are a problem for nurses to address; instead, the studies assign responsibility for the current situation of nurses' work and the threat of a system-wide shortage of nurses to governments, employers, and professional organizations.

Strategies to overcome the existing barriers to resolving issues that arise from the nature of nurses' work are those that "enable nurses to practice in a way that optimises the use of their knowledge and expert judgment" in their practice (Laschinger et al., 2001, p. 240). "Work environments that provide opportunities to learn and grow" and "support creative strategies" in nurses' work are those that will be considered health promoting for nurses and those to whom they provide care (p. 240). Strategies increasing "decision-making latitude" (the extent to which a worker has control over the job and how it is done) will "moderate the effects of high levels of psychological demands" (p. 239) and enhance the quality of nurses' work lives.

In her research on work overload, Gaudine (2000) stressed the importance of administrators listening carefully to the accounts of nurses' experiences of workload as part of verifying what a particular workload might be. Although one can make use of the tools available to get some indication of workload, one should not interpret the findings of such tools without considering the particularities of the nurse or nurses involved. An additional insight gained from Gaudine's study was that even in situations in which it is not possible to alter the workload or change the conditions at that particular time, taking the time to understand a particular nurse's experience of workload or work overload can make a contribution to the quality of a nurse's work life through validation and support.

In the United States and elsewhere, research on magnet hospitals (i.e., hospitals that embody a set of organizational attributes that nurses find desirable and that are conducive to better patient care [Aiken,

Smith, & Lake, 1994]) may provide valuable direction for strategies to mediate some of the issues arising from the nature of nurses' work. Kramer and Schmalenberg (1988, p. 13) suggest "magnet hospitals may be dealing effectively with the nursing shortage by creating organizational conditions conducive to eliminating the shortage." They identified the following attributes of magnet hospitals:

- Innovative policies and practices
- Intelligent use of staff (nurses are not treated as replaceable parts in the bureaucratic machinery; rather, they are moved in teams)
- Informal communication lines and open-door policies
- Pervasive and deliberately promoted and promulgated quality care values, including (1) advocacy of education, (2) drive for quality, and (3) importance of autonomy (includes freedom to act and freedom to act and fail)

Aiken and colleagues (1994) extend the work on magnet hospitals, which they identify as "like other hospitals except in the organization of nursing" (p. 784). They produced evidence to show that the magnet hospitals in their study had lower mortality rates, suggesting that factors such as the organization of nursing care can be linked to better patient outcomes. Research is one of the most convincing strategies to support the link between nurses' work and positive patient outcomes.

In making reference to the many challenges and limited benefits that nursing offers today, the report of Baumann and associates (2001) on the benefits of a healthy work experience for nurses predicts that if nursing is to "remain a viable profession, its status must be enhanced and the welfare of nurses promoted" (p. 13). In their policy synthesis on the benefits of a healthy work experience for nurses and the patients they care for, Baumann and associates (2001) stressed that governments, professional organizations, employers, educators, and researchers must act together to promote patient welfare by facilitating healthy work experiences for nurses. What follows are a selection of the key points identified by this research team (Baumann et al., 2001).

Key points for governments include the following:

- Revise funding formulas to better support the many dimensions of nursing practice.
- Set rules for using the funds, and monitor how they are spent.
- Support the welfare of nurses by providing funds to increase staff so managers can assign workloads that consider the acuity and complexity of patient care.
- Ensure the supply of nurses in the future by investing in continuing education, including baccalaureate and postgraduate education.

Key points for professional associations and councils include the following:

- Continue to advocate for nurses, and advise governments and employers to allow nurses to practise to their full scope.
- Share recruitment and retention strategies, and promote nursing through advertising and marketing strategies.

Key points for employers include the following:

- Address staffing issues by hiring sufficient nurses to ensure a reasonable workload.
- Address issues of staff mix and full-time and part-time statuses.
- Work with unions to develop flexible scheduling that suits both nurses and employers.
- Engage nurses on units in the recruitment and hiring processes.
- Adopt the most effective tools for measuring and allocating workload.
- Recognize effort and achievement with economic remuneration and other rewards.
- Support nursing leadership and professional development.
- Monitor nurses' health.
- Promote recruitment and retention of graduates into the workforce.

Key points for educators include the following:

- In partnership with employers, governments, and nursing associations, integrate new nurses into the workplace through such strategies as clinical internships and cooperative programs.
- Ensure a match between the curriculum and the skills required in the workplace.
- Teach leadership skills, health care policy, and work–life health issues for nurses.
- Work with nursing associations on scope-of-practice issues.

Key points for researchers include the following:

- Develop databases, workload-measurement instruments, and human resources forecasting tools.
- Conduct studies to evaluate the effectiveness of strategies to improve nurses' well-being.

The strategies suggested in this chapter are directed toward individuals and groups with the power to sustain or to revise the structures and ideologies that underlie the issues arising from the nature of nurses' work. Societal and cultural analysis, in particular, helps us to recognize that the burden for the resolution of these issues does not rest with individual nurses but with governments, professional groups, employers, and labor groups.

What, then, is the role of the individual nurse in coping with and contributing to the establishment of a healthier work experience for nurses and, subsequently, to improved patient care? Perhaps the most powerful action that individual nurses can take is to disrupt or to interrupt the dominant discourse in health care and in society regarding the versatility and subservience of nurses. When given the opportunity, nurses can make their voices heard with governments, professional associations, and labor groups by broadcasting the issues of justice and health arising from the nature of nurses' work as it is currently experienced.

■ SUMMARY

Although historically the nature of nurses' work has been less than ideal, the changes in nurses' work and the issues that have arisen from this work in the past decade have seriously compromised nurses' ability to provide quality care in some circumstances and even adequate care in others. Nurses' work has undergone dramatic changes without corresponding support to moderate the effect of these changes. Increased workloads and work overload, higher patient acuity and care complexity, and increased job insecurity in the workplace have had an overwhelming effect on how nurses experience their work. The impact of the issues that arise from the nature of nurses' work can be seen in the way nurses care for their patients and ultimately contributes to both the quality of nurses' work and the quality of care they are able to provide.

There is significant research evidence presented in this chapter to support the links between nurses' work, nurses' health, quality of nursing care, and patient outcomes. Studies support the link between the practice of nursing and hospital mortality and nurses' work satisfaction with better patient care (Aiken et al., 1994; Laschinger et al., 2001).

Barriers to resolving the issues arising from the nature of nurses' work are many, but the need to overcome these barriers and begin to address these issues has never been more urgent. Strategies for resolution involve the cooperation of governments, professional organizations, employers, educators, and researchers. The time to act is now.

Online Resources

Add to your knowledge of this issue:

Canadian Federation of Nurses Unions   **www.nursesunions.ca**
Canadian Nurses Association   **www.cna-nurses.ca**
International Council of Nurses   **www.icn.ch**

Provincial and Territorial Organizations

Alberta Association of Registered Nurses	www.nurses.ab.ca
Association of Nurses of Prince Edward Island	www.anpei.ca
Association of Registered Nurses of Newfoundland and Labrador	www.arnn.nf.ca
College of Nurses of Ontario	www.cno.org
College of Registered Nurses of Manitoba	www.crnm.mb.ca
College of Registered Nurses of Nova Scotia	www.crnns.ca
Nurses Association of New Brunswick	www.nanb.nb.ca
Ordre des Infirmières et Infirmiers du Québec	www.oiiq.org
Registered Nurses Association of British Columbia	www.rnabc.bc.ca
Registered Nurses Association of the Northwest Territories and Nunavut	www.nwtrna.com
Registered Nurses Association of Ontario	www.rnao.org
Saskatchewan Registered Nurses' Association	www.srna.org
Yukon Registered Nurses Association	www.yrna.ca

REFLECTIONS on the Chapter . . .

1. From your own experiences in practice, describe situations that support or challenge what you have read about the nature of nurses' work.

2. How do you account for the current issues arising from the nature of nurses' work in your practice or practicum areas? Who might you ask or where might you look to gain an understanding of these current issues?

3. Researchers have located the responsibility for the issues arising from the nature of nurses' work with governments, employers, and professional organizations. Support or challenge this view.

4. Identify additional barriers to resolving issues related to the nature of nurses' work.

5. What other strategies might you suggest for resolving issues related to the nature of nurses' work?

References

Aiken, L., Sloane, D., & Sochalski, J. (1998). Hospital organization and outcomes. *Quality of Health Care, 7*(4), 222–226.

Aiken, L. H., Smith, H. L., & Lake, E. T. (1994). Lower Medicare mortality among a set of hospitals known for good nursing care. *Medical Care, 32*(8), 771–787.

Baumann, A., O'Brien-Pallas, L., Armstrong-Strassen, M., et al. (2001). *Commitment and care: The benefits of health workplaces for nurses, their patients and the system. A policy synthesis.* Canadian Health Research Foundation. Ottawa: Government of Canada.

Blegen, M. A., Goode, C. J., & Reed, L. (1998). Nurse staffing and patient outcomes. *Nursing Research, 47*(1), 43–50.

Blythe, J., Baumann, A., & Giovannetti, P. (2001). Nurses' experiences of restructuring in three Ontario hospitals. *Journal of Nursing Scholarship, 33*(1), 61–68.

Burke, R. J., & Greenglass, E. R. (2000). Effects of hospital restructuring on full time and part time nursing staff in Ontario. *International Journal of Nursing Studies, 37*(2), 163–171.

Canadian Nurses Association. (1996a). *Chief executive officer.* Ottawa: Author.

_____. (1996b). *Nursing leadership.* Ottawa: Author.

_____. (2001). *Position statement: Quality professional practice environments for registered nurses.* Ottawa: Author. Retrieved April 19, 2005, from http://www.cna-nurses.ca/CNA/documents/pdf/publications/PS53_Quality_Prof_Practice_Env_RNS_NOV_2001_e.pdf

_____. (2002). *Code of ethics for registered nurses.* Ottawa: Author.

Ceci, C., & McIntyre, M. (2001). A "quiet" crisis in health care: Developing our capacity to hear. *Nursing Philosophy, 2*(2), 122–130.

Cockerill, L., & O'Brien-Pallas, L. (1990). Satisfaction with nursing workload systems: Report of a survey of Canadian hospitals. Part A. *Canadian Journal of Nursing Administration, 3*(2), 17–22.

Davies, C. (1995). *Gender and the professional predicament in nursing.* Philadelphia: Open University Press.

Donner, G., Semogas, D., & Blythe, J. (1994). *Towards an understanding of nurses' lives: Gender, power and control.* Toronto: Quality of Nursing Worklife Research Unit.

Gaudine, A. P. (2000). What do nurses mean by workload and work overload? *Canadian Journal of Nursing Leadership, 13*(2), 22–27.

Gibbon, M., & Mathewson, M. (1947). *Three centuries of Canadian nursing.* Toronto: MacMillan.

Kramer, M., & Schmalenberg, C. (1988). Magnet hospitals: Part 1, Institutions of excellence. *Journal of Nursing Administration, 18*(1), 13–24.

Kristensen, T. S. (1999). Challenges for research and prevention in relation to work and cardiovascular diseases. *Scandinavian Journal of Work, Environment and Health, 25*(6), 550–557.

Laschinger, H. K. S., Finegan, J., Shamian, J., et al. (2001). Testing Karasek's demands-control model in restructured health care settings: Effects of job strain on staff nurses' quality of worklife. *Journal of Nursing Administration, 31*(5), 233–243.

McGirr, M., & Bakker, D. (2000). Shaping positive work environments for nurses. *Canadian Journal of Nursing Research, 13*(1), 7–14.

O'Brien-Pallas, L., Irvine, D., Peereboom, E., et al. (1997). Measuring nursing workload: Understanding the variability. *Nursing Economics, 15*(4), 171–182.

O'Brien-Pallas, L., Thomson, D., Alksinis, C., et al. (2001, May). The economic impact of nurse staffing decisions: Time to turn down another road? *Hospital Quarterly, 4*(3), 42–50.

Purkis, M. E. (2001). Managing home nursing care: Visibility, accountability and exclusion. *Nursing Inquiry, 8*(3), 141–150.

Scharff, J. (1998). The distinctive nature and scope of rural practice: Philosophical bases. In H. J. Lee (Ed.), *Conceptual basis for rural nursing* (pp. 19–38). New York: Springer.

Shullanberger, G. (2000). Nurse staffing decisions: An integrative review of the literature. *Nursing Economics, 18*(3), 124–132, 146–148.

Sochalski, J. (2001). Nursing's valued resources: Critical issues in economics and nursing care. *Canadian Journal of Nursing Research, 33*(1), 11–18.

Stuart, M. (1993). Nursing: The endangered profession. *Canadian Nurse, 89*(4), 19–22.

Taft, K., & Steward, G. (2000). *Clear answers: The economics and politics of for-profit medicine.* Edmonton: Duval House.

Viens, C. (1996). The future shock of nursing graduates. *Canadian Nurse, 92*(2), 40–44.

White, J. P. (1997). Health care, hospitals, and reengineering: The nightingales sing the blues. In A. Duffy, D. Glenday, & N. Pupo (Eds.), *Good jobs, bad jobs, no jobs: The transformation of work in the 21st century.* Toronto: Harcourt & Brace.

Winters, C., and Mayer, D. (2002). Special feature: An approach to cardiac care in rural settings. *Critical Care Nursing Quarterly, 24*(4), 75–82.

As a way of engaging with the ideas in this chapter, consider the following:

1. How do you understand the difference between the mandate for collective bargaining organizations and professional associations/colleges?

2. What assumptions do you hold about the relationship between nursing as a profession and nurses as members of collective bargaining units?

3. Attitudes toward collective bargaining vary significantly from province to province and territory to territory in Canada. What do you already know about the nature of your province/territory that might influence these attitudes?

4. Another significant difference is the way in which the nature of collective bargaining seems to be changing over time. Consider what changes within society and in the nursing profession as you understand it might contribute to the changing face of unions and collective bargaining.

CHAPTER

17

Marjorie McIntyre
Carol McDonald

Unionization: Collective Bargaining in Nursing

In many cases, collective ▶ action leads to collective bargaining. Here, the Saskatchewan Union of Nurses (SUN) shines a bright light on nurses' working conditions.

Chapter Objectives

After completing this chapter, you will be able to:

1. Understand the significance of issues related to collective bargaining for nurses.
2. Describe the breadth and scope of collective bargaining groups and the issues they address for nurses.
3. Explore personal, professional, and societal assumptions about unionism.
4. Discuss the events that led to the separation of professional organizations and collective bargaining groups.
5. Identify legislation that has shaped nurses' collective action.
6. Discuss the influence of public support on nurses' collective bargaining.

This chapter highlights issues that arise from nurses' unionization and collective bargaining activities. It introduces collective bargaining and the issues that arise from nurses' relationships with unions and unionization. It also presents a selection of issues that arise for nurses within the context of unions and collective bargaining, along with their significance. It presents a framework by which to analyze issues that draws on historical, social-cultural, political, ethical-legal, critical feminist, and economic perspectives. And, this chapter addresses barriers to nurses' participation in the collective bargaining process as well as strategies to increase nurses' understanding of the issues that surround unions and collective bargaining.

The intent of this chapter is to make visible the current situation for nurses in collective bargaining in Canada and to provide nurses with a framework by which to analyze these issues. Although nurses' collective bargaining procedures affect many people, the principal participants in collective bargaining include two groups: "nurses and their unions" and "employers and their organizations" (Hibberd, 1999, p. 506). Governments also are involved; they "fund hospitals and community health-care agencies," create labor laws, and are responsible for protecting the public interest (p. 506).

In Canada, the direction for union certification comes from provincial labor legislation. The labor relations system is decentralized much like that of the health care system, leaving responsibility for collective bargaining mostly with the provinces. Because each province and territory has its own labor legislation, the formation of unions and collective bargaining procedures tend to vary from province to province, which is "why nurses are entitled to strike in some provinces and not in others" (Hibberd, 1999, p. 506; Box 17.1).

■ COLLECTIVE BARGAINING

Collective bargaining refers to the activities that nurses and their unions are involved in to negotiate working conditions and remuneration. A collective agreement, the product of collective bargaining, is a "contract of employment" (Hibberd, 1999, p. 506).

In most situations, unions now act as the bargaining agents for many nurses in Canada. Before the establishment of independent unions for nurses, collective bargaining took place through nurses' provincial or territorial professional associations. Before the establishment of professional organizations, nurses were self-employed and singularly negotiated salary and work conditions with their employers. Independent unions certified by provincial labor relation systems have now been in place for nurses in each of the provinces and territories in Canada for more than 3 decades (Table 17.1).

The board of the Canadian Federation of Nurses Unions (CFNU) includes elected representatives from each of the provincial member unions except Quebec. The CFNU represents 122,000 nurses, including registered nurses, registered psychiatric nurses, and licensed practical nurses, and is the largest organization of nurses in Canada. Founded in 1981, the CFNU provides a national voice for the concerns of Canadian nurses as well as resources to support provincial union activities (Connors, 2002).

BOX 17.1	Glossary: Terms of Labor

Arbitration—process by which a final decision is made by a third party.

Collective agreement—a contract of employment.

Collective bargaining—the procedures and processes that all nurses are involved in to negotiate working conditions and remuneration.

Grievance—a claim that one or more of the provisions of a collective agreement have been violated, accompanied by a request for compensation.

Lockout—the employer locks employees out of the work setting.

Mediation—process by which all parties involved in conflict agree to reach a decision that all parties can accept.

Negotiation—give-and-take process in which multiple parties meet to discuss issues, present requests, and settle demands.

Ratified agreement—contractual process in which the provisions in a contract are agreed on by both parties and by which both parties are duty-bound to honor until such time as a new contract is negotiated.

Strike—withdrawl of services; a *legal strike* involves action permitted by existing labor laws; an *illegal strike* involves action in defiance of existing labor laws.

Work-to-rule—job action taken to challenge contract provisions, such as refusal to work overtime, restriction of activities to the practice of nursing, and refusal to do non-nursing work.

Source: Hibberd, J. (1999). Working with unions. In J. Hibberd & L. Smith (Eds.), *Nursing management in Canada* (2nd ed., pp. 505–524). Toronto: W. B. Saunders. Used with permission.

Issues Arising From the Unionization of Nurses

The impetus for this chapter is the assumption that many nurses experience ambivalence regarding participation in, and support of, collective bargaining. Nurses' ambivalence is assumed to link to complex unresolved issues within the collective bargaining process. Selected issues are identified and discussed below.

1. Nurses experience tension between unionism and professionalism.
2. Conflict exists over participating in job action that involves the withdrawal of services.

TABLE 17.1	Formation of Canadian Nurses' Unions

Province	Union	Date of Independence
Alberta	UNA	1977
British Columbia	BCNU	1981
Manitoba	MNU	1975
New Brunswick	NBNU	1978
Newfoundland and Labrador	NLNU	1974
Nova Scotia	NSNU	1976
Ontario	ONA	1973
Prince Edward Island	PEINU	1988
Quebec	FIIQ	1987
Saskatchewan	SUN	1974

Source: Jensen, P. (1992). The changing role of nurses' unions. In J. Larsen & A. Baumgart (Eds.), *Canadian nursing faces the future* (pp. 557–572). Toronto: Mosby. Used with permission.

3. Nurses face alienation from coworkers whose views differ from theirs.
4. Conflict-of-interest legislation divides nurses and their leaders.
5. Ambiguity exists as to what constitutes "essential services."
6. Pay equity (equal pay for work of equal value) is an issue.
7. Knowledge of collective bargaining, its history, and its legislated authority is inadequate.
8. The nature of relationships among nurses' unions, governments, and employers is adversarial.

Tension Between Unionism and Professionalism

Nurses' ambivalence also can be understood as a tension between unionism and professionalism. Conflict is created for individual nurses who hold memberships in union and professional organizations. These organizations hold differing mandates that occasionally could be seen as at cross-purposes. The central focus of nursing unions is its members' remuneration and working conditions, whereas the central focus of professional associations is the maintenance of standards of care and the protection of the public (Table 17.2).

The history of nursing reflects nurses' unresolved tensions between the interests of quality care for patients and the interests of a quality work life for nurses who provide that care. In a study exploring nurses' perceptions of the coping of colleagues during the fallout from a strike, Hibberd and Norris (1991, p. 52) reported that nursing strikes and other forms of job action "place nurses in the dilemma of having to choose between loyalty to patients in providing uninterrupted services, and loyalty to peers in collectively pursuing improvements to working conditions and socio-economic status." In a practice discipline in which interpersonal relationships

TABLE 17.2   Differences Between Unions and Professional Associations

	Professional Association	Union
Membership	All registered nurses in the province	Excludes management and administration
Legislative authority	Health Professions Act	Provincial Labor Relations Boards
Mandate	To promote the profession of nursing and to protect the public interest	To advance social, economic, and general welfare of nurses
Roles	Registration of members	Regulation of relations between nurses and their employers
	Regulation and discipline of members	Negotiation of written contracts with employers
	Scope of practice; standards of care and competency	Promotion of the knowledge of nurses through education and research
	Represents the concerns of its members to government, the public, and allied health professions	Promotion of the highest standards of health care
	Provision of educational loans and scholarships	Promotion of unity within the labor movement, the nursing profession, and other allied fields
		Promotion of occupational health and safety

Information modified from data provided by United Nurses of Alberta, at www.una.ab.ca.

between colleagues can affect the delivery of quality of care, it is important to consider the effects of conflicting feelings both within the individual nurse and in relationships with peers.

Conflict Over Participating in Job Action That Involves the Withdrawal of Services

Despite the increasing unity of nurses regarding the need for collective bargaining, nurses remain divided when it comes to making decisions about job action. Nurses' dissonance on this issue can be linked to the adversarial nature of this discourse in media coverage, in collective bargaining legislation, and in the message heard in day-to-day life (Hibberd, 1992). Some of this dissonance can be traced to 1944, when the Canadian Nurses Association (CNA) approved collective bargaining for practicing nurses but rejected the idea that nurses would even consider the withdrawal of services (Jensen, 1992). Since that time, provinces have taken different and fragmented stands based on the differing provisions of provincial legislation. As a result, nursing organizations have been fragmented and the possibility of solidarity for Canadian nurses as a group has been disrupted. Despite the increasingly unified stand of nurses regarding the need for collective bargaining, there remains less solidarity over what constitutes acceptable job action (Kerr, 1996).

Nurses Face Alienation From Coworkers With Differing Views

Nurses identified the importance of aligning their views with colleagues, coworkers, and nurse leaders out of "fear of alienation" from them. In Hibberd and Norris' (1991, p. 50) study, nurses identified the most powerful reason for joining a strike as "fear of peer pressure and possible retribution" if they chose to cross their own picket lines. Nurses in this study also feared that not aligning with a majority decision could result in adverse personal consequences. One nurse expressed her concern in this way: "If you ever cross the picket line, they [coworkers] never let you forget it. The people you work with will never, ever forget that you crossed" (p. 50). Given the centrality of interpersonal relationships in nurses' work, these tensions are extremely important to nurses and their workplace environments.

Conflict-of-Interest Legislation

Conflict-of-interest legislation has divided staff nurses from administrative nurses, leaving the staff nurses without managerial support and managers without the security of a collective agreement. In 1973, a controversy erupted over who would be certified as the official bargaining unit for a group of Saskatchewan nurses. Before this time, the professional organizations, which included nurse managers, had carried out collective bargaining. A question was raised of whether the staff nurses' association, part of the professional association, should continue as the bargaining agent or if independent unions should be formed. The controversy was resolved in favor of a union. A 1973 Supreme Court ruling "ultimately required that a separate and completely independent nursing union or unions be formed to assume the collective bargaining function for general staff nurses" (Ross-Kerr, 1998, p. 274). By 1981, the "transition from responsibility vested in professional associations to responsibility vested in independent nursing unions had taken place in every province in Canada" (p. 274). The tension for nurses created by this change from professional organizations to unions as their collective bargaining agent remains.

On one hand, the conflict-of-interest concern of nurse managers evaluating staff nurses is defensible. Nurses need to be able to bargain independently of administrators. On the other hand, this legislation has the potential to create a rift between staff nurses and their leaders (McPherson, 1996). Nurse leaders, in their capacity as representing employers and acting on their behalf, were cut off from the larger group of nurses. One could even argue that unionization divided the group that the professional association had contained. A further concern that can be linked to much of the current ambivalence to the 1973 legislation is the vulnerability of nurse leaders to lose their positions in cost-containment strategies and the fragmenting effects of these cuts in staffing on nursing and on nurses as a group. This is not a comment for or against nurse unions but rather a reminder for nurses to be cognizant of the effects of this legislation.

Ambiguity About What Constitutes Essential Services

From the inception of collective bargaining in nursing, the understanding that essential services would be in place and would not be compromised by any job action has been a given. What complicates this tenet of collective bargaining agreements is that it is "not inherently obvious" (Ross-Kerr, 1998, p. 280) which services are essential. Even in those provinces where there is some agreement as to what constitutes such services and guidelines are in place to identify "how essential services should be put in place in the event of a strike," conflicts can and still do occur (p. 280). Ambiguity as to what constitutes "essential services" complicates nurses' decision making about supporting strikes and about how to act during a strike.

Pay Equity: Equal Pay for Work of Equal Value

The issue of pay equity, equal pay for work of equal value, both complicates and is complicated by negotiations involving the gendered nature of nurses' work (Day, 1993). Despite general agreement by most members of society that women generally and nurses particularly have the right to equal pay for work of equal value, salary inequities remain the reality for many Canadian nurses. The major challenge of pay equity is and always has been the lack of clarity about what constitutes nurses' work. Once the nature and scope of nurses' work is agreed on, there is the added difficulty of finding a comparable group in which the dominant gender is male to assess equity (Schriber & Nemetz, 1992). As long as the values associated with nursing and nurses' work are not made explicit, both nurses and their employers go on accepting the way things are. However, with pay equity legislation forcing "nurses to articulate the value of nurses' work" (p. 19) and forcing administrators to make explicit "how much (or how little) they value nursing work" (p. 19), this will need to change.

Nurses' Inadequate Knowledge of Collective Bargaining, Its History, and Its Legislated Authority

Interviews conducted with nurses during strikes suggest that an important issue for the nursing unions is lack of understanding about collective bargaining, its history, and its legislated authority (Day, 1993). Nursing curricula have been slow to provide this knowledge—and its place in the nurse's work life (Day, 1993).

Despite significant public relations work by unions and professional associations, practicing nurses do not always understand the need to belong to both a professional organization and a union. Such misunderstanding can be traced to nurses' lack of familiarity with the legislation that mandated the need for independent unions and professional associations and the scarcity of information about political and historical collective bargaining in nursing curricula. Even today, nurse educators are ambivalent about the place of collective bargaining in nursing and the role of unions in the profession. This, of course, can result in differences in the way this knowledge is presented, or not presented, to students. Also, until very recently, many textbooks for nursing programs were American and were more reflective of the American labor situation.

Even when nurses understand the diverse purposes of unions and professional organizations, the resistance to accepting the need for two organizations may arise from the burden of paying dues to both. Another possible reason for some nurses' ambivalence is that nurses may not comprehend the breadth and scope of what unions have to offer. Typically, many nurses—and the public—equate unionism with strike action and financial remuneration.

A review of national and provincial Web sites reveals that nursing unions across Canada are taking action to raise awareness of recruitment and retention issues, increase nursing seats in educational institutions, and increase nurses' autonomy, power, and control in the workplace. Union leaders are speaking out on issues of access to quality basic care, Medicare, and the universality of the health care system. Union organizations are developing strategies to partner with professional organizations, employers, and governments to address issues of nurses' work lives and to improve nurses' relationships with employers.

Adversarial Nature of Relationships Among Nurses' Unions, Governments, and Employers

Talk of cost containment and rollback of nurses' salaries is common at collective bargaining tables across the country. It is difficult for nurses and their unions to get ahead when they need so much energy just to maintain the collective agreement provisions they already have achieved. Despite gains for many Canadian nurses at bargaining tables from 1998 to 2001, constant governmental talk of cost containment and restructuring is and always has been accompanied by the possibility of the loss of significant gains for nurses.

Nurses and their unions, particularly in provinces that have removed the right to strike, put themselves, their union, and their certification to bargain as a group at risk when they engage in illegal strikes. However, when nurses see themselves as losing what they have gained through 3 decades of past collective bargaining, it is not that difficult to understand their willingness to take such risks.

In the United Nurses of Alberta's (UNA) illegal strike of 1988, the employer was poised to roll back a significant percentage of the salary increases and contract provisions gained in previous collective bargaining. Although faced with heavy fines for an illegal strike, on January 25, 1988, some 11,000 nurses from 96 hospitals left their work and picketed for 19 days in −30°C weather (Ross-Kerr, 1998). The union paid the fines but also stopped the rollbacks and other provisions that employers were negotiating to take away. Nurses made other gains on this illegal strike: The public strongly supported the nurses' collective bargaining despite the disruption it created, and nurses who had previously not participated in strike actions (because they were illegal in their places of employment) joined the picket lines. Strategically planned on the eve of the Calgary Winter Olympic games, the strike by the UNA nurses showed that they would not tolerate unjust treatment. Yet while it is true that "illegal strikes by unions are becoming more common, that nurses have been willing to engage in them has been shocking to many" (p. 283).

Although the issues overlap and are not representative of all issues that arise for nurses in the collective bargaining process, they are issues that have been present in nurses' collective bargaining since its inception (McPherson, 1996). The multiple tensions that exist for nurses are further complicated by society's expectations of nurses and the media's questionable accounting of these expectations (Day, 1993). In many cases, nurses' ambivalence toward collective bargaining can be traced to their reluctance to be involved in strikes or other forms of job action involving withdrawal of services. In other cases, however, particularly in the past, the ambivalence can be linked to the somewhat naïve belief still held by some nurses that employers will treat nurses fairly without such action (Jensen, 1992).

Significance of Addressing Collective Bargaining Issues

The restructuring of the health care system throughout the 1990s has shifted the priorities for nurses and significantly affected the conditions in which nurses work. Although nurses have made notable gains in their salaries in many provinces, shifting priorities within provincial health care systems in recent decades have influenced working conditions in ways that are reminiscent of nurses' working conditions in much earlier times. Canadian nurses continue to struggle with their work being recognized and valued in society, with the establishment of safe and healthy work environments, and with reasonable work–life demands.

In the past, nurses were more able to rely on the leadership and mentorship of senior nurses. In many instances, these long-established relationships were eroded in the restructuring of health care workplaces. Although one could argue that leadership within unions is a constant support for practicing nurses, the need remains for every nurse to understand the contribution that she or he can make to the resolution of the issues that are addressed through collective bargaining. Further, there is need for some form of connection between the collective bargaining engaged in by nurses, their provincial professional associations, and the national professional association.

■ FRAMEWORK FOR ANALYZING COLLECTIVE BARGAINING ISSUES

A framework for analysis highlights how the issues surrounding nurses' ambivalence are constituted for nurses in relation to the collective bargaining process. In some instances, nurses' ambivalence can be linked to the history of nursing and of collective bargaining itself. Nurses' ambivalence reflects prevailing societal attitudes about women's work, nurses' work, and the gendered nature of workplace realities (Stuart, 1993). This framework for analysis draws on historical, social–cultural, political, ethical–legal, critical feminist, and economic discourses. These discourses are more than ways of thinking; they reflect the practices and social values that contribute to our understandings of nurses' experiences of collective bargaining (Thorne, McCormick, & Carty, 1996).

Historical Analysis

Historical analysis helps to identify the events and conditions that have led to the development of the issue. Nurses' living and working conditions in the early 20th century can best be described as deplorable. Hospitals were almost completely staffed by student nurses, and in situations in which graduate nurses were hired, they were treated as students. Salaries, holidays, sick time, and benefits were almost nonexistent, as were standards of practice and regulation of working conditions. Nurses often worked in private homes and relied on their employers' goodwill for their well-being. Some nurses worked for only room and board. Nurses were vulnerable to workplace discrimination rooted in "age, physical attraction and ethnicity" (Jensen, 1992, p. 558).

Faced with abysmal working conditions and unsympathetic employers, nurses had little choice but to organize collectively. Although practicing nurses at the time recognized the need for a collective voice, the idea of collective organization generated ambivalence in many nurses from the outset. As a group of women, nurses found an uncomfortable fit with both the idea of lobbying government for the legislation needed to form a professional organization and the thought of aligning themselves with labor unions. Nurses first organized themselves collectively in the late 1920s into professional organizations. Although these professional organizations were able to influence schools of nursing and the regulation of nurses, they had little influence on issues of nurses' remuneration and working conditions (Jensen, 1992). In 1944, a full 2 decades after the formation of professional organizations, the CNA approved the involvement of professional associations in collective bargaining. Despite this approval, the national organization strongly opposed strike action or any form of job action that involved withdrawal of services by nurses. In 1946, the professional association of British Columbia was the first to be certified as a bargaining agent (Jensen, 1992). Throughout the middle decades of the 1900s, professional associations represented nurses in the collective bargaining process.

Emergence of Unions

Although collective bargaining units within professional organizations made considerable gains, the success of professional associations in the collective bargaining process was compromised by the competing interests of bedside nurses and nurses in management and administrative positions, all of whom were legitimate members of the professional associations. This inherent bias came to prominence with the 1973 Supreme Court challenge mandating the separation of bargaining units from organizations in which administrators were members. This challenge was intended to address the many situations in which managers had conflicts of interest with the requests of staff nurses. This separation of nurses from their nursing leaders also has contributed to their ambiguous support for unionization. The separation process divided the membership: Nurse leaders were excluded; today, they still remain unprotected by collective bargaining.

Historically, the relationship between nurses and their leaders was one of solidarity. Conflict between nurses and their managers, according to McPherson (1996), was mitigated by shared experiences of education and practice. Divisions among nurses "were reflected but also resolved within the organizational structures they supported" (p. 261). Professional nursing associations, which combined trade union activity with professional organizational duties, created solidarity among its members—"a solidarity built in part on the gender of its members" (p. 262).

Social and Cultural Analysis

According to Jensen (1992), nursing is steeped in a tradition of nurturing and care for others, with less attention given to meeting assertively nurses' own needs. Some nurses continue to associate unionization with labor unrest when, in actuality, unions have worked to address and improve working conditions for nurses for more than 3 decades. This history of nurses as selfless caregivers has, however, made it difficult for nurses to conceive of themselves as adversarial participants in unionism. "Paradoxically, under labor law, the process of coming to agreement is structured as adversarial and promotes conflict rather than resolution. By law, unions must take the initiative in the process and, as a result, tend to be blamed when two parties fail to come to agreement" (Jensen, 1992, p. 558). This adversarial stance continues to fuel the flames of conflict between nurses and their unions, between unions and nurses' professional organizations, and between both of these groups and provincial governments. It is important not to locate this adversarial stance with unions but to look to the legislative authorities behind it.

Labor legislation also plays a role in nurses' pay equity issues. Some segments of society have made progress regarding work equity and the rights of workers, but the gendered nature of nurses' work continues to confound nurses' collective bargaining efforts. Although one could argue that nurses have made tremendous gains, particularly in the area of wages, nurses continue to be frustrated with only minimal gains for improved conditions of their work and workplaces. The progress that has been made has not been without personal angst for nurses, originating in prevailing attitudes of society. This tension pits nurses against other nurses, their leaders, and the public and, more importantly, creates an inner turmoil for nurses. The ultimate struggle for nurses is being caught between knowing that improving their own working conditions will positively affect patient care and the concern that society will see their efforts as self-serving.

Political Analysis

Political analysis is useful to highlight the ways in which nurses influence others, particularly those with the power to make changes. Nurses are well positioned with their privileged access to patients' experiences within the health care system to know what needs to change within this system. In this capacity, nurses have been able to make many significant contributions. However, nurses have been less successful in convincing governments that the conditions of nurses' work and the quality of work environments significantly influence the quality of care that patients receive. If nurses' salaries are not competitive with other choices nurses can make, the recruitment and retention of qualified experienced nurses will be impossible.

Nurses and their unions have brought these issues to the bargaining table time and time again. It is these issues that influence nurses to participate in illegal strikes. Nurses, more than other members of society, recognize that unless salaries and working conditions are comparable with other work of equal value, there will be no nurses. Although nurses have used many ways to communicate this message and to influence decision makers to make changes, some would argue that it has been through strikes—legal and illegal—that nurses have been most able to inform Canadians of these issues and exercise influence in these changes.

Ethical–Legal Analysis

Ethical–legal analysis highlights the laws, legislative acts, and professional codes that inform, constrain, or otherwise influence an issue. The issue of nurses' ambiguous relationship with unionization is fueled by the tension between and among legislative acts, codes, and laws. For example, unions have traditionally drawn on the Charter of Human Rights to support job action as an essential right in collective bargaining, which, for nurses and others deemed to be providing essential services, was countered by a Supreme Court of Canada ruling in 1987. The CNA's *Code of Ethics* (1997) has recognized nurses' right to collective bargaining action on the condition that steps are taken to ensure the reasonable safety of clients. Despite the amazing efforts of nurses to provide essential services and to participate in strikes, nurses have lost the right to strike in many provinces.

When nurses face conflicting directions from their professional organizations, unions, and the legal system regarding the ethicality of collective bargaining and job action, the situation is confounded. Nurses cannot resolve their positions based on consistent and clear external leadership. What further contributes to nurses' ambiguity is the knowledge that some of the most successful collective bargaining enjoying resounding public support has taken place as "illegal" action. One could argue that existing legislation not only confounds this situation but also is at the heart of the difficulty. Do existing laws make fulfilling nurses' ethical obligations to provide competent care impossible?

Critical Feminist Analysis

Feminist analysis helps us to understand the structures and ideologies that foster misrepresentation of women's and nurses' (women and men) experiences. Nurses' reluctance to become involved in union activity can be tied to the patriarchal nature of their relationships with their employers, the gendered nature of nurses' work as feminine, and the gendered nature of labor unions as masculine. Nurses have had difficulty in "identifying with the male-dominated, working-class labour union movement" (Jensen, 1992, p. 559). In its place, nurses have relied on the benevolence of their employers, believing that, if they worked hard as loyal employees, they would be rewarded justly.

According to Day (1993), women face a work–life dilemma: They are trained to be responsible on the one hand and made to feel guilty on the other. Despite the propensity of health care facilities to lay off workers and eliminate jobs regularly, despite the consequent overcrowding of hospital emergency rooms and growing surgical waiting lists, the nurses (mostly women) who protest such conditions by leaving their jobs are censored for abandoning services considered to be "essential." What's more, the "media blame the women for lack of care" (p. 93). This is the hallmark of patriarchal thinking, and this is where a critical feminist analysis is most needed in nursing.

Economic Analysis

Nurses' salaries have been and continue to be the pivotal point both for nurses' unions and employers' organizations in negotiating a collective agreement. For the nurses, equitable salaries indicate the value attributed to their work; to employers, salaries are the largest item on their budgets. The political and economic environment is also likely to have a significant influence on how nurses and employers approach collective bargaining. In an economic recession, nurses and their unions are likely to make job security, rather than salary increases, a priority. Employers involved in collective bargaining in a recession are more likely to be looking for wage concessions or rollbacks.

In many instances, economic considerations dominate collective bargaining processes and agreements. When significant salary increases are gained, concerns are raised about how existing budgets can accommodate this and how increased salaries for nurses could mean fewer available positions. In these cases, the decision to cut positions rather than reassess budget allocations suggests that decisions are based on what governments have budgeted versus what is needed to provide safe and competent nursing care to Canadians.

Alberta is a good example: Budgets have been called into question for creating the impression that there was a shortfall when in reality no shortfall existed (Taft & Steward, 2000).

■ BARRIERS TO RESOLUTION

One of the greatest barriers to resolving nurses' ambivalence in participating in the collective bargaining process is the failure of nurses to comprehend fully the scope and role of unions. Although one can make a strong argument for the participation and support by nurses of union work when collective bargaining agreements are being renegotiated, one cannot overlook the importance of the work that needs to be done by unions going forward. Nurses' involvement ensures that issues addressed in collective bargaining are the issues that nurses see as relevant. Nurses need access to such knowledge and to ways of conceptualizing issues for their own practice. To increase their interest and participation in union activity, they can also benefit from knowing the history of collective bargaining in nursing, the legislation that authorizes nurses' unions to engage in collective bargaining, and the societal structures and ideologies that shape nurses' views of collective bargaining.

A second barrier concerns the many different realities of nurses' collective bargaining. Nurses' collective bargaining is a provincial matter; hence, the provisions of the collective agreement vary significantly across provinces and territories. The solidarity that could be achieved through the national organization, the CFNU, is compromised by the differences in provincial provisions in collective bargaining. Even provincial unions do not represent all nurses in the provinces. Federal union groups represent nurses who work for federal institutions. Federal labor codes direct these unions, contributing to further fragmentation of Canadian nurses.

As discussed earlier, nurses' collective bargaining excludes nurse leaders. Nurse leaders, often the most highly educated nurses in Canada, work across the bargaining table from staff nurses; the best of nursing expertise is in an adversarial position to the nurses who perform the day-to-day work of nurses. Nurse leaders speak with a knowledge grounded in practice, but they do not speak for practicing nurses. Nurse leaders have been co-opted to speak for employers who have different goals and purposes in the collective bargaining process. Sometimes, they speak for practice, but no one hears them. If they are heard, their own jobs are in peril. Our leaders are positioned as the adversaries of nurses and their unions. They are expendable. They are vulnerable. As stated earlier, in our current system, nurse leaders and their positions are unprotected by collective bargaining. Nurses and nursing are divided by this system. Nurse leaders are lost to practicing nurses and to the patients they care for.

A third barrier for nurses and their unions is isolation. The interests of unions, by virtue of legislative mandates, are in conflict with the interests of nurses' professional organizations because professional associations include nurses involved in evaluating staff nurses. The interests of nurse unions are in conflict with the interests of government agencies that are positioned in opposition to nurses as they carry out their role of protecting the public interest. Although one can convince a government representative that nurses' working conditions are connected to and inseparable from nurses' work with patients, elected representatives are vested to spend public funds wisely. Put another way, elected officials are influenced by structures of power in which nurses' working conditions and the quality of patient care are important but not central to decision making.

A final barrier for nurses is a certain naïveté about unionization and the collective bargaining process. Despite abundant evidence to the contrary, a considerable number of nurses have operated and continue to operate under the assumption that dedicated and loyal employees will be adequately recognized and rewarded. There are many examples of nurses' unconscious complicity in ideologies that sustain nurses' work as service, that support prevailing societal attitudes about nurses' work as women's work and labor unions as working-class male organizations (McPherson, 1996). The literature holds countless examples that call nurses to join in solidarity, that invite the 250,000 Canadian nurses to speak with one voice, to listen to one another, to empower themselves and one another, to collaborate with others, and to think about alternatives to strike action (Ritchie, 1990). Regardless of how well intentioned such messages are, this professional rhetoric creates barriers to our understanding of what has to change. Collective bargaining has become part of what many nurses do to improve the quality of care they provide and the places in which they work. Although many barriers exist for nurses in resolving issues in and related to the collective bargaining process, the major barrier is nurses' ambivalence about collective bargaining.

■ STRATEGIES FOR RESOLUTION

One of the first and more important strategies to resolve issues surrounding nurses' involvement in collective bargaining is education. In the case of nursing students, nursing curricula need to include the various viewpoints of those involved in nurses' collective bargaining: nurses' views, nurses' unions' views, professional associations' views, employer organizations' views, government agencies' views, and consumers' views. Students need opportunities to understand and to learn to critique the structures and ideologies that dominate their lives as men and women.

In the case of graduate nurses, the same materials need to be made available through continuing education workshops, conferences, and in-service speakers. Scholarship in the field of unionization needs to be further developed to include feminist approaches to the conceptualization of nurses' work to highlight the value attributed to nurses. Work and the gendered nature of nurses' work must be understood as located within relationships of power, and nurses need opportunities to explore collective bargaining as well as other strategies to engage in such relationships.

A second strategy that would move this very complex issue toward resolution involves efforts to make collective bargaining activities by all participants more transparent. That is, decisions and the reasons behind particular decisions need to be made explicit. Nurses and their unions can make public the accomplishments of unions. They can also publicize the need to maintain the tension with bargaining units to accomplish and then to maintain the provisions of collective agreements.

A third strategy is to foster partnerships among unions, governments, and professional associations with a goal of understanding the different perspectives that each brings to the bargaining table. The differences between nurses' professional organizations and nurses' unions are often oversimplified. Professional organizations do focus on the safety of the public, and unions and organizations do focus on remuneration and the work lives of nurses. What is even more important to highlight but more difficult to articulate are the ways in which these two organizations work and have the potential to work even more smartly on common areas of interest. Governments also stand to benefit from partnering with nurses' professional organizations and their unions. Although much of the rhetoric from the media would suggest that these three groups are always and already positioned in adversarial positions, an argument could be made that the health of Canadians might be better served through the partnering of these groups. Given that the media has become a powerful influence on public awareness, the ability of such partnerships to bring the media onside to support the outcomes of this partnering is pivotal.

■ SUMMARY

This chapter explores the realities of today's nurses and their unions in an overview of nurses' experiences with collective bargaining. Significant dates, events, and legislation are discussed. Central to these discussions are the issues that collective bargaining and unionization present for nursing. Although several issues thought to arise in collective bargaining and unionization for nurses are presented, these issues cohere and overlap around one central theme: nurses' ambivalence on the one hand and a growing awareness of the need for solidarity to influence change on the other.

A framework for analyzing these issues uses historical, social–cultural, political, ethical–legal, and critical feminist approaches. Questions are raised about the barriers to resolving these issues, and strategies are presented to begin to move these issues toward resolution.

A review of the excellent scholarship on unionization in the Canadian nursing literature suggests that more research and more writings of a critical interpretive nature are needed. Despite this, what has been written points the way to an exciting future for nurses.

Nurses are reclaiming their connection with their feminist past and forging the way to a future where nurses' unions and nurses' professional organizations will create the collective needed to improve the quality of the care nurses provide and of the workplaces where this care is provided.

Nurses can and must speak in one voice to challenge those structures and ideologies that impede our progress. Success depends on nursing's ability as a profession to create a rightful space for nurses and their unions.

Online Resources

Add to your knowledge of this issue:

British Columbia Nurses' Union	www.bcnu.org
Fédération des infirmières et infirmiers du Québec	www.fiiq.qc.ca
Manitoba Nurses' Union	www.nursesunion.mb.ca
New Brunswick Nurses' Union	www.nbnu-siinb.nb.ca
Newfoundland and Labrador Nurses' Union	www.nlnu.nf.ca
Nova Scotia Nurses' Union	www.nsnu.ns.ca
Ontario Nurses' Association	www.ona.org
Saskatchewan Union of Nurses	www.sun-nurses.sk.ca
United Nurses of Alberta	www.una.ab.ca

REFLECTIONS on the Chapter . . .

1. In 1944, the CNA approved the principle of collective bargaining for nurses. What legislation that was passed just before this influenced this approval?

2. How might you account for the slow response of the provinces to act on this approval of collective bargaining by the national body?

3. What finally prompted Alberta nurses to move to have the Registered Nurses Act amended in1966 to allow for collective bargaining between staff nurses' associations and their employers?

4. Two Supreme Court of Canada rulings (in 1973 and 1987) have significantly influenced the nature of nurses' collective bargaining. State the rulings and discuss their effects on nurses' collective bargaining.

5. In nurses' collective bargaining, pay equity has been an issue. What is the nature of this issue?

6. How do nurses describe the dilemma that the issue of strikes and withdrawal of services presents for them?

7. Nurses' salaries are and continue to be central in collective bargaining between nurses' unions and their employers. Discuss the different viewpoints held by nurses and their employers on nurses' salaries.

8. Despite the significant increases in wages gained through the collective bargaining of nurses' unions, there continues to be a proliferation of strikes by nurses. How might you account for that?

9. Why is it that nurses can strike in some provinces but not in others?

References

Canadian Nurses Association. (1997). *Code of ethics for registered nurses.* Ottawa: Author.

Connors, K. (2002, May 28). Values guided care: Evidence based decision. Presentation to the Future of Health Care in Canada. Retrieved June 19, 2002, from http://www.nursesunions.ca/cb/index/shtml

Day, E. (1993). The unionization of nurses. In P. Armstrong, J. Choinere, & E. Day (Eds.), *Vital signs: Nursing in transition* (pp. 242–265). Toronto: Garamond Press.

Hibberd, J. (1992). Strikes by nurses: Incidence, issues, and trends. *Canadian Nurse, 88*(3), 26–31.

_____. (1999). Working with unions. In J. Hibberd & L. Smith (Eds.), *Nursing management in Canada* (2nd ed., pp. 505–524). Toronto: W. B. Saunders.

Hibberd, J., & Norris, J. (1991). Strikes by nurses: Perceptions of colleagues coping with the fallout. *Canadian Journal of Nursing Research, 23*(4), 43–54.

Jensen, P. (1992). The changing role of nurses' unions. In A. Baumgart & J. Larsen (Eds.), *Canadian nursing faces the future* (pp. 557–572). Toronto: Mosby.

Kerr, J. (1996). Unionism and professionalism: Conflicting or compatible processes? In J. Kerr and J. MacPhail (Eds.), *Canadian nursing: Issues and perspectives* (3rd ed., pp. 282–288). Toronto: Mosby.

McPherson, K. (1996). The price of generations: Canadian nursing under Medicare (1968–1990). In *Bedside matters: The transformation of Canadian nursing* (pp. 248–349). Toronto: Oxford University Press.

Ritchie, J. (1990). Feeling empowered. *Canadian Nurse, 86*(1), 3.

Ross-Kerr, J. (1998). The rise of unions in Alberta. In J. Ross-Kerr (Ed.), *Prepared to care: Nurses and nursing in Alberta, 1859–1996.* Edmonton: University of Alberta Press.

Schriber, R., & Nemetz, E. (1992). Pay equity for Ontario nurses. *Canadian Nurse, 88*(9), 17–19.

Stuart, M. (1993). Nursing: The endangered profession. *Canadian Nurse, 89*(4), 19–22.

Taft, K., & Steward, G. (2000). *Clear answers: The economics and politics of for-profit medicine.* Edmonton: Duval.

Thorne, S., McCormick, J., & Carty, E. (1996). Deconstructing the gender neutrality of chronic illness and disability. *Health Care International for Women, 18*, 1–16.

Critical Questions

As a way of engaging with the ideas in this chapter, consider the following:

1. What knowledge do you already have of ethics that will inform your reading of this chapter?

2. Reflecting on what you already know about the nurses' *Code of Ethics*, what ethical issues do you imagine might arise for nurses in practice?

3. How might we account for the increasing interest in ethical dilemmas among nurses in practice?

CHAPTER
18

Laurie Hardingham

Ethical and Legal Issues in Nursing

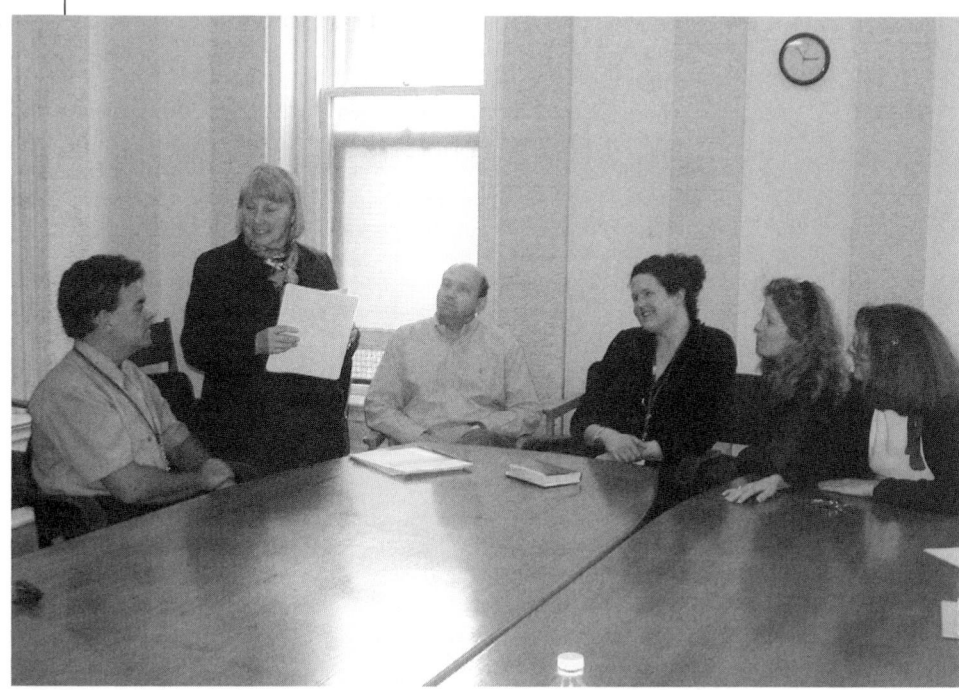

Laurie Hardingham, nurse and senior fellow in Clinical Ethics, with members of the Clinical Ethics Group, the Toronto Rehabilitation Institute/ University of Toronto Joint Centre for Bioethics. Used with permission.

After completing this chapter, you will be able to:

1. Defend the importance of ethical and legal issues for nursing practice.

2. Describe the difference between ethical and legal issues.

3. Articulate relevant ethical and legal issues.

4. Understand the implications for individual nurses and for the nursing profession when ethical and legal issues are not resolved.

5. Identify some of the barriers to, and strategies for, resolving ethical and legal issues.

6. Identify some of the ethical and legal resources available to nurses.

This chapter introduces readers to some ethical and legal issues in nursing and provides an overview of their significance to nursing practice. Specifically, readers are given a case along with its legal and ethical issues. Examining the case will help readers to discern, explore, articulate, analyze, and generate resolutions to the issues. This chapter also focuses on bioethical issues, with a particular emphasis on those that arise for nurses and in the nursing profession.

■ STORY: THE WINNIPEG NURSES

Chapter 1 of the *Report of the Manitoba Pediatric Cardiac Surgery Inquest* (Sinclair, 2000, p. 3) begins:

Pediatric cardiac surgery is one of the most professionally difficult and personally satisfying medical disciplines in which to work. It demands precision and accuracy from the surgeon, as well as a high degree of efficiency and teamwork from other doctors, nurses, and technicians who form its operating-room teams.

Sometimes called the Sinclair Report, the inquest report tells the story of 12 children who died and the health care providers who worked with them during 1994 in the pediatric cardiac surgery program at the Winnipeg Health Sciences Centre.

The program was suspended in February 1995, following an external review. When many parents of the children who died demanded a public inquiry into their children's deaths, the chief medical examiner for the province of Manitoba ordered an inquest, which commenced hearings in December 1995. The hearings lasted until the fall of 1998; the report was released in the fall of 2000.

The 900-plus page report found that the program had a mortality rate more than twice as high as similar programs. Two of the four central themes recorded at the inquest were the heartrending narratives of the children and their parents and the stories about the treatment of nurses.

History of the Program and Nursing Concerns

When the cardiac surgery program was restarted in 1994, after a break due to the previous surgeon leaving for Winnipeg, the operating room and intensive care nurses began to have concerns about the lack of preparation, about the problems in surgery, and about the many complications the young patients were experiencing. As the deaths of infants began and continued, the nurses voiced their concerns to their supervisor, to physicians and surgeons, and to the director of nursing.

The nurses "were never treated as full and equal members of the surgical team" (Sinclair, 2000, p. viii). Their concerns were ignored, and the program continued. The nurses continued to keep notes and speak out to their supervisors. Finally, after the twelfth child died, the program was suspended.

Inquest Findings

The report found that the nurses did nothing wrong; in fact, they did many things that were right. However, the nurses continue to wonder if events might have been different had they acted differently.

After several children had died, one of the nurses, Carol Youngson, decided to attempt to limit her contact with parents. She would no longer take the children from their parents' arms into the operating room. She told the officials at the inquest that she had considered telling parents to "take your baby and run" (Sinclair, 2000, p. 355). When asked why she did not warn the parents, she stated that had she done so, "all hell would have broken loose." She felt that she would have been perceived as overly emotional and that, although she could have perhaps saved one child, there would have been more children coming in, and nothing would have changed. She would have lost her job. Less experienced nurses would be hired, and the program would continue; it would not have been stopped (Sinclair, 2000, p. 355).

Using this story as a background for analysis, nurses can examine relevant ethical and legal issues and try to uncover what it means to practise ethically and legally in the difficult environment that is health care today. Although the story of the nurses in the Winnipeg Pediatric Cardiac Surgical Program is a particularly dramatic one, it raises many issues that concern nurses across the country on a daily basis.

■ WHAT IS ETHICS? WHAT IS BIOETHICS?

Ethics is the philosophical study of morality, the study of what is right and wrong behavior. Studying ethics enables us to examine the things that influence our moral decisions, our obligations and duties to others, our character, the nature of "good," and the underpinnings of what makes a good society.

A subset of ethics is applied ethics, in which ethical theory is applied to real-life situations. This can be divided into various categories, such as bioethics (the study of ethics in the life sciences), business ethics (the study of ethics in the business world), and environmental ethics (ethics related to the natural world and our relationship to it).

Bioethics can be broken into several subspecialties, for example, biomedical ethics (the study of ethics in the medical profession), health care ethics (ethics in the health care setting), nursing ethics (applied ethical theory in nursing), or clinical ethics. Clinical ethics concerns issues that are morally sensitive that arise within the context of patient care and the relationships between the people involved. Clinical ethics involves a process of critical reflection on moral and ethical problems faced in health care settings which helps people to:

- Decide *what* we should do (what actions are ethically right or acceptable)
- Explain *why* we should do it (giving reasons or justifying our decision in ethical terms)
- Describe *how* we should do it (the method of our response; B. Secker, personal communication, 2002. This definition is adopted from Dr. Secker's definition.)

This is a process we should all participate in, because ethical decisions are made by everyone on a daily basis.

■ RECOGNIZING ETHICAL ISSUES

Because ethics is the study of right and wrong behavior, it involves the analysis of what we "ought" to do, what our duties and obligations are to other people, and what kinds of behavior we should expect from others.

What guides this analysis? How do we determine what is the right (and the wrong) action in specific situations? When other people think differently about what actions are morally right, how do we defend our beliefs and question others about theirs? And should we do this?

Moral philosophers and ethicists are not moral experts claiming to have the answers to these questions. They can, however, be a resource to health care professionals, offering rational grounds or bases for our moral beliefs and helping us sort out difficult problems. They can help the decision makers in a situation to make the best decisions possible. Although they cannot be the "moral conscience" of society, ethicists have knowledge of moral theory, which is the systematic, critical study of the basic underlying principles, values, and concepts used in thinking about moral life (Boetzkes & Waluchow, 2000).

■ IDENTIFYING AND ARTICULATING ETHICAL ISSUES

The identification of an ethical issue is not always a straightforward activity. For example, when consent for surgery was obtained but the problems in the pediatric cardiology surgery program were not divulged, the surgeon might have justified the situation by claiming that he was maintaining public confidence in the program. And perhaps the administrators viewed the issue as one of risk management. The nurses, on the other hand, saw the problem as an ethical issue. They believed that the parents were not given all the information they needed to give an informed consent which was consistent with their values and beliefs. This is, in fact, what made it an *ethical* issue—it concerned deeply held values and beliefs about how we treat other people and about the values and beliefs of the children's parents and of the health care professionals who were involved.

The issue of informed consent was identified both by the nurses and later by the Sinclair Report as an important ethical issue in the Winnipeg situation. This issue can be examined in greater detail to see how ethical analysis can help in identifying difficult problems.

Informed Consent: Example of an Ethical Issue

One of the major issues explored in the report was whether the families of the deceased children were fully informed of risks and benefits of surgery before giving their consent to the surgical procedures involving their children. The following story is told in the report:

Mary Jane Wasney's nephew was scheduled for cardiac surgery in June 1994 at the Health Sciences Centre (HSC). Mary Jane, a surgical nurse at HSC, had heard about the deaths of a number of children undergoing cardiac surgery, and she knew that operations were taking longer than expected. Concerned, she spoke with Carol Youngson, the senior nurse in charge in cardiac surgery. Carol advised her to speak with Joan Borton, a nurse clinician at HSC. Mary Jane went to Joan in tears, worried that her nephew was going to die. Joan suggested that Mary Jane could get her nephew "referred out of the province" and advised her to talk to the acting section head of pediatric cardiology. The cardiologist acknowledged that there was a "learning curve in any new program" but stated that he was confident that Dr. Odim could do the nephew's surgery.

Still concerned, Mary Jane asked several of the anesthetists in the program for advice. In her testimony at the inquest, she recalled that all three anesthetists she spoke with recommended against having the operation done in Winnipeg. In the end, her nephew was operated on in Saskatoon (Sinclair, 2000).

Many people do not have access to the information that Mary Jane had. If you were the parents or a close relative of this child, would you have wanted to be informed about the problems in the surgical program? The inquest judge thought that you would and went on to make several recommendations regarding informed consent that, if adopted, would change our thinking about what is sufficient information needed by people to give truly informed consent.

The Right to Be Informed

It is now widely recognized that a capable patient has the right to be informed about a proposed treatment and to decide whether to consent to that treatment. For consent to be valid, it must have the following attributes:

▧ It must be provided by a competent person.
▧ It must be informed (i.e., appropriate and sufficient information must be given in a way that the patient understands, and the informer must be satisfied that the patient understands).
▧ It must be voluntary (i.e., without undue coercion or pressure).

How much information must a physician provide? Until recently, the courts recognized a professional standard: Physicians must provide the amount of information that the average, prudent, reasonable physician would provide in a similar situation. Physicians would have fulfilled their legal obligations if they provided information to a patient in accordance with the practices among their colleagues. However, the law of medical consent has changed recently. The current standard appears to be patient centered. The information provided is sufficient if it meets the standard that a reasonable, average patient in that patient's situation would expect (Baylis et al., 1995).

The Sinclair Report (2000) reviews recent case law that suggests it is not only the patient (rather than the physician) who should decide whether medical treatment will be performed (and where and by whom it will be performed) but it is also a doctor's duty to inform the patient of all material risks. What is material is determined by asking the question "What would a reasonable patient want to know?" Material risks are also those risks that pose a real threat to the patient's life, health, or comfort.

Merely having a signed consent form in which it is acknowledged that the nature of the operation has been explained to the patient does not necessarily prove that the duty to inform has been observed. For example, in an Ontario case, a surgeon had failed to disclose to his patient that he had little experience with the technique being used. In this case, the trial judge held that the surgeon failed in his duty to his patient by not disclosing his inexperience and by failing to give his patient the opportunity to have the procedure performed by another, more experienced surgeon.

In light of such cases, the report states that when a person has been deprived of the opportunity to make a proper decision regarding treatment and when there is a significant risk that would affect the judgment of a reasonable patient, then in the normal course, it is the responsibility of the physician to inform the patient of that significant risk—if the information is needed by the patient to determine for himself or herself what course he or she should follow (Sinclair, 2000).

The report concludes that the evidence suggests that the parents of the children involved in the Winnipeg cases were not as fully informed as they were entitled to be. The report made several recommendations to both the Manitoba Department of Health and the hospital aimed at improving the process of consent and communication with families. These recommendations suggest that the information required is much more than is commonly given; it is the kind of information that the Winnipeg nurses wanted to give to the parents.

Increasing the standard for informed consent certainly involves not only physicians but also others in the health care environment. Those who recognize problems with consent in specific cases have a moral obligation, if not a legal obligation, to ensure that fully informed consent is obtained.

Ethics Informs Law

The last chapter in the *Report of the Manitoba Pediatric Cardiac Surgery Inquest* concludes (Sinclair, 2000, p. 466):

The thrust of the recommendations in this chapter is not punitive. The need is to improve the health-care system so as to prevent the recurrence of events that occurred in 1994. It is necessary to accept that the health-care system will not improve if people act solely on the basis of a fear of consequences for themselves or their careers. Instead, the recommendations are intended to establish a structure within which highly skilled and talented people can establish a health-care team that continually works together to provide a high standard of care. All of the comments and recommendations in this chapter are intended to fulfill this objective.

The report also clearly points out that often nurses are the first people on the health care team to perceive a problem in the informed consent process. This is because nurses have access to information about health care professionals, programs, and institutional problems that most patients do not. Because they usually are more familiar with patient and family values, nurses can appreciate when these patients and families need to know more to make an informed and reasoned decision about medical care.

The law is ethics codified, or shaped by what a society believes is ethical. Because it takes so long to enact laws, the legal system tends to lag behind society's ethical thinking. Usually what the law requires us to do is the minimum, with ethical obligations over and above what is required by law.

The standards of informed consent imposed by recent court decisions and recommended by the Winnipeg inquest report have implications for nurses. Nurses need to be aware of the requirements for informed consent and the kinds of disclosure that are seen as relevant by the courts (Hardingham, 2001a, 2001b). The inquest report also recommended that laws be put in place to protect whistle-blowers in health care, an action that, although most citizens would agree is needed, has not yet been accomplished.

Legal Responsibilities of Nurses

What legal responsibilities do nurses have regarding informed consent? To answer this question, it is important, first of all, to distinguish between two kinds of situations:

- Getting patient consent for what nurses do
- Participating in the consent process for what other health care professionals do

For the first kind of situation, the Canadian Nurses Protective Society (CNPS) cautions: "A nurse carrying out an invasive nursing procedure should provide an explanation and document that the explanation was given and consent obtained" (CNPS, 1994, p. 13). Further, the CNPS states:

Any touching of a client requires verbal, and in some cases, written consent. Legal experts suggest that the person carrying out the treatment should provide the relevant information to the client. So, nurses should be aware of disclosure and consent requirements, and they should be sure to chart that these requirements were met. Failure to obtain consent can result in professional sanctions, civil liability and/or criminal charges (p. 13).

For the second type of situation (e.g., when nurses witness the signing of a consent form for a surgical or medical procedure to be performed by a physician), nurses are not responsible for providing information. The physician, as the caregiver performing the treatment, must provide this. Nurses do, however, have an ethical responsibility to inform the physician when there is evidence that the patient does not have enough information to make an informed decision or that the decision is otherwise not fully informed. If the physician does not remedy the situation, nurses have a role to play as patient advocates. Under both the *Code of Ethics* and the nursing practice standards, each nurse as an individual practitioner has responsibilities to the patients in his or her care. For example, under the value of "choice," the *Code of Ethics* (CNA, 2002) states:

Nurses provide the information and support required so that clients, to the best of their ability, are able to act on their own behalf in meeting the health and health care needs. Information given is complete, accurate, truthful, and understandable. When they are unable to provide the required information, nurses assist clients in obtaining it from other appropriate sources.

These ethical responsibilities may become legal responsibilities if the provincial nursing practice standards or the *Code of Ethics* (CNA, 2002) are recognized by a court of law as guidelines for what a reasonable nurse would do in a specific situation.

■ ETHICAL OR LEGAL ISSUE? ALIKE BUT DIFFERENT

As the preceding analysis points out, ethical and legal issues are closely linked. A legal action and an ethical action one might consider taking may be the same action—but not necessarily. For example, a nurse working in an emergency setting might be reluctant to report suspected child abuse to the authorities, which is required by law, because by doing so she might lose the trust of the family and in turn discourage them from seeking needed medical help for their child or children in the future. The nurse's values suggest that the ethical thing to do would be to work with the family as long as possible to determine whether there is actual abuse or to refer the family to appropriate resources to help them resolve significant problems.

Like all professionals, however, nurses operate within a framework of legal as well as ethical rules and guidelines. (See Box 18.1 for a review of informative resources.) The legal rules that nurses must follow include those that apply to all members of society. In addition to these, nurses as professionals have legal and ethical duties that flow from their obligation to serve the public interest and the common good (Keatings & Smith, 2000). Having a unique body of knowledge, skills, and expertise, nurses have been granted certain rights and privileges by society. In return for this, society holds nurses to high standards of professional, moral, and ethical competence. To balance these responsibilities, nurses must be familiar with the legislation that governs nursing practice and the relevant policies, codes, and standards of practice, as well as with their rights and privileges as professionals.

The Need to Understand Legal Requirements

There are four reasons why nurses should be familiar with the law and have a basic understanding of Canada's legal system. First, the CNA *Code of Ethics* and each provincial regulatory body impose certain requirements with respect to nurses' levels of professional knowledge and skill. If nurses do not meet these requirements, they are open to disciplinary action from their professional governing bodies and, if the conduct is serious enough, the courts.

Second, nurses have access to drugs that are regulated both by legislation and hospital procedures governing their use, dispensation, and handling. They need to know the relevant laws and policies that apply to drugs.

Third, nurses need to be familiar with legal requirements because everyday actions and decisions made by nurses affect the basic rights of their patients. Nurses need to know what those rights are and how to respect and protect them.

Finally, nurses have access to confidential information about individual patients, and they are both legally and ethically obligated to keep such information confidential and not divulge it without patient consent. In some cases, however, nurses are required to divulge such information in court—in the form of testimony—or to report information, such as that related to child abuse (Keatings & Smith, 2000).

The legal system is founded on rules and regulations that guide society in a formal and binding manner. Although constructed by individuals and capable of being changed by the judiciary or legislative enactments, the legal system is a general foundation that gives continuing guidance to health care professionals regardless of their personal views and values systems. For example, the law recognizes the competent patient's right to refuse treatment. A patient has this right whether or not the health care providers agree with the patient's choice. This right, however, is not absolute. If there are overriding state interests, treatment may be mandated against a patient's or parent's wishes. Some examples of this are a court order to fluoridate the water supply or to perform a blood transfusion for a child whose parents refuse such treatment because of religious beliefs. One may have difficulty reconciling law and ethics in areas that transect both, such as issues of death and dying, abuse of others, or futility of health care; legal and ethical issues are often entwined.

One way of differentiating between legal and ethical issues is that laws may be seen as external to oneself, being imposed from the outside. Ethics, on the other hand, can be viewed as something internal. Although this is often true, there are exceptions. Professional codes of ethics may be seen by some as imposed externally,

| **BOX 18.1** | Book Review |

The following resources are suggested for increasing knowledge and skills for legal and ethical practice.

■ Keatings, M., & Smith, O. B. (2000). *Ethical and legal issues in Canadian nursing* (2nd ed.). Toronto: W.B. Saunders Canada.

This book explores the ethical and legal challenges that nurses meet in everyday practice. It is a good resource for nurses on the Canadian legal system, how nursing is regulated in Canada, and professional conduct, misconduct, and malpractice.

■ Yeo, M., & Moorhouse, A. (Eds.). (1996). *Concepts and cases in nursing ethics* (2nd ed.). Peterborough: Broadview Press.

Focusing on the ethical dilemmas faced by nurses who work in the "front lines" of the health care system, this book has many excellent case studies that illustrate how ethical theory can be applied in nursing practice.

■ Boetzkes, E., & Waluchow, W. (2000). *Readings in health care ethics*. Peterborough: Broadview Press.

This anthology contains an excellent introductory chapter on ethical justification and theory, "Ethical Resources for Decision Making," as well as a well-chosen selection of readings, both well known and newly written, in the main areas of health care ethics.

■ Thomas, J., & Waluchow, W. (1998). *Well and good: A case study approach to biomedical ethics* (3rd ed.). Peterborough: Broadview Press.

This text uses a case study approach to health care ethics, with a brief but good discussion on ethical theory. Included are some well-known Canadian cases, such as the "mercy killing" by Robert Latimer, the assisted suicide of Sue Rodriguez, and the pregnancy solvent-abuse case of Mrs. G., as well as little-known real-life cases.

■ Canadian Nurses Association. (2002). *Ethical research guidelines for registered nurses*. Ottawa: Author.

This document links ethical guidance for nurses involved in research with humans to the ethical guidance offered by the *Code of Ethics for Registered Nurses* (CNA, 2002).

■ Canadian Nurses Association. (2003). *Everyday ethics: Putting the code into practice* (2nd ed.). Ottawa: Author.

This updated study guide is intended to be used along with the *Code of Ethics for Registered Nurses* (2002). It is a practical tool that brings the code to life, with case studies and suggestions for using the *Code of Ethics*.

■ Chambliss, D. F. (1996). *Beyond caring: Hospitals, nurses, and the social organization of ethics.* Chicago: University of Chicago Press.

This book, written by a sociologist, is based on more than 10 years of field research and shows how nurses, patients, and others become objects of the bureaucratic machinery of the health care system.

■ Storch, J. L., Rodney, P., & Starzomski, R. (Eds.). (2004). *Toward a moral horizon: Nursing ethics for leadership and practice*. Toronto: Pearson Prentice Hall.

This recently published Canadian book is written by current leaders in researching nursing ethics and is for the study of ethics at an advanced level. It relates the application of moral knowledge to ethical problems in everyday nursing practice, education, research, and management of nursing care.

although the aim might be to have nurses internalize their professional ethics during their education. If people agree with the laws of society, they may have internalized them. Someone might believe that it is always ethical to obey the laws of the society in which they live. Another distinction might be that one might obey the law because it is prudent to do so, that actions that disobey the law might result in some harm. Ethical actions, on the other hand, are done not out of fear of punishment but because they are the right things to do.

The Need to Incorporate Law and Ethics Into Practice

In the story at the beginning of this chapter, the Winnipeg nurses advocated repeatedly for their patients but seemed to get nowhere. Here we might ask the following question: If nurses are unable to fulfill the requirements in the *Code of Ethics* and their nursing practice standards, are these requirements then empty ones? Because if they are not empty, then nurses must be able to incorporate them into their nursing practice.

However, a nurse who chooses to be a patient advocate by disclosing directly to a patient that there are problems with a specific health care professional or program may be legally open to a charge of defamation. If following the requirements means that nurses must perform heroic acts, such as putting their jobs at risk by repeatedly taking their concerns to upper management or by blowing the whistle (informing) on wrongdoers or on unsafe practices or conditions, then, for most nurses, the requirements may seem to be empty. Is this an unsolvable problem for nurses?

■ ISSUES OF MORAL INTEGRITY

A major issue that arises for nurses facing difficult situations is how they can maintain moral integrity, or a sense of moral wholeness, when their values go unheeded and they see themselves as powerless to influence change. As Redman and Fry (2000, p. 360) point out:

It is no surprise that nurses experience ethical conflicts while providing care. They are individuals with personal and professional values; they ply their skills in institutions in conjunction with other professionals— all of whom have different values. They provide nursing care to patients who may have religious, cultural, and moral values quite different from their own.

These value conflicts often lead to problems within the health care setting. In an analysis of five studies on ethical conflicts faced by nurses, Redman and Fry (2000) found two underlying themes:

1. Evidence of widespread conflict between professional, corporate, and societal definitions of adequacy of care.
2. Evidence of differences in the philosophical orientations of the various health professions. For example, some nurses believe that they value patient autonomy more than physicians value patient autonomy.

Redman and Fry ask two questions: Will the differences and the concerns of nurses be seen as worthy of attention? In practice settings, what kind of moral agency of nurses will be supported? These are important questions because nurses make daily decisions in their work with patients. Some of these are moral decisions, and when nurses act deliberately on moral decisions, they are moral agents. As moral agents, nurses are required to examine, or reflect on, their actions.

Familiar to anyone who has taken a philosophy course, Socrates' assertion that "the unexamined life is not worth living" indicates how important thinking, self-analysis, and reflection are to understanding the world and our part in it. When feelings of distress arise, almost everyone examines the choices they have made and wonders if things would have turned out differently if they had made different decisions or pursued different actions.

Health care professionals do this a lot and, in fact, are encouraged to do so. For example, the Alberta Association of Registered Nurses (AARN) requires, in their Continuing Competence Program, that nurses conduct a "review of one's own nursing practice to determine learning needs and incorporate learning to improve one's own practice." The key to this process is "reflection on your practice against the Nursing Practice Standards" (AARN, 2000, p. 8). In other words, nurses are asked to reflect on the extent to which their practice meets the standards.

Reflection is serious thinking about something, thinking that "reflects" back to us what we believe or value, so that we can understand better why we think that way. If we can find no good reasons for our beliefs, then we may need to think about whether we should change them.

Thomas and Waluchow (1998) use the notion of "reflecting" in their description of three levels of response to a moral question or problem:

1. The expressive level
2. The pre-reflective level
3. The reflective level

At the expressive level, responses are unanalyzed expressions or feelings, which, in themselves, do not constitute any kind of justification or reason for the response. The emotional response "this is just not right!" is an example of the expressive level.

At the pre-reflective level of response, justification is given by reference to values, rules, and principles that are accepted uncritically. Most often, justification is made by reference to a "conventional" or commonly agreed-on standard or rule. We do not stop to think why we should act or base our judgments on these rules or whether they are good standards to adopt. For example, a nurse might say, "This is not right because it goes against hospital policy."

At the reflective level of response, moral judgments are based not entirely on blindly accepted conventional norms but rather on principles, rules, and values to which we ourselves consciously subscribe. A rational moral agent operating at the reflective level should be prepared to offer a reason for a moral judgment. Thus, moral reflection serves to concentrate one's thoughts back on a problem or an idea. This is not a new activity; it is something most of us have been doing all our lives. However, as moral agents, we need to continuously and consciously think in a reflective way about constructing and evaluating the reasons for our rules and beliefs and to set out standards we can use to judge these reasons as good or poor ones. We need to direct our attention explicitly toward things that we normally take for granted, to examine carefully our beliefs and opinions and the evidence we have for them.

Reflection and Integrity

May (1996) includes critical thinking as an important aspect of moral integrity. Integrity means completeness or wholeness, and when we refer to our moral integrity as a person and as a professional, we think about the relationship of our actions to our beliefs. This relationship is very important to our self-concepts.

According to May, the development of a critical point of view means that we need to view moral integrity not as holding steadfastly to a code of conduct or rules that others have provided—even if we approve of the code or rules—but rather "as a form of maturation in which reflection on a plurality of values provides a critical coherence to one's experiences" (May, 1996, p. 16). Achieving integrity means developing a critical perspective, a standpoint from which one can examine and then endorse or reject new social influences.

Implicit in this view is the requirement that our choices must be our own. We mature not merely by being socialized to accept certain values and beliefs but also by becoming committed to certain values and beliefs as a result of critical reflection. When our actions are in harmony with those values and beliefs, we have personal integrity. Acting at the pre-reflective level is a type of externally directed behavior, the blind following of standards or norms set by someone else. Although not necessarily bad (sometimes conventional norms are capable of reasoned defense and can be fully justified morally), our conventional standards and rules must always be subject to scrutiny. Perhaps there are much better rules that we should try to persuade others to adopt, or perhaps existing conventions are morally objectionable.

What happens when moral integrity is compromised? Webster and Baylis (2000) distinguish among three kinds of experiences:

Moral uncertainty occurs when one is unsure what moral principles or values apply, or even what the moral problem is. Sometimes all that is required is more information to resolve the uncertainty, but, at other times, the uncertainty can persist.

Moral dilemmas arise when there are obligations to pursue two or more conflicting courses of action and no obvious reason to prefer one course over the other. Moral dilemmas can also arise when some evidence suggests that a particular course of action is morally right, other evidence suggests that it is morally wrong, and in each case the evidence is inconclusive.

Moral distress is experienced when there is an inconsistency between one's beliefs and the actions that one takes. This inconsistency is usually because the person knows what the right thing to do is, but fails to do it (or fails to do it to his or her satisfaction) for such reasons as an error of judgment, a personal failing (e.g., a weakness or crimp in one's character, such as a pattern of "systemic avoidance"), or other circumstances beyond one's control, such as when one lacks the authority to act.

Redman and Fry (2000) found that studies of nurses and ethical conflicts show that moral uncertainty is rare. Most nurses believe that they understand the nature of the conflict; however, about one third of the nurses studied experienced moral distress. Nurses also perceived an organizational disinclination to deal with physicians when the ethical conflicts involved physicians, making nurses believe that these kinds of conflicts were unresolvable.

When situations that contribute to moral distress are not resolved, the result can lead to *moral residue*, "that which each of us carries with us from those times in our lives when in the face of moral distress we have seriously compromised ourselves or allowed ourselves to be compromised" (Webster & Baylis, 2000, p. 218). Moral residue results from the lingering distress that accompanies times when people compromise their basic values and principles. Moral residue can be profound and lasting, concentrated in our thoughts, and usually very painful because it threatens and sometimes betrays deeply held and cherished beliefs and values.

Carol Youngson, the Winnipeg nurse who could no longer take the children from their parents' arms into surgery, experienced profound moral distress, which remains with her as moral residue (Armstrong, 2001). Youngson and the other nurses involved in the pediatric cardiac surgery program found that their personal moral integrity was compromised because a combination of fear, uncertainty, and doubt led them to question their values and their actions. They set aside actions that they might have performed, such as warning the parents or going to the press, because these actions did not appear to be open to them at the time.

Unfortunately, in today's health care system, each professional may not have the time and the environment for the kind of critical reflection on values that might be required. And it is not clear that a distinction can be drawn between personal and professional integrity. In the same way, it is difficult to distinguish between errors caused by individual actions and errors resulting from systemic causes. However, in both situations, the individual is harmed when she or he experiences serious moral compromise. As May (1996) and Webster and Baylis (2000) point out, compromised integrity irreversibly alters the self. "One does not experience serious moral compromise and survive as the person once was" (Webster & Baylis, 2000, p. 224). When such change prompts the person to know with greater clarity what actions or situations he or she will or will not tolerate or cooperate with in the future, then it can be change for the better. The change can be harmful, however, if the person adapts by constantly shifting his or her values. As time passes, the person's values become so changeable that it is nearly impossible to articulate what she or he sincerely believes. The person then becomes desensitized to wrongdoing and willing to tolerate morally questionable or morally impermissible actions.

Webster and Baylis (2000) also suggest that moral residue may actually lead to error. Commonly, the error will take one of three forms:

1. Denial of the incoherence between beliefs and actions
2. Trivialization of the incoherence between beliefs and actions
3. Unreflective acceptance of the incoherence between beliefs and actions

Very often, the structure and culture of the clinical setting are factors that contribute to such errors. For example, ethical issues can be camouflaged in the ordinariness of things, when familiar nonmoral language and categories are used to describe normative issues. The culture can appear to be willing to dismiss or trivialize certain ethical concerns and overlook or sidestep others. Therefore, we need to ask not only about the quality and clarity of thinking in terms of knowledge and analytical skills but also about whom we are in situations that arise and about the relationships we have, or expect to have, with colleagues and the wider health care community.

Moral Dilemmas

Bruce Jennings (1996) makes a useful distinction between two types of moral dilemmas. There are those moral dilemmas inherent in the human condition, such as the fact that all people die sooner or later. And there are those moral dilemmas created by institutional structures, such as policies that prohibit us from doing what we think is the right thing. The first type of dilemma, Jennings says, is unavoidable. The second type can often be avoided by altering institutional structures. Jennings claims that an important part of professional ethics is to be open to the possibility of avoiding some moral dilemmas by modifying the institutions within which professionals work. In other words, we need to identify whether the moral dilemmas that we face are somehow inherent in our moral agency itself or whether the dilemmas are artifacts of specific institutional structures.

Those types of moral dilemmas that are artifacts of specific institutional structures require change in those structures. Both the *Code of Ethics* and the many nursing practice standards recognize this, calling attention to the value of practice environments conducive to safe, competent, and ethical care and to the organizational supports needed in the practice setting. What is implicit in both the *Code of Ethics* and standards of practice documents is that professional nurses working in institutional settings cannot practise ethically without the required support.

Does this let nurses off the hook? Not exactly. First of all, even if nurses recognize that without change in the institutional structure they cannot practise ethically, they are still in a difficult situation, often facing severe moral distress. The Winnipeg nurses agonized over the deaths of the children. They continued to press for change, despite sarcasm and criticism from other members of the health care team (Sibbald, 1997). Second, the *Code of Ethics* explicitly states that nurses must work both individually and in partnership with others to improve practice environments and to address unsafe practice issues (CNA, 2002).

Nurses and Professional Integrity

Many bioethicists make a strong argument that such moral concepts as integrity and responsibility need to be understood as embedded in social structures (May, 1996; Sherwin, 2000; Webster & Baylis, 2000). For a professional, this means that professional ethics not only are embedded in an individual conscience but also result from interactions between persons. Thus, to have moral integrity as a professional, an individual must do more than simply adhere to what his or her conscience says. The person needs to evaluate critically the standards that he or she as a professional is required to follow both as an individual and collectively with others in the profession.

As we saw earlier, acting at the pre-reflective level is a type of "externally directed behaviour," whereby standards or norms set by someone else are followed blindly (Thomas & Waluchow, 1998). This is not necessarily bad. Sometimes, conventional norms are capable of reasoned defense and can be fully justified morally and, therefore, would be good standards to adopt. However, our conventional standards and rules must always be subject to scrutiny. Perhaps there are much better rules, and we should try to persuade others to adopt them, or perhaps existing rules are morally objectionable. For example, the convention—followed until fairly recently—whereby nurses always deferred to physicians and obediently complied with their orders, never questioning them, is now seen as unacceptable and archaic. Most nurses would agree now that some orders, if the nurse feels they are not right for the patient, should be questioned.

To have moral integrity, nurses need to assess the standards, codes, and rules that they are asked to follow in their practice. They must have good reasons for accepting them. This requires not only reflection on whether their practice follows codes of ethics and nursing practice standards but also reflection on the codes and standards themselves. Nurses ought to determine whether they are genuinely in accord with them and why. Reflective practice means thinking about standards, codes, and practices from a critical point of view and sharing this responsibility with other nurses.

Reflective practice takes time! It takes time to become familiar with the standards and practices nurses are asked to follow in their professional lives as well as to subject these standards and practices to a critical point of view. Nurses do not always have time for reflective practice, but they need to find space for reflection because nurses are morally and legally required to do so. Reflective practice might be time-consuming and frustrating, yet it offers the best hope for nurses' work to be responsive to the needs of their patients and society.

■ BARRIERS TO RESOLVING ETHICAL AND LEGAL ISSUES

Nurses are accountable to individual patients, their families, health care team members, employers, the profession, and society as a whole. As well, they also have rights as professionals. These multiple obligations can present difficulties and complicate the identification of barriers to the resolution of problems.

Lack of Workplace Supports

Kelly (1998) carried out a study that describes, explains, and interprets how new graduate nurses perceived their adaptation to the "real world" of hospital nursing. This study examined the major influences on the new graduates' moral values and ethical roles in the 2 years after their graduation. Kelly found that the nurses went through a complex psychosocial process to preserve moral integrity and maintain a valued professional identity. This process resulted in a struggle that led to moral distress. Kelly concluded that the self-doubt and confusion from intense stress resulted in greater reliance on others as references for self-evaluation. She found also that individual ethical standards are influenced by group norms and that the environment in which nurses work and the practice and support of their more experienced colleagues are very important in the maintenance of professional values and a professional identity. With the results of Kelly's work in mind, it is very important to have a practice setting that some authors have described as a "moral community" (Storch, 1999, Webster and Baylis, 2000). A moral community is one in which (Webster & Baylis, 2000, p. 228)

there is coherence between what healthcare institutions publicly profess to be—namely, helping, healing, caring environments that embrace the virtues intrinsic to the practice of healthcare and what employees, patients, and others both witness and participate in.

Without this coherence, it is very difficult for individual practitioners to practise with *integrity,* a word that means "wholeness." When there is an incoherence between how professionals say they behave and the way they actually behave and practise, it is very difficult to maintain wholeness, or integrity. The person with integrity can be relied on to act in a way that is responsive to a well-thought-out view of the relation between his or her beliefs and actions. But for people who practise in health care institutions, the ability to have integrity rests within the kind of society we are a part of and can be said to be a relational concept. This is because when we work in a large institution, we rely on and have obligations to many other people, not just to our patients. Thus, gaining and maintaining our integrity is a relational process in which we need to reflect within ourselves and with others we work with (Hardingham, 2004a).

Conflict: Ambivalent Views and Approaches to Issues

Another barrier exists in the ways that society views health care hierarchies and concepts. For example, the notion of respect for patient autonomy, broadly recognized as the principle that patients have the authority to make their own decisions about their health care, occupies a prominent place in bioethics. However, Sherwin (2000) points out that feminists and others feel deeply ambivalent about the autonomy ideal. Although it is woven throughout many feminist approaches, Sherwin points out that this is something in need of a specifically feminist analysis.

Although there are many good reasons why respect for personal autonomy is important, there are also many problems with the autonomy ideal. For many feminists, the main problem is the focus on the individual that it usually takes, because life, especially for women, is not lived in a vacuum in which the decision maker acts in isolation. Decisions are made taking into consideration the relationships to other human beings, whether they are close relationships, such as those with parents, children, and partners, or less intimate relationships, such as those within communities or in professional–client relationships.

Sherwin proposes an alternative conception of autonomy, which she calls "relational autonomy." Although not denying that autonomy ultimately resides in individuals, Sherwin's concept takes into account the impact of social and political structures, especially sexism and other forms of oppression, on the lives and opportunities of individuals. "It realizes that the presence or absence of a degree of autonomy is not just a matter of being offered a choice. It also requires that the person have the opportunity to develop the skills necessary for making the type of choice in question, the experience of being respected in her decisions, and encouragement to reflect on her own values" (Sherwin, 2000, p. 79).

Applying the term *relational autonomy* to the full range of human relations, both personal and public, allows a political dimension to come in. It "makes visible the importance of considering how . . . social factors affect women's decision making" (Sherwin, 2000, p. 82) and how the place of nurses within the institutional context influences their ability to provide good nursing care.

Looking again at the Winnipeg nurses' story, the notion of relational autonomy is an excellent one. The nurses were concerned about their relationships with the children who were their patients, with the parents and families, with other members of the health care team, and with the wider community. In their decision making, they considered all of these groups, as well as the kinds of authority and influence that nurses had within the team, and decided that such actions as quitting or going public with their concerns would not be helpful. They continued to press for change through the proper channels but remained distressed about taking the children into the operating room. Their worry that the parents didn't know enough about the program to make good decisions for their children's treatments was a constant source of pressure for them. On the other hand, the nurses realized the complexity of the relationships in health care and that the relationships depended on trust and cooperative action. Warning the parents or going to the press could do irreparable damage to trust and cooperation. The nurses felt that their own autonomy was diminished when their concerns went unheeded, leading some of the nurses to "silence themselves" (Sinclair, 2000, p. 478).

Sherwin (2000) also agrees that the moral community in which health care professionals work is important. Relational autonomy demands that appropriate structural conditions be met.

Limited Resources

Relational theory reminds us that material restrictions, including very restricted economic resources, "constitute real limitations on the options available to the agent. Moreover, it helps us to see how socially constructed stereotypes can reduce both society's and the agent's sense of that person's ability to act autonomously. Relational theory allows us to recognise how such diminished expectations readily become translated into diminished capacities" (Sherwin, 2000, p. 79).

The diminished capacities of the Winnipeg nurses resulted from, among other things, the lack of vehicles through which nurses could report incidents and concerns without risk of professional reprisal, the subservient position that nursing occupied within the organization, and the failure to involve nurses in the planning process of the pediatric cardiac surgery program (Sinclair, 2000).

■ STRATEGIES FOR RESOLUTION OF ETHICAL AND LEGAL ISSUES

Once an ethical or legal issue for nurses is identified and analyzed, many strategies can be implemented to address and resolve it. Strategies include, but are not limited to, the following:

- Review the *Code of Ethics*. The code is reviewed every 5 years, and nurses' input is invited for this process. If you identify an issue that does not seem to be addressed, you could volunteer to contribute to the code's review.
- Become familiar with the legislation, standards, and policies that apply to nursing practice. When you cannot conform to them, document the problems. Incident report forms, professional responsibility forms, and other ways of reporting and discussing concerns should be utilized as often as possible to draw attention to unsafe and unethical practice.
- Ask for advice and support. Nurses' stories are of immediate interest in the political sphere, especially those that deal with ethical issues. Respect confidentiality, but try to find ways to broaden the approach to your issues. For example, contact your professional association or union for advice, support, and assistance to resolve concerns.
- Work to establish a moral community in your workplace. Participate actively on ethics committees, ethics rounds, and the like in hospitals and health care organizations. Most hospitals have an ethics committee, an ethics consultation service, or other ways of dealing with ethical issues for accreditation purposes. Bringing instances or concerns forward can often bring them to the attention of people who can take action to resolve them. Suggest a nursing ethics interest group or brown-bag lunch in your workplace to learn more about ethics and to discuss problems.
- Identify what you can do both as an individual and as part of a group to build a supportive moral community in your workplace. Research shows that the culture, the amount of support from colleagues, and the kind of environment in which nurses work are important components to ethical practice (Kelly, 1998).
- Bring up ethical concerns with your colleagues and with the interdisciplinary team. Chances are that if you have a concern about something, other people in your workplace may as well. Remember, ethics is not just something you read about or study, but a practice, something you do. It requires dialogue and reflection on right action among members of a community; it also requires self-reflection. Organize a journal club or request educational sessions on ethical issues that arise.
- Call the risk management committee's or coordinator's attention to a legal problem or a potential legal problem in a hospital or other health care facility where you work. This alone may be enough to have action taken. Also, for legal issues, expertise and assistance are available from professional nursing organizations.
- Review ethically troubling cases retrospectively with colleagues. Take time to get together after a difficult case to discuss feelings, values, and beliefs about the case as well as what might be done differently the next time a similar case arises. Consider doing "preventive ethics" to put processes and procedures in place that might prevent ethically troubling situations (Hardingham, 2004b).

■ SUMMARY

Consider again the distress of the Winnipeg nurses in the pediatric cardiac surgery program. They were not facing moral uncertainty. They did not have a moral dilemma: They knew what the right thing to do was, and they did it. However, their concerns and attempts to use proper process did not help. They could have said, "We followed the policies, we took our concerns to the people we were supposed to report to, and so our responsibility is ended." But they did not: They continued to reflect on their concerns and continued to speak up for their patients. They decided that whistle-blowing or warning the parents might cause more problems. They thought it better for the children if they remained on the job and continued to try to work for institutional change. Carol Youngson and the other nurses suffered moral distress, and the resulting moral residue remains with them, possibly forever (Armstrong, 2001).

The issues around informed consent are not the only legal and ethical issues arising out of the Winnipeg story. Other issues include those of truth telling, whistle-blowing (going outside of the organization with information about harms or wrongdoing), nurse–patient relationships, conflicts between members of the health care team, and gender issues. However, the analysis presented around informed consent may act as a prototype that gives the reader a sense of what approaches to take to other issues.

Legal and ethical issues are significant to nurses, and they should be familiar with laws, codes, standards, and policies that apply to nursing practice.

Additionally, nurses should be able to identify, articulate, and understand ethical and legal issues and the problems that result when they are not able to do so. Identifying barriers to ethical and legal nursing practice is an important step for nurses to take.

The task of overcoming those barriers is one that cannot be undertaken only by individuals. Nurses are vulnerable when faced with legal and ethical issues. They require knowledge about the law and about ethics as well as the realization that they need to work individually and collectively to move identified issues toward resolution.

Online Resources

Add to your knowledge of this issue:

Canadian Nurses Association (CNA)	**www.cna-nurses.ca**
Canadian Nurses Protective Society (CNPS)	**www.cnps.ca**
Bioethics for Clinicians	**www.cmaj.ca/cgi/collection/ bioethics_for_clinicians_series**
NursingEthics.ca	**www.nursingethics.ca**
University of Toronto Joint Centre for Bioethics	**www.utoronto.ca/jcb**
The Canadian Bioethics Society (CBS)	**www.bioethics.ca/english**

REFLECTIONS on the Chapter . . .

1. From your practice experience, identify examples of ethical and legal issues. How do you know that they were either ethical or legal issues? Were the two categories intertwined? If so, how, and how did you approach them?

2. Have you experienced moral uncertainty? A moral dilemma? Moral distress? What steps did you take? Looking back, what, if anything, would you do differently?

3. Think of the resources that are available to you to help you with ethical and legal issues. How would you go about accessing them?

4. Identify at least one ethical issue that seems to be prevalent in nursing practice. Is this issue one that is discussed publicly? What are the barriers to effective resolution of this issue? How are nurses approaching this issue and the problems it presents?

5. This chapter focuses on bioethical issues, with a particular emphasis on those that arise for nurses and in the nursing profession. What other approaches to ethics might inform nursing practice?

References

Alberta Association of Registered Nurses. (1999). *Nursing practice standards.* Edmonton: Author.

_____. (2000). *Continuing competence document.* Edmonton: Author.

Armstrong, S. (2001, March). The crying shame. *Chatelaine,* pp. 86–94.

Baylis, F., Downie, J., Freedman, B., et al. (1995). *Health care ethics in Canada.* Toronto: Harcourt Brace Canada.

Boetzkes, E., & Waluchow, W. (2000). *Readings in health care ethics.* Peterborough: Broadview Press.

Canadian Nurses Association. (2002). *Code of ethics for registered nurses.* Ottawa: Author.

Canadian Nurses Protective Society. (1994). *Consent to treatment: The role of the nurse.* Ottawa: Author.

Hardingham, L. B. (2001a). Ethics in the workplace: Raising the standards of informed consent. The Winnipeg Inquest. *Alberta RN, 57*(1), 22–23.

_____. (2001b). Ethics in the workplace: Nurses and informed consent: Lessons from the Winnipeg Inquest. *Alberta RN, 57*(2), 22–23.

_____. (2004a). Integrity and moral residue: Nurses as participants in a moral community. *Nursing Philosophy, 5,* 127–134.

_____. (2004b). Managing ethically. In A. Crowther (Ed.), *Nurse managers: A guide to practice* (pp. 23–36). Melbourne, Australia: Ausmed Publications.

Jennings, B. (1996). The regulation of virtue: Cross-currents in professional ethics. In R. A. Larmer (Ed.), *Ethics in the workplace: Selected readings in business ethics* (pp. 397–404). Minneapolis/St.Paul: West Publishing.

Keatings, M., & Smith, O. B. (2000). *Ethical and legal issues in Canadian nursing* (2nd ed.). Toronto: W. B. Saunders Canada.

Kelly, B. (1998). Preserving moral integrity: A follow-up study with new graduate nurses. *Journal of Advanced Nursing, 28*(5), 1134–1145.

May, L. (1996). *The socially responsive self: Social theory and professional ethics.* Chicago: University of Chicago Press.

Redman, B. K., & Fry, S. T. (2000). Nurses' ethical conflicts: What is really known about them? *Nursing Ethics 2000, 7*(4), 360–366.

Sherwin, S. (2000). A relational approach to autonomy in health care. In E. Boetzkes & W. Waluchow (Eds.), *Readings in health care ethics.* Peterborough, ON: Canadian Nurses Protective Society, Broadview Press.

Sibbald, B. (1997). A right to be heard. *Canadian Nurse, 93*(10), 22–28, 30.

Sinclair, C. M. (2000). *Report of the Manitoba pediatric cardiac surgery inquest* [Online]. Winnipeg: Manitoba Provincial Court. Available: http://www.pediatriccardiacinquest.mb.ca

Storch, J. (1999). Ethical dimensions of leadership. In J. M. Hibberd & D. L. Smith (Eds.), *Nursing management in Canada* (2nd ed., pp. 351–367). Toronto: W. B. Saunders Canada.

Thomas, J., & Waluchow, W. (1998). *Well and good: A case study approach to biomedical ethics* (3rd ed.). Peterborough, ON: Broadview Press.

Webster, G. C., & Baylis, F. (2000). Moral residue. In S. B. Rubin & L. Zoloth (Eds.), *Margin of error: The ethics of mistakes in the practice of medicine.* Hagerstown, MD: University Publishing Group.

As a way of engaging with the ideas in this chapter, consider the following:

1. How have you come to hold the views you hold of gender and gendered roles?

2. How is it that historically some work has been thought of as women's work?

3. How does value get assigned to particular work?

CHAPTER
19

Carol McDonald

Issues of Gender and Power: The Significance Attributed to Nurses' Work

The identification of nursing as a gendered occupation is nothing new. A man who chooses nursing as a profession is inevitably identified as a "male nurse," whereas a woman is rarely referred to as a "female nurse." In nursing practice today, the concept of a profession as gender specific is rarely validated. Rather, the attributes of knowledge, skill, effectiveness, and care empower all nurses. Photograph by Larry Arbour. Used with permission from Faculty of Nursing, University of Calgary.

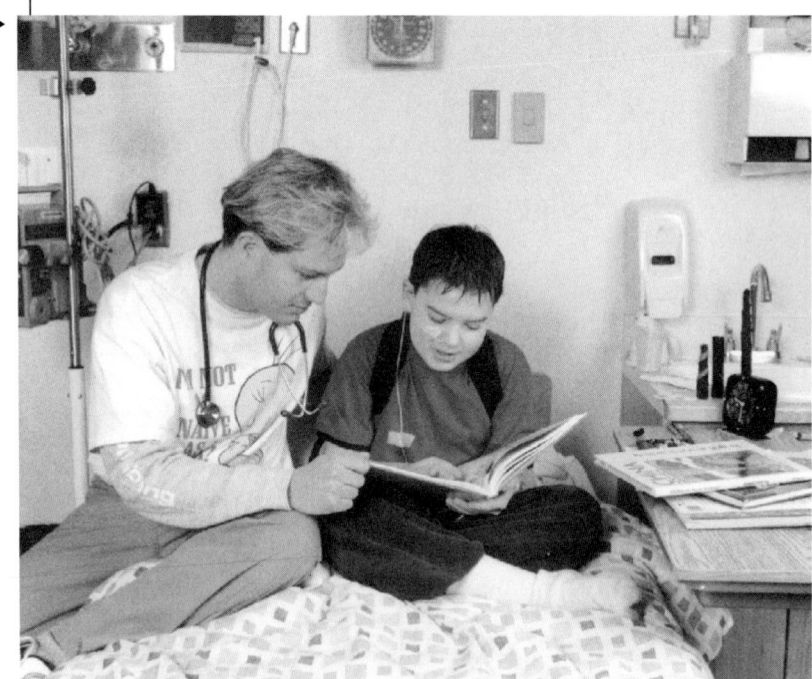

After completing this chapter, you will be able to:

1. Identify ways of thinking about power structures, including ideologies, social discourses, and the discursive process.

2. Understand the conceptualization of gender as socially constructed, the process of naturalizing knowledge, the idea that gender resides both within and beyond the individual, and the ways in which gender knowledge is bound by cultural, temporal, and social realities.

3. Recognize gender as one of a number of intersecting identities, including race, class, age, ethnicity, and sexual orientation, through which we are uniquely constituted as persons.

4. Articulate the nature of nurses' work, nurses' knowledge, and nurses' public representation as gendered, and discuss the historical social discourses of women's work and nurses' work that have contributed to this understanding.

5. Discuss the barriers that interfere with the resolution of issues that arise from relations of power and gender and the significance attributed to nurses' work.

6. Identify strategies that will serve to interrupt the taken-for-granted notions of gendered work that underlie the devaluing of nurses' work.

This chapter presents opportunities to consider the idea that societally derived concepts about gender are inherent in claims about the value of nurses' work and the importance of nursing knowledge. The chapter challenges readers to look beneath the taken-for-granted assumptions about what is called women's work in general and nurses' work in particular. In reconsidering what we think we know, we come to see the web of social discourses through which work, knowledge, and nursing itself are inscribed with meanings of gender.

Ideas about women and women's work and whether this work requires significant knowledge, responsibility, and skill contribute to the devaluing of nurses' work by society. This chapter examines historical changes in the valuing of work that is ordinarily performed by women. It suggests that the devaluing of nurses' work and knowledge stems from cultural power arrangements. The impact of discourses of care, or ideas about care as central to nursing practice, on the value attributed to nurses' work are examined as well (Box 19.1).

■ GENDER AND POWER: ARTICULATING THE ISSUE FOR NURSING

How do concepts of gender and power arise in a discussion of the issues currently affecting Canadian nurses in education and in practice? Gender is a concept in our society that is simultaneously taken for granted and poorly understood. In this chapter, *gender* refers to the ways in which a person lives her or his life that demonstrate or reflect masculinity and femininity. As the chapter explores, gender can be thought of as constructed through social influences outside of a particular individual. And although there is undoubtedly some interrelationship between biologic sex and gender, this chapter addresses gender as distinct from the categories of biologic sex.

As nurses, we seldom think about the preponderance of practicing nurses who are women. When we do reflect on the gender division in nursing, we may think no further than "the numbers," that is, the distribution of genders in the profession. However, the issues of gender and power, as they relate to nursing, are more complicated than the biologic sex of those who practise nursing. Moreover, gender itself is not an "issue" in nursing. The fact that most practicing nurses are women is not in itself problematic. What is

BOX 19.1   Glossary of Terms and Definitions

This list describes the way some terms are used in the content of this chapter. They should not be taken as absolute definitions of the words.

Complicity—our own participation in, for example, supporting or reinforcing societal norms that undermine the value of women's work.

Essentializing—seeing something as representative of all members of a particular group or category. For example, essentializing nurses' work in a woman's domain implies that there is something about nursing that could only be performed by women.

Discourses—social practices, values, and cultural beliefs that prevail in a given culture or sub-culture at a specific historical moment and shape a collective sense of what is right, proper, worthwhile, or valuable (Thorne, McCormick, & Carty, 1997, p. 2).

Discourses of care—the ways in which ideas about care have been represented in nursing, particularly the values and beliefs that have placed care central to nursing practice.

Discursive process—how we learn to be and to behave in particular ways through the messages received in social discourses.

Gender—the ways in which femininity and masculinity are reflected in the lived life. Gender is distinct from the biologic sex of a person. Culturally, there is value attached to particular genders and the way in which that gender is performed.

Ideologies—not merely ideas, but a powerful and authoritative voice in society that tells us who we are and how we are to behave.

Location of gender—gender is constructed through the interaction of the person with the social realities, values, and beliefs of a culture at a particular time in history. In this sense, gender resides both within and beyond the individual.

Naturalized—when some quality is taken to be innately, or obviously "the way it is," without questioning the beliefs on which that assumption is formed. For example, the symbol of a "woman" (wearing a dress) and a "man" (wearing pants) have become naturalized in our culture to represent the washrooms in public places to be used by women or men. Although there is nothing innately natural about these symbols representing men or women, we have come to interpret them unquestioningly in this way (see Figure 19.1).

Reinscribing—reinforcing or reproducing a concept or belief, at times without the thoughtful intention of doing so.

Social construction—ideas, concepts, and roles that are understood to be formed or built up through the agreed-on ideologies of a society.

Transparency—the ways in which we can see something clearly, or obviously (high transparency), or in which something is obscured from our view. For example, increasing our awareness of material and social realities that contribute to gendering of nurses' work will improve our ability to see, or make transparent to us, the manner in which nursing is undervalued because it is "women's work."

problematic for the profession is that gender is inextricably linked to relations of power. This connection of gender and power underlies and fuels issues related to the devaluing of nurses' work and the subordination of nurses' knowledge.

The discussion of power, and particularly relations of power as they affect nursing, may rouse a certain discomfort within nurse-readers in view of the societally ingrained reluctance to examine our own power (Falk Rafael, 1996). However, because nursing as a profession has been largely composed of women, who are socialized to avoid discussions of power, we must venture into this deliberation.

This chapter explores and raises questions about value and worth, particularly the value and worth attached to the gendered nature of work, of knowledge, of nursing. These concepts of value and worth are the commodities of power. When we talk about the value of nurses' knowledge or the ways in which work that is called women's work is devalued, we are talking about power.

In exploring the significance of gender in relation to nursing practice, nursing knowledge, and nurses themselves, we may begin by acknowledging the complexity of gender *per se*. Then we need to explore ways of thinking about gender beyond distribution, beyond the numbers of nurses who are female or male. These ways of thinking about gender will anchor us in the world of social realities where nursing is practised and where concepts of gender and gender practices are formed.

The first section of this chapter explores the theories that support an understanding of the gendered nature of work, knowledge, and the individual nurse. Grounded in feminist thought, this way of conceptualizing gender and its effects in the social world is useful in understanding the significance of nurses' work.

Understanding Gender

As concepts, gender, women's work, and nursing itself derive their meaning in society through social construction. Social construction means that ideas, concepts, and roles are understood to be formed or built up through the agreed-on ideologies of a society. Ideologies, in this sense, are not merely ideas; they are imbued with power. They become the authoritative voice in society through which we come to understand ourselves. Ideologies tell us who we are, what we are to think, and how we are to behave (Althusser, 1971).

The power of ideologies lies in the authority that has us view much of our world as "natural" (obvious). *Nurse,* for example, is not a naturally occurring phenomenon, but the concept of *nurse* may become naturalized through ideologies about what constitutes or makes up the role of nurse. Although we may acknowledge intellectually that there is no natural role or personality attributable to *nurse,* we often, unthinkingly, act as if the opposite is so. The opportunity and the challenge in considering the social construction of nursing, gender, and "women's work" is twofold:

■ To disrupt the thinking that supports taken-for-granted notions
■ To question the source of ideologies on which the "natural facts" are based

Thinking in a way that interrupts that which is taken for granted helps us to recognize our own participation and complicity in supporting (reinscribing) ideologies that contribute to the undervaluing of nurses' work and nursing knowledge (Figure 19.1).

Gender as Social Construction

What does it mean to think of gender as socially constructed? How does this way of understanding gender benefit one's thinking about issues of gender and power in nursing as a profession and in nursing practice?

That people are gendered is taken for granted in everyday life and, although central to our experience of the world, is seldom thought about beyond the surface level. The lack of clarity between concepts of gender and biologic sex supports the tendency to keep our understandings of gender superficial. From the moment of birth, the biologic sex of the newborn is announced in a public way. This proclamation, biologically driven, determines much of the future of the child's life. Or does it?

In *Revisioning Gender*, Nakano Glenn notes that "feminist scholars adopted the term *gender* precisely to free our thinking from the constrictions of naturalness and biological inevitability attached to the concept of sex" (2000, p. 4). In this sense, gender moves us to a broader understanding of what it is to live one's life in ways that reflect masculinity and femininity. Butler (1990), a prominent feminist thinker, discusses

FIGURE 19.1 The symbols of a "woman" (wearing a dress) and a "man" (wearing pants) have become naturalized in our culture to represent the washrooms in public places to be used by women or men. Although there is nothing innately natural about these symbols representing men or women, we have come to interpret them unquestioningly in this way.

gender not as the expression of an internal identity but rather as a performance in which the person acts a script that is written in and through social discourses. In this context, discourses are "social practices, values and cultural beliefs that prevail in a given culture or subculture at a specific historical moment and shape a collective sense of what is right, proper, worthwhile or valuable" (Thorne, McCormick, & Carty, 1997, p. 2).

Through these social discourses, we are inscripted with the knowledge of what it is to live a particularly gendered life. Although Butler maintains "that there is nothing about a binary gendered system that is given" (1990, p. 282), the scripts that are currently provided and normalized through social discourses offer little alternative to the categories of male and female. A concept of gender that surpasses biologic determinism provides the possibility, at least, of recognizing and valuing the masculine and the feminine that reside within each of us.

Crucial to this understanding is what may be called the *location of gender*. Although the biologic anatomy of an individual resides with that person, gender as a social construction is located in a more complex way, both within and beyond the individual. The construction of gender, meaning the ways in which gender identities are acted out and the value attached to gender, originates outside of the individual person, in society. Notions of gender are constructed through the ideologies of the culture; they become known to us through social discourse. Gender knowledge is situated in particular temporal and social realities that are largely taken for granted by members of the culture. This taken-for-grantedness reflects our participation in the ideologies of the society in which we reside. In other words, we are complicit in reinforcing the ideas that define and structure what are accepted as normal, gender-appropriate behaviors and beliefs in our immediate culture and time.

The often-unexamined evidence of the ways in which gender knowledge is bound by cultural, temporal, and social realities surrounds us. When a child is born, how others respond to "It's a girl!" or "It's a boy!" is heavily influenced by the gender knowledge of the particular culture in a particular time in history. The proclamation communicates not only the sex of the child but also the meaning and value that is held for this young gendered life. Through the powerful ideologies of the culture, parents, family members, and strangers take up the life of the child as gendered, in effect, teaching the child to be in the world in gender-appropriate ways. As adults, we come to perform our gender roles, in large part, as they are prescribed through these social discourses.

Gender as Part of Identity

In recognizing how dominant social discourses influence who we are to be, the production of identity becomes a discursive process (Scott, 1992). The term *discursive process* refers to how we learn to be, in particular ways, through the messages we receive in social discourses. Our concept of ourselves as gendered is one way in which we become subjects with particular identities. As we move on to consider some of the implications of what it means to be gendered subjects, we need to bear in mind that gender is but one component of our identity that is formed through discursive processes.

The gendered self is one of a number of the selves or identities through which we are uniquely formed as people. The gendered self intersects with other identities, such as race, class, age, ethnicity, and sexual orientation, in the constitution of each individual. The experience of living one's life as a black, young, middle-class, heterosexual, male, nursing student may be quite different from the experience of living as a white, middle-aged, poor, lesbian, single mother, nursing student. The difference of experience, although influenced by gender and what it means to be gendered in particular ways, is constructed through the material realities, such as economics and availability of social resources, as well as through the influence of dominant social discourses.

The idea of the intersecting identities of nurses is addressed in Reverby's (1987) historical critique of American nursing. In her exploration of some of the historical unrest in the discipline, Reverby suggests that class differences among individual nurses and between groups of nurses with diverse training contributed to an internal hierarchy within nursing. Although the oppression of women was a reality for these nurses, they were also bound by their own participation in classist assumptions and ideologies. In this case, the "commonalities of the gendered experience could not become the basis for unity as long as hierarchical filial relations, not equal sisterhood, underlay nurses' lives" (Reverby, 1987, p. 201). Reverby describes a situation in which the class identities of these nurses held more influence than their shared gender identity.

In essence, ideologies that become imbued with power carry societal authority to tell us who we are. Allen, writing of the postmodern critique in nursing, calls us to notice and to question "the ways in which discourses function as regimes of power, where knowledge and power interact to normalize or legitimate specific interests" (1992, p. xiv). The power attributed to particular social positions and particular identities, including gender, is neither random nor benign. Collins, a black feminist scholar, reminds us that "race, gender, social class, ethnicity, age and sexuality are not descriptive categories applied to individuals. Instead these elements of social structure emerge as fundamental devices that foster inequity in resulting groups" (1997, p. 376). This reminder challenges us to question the centrality of power in gendered identities as they are formed through the discursive process.

■ THE EFFECTS OF GENDER IN NURSES' LIVES

Once we think of people as gendered through a discursive process influenced by the social and material realities of a culture at a particular time, we can see that the gendering process extends beyond individuals—to institutions, organizations, and bodies of knowledge. Although it may be obvious that gender does not explicitly reside in these locations, it is also true that gender attributes are assigned to, or play themselves out in, various institutions. In this way, particular work becomes gendered in our minds. The implications of gendered institutions and gendered knowledge are profound. Gender in our society is not value neutral; thus, the gendered nature of knowledge, work, and institutions impacts the value given to that knowledge or work in our society.

The Gendered Nature of Work

"The gendered division of labor in the home and in the work place is part of a negotiated order that is accomplished within the social context of a prevailing set of normative conceptions or ideologies, about what activities are appropriate for men and women" (Angus, 1994, p. 24).

In exploring the working lives of Canadian women, Angus notes that the "labor force is characterized by marked horizontal (occupational) and vertical (hierarchical) gender divisions" (1994, p. 32). What this means is that women in preponderate numbers enter a limited subdivision of the workforce: a subdivision understood to be gender-typed as "women's work." Among these occupations is nursing, which composes part of about 80% of women workers who are "employed in labor-intensive occupations . . . concentrated in the public sector . . . where cost containment has produced additional burdens and frustration" (Angus, 1994, pp. 32, 38).

Angus' (1994) work also comments' on the vertical division of labor by gender in certain occupations. This refers to the socially created reality that occupations dominated by men are better rewarded than those dominated by women. According to Angus (1994), this is attributable to the dominant discourses in our society that support the valuing of technical skill over interpersonal skill. It is also evident that, within many occupational groups, women are less likely to be promoted to administrative positions or to be financially rewarded as generously as their male counterparts.

Although this argument within the nursing profession is open to debate, the challenges that women often negotiate as the primary caregivers in their personal or familial situations along with the demands of professional nursing practice are rigorous. The requirements of personal responsibilities may be experienced as incompatible with the additional demands of administrative work or participation in professional or union organizations, thus limiting the participation of nurses—in particular, women nurses—from positions of power and politics (Angus, 1994). This is not to suggest that men in nursing may rise to particular positions by virtue of being men, but it does open questions about the social landscape on which the realities of the demands of labor reside. Other questions may be raised as well. How do these social arrangements contribute to what some have called an "over-representation (of men) in top positions compared with their minority status in the profession" (Davies, 1995, p. 9)?

A feminist critique would suggest that we resist the temptation to assign responsibility for the work-life choices that women are forced to make to the individual nurse. Instead, we might examine the social conditions of nurses' lives, such as primary caregiving responsibilities and a lack of child-care resources, and the incompatibility of these social realities with the career demands of nursing.

Nursing practice has long been equated with "female virtues"—the virtues of care, nurturance, and altruism. In an exploration of classism, genderism, and racism in nursing, Turkoski notes that, historically, nursing has been "described in purely genderised terms as: 'women's mission, ministry, humanitarian service,' a 'service of womanly duty and conscience' and 'the noblest and most womanly of professions'" and reminds us that these descriptions "reinforced the assumption that nursing is essentially related to one's biological makeup" (1992, p. 162). "Gentleness and quietness were required of Nightingale's nurses, and many nurses in today's work force that 'trained' in the 1960s and earlier can attest to the importance attached to those virtues" (Falk Rafael, 1996, p. 9). Some of those nurses, who are still in practice, were expected to demonstrate as their "professional" behavior unquestioning deference to physicians, for example, standing when physicians entered the room, vacating chairs and opening doors for them, as well as obediently, even unthinkingly, carrying out physicians' orders. Abbott and Wallace argue that although "nurses no longer see themselves as handmaidens to doctors, they have remained trapped in their status as subordinate to doctors" (1990, p. 22). In support of this argument, Abbott and

Wallace remind us of nurses being accountable for administering medication that they are not authorized to prescribe.

In an article discussing the tensions between power and caring in the nursing profession, Falk Rafael itemizes the characteristics traditionally associated with femininity and masculinity as follows (1996, p. 5):

Femininity	*Masculinity*
Submissiveness	Strength
Helplessness	Aggression
Dependency	Mastery
Tenderness	Independence
Nurturance	Logic
Altruism	Being unemotional
	Competitiveness
	Ambition

Falk Rafael (1996) notes that these traditional notions of femininity and masculinity have been constructed in a way that associates the masculine with power and the feminine with care. She reminds us that knowledge is developed and propagated in particular ways to maintain power. The "scientification" of knowledge over the past several hundred years demonstrates the systematic devaluing of the feminine. The "denigration of women and that which is feminine has been entrenched in all of civilisation's major institutions" (Falk Rafael, 1996, p. 6). In this conceptualization, *care* is constructed as a female virtue and one that holds little esteem in Western society. How do we reconcile this devaluing of care with the centrality of it to the nursing profession?

Fisher, in exploring gender and power in nursing, locates a discourse of care as having "played a central role in the constitution of nursing as a gendered profession" (1993, p. 117). The association of nursing with care is complicated by the social belief in care as an innately female quality. When viewed as natural or essential—meaning innately residing in all women—the idea of care may contribute to undermining the value of nurses' work. When care is undervalued, as a feminine virtue, the devaluation extends beyond the individual nurse, be that nurse a woman or a man, to the work itself.

How is it that the value of care has been so compromised by society? A feminist historical analysis connects the value attached to work ordinarily performed by women in the public sphere to the changing value attached to work performed by women in the private sphere (Bunting, 1992). In preindustrial times, before the advent of large-scale productivity and commercialization, the work ordinarily performed by women was associated with the maintenance and care of home and family and was more closely aligned, in worth, to the work ordinarily performed by men. The refocusing of modern society on a production- and wage-oriented economy resulted in a devaluation of the care-work ordinarily performed by women in the private sphere. Women were placed in the "position of performing services and producing products for the family that have no recognised market value" (Bunting, 1992, p. 58). Along with Bunting, we might wonder about the "connections between the devaluing of women's care in the home and the difficulty of gaining recognition for *nurses'* contributions of care" (1992, p. 60). Bunting (1992) finds a relationship between the invisibility and taken-for-grantedness of caregiving in the private sphere, based on the absence of financial remuneration, and the low status of nursing as a profession. Are there, then, in the social discourses of care, blurred boundaries between work that is "recognised, valued, and paid for . . . [and] work [that] is treated as a labor of love or duty" (Bunting, 1992, p. 61)?

Condon suggests we consider the feminist understanding of Fisher and Tronto that appreciates caring as a "positive dimension of our lives that has been socially devalued by a patriarchal and capitalistic order" (Condon, 1992, p. 73). In this way, the concept of care continues to be valued, and the effort is directed toward interrupting the social discourses that contribute to the devaluing of care. In contrast to duty and calling, which she calls "old masculine metaphors," Condon maintains that care provides an "infinitely more authentic metaphor grounded in the experience of women and capable of being practiced by anyone who chooses it as a social, as well as a professional, ethic" (1992, p. 81).

The Gendered Nature of Knowledge

"Ideas about women, about women's work and how it does or does not require significant knowledge, responsibility, and skill are embedded in nursing and become part of nursing's taken-for-granted reality" (Ceci & McIntyre, 2001, p. 121).

In considering the gendered nature of knowledge, and particularly the impact of gendered knowledge on nursing practice, we may ask, What counts as knowledge? Who decides what counts as knowledge? How might we understand the significance of knowledge gendered in particular ways? McIntyre suggests that "nursing knowledge is inextricable from the assumptions and values underlying its generation. Explicating the assumptions underlying different approaches to knowledge generation in nursing . . . helps nurses avoid unquestioning conformity to existing knowledge" (1999, p. 46).

Through time, nurses have been influenced by the discourses around several bodies of knowledge. Before the industrialization of nursing, women healers and caregivers were privileged to gynocentric (feminine-centered) knowledge, for example, midwifery and herbal pharmacology, as well as the knowledge necessary for the care of home and family (Ginzberg, 1999). These areas of knowledge have lost value in the foreground of Western science and scientific knowledge, which was produced with an androcentric (masculine-centered) focus. Critiques of science in the 20th century suggest that "knowledge produced by the sciences is part of the social and political tradition within which it is produced" (Welch, 1999, p. 423). Such critiques support the notion that particular "women's activities haven't been called 'science' for *political* reasons, even when those activities have been model examples of inquiry leading to knowledge of the natural world" (Ginzberg, 1999, p. 441).

In her work *Gender and Science*, Fox Keller, a scientist and feminist, explores the "historically pervasive association between masculine and objective, more specifically between masculine and scientific" (1999, p. 427). She addresses this notion as having reached near-mythical status as "it has simultaneously the air of being 'self-evident' and 'nonsensical'—the former by virtue of existing in the realm of common knowledge and the later by virtue of . . . conflicting with our image of science as emotionally and sexually neutral" (Fox Keller, 1999, p. 427). She cautions, however, of the potential for unexamined myths to affect subversively our thinking. How, for example, might the masculinity associated with the knowledge we call science influence what counts as nursing knowledge?

The kinds of knowledge that are valued and prioritized in nursing education are clearly reflective of the gendered nature of the profession. The association of early nursing education with "womanly virtues," as discussed earlier, continues to be relevant in what Rafferty calls the "intellectual and social subordination of nurses" (1996, p. 1) and in the "deep anti-intellectual prejudice attached to woman's work in general" (1996, p. 1). The concept of the mandate of nurses' education toward producing graduates of a particular moral character remains covertly present in social discourses and reinforces the location of nursing within the "natural" domain of womanhood.

In discussions of Project 2000, regarding nursing education in Britain, Davies found among healthcare professionals the "distinct echoes . . . of the historical equation of nursing with the female sex, of the view that a good nurse is born, not made, that a good woman is a good nurse" (1995, p. 114). Davies (1995) reports, in her gender analysis of the profession, on the belief held by nurses and other health care professionals that the work of nursing is a practical skill that does not require advanced education in the sciences or in theory but is best developed through an apprenticeship model of learning. Mackay also argues that there is a "tension between a vocational and a professional view of the nurse" (1998, p. 62) in Britain. She notes that although this may not be directly acknowledged by nurses, the "concept of vocation is embedded in many of the accepted practices and attitudes within nursing, such as being of service to others and putting others first" (Mackay, 1998, p. 63).

Is this discussion relevant to Canadian nurses and to the education of nursing students in Canada? Although some may argue that the Canadian Nurses Association has advocated the baccalaureate entry to practice since 1993, the view of nursing as a vocation may be held by numbers of nurses in practice. In discussing the situation in Canada, Armstrong (1993) presents student nurses as apprentices and points out the financial inequities between these students and apprentices in male-dominated occupations. Despite the endorsement of baccalaureate entry to practice and the increasing academic preparation of nurses, the gender issues of nurses remain.

These conflicted ideals regarding the meaning and methods of nurse education raise resounding questions. Whose purpose is being served through the deintellectualization of nurses' education? How does the apprenticeship model serve the economic and labor needs of hospitals and the health care system? What is the meaning for nurses of an education that prepares them to develop "character" and practical skills while undervaluing the development of intellectual pursuit in independent thinking, analysis, and problem solving, to say nothing of the theoretical knowledge underlying the practice of manual or technical skills? How does the intellectual devaluing of nurses' knowledge, reinscribed by particular health care professionals, contribute to the marginality of the nurse's position in the health care system?

The Gendered Nature of the Nurse

"Nursing has always been a much conflicted metaphor in our culture, reflecting all the ambivalences we give to the meaning of womanhood" (Reverby, 1987, p. 207).

At any given point in time, there may be multiple discourses participating in the construction of the nurse as subject. Put another way, social discourses present an image of what it is to be and to practise as a nurse. "Just as the cosmetic and fashion industries created the 'ideal woman,' so nursing texts, be they in popular press, television, or textbook form, create images of the ideal nurse" (Cheek & Rudge, 1994, p. 589). These idealized images of nurse are by no means unified. Part of the complexity of attaining the ideal is that it comprises mixed and conflicting messages and changes over time.

Regardless of the variables that form this ideal—including race, ethnicity, age, and sexuality—"both the nurse and the work of nursing are firmly associated in the public mind with the female sex" (Davies, 1995, p. 2). The naturalness of a woman performing as a nurse is reflected in the fact that "a man in the same job will be described not just as a nurse but as 'male nurse'" (Davies, 1995, p. 2). As suggested by Davies in the introduction to her text *Gender and the Professional Predicament in Nursing*, "a closer acquaintance with nursing, however, shatters any cozy image of women doing work that is somehow *natural* to them and hence being entirely comfortable in and satisfied with the role they have chosen" (1995, p. 2; emphasis added).

A current American television portrayal of an emergency room nurse as an autonomous, independent, respected, and compassionate professional conveys a particular appeal to nurses entering the profession. The actual social and material realities of this nurse's professional world may, in fact, be as much of a fabrication as the professionally submissive representation of the fictional Dr. Welby's nurse several decades ago. Both of these media portrayals of the nurse reflect an idealized image of "woman" formed through the prominent social discourses of the day. Although these images differ vastly from one another, they both present an idealized image of nurse-woman.

Is it possible that the public propagation of these ideals serves to undermine a more accurate representation of the nurse's lived experience, both in the eyes of the public and in the eyes of nurses themselves? Kalisch and Kalisch (1987) would concur that through the 19th and 20th centuries, media representations of the nurse have contributed to a narrow and undervalued image of nursing, drawing strongly on a received view of the nature of woman. We are challenged by nursing scholars to "raise questions about those discourses and ways of thinking, in the world or in us, which diminish nursing" (Ceci & McIntyre, 2001, p. 121). Among the discourses that require our ongoing interrogation are those that present a gender-idealized image of the nurse.

■ BARRIERS TO AND STRATEGIES FOR ISSUE RESOLUTION

Several barriers to resolving the issue of gender-related devaluing of nursing practice and the nursing profession need to be identified before strategies for change can be devised.

Identifying Barriers: Furthering Our Understandings

"The dilemma of nursing is too tied into the broader problems of gender and class in our society to be solved solely by the political efforts of one occupational group" (Reverby, 1987, p. 207). The barriers to the resolution of issues of gender and power in nursing are embedded in societal ideology. As nurses, we require both the knowledge and the willingness to critique and to challenge these social discourses. In particular, we can consider the following barriers that impair movement toward understanding the issues:

1. The gendered nature of work in general, and nurses' work in particular, is concealed—or implicitly present—in nursing practice. Although the effects of gendering on nursing practice are part of our experience, there is a lack of discussion that identifies these experiences as the problematic effects of gender and power.
2. The effects of power and gender in nurses' work and nursing knowledge are taken for granted in nurses' practice and education. The lack of transparency regarding the gendered nature of nurses' work (see barrier 1) contributes to our inability to question the embedded assumptions regarding gender and nurses' work.
3. Historically, nurses have lacked a critical feminist analysis that provides a framework to critique and question the taken-for-granted social discourses of gender, nurses' work, and the valuing of care in society.
4. Although the gendered divisions of labor have long been ingrained in society, only recently has the gendered nature of work been called into question in academic discourses that are accessible to nursing.
5. Understandings of the gendered nature of nurses' work are impaired by the larger lack of clarity and articulation of the nature of nurses' work in general. The inaccurate and limited public representations of the nurse and nurses' work contribute to the limited understanding and devaluing of nurses' work and nursing knowledge.
6. Individual efforts to disrupt the taken-for-granted ideas of gender require one to challenge social discourses and dominant views. This necessary strategy produces a barrier for the individual by placing her or him in a tension with commonly held societal views.

Devising Strategies: Voice and Action

1. Several of the barriers to resolving issues of gender and power, and their impact on the significance attributed to nurses' work, could be broken down by providing knowledge regarding the gendered nature of nurses' work both historically and as it is currently embedded in nursing practice. The knowledge necessary for a thorough understanding of gender and power issues is complex and requires familiarity with a structure that can be used to critique and challenge the taken-for-granted assumptions embedded in these issues. Knowledge of the gendered nature of nurses' work may be supported by feminist analysis, which focuses on the idea of power embedded in ideologies and the formation of gendered subjects through social discourses. This knowledge and the means to illuminate and question assumed truths belong in nursing curricula early in undergraduate nursing education. Much of the complexity of this knowledge lies in our lack of familiarity with concepts of gendering and social construction. As nurses become fluent in knowledge and language, the transparency regarding the gendered nature of nurses' work will be improved.

2. As identified in the aforementioned barriers, there is a tension generated between the origin of social discourses of gender and the value of particular types of work in society, and the disruption of these discourses must begin at an individual level. Important strategies to interrupt discourses that undermine the significance attributed to nurses' work begin with increasing our own awareness of these taken-for-granted discourses in our daily lives. Influencing these discourses in ways that call into question the way things have always been or the way things have always been done requires confidence and courage for the individual nurse.

3. The action required to change or disrupt large social ideologies can begin with wondering about the following:
   - What it is we think we "know"
   - The effects of taken-for-granted "truths" on the valuing of nurses' knowledge and practice
   - The ways in which we reinscribe social discourses of gender in our own practice

4. As members of society, nurses and women have been socialized to suppress difference. To challenge effectively what is taken for granted about the role of gender and its powerful influence on nurses' work, we must be willing to notice difference and to acknowledge the way that differences, such as gender, class, race, ethnicity, and sexual orientation, matter in the ways our identities are lived and viewed by the world.

5. Social discourses of gender are more than ideas. They are intimately connected to the social and material realities of our lives. Exerting influence that will change or disrupt discourses of gender necessitates action that will improve, in particular, the material realities of women's lives. This means, for example, advocating for changes in the workplace that support the lives of women as they negotiate family and work responsibilities and demands. Adequate resources for child care and family responsibilities are gendered workplace issues. Attending to these needs influences the value and respect attributed to women's multiple roles, including the significance attributed to nurses' paid work.

■ SUMMARY

This chapter explores multiple issues associated with the gendered nature of nurses' work, of nursing knowledge, and of the public representation of the nurse. Central to the issue are the social discourses about gender that are inherent in the value attributed to nurses' work and the importance attached to nurses' knowledge.

One question examined is this: Is the value accorded to nurses' work representative of the societal devaluing of work that is ordinarily performed by women? The exploration extends our understanding of gender and power in nursing beyond the idea of the distribution of gender in the profession. The significance of nurses' work and the value accorded this work are steeped in societal structures and ideologies that surpass the particular gender of the nurse who is performing the work.

The gendered nature of nurses' work and education has been with us since the inception of nursing. The gendered division of labor has historically placed nursing in the realm of women's work, a division that was supported through the early educational program for nurses that focused on "womanly virtues" and "moral character." The legacy of this account of nursing has been the conceptualization of care as both an innately feminine virtue residing in all women and a discourse central to nursing practice. The significance of nurses' work parallels the devaluing of care in a society that has increasingly valued science and a production-focused economy.

Given the early image of nursing as a natural extension of feminine virtues, we may be tempted to assign responsibility for "gendering" to the pioneering women of nursing practice and education. This chapter argues that the gendering of work occurs not with particular individuals but through society's discourses, which are embedded with ideologies.

The current and perhaps more difficult challenge is to recognize the less overt but no less present discourses of gender that structure current nursing practices. These discourses of gender—the nature of the work called "women's work" and the value that is afforded to caregiving in our society—underlie the significance of nurses' work.

In locating the discourses of gender in society, we need not look beyond ourselves. Our complicity is evident as we participate in the reinstatement of gendered discourses birthed in the societal ideologies from which we cannot extricate ourselves. The challenge, then, is to look for opportunities to recognize and to disrupt the taken-for-granted notions that define and constrain the possibilities for gendered people who are practising and being nurses.

REFLECTIONS on the Chapter . . .

1. How do you understand gender as socially constructed? What are the implications of your understanding for nurses, for nurses' work, and for nursing as a profession?

2. What does a feminist analysis of gender add to our understanding of the value and conditions of nurses' work?

3. What are the benefits and limitations of placing gender in a central place in our analysis of nurses' work? How does gender intersect with other realities and conditions of nurses' lives?

4. From your own nursing experience, provide an example of your participation in a taken-for-granted, socially sanctioned norm regarding gender. In retrospect, how might you have acted to interrupt this particular social discourse around gender?

References

Abbott, P., & Wallace, C. (Eds.). (1990). *The sociology of the caring professions.* London: Falmer Press.

Allen, D. (1992). Introduction. In J. Thompson, D. Allen, & L. Rodrigues-Fisher (Eds.), *Critique, resistance and action: Working papers in the politics of nursing* (pp. xi–xvi). New York: National League for Nursing Press.

Althusser, L. (1971). Ideology and ideological apparatuses. In B. Brewster (Trans.), L. Althusser (Ed.), *Lenin and philosophy and other essays* (pp. 123–172). London: New Left Books.

Angus, J. (1994). Women's paid/unpaid work and health: Exploring the social context of everyday life. *Canadian Journal of Nursing Research, 26*(4), 23–42.

Armstrong, P. (1993). Women's health care work: Nursing in context. In P. Armstrong, J. Choiniere, & E. Day (Eds.), *Vital signs: Nursing in transition.* Toronto: Garamond Press.

Bunting, S. (1992). Eve's legacy: An analysis of family caregiving from a feminist perspective. In J. Thompson, D. Allen, & L. Rodrigues-Fisher (Eds.), *Critique, resistance and action: Working papers in the politics of nursing* (pp. 53–68). New York: National League for Nursing Press.

Butler, J. (1990). Performative acts and gender constitution: An essay in phenomenology and feminist theory. In S. Case (Ed.), *Performing feminisms: Feminist critical theory and theatre* (pp. 270–282). Baltimore, MD: Johns Hopkins University Press.

Ceci, C., & McIntyre, M. (2001). A "quiet" crisis in health care: Developing our capacity to hear. *Nursing Philosophy, 2*(2), 121–127.

Cheek, J., & Rudge, T. (1994). The panopticon revisited? An exploration of the social and political dimensions of contemporary health care and nursing practice. *International Journal of Nursing Studies, 31*(6), 583–591.

Collins, P. H. (1997). Comment on Hekman's "Truth and method: Feminist standpoint theory revisited": Where's the power? *Signs: Journal of Women in Culture and Society, 22*(2), 375–381.

Condon, E. (1992). Nursing and the caring metaphor: Gender and political influences on an ethics of care. In J. Thompson, D. Allen, & L. Rodrigues-Fisher (Eds.), *Critique, resistance and action: Working papers in the politics of nursing* (pp. 69–84). New York: National League for Nursing Press.

Davies, C. (1995). *Gender and the professional predicament in nursing.* Philadelphia: Open University Press.

Falk Rafael, A. (1996). Power and caring: A dialectic in nursing. *Advances in Nursing Science, 19*(1), 3–17.

Ferree, M. M., Lorber, J., & Hess, B. (Eds.). (2000). *Revisioning gender.* New York: AltaMira Press.

Fisher, S. (1993). Gender, power, resistance: Is care the remedy? In S. Fisher & K. Davis (Eds.), *Negotiating at the margins: The gendered discourses of power and resistance* (pp. 87–121). New Brunswick, NJ: Rutgers University Press.

Fox Keller, E. (1999). Gender and science. In E. C. Polifroni & M. Welch (Eds.), *Perspectives on philosophy of science in nursing: An historical and contemporary anthology* (pp. 427–439). Philadelphia: Lippincott Williams & Wilkins.

Ginzberg, R. (1999). Uncovering gynocentric science. In E. C. Polifroni & M. Welch (Eds.), *Perspectives on philosophy of science in nursing: An historical and contemporary anthology* (pp. 440–450). Philadelphia: Lippincott Williams & Wilkins.

Kalisch, P., & Kalisch, B. (1987). *The changing image of the nurse.* Menlo Park, CA: Addison-Wesley.

Mackay, L. (1998). In P. Abbott & L. Meerabeau (Eds.), *The sociology of the caring professions* (2nd ed.). London: University College of London Press.

McIntyre, M. (1999). The focus of the discipline of nursing: A critique and extension. In E. C. Polifroni & M. Welch (Eds.), *Perspectives on philosophy of science in nursing: An historical and contemporary anthology* (pp. 46–54). Philadelphia: Lippincott Williams & Wilkins.

Nakano Glenn E. (2000). The social construction and institutionalization of gender and race: An integrative framework. In M. M. Ferree, J. Lorber, & B. Hess (Eds.), *Revisioning gender* (pp. 3–43). New York: AltaMira Press.

Rafferty, R. (1996). *The politics of nursing knowledge.* London: Routledge.

Reverby, S. (1987). *Ordered to care: The dilemma of American nursing, 1850–1945.* Cambridge, UK: Cambridge University Press.

Scott, J. (1992). Experience. In J. Butler & J. Scott (Eds.), *Feminists theorize the political* (pp. 22–40). London: Routledge.

Thorne, S., McCormick, J., & Carty, E. (1997). Deconstructing the gender neutrality of chronic illness and disability. *Health Care for Women International, 18*(1), 1–16.

Turkoski, B. (1992). A critical analysis of professionalism in nursing. In J. Thompson, D. Allen, & L. Rodrigues-Fisher (Eds.), *Critique, resistance and action: Working papers in the politics of nursing* (pp. 149–166). New York: National League for Nursing Press.

Welch, M. (1999). Science and gender. In E. C. Polifroni & M. Welch (Eds.), *Perspectives on philosophy of science in nursing: An historical and contemporary anthology* (pp. 423–426). Philadelphia: Lippincott Williams & Wilkins.

PART 5

SOCIETAL ISSUES:
Challenges for Nursing Practice

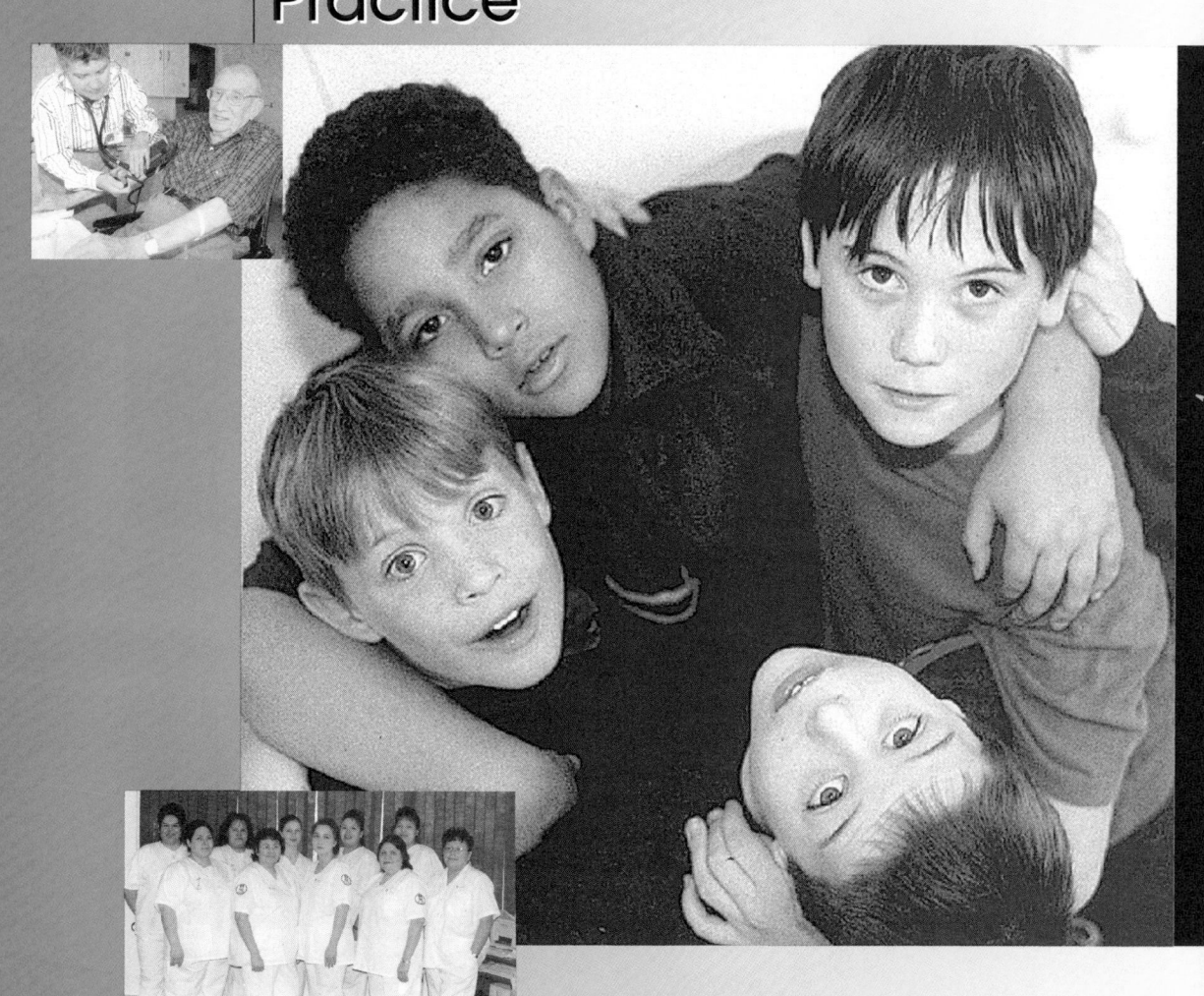

Critical Questions

As a way of engaging with the ideas in this chapter, consider the following:

1. As a consumer, what do you assume are your rights or the rights of your family in the Canadian health care system?

2. How do you imagine that consumers who have concerns about the provision of health care are able to have these concerns heard and addressed?

3. How important do you think the consumer movement is to Canadian health care?

CHAPTER
20

Isobel Boyle

The Consumer Movement

Used with permission from the Faculty of Nursing, University of Calgary.

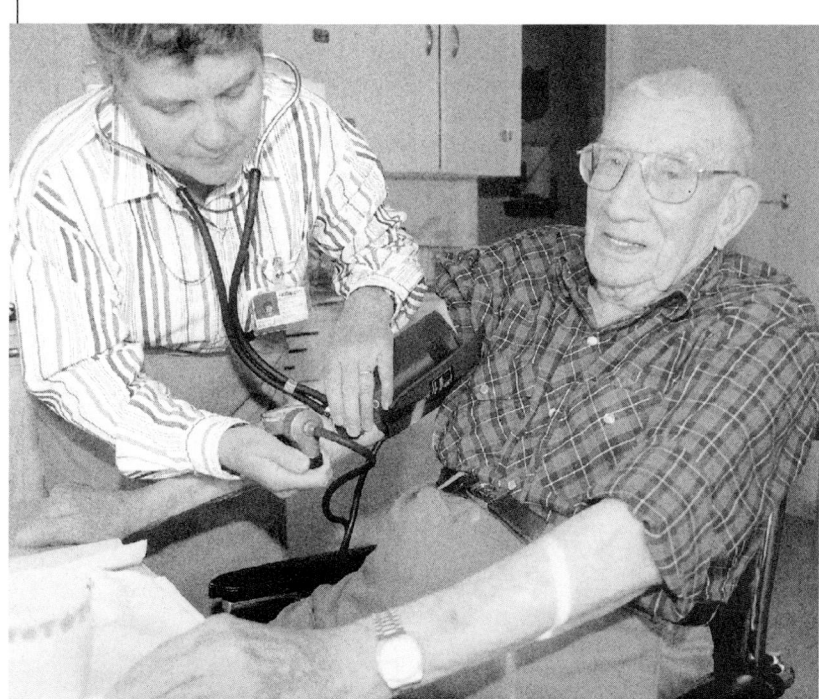

Chapter Objectives

After completing this chapter, you will be able to:

1. Understand the evolution of the consumer movement in health care.

2. Explore societal influences on the consumer movement in health care.

3. Discuss patients' rights for informed consent.

4. Analyze the trends, issues, and barriers to public participation.

5. Articulate the role of nurses as advocates.

6. Examine the effects of the consumer movement on nursing.

7. Identify future trends in the consumer movement in health care.

A consumer may be defined as a person who purchases and/or uses goods (such as food and clothing) or services (such as health services) to satisfy various needs. A consumer has both rights and responsibilities. In respect to rights, a consumer is entitled to receive the full goods and/or services that he or she has purchased or been promised. In respect to responsibilities, a consumer is responsible for being well informed before buying or using goods and services, for making sure that those goods and services are delivered and are what the consumer contracted for, and for initiating action so problems related to consumed goods or services are resolved quickly and satisfactorily. Consumer rights and demands are important forces for any change.

The demand for health care is affected by the illnesses consumers experience, their tastes and preferences, their income, and their knowledge about health care (Milburn & Griffith, 1991, p. 111). Consumerism in health care occurs at both the individual and collective level. At an individual level, treatment decisions may be made, whereas collectively, consumerism may influence health services and policy. It has been argued that "consumerism" is one of the main influences on health policy (Calnan & Gabe, 2001, p. 119). Groups, such as wellness advocates and those comprising self-help and women's health movements, have heightened awareness of the rights of consumers and the desire for greater public accountability in health care decision making.

■ HISTORY OF THE CONSUMER MOVEMENT

The Consumers' Association of Canada (CAC) formed in 1947 and continues today. The CAC focuses on a broad range of topics including food safety, health, trade, financial services, communications industries, and other marketplace issues as they emerge. The CAC brings consumers together to establish standards to ensure that safe, high-quality goods and services are available in Canada at affordable prices (Consumers' Association of Canada, 2001).

Consumer Rights and Responsibilities

The CAC, along with professional associations such as the Canadian Medical Association and the Canadian Nurses Association, lobbied successfully for the passage of Canada's Health Act (1962) and universal Medicare (1966). Consumer rights in health care were defined as early as the 1970s. These rights included:

> *...the right to be informed, the right to be respected as the individual with the major responsibility for his own health care, the right to participate in decision-making affecting his health, and the right to equal access to health regardless of the individual's economic status, sex, age, creed, ethnic origin and location (Storch, 1982, p. 186).*

The establishment of these rights in health care has been viewed as the beginning of the health care consumer movement in Canada. The balance between benefits and costs determines health care preference, and, although benefits include collective goals, personal costs are notably the dominant factor (Singer, 1995). To achieve these consumer rights, it became incumbent on governments, health administrators, health professionals, and consumers to work collaboratively in establishing legislation and policy.

Consumers are more than mere recipients of goods and services, particularly in health care. They want and need to be partners in seeking and obtaining appropriate health care services directed toward helping themselves. There is a need for an interdependent relationship in which consumers of health care are advised and consulted rather than the historical relationship wherein consumers depended on the decisions of health care professionals.

Today, the CAC defines the needs of consumers in the areas of protection, safety, information, education, choice, participation, compensation, and environment. The CAC has many national issues' committees, networks, and task forces that have consumer representation to establish policies within a set of general, consumer-oriented principles. Foremost among these principles are the rights to choose and to be heard as consumers. Examples of these committees include the Environmental Network, the National Health Council, the Policy Advisory Group, the Standards Task Force, Food Labelling, and Health Care Services.

Many individual health care institutions have developed or adopted patient's bills of rights. In the United States, the American Hospital Association's (AHA) Patient's Bill of Rights is used nationally. In this document, consumer rights are similar to those articulated by the CAC. The AHA Patient's Bill of Rights strives to ensure that all patients

- Know what their medical choices are
- Are aware of any risks from procedures and treatments
- Understand how they may be involved in research and how this may affect them

Respectful communication between consumers and health professionals is expected. Obtaining complete information in understandable terms is emphasized.

Factors Influencing Rights and Responsibilities

On a societal level, demographic factors such as affluence, education, and the age of the population influence demand for health care. Increased coverage of medical topics in the popular media as well as the availability of medical information on the Internet has created a more knowledgeable public. Across Canada, telephone lines staffed by health professionals offer free health advice and information 24 hours a day, 7 days a week (Table 20.1). The objectives of these lines include increasing health education of the public and improving consumer satisfaction. A cross-Canada synopsis shows an increase in both the number and use of these lines. There continues to be an increasing demand, indicating that people want to be empowered and to take charge of their health care. Blomqvist (1979, p. 10) noted that "the market mechanism provides an effective signalling device through which consumers' relative valuation of different goods and services is transmitted to producers, and the allocation of productive resources is indirectly guided by individual preferences of the consumers."

Consumers are demanding quality care, courteous service, and personal concern from health care providers. They want to have access to quality services, knowledgeable professionals, and accurate and current health information. They want to have choices to ensure that the drive for excellence in health care continues.

Consumerism Worldwide

The World Health Organization's (WHO) vision, as articulated in the 1986 Ottawa Charter, was an attempt to emphasize health promotion and disease prevention. The report, *Achieving Health for All by the Year 2000,* focused on the need for greater individual involvement in developing a healthy lifestyle, satisfactory relationships, and interdependency with professionals. "The WHO 1986 conference changed the model of health

TABLE 20.1

Province	Public Information 24-Hour Telephone Lines	Comments
British Columbia	BC NURSELINE	Provincewide nurse access line continues to increase links to other health information lines
Alberta	Health Link Alberta	Launched in 2000; over 940,000 calls received
Saskatchewan	HealthLine	Launched in August 2003
Manitoba	HealthLink-Info Sante	Six-station call center in 1994 to 35-station call center in 2004; 100,000 annual inquiries, expected to increase to 250,000 to 300,000 calls annually
Ontario	TeleHealth Ontario	Provincewide launch in 2001; over 1 million calls by December 2002 and over 3 million calls by December 2003
Atlantic Provinces	Telecare Line	Submission to expand Telecare line already in existence in New Brunswick

service delivery from the biomedical to a social model of care, recognizing that community members have been excluded not only from consultation about individual health issues, but from health service policy making in general" (Crichton, 1997, p. 66). This model of health and the ensuing activity is referred to as the *wellness movement.*

However, the largest health expenditures continue to be focused on acute care and the treatment of illness. Although there is some movement toward healthy lifestyle changes, consumers with chronic illnesses still demand the majority of treatment and care, leaving little money for prevention strategies. Attempts throughout the 1990s to restructure the health care system with a greater emphasis on health promotion have been restricted and financially driven to save money. As a result, services and the number of beds for acute care have been reduced. At the same time, the demand for services and beds has increased as more sophisticated diagnostic measures have been developed and implemented and as more people live longer. Krueger Wilson and Porter-O'Grady, in their 1999 book, entitled *Leading the Revolution in Health Care: Advancing Systems, Igniting Performance,* state that, to change the health care system, we must put greater emphasis on life management processes instead of just illness treatment. This shift will demand a more dynamic relationship between consumers and health care providers.

■ INFLUENCES ON THE CONSUMER MOVEMENT

A number of sociologic factors have influenced the consumer movement in health care. These include the women's movement, an aging population, and the emergence of self-help groups and patient representatives. Traditional assumptions have been challenged as greater demands have been placed on the health care system.

The Women's Movement

In an edited collection of papers related to health care and women, Gallant, Puryear, and Royal-Schaler (1997) describe how the influence of the women's movement has broadened the definition of women's health beyond women's health care and educated women to become informed consumers when making health care decisions. The focus on women's health has intensified over the past 2 decades. Women who previously accepted any medical recommendation at face value began to ask health care professionals about the availability of alternate treatments. For example, radical mastectomies were frequently the norm for women in the 1960s and early 1970s, but, as more information about breast cancer became available, women began questioning their physicians and advocating for less deforming surgeries. Maharaj (1999) explains the role of women's advocacy groups in shaping the Canadian health care system and describes these groups as agents for change and system "watchdogs" (p. 260).

The concern about issues in woman's health continues to grow. To meet the goal of improving and advancing women's health, women's health council groups have been established in most Canadian provinces. Largely because of partnerships and collaboration with consumers, health care groups, governments, and other public and private groups, advancements in women's health have been stimulated and changes are occurring.

Although the changes in health services for women are positive, evidence of inequities in the conduct of research for women's health issues continues to exist. The recent formation of the Centres of Excellence in Women's Health (2001), funded by Health Canada, is an attempt to strengthen policy-focused research on women's health in Canada. These centers are directed to making the Canadian health system more responsive to the needs of women. Opportunities for collaboration among community-based women's health groups, service providers, and academic researchers are encouraged in the interest of promotion of women's health.

An Aging Population

In the consumer movement, the influence of the "baby boomers" has been significant, particularly in health care. Baby boomers represent the population born in the 20 years from 1947 to 1966 (Foot, 2000, p. 15). This largest cohort of the population makes decisions not only for themselves but also for their parents and children. Maloney and Paul (1991), in their essay, "The Consumer Movement Takes Hold in Medical Care," state that baby boomers want more information, involvement, control, and choice regarding the services they buy (including medical care) than do previous generations. This influence was evidenced by increased family participation in obstetric and pediatric units in the late 1970s and early 1980s. Participation by fathers or significant others in the delivery room became a norm. Parents demanded to be with their children in hospitals and to be part of the decision-making process in the treatment of their children. Consumer advisory groups have become an expected component within hospitals and community health organizations. Consumer input is now standard within many institutions. Community involvement has been incorporated into the Canadian Council of Health Services Accreditation Standards (2001).

"An older population is more demanding and more knowledgeable about the products and services it needs and is less willing to tolerate poor service" (Foot, 2000, p. 223). Advances in medical science have improved the life expectancy of Canadians. Despite these advances and public health initiatives, as the baby boomers grow old, the burden of chronic illness grows as well, and the demand for a more responsive health care system increases. Then, as the demand for health services grows, so grows the fear that the health care system will be unable to meet the demands. It will be incumbent upon this group of consumers to participate in the system at all levels.

More than half of the nurses in the workforce today are members of the baby boomer generation. These nurses are beginning to retire and will continue to do so over the next 20 years. Meanwhile, proportionately fewer nurses are entering the workforce. Nurses are involved as professionals in the health care system, but, on a personal level, they are among the consumers demanding services for their children, their parents, and themselves. Meeting these demands is the challenge for governments, nursing associations, and administrators.

Self-Help Groups

Self-help groups exemplify increased consumerism in health care. Peer self-help groups offer guidance, information, and support to individuals experiencing a variety of medical, societal, or behavioral conditions. Frequently they have formed as groups seeking support and are typified by their absence of professional leadership. Professionals are consulted but do not take the leadership role. In addition to providing information and support to others, these groups discuss issues and develop strategies for action and interaction with health professionals and the health care system. Some groups lobby the health care system and governments in the interest of advocating for members of the group represented. These groups identify their own issues rather than rely on the agendas of the health care community (Leigh, 1994).

Self-help groups are available for most diseases, particularly those of a chronic nature. They are becoming more prevalent with increased numbers of patients using the Internet for information and communications. The American Self-Help Group Clearinghouse provides a database of more than 900 national and international self-help support groups for various health problems. These groups range from those advocating and supporting persons with disabilities to those providing support and information on such diseases as rare blood disorders. The medical community has raised some concern regarding the value of these groups. Criticisms by some physicians and others include the potential for providing misinformation, promoting a strong emphasis on illness, and potentially encouraging unconventional therapies. However, others value self-help groups for the experience and the support that individuals in the group provide to other group members.

Among the most prevalent self-help groups are those associated with cancer. People with cancer are demanding that nonmedical support services become an integral part of cancer care (Leigh, 1994). The increased information available on early detection and treatment options has increased long-term survival rates for people with cancer. While supporting one another, these survivors—and groups identified with other chronic conditions—advocate for effective communication, appropriate information, and care. They are active participants in identifying issues related to their diseases. They also seek help from health professionals, politicians, or whoever may be in the best position to assist them. Moreover, they demand accountability not only from professionals but also from the health care system.

Patient Representatives

During the 1970s, a new group of hospital workers emerged. Known as patient representatives, these hospital workers help patients and their families to address special needs that may arise in the course of treatment. Patient representatives are not only involved in advocacy but they also pinpoint potential problem areas and get involved in conflict management and dispute resolution (Beardwood et al., 1999, p. 371).

Responsibilities of patient representatives will vary from hospital to hospital but generally include:

- Providing information on patients' rights
- Acting as an intermediary between the hospitals/departments and patients and their families to bring about the most effective health care treatment
- Investigating and directing inquiries and complaints to appropriate staff
- Advocating for patients and their families

Patient representative positions were first evident in children's hospitals throughout Canada and the United States but are now established in most hospitals and medical care centers. There are no official, specific requirements for this position: Hospitals and other employers establish their own educational and work experience requirements to meet specific needs of the settings in which the representatives will work. Many of these workers have backgrounds in health care, education, human resource services, or communications.

Patient representatives have been effective in participating in the change of hospital policies, procedures, and services to health care consumers.

■ ISSUES FOR HEALTH CARE CONSUMERS

Health Care Reform

Health care reform in Canada has generally been viewed as a cost-saving measure rather than a real reform or change to the way health care is delivered. Each province has attempted to incorporate different ways of accommodating the increasing demand for health care spending and the reduced federal budgeting for health care. District or regional authorities were formed, inpatient beds were eliminated, and every health care sector was restructured. Reform included the incorporation of many hospitals and other health care units. Rewards to authorities/districts were based on meeting budgets rather than on the quality of health care delivery. Emergency room backups, waiting lists for surgery, and other concerns related to effective and safe delivery of health care were reported in the media daily. Consumers continue to voice concerns that health care is not just a social right but also a consumer right—a right for the individual (Beardwood et al., 1999).

Health care reform has created mixed meanings and diverse intentions. Consumers are no longer passive recipients of health care. They demand information and quality in health care delivery. There is also a movement to involve consumers in decision making that will have system-wide repercussions. Members of the public as well as officials who govern professional associations are being elected to regional health boards.

Informed Consent

An inherent health consumer's right is that of informed consent. Giving informed consent to a health procedure or treatment means that a patient or a responsible caregiver (if the patient is incapacitated) has received and understands all the information that he or she needs to make a decision regarding treatment or nontreatment. Informed consent implies both a legal and moral obligation on the part of patients and health professionals. The patient's signature on a form denotes the legal responsibility he or she accepts. In turn, health professionals have a legal and moral obligation to give adequate health information. True informed consent allows patients to make an autonomous decision about treatment based on the information they receive. This process involves more than the giving and receiving of information. Many patients want to be a partner in the decision-making process. Key issues of informed consent include

- Understanding treatment options including the associated risks and benefits
- Appropriate communication
- Respect for the decisions that patients make

O'Connor (1997, p. 8), in her analysis of decision support for patients, notes that "the rise of consumerism and patient empowerment has shifted the emphasis from the more passive informed consent to informed choice."

Switankowsky (1998, p. 119) describes informed consent as being at a "crossroads between the traditional, paternalistic, harm-avoidance model and the autonomy enhancing, patient-focused model." The harm-avoidance model may be viewed as paternalistic and one in which the patient consents to treatment by passively accepting the treatment prescribed by physicians or other health care providers. In the autonomy-enhancing model, both the patient and the physician or other health care provider must be viewed as contributing to the process. There is growing recognition that a patient's values, preferences, and lifestyle must be incorporated into the process of informed consent. This process involves a partnership in which both parties have something essential to contribute to the process of being informed. The provider has expertise in a particular area of treatment, whereas the patient possesses self-knowledge. This knowledge may be about

BOX 20.1

Questions to Ask Your Doctor Before You Have Surgery

■ Why do I need this surgery?
■ What alternatives to surgery are available?
■ What is the surgeon's experience?
■ What kinds of anaesthesia are available?

Adapted from the Agency for Healthcare Research and Quality, 2001.

the medical condition, family values, or other personal idiosyncrasies affecting the patient's ability to make an informed decision.

Consumers of health care increasingly seek knowledge to inform their consent—or dissent. In addition to health care providers, sources for information include family, friends, the popular media, available literature, and the Internet (Box 20.1). The completeness and accuracy of this information vary and challenge health care providers to ensure that patients obtain the best possible information. Adequate information is required before patients can be meaningful participants in their own care.

Privacy and Confidentiality

As more patient information becomes available electronically, there is concern about access to personal information. Concerns about preserving a patient's right to privacy and limiting access to patient data have given rise to both federal and provincial legislation, such as the Manitoba Provincial Health Information Act (PHIA) or the Ontario Municipal Freedom of Information and Protection of Privacy Act (MFIPPA). Patients have advocated for and must be able to expect that access to their information will have appropriate, reliable, and consistent standards. With increased technology, such as electronic records used to communicate patient information, the issues of privacy and confidentiality present new challenges.

Privacy Legislation and Its Implication

The federal government enacted the Personal Information and Protection and Electronic Documentation Act (PIPEDA) on January 1, 2001, with phased-in application of various provisions. As of January 1, 2004, the federal PIPEDA applies to all organizations that collect, use, or disclose personal information in the course of commercial activities, unless provinces have legislation deemed federally to be substantially similar. Quebec, British Columbia, Alberta, and Ontario have adopted legislation deemed to be similar.

What are the implications of this legislation for health care organizations and consumers of health care? For health care organizations, it is necessary to identify the purpose for which all personal health information is collected and to obtain expressed consent for the collection, use, and disclosure of personal health information. Information can only be collected and used for the purposes that have been identified. It is imperative that information collected is accurate. The consumer has the right to know how the information collected will be used, the practices of the organization to protect this information, and how this information can be accessed for review.

Consumer Participation

The National Forum on Health (1997) noted the concern Canadians have regarding the erosion of the health care system. Consumers are not mere recipients of health services. A consumer-based approach to health care implies that consumers become active participants in decisions related to health care. "The concepts of community empowerment and participation reflect a commitment to such precepts as the common good and shared responsibility for health" (Minkler, 1994, p. 406). Consumers act as partners in both the definition of issues and the development of solutions to address these issues.

The concept of community participation has been endorsed at many levels within the health care system. Community representation is seen on hospital boards, community health organizations, and boards of professional organizations. Higgins (1999) notes that many sources support public participation in both health promotion and community development. Consumer representation on health and health-related boards and committees provides a unique perspective. Many boards are now required by law to include public representation. These members are chosen either by governments to represent constituents, socioeconomic groups, regions, or the public at large, or they are chosen by a general assembly. This is exemplified across Canada by the appointment of consumers to the provincial professional nursing boards.

Consumers are now viewed as major stakeholders in health care. The increasing need for broad involvement comes at a time when Canadians, as a population, are adopting a broader definition of health and acknowledging the wide range of factors that contribute to the health of the population. Studies have demonstrated that consumers can be influential in both improving their own health outcomes and influencing policy issues. "Consumers reap the benefits, but also bear the financial and clinical burdens, of research and medical practice" (Hiller, Landenburger, & Natowicz, 1997, p. 1280).

However, what public participation really means remains ambiguous. Who are the public representatives? Whom do they represent? What information do these representatives need to give meaningful input to the decision making? What is the level of participation by these individuals? Individuals chosen as public representatives are often characterized by "their skill in public speaking, ability to understand policy and technical language, familiarity with meeting etiquette and professional status that motivates and enables them to become involved" (Higgins, 1999). The question remains as to their ability to understand and represent the issues of the public they represent.

Controlling health care costs is now a top priority for both the federal and provincial governments. The federal government has increased the shift of fiscal and moral responsibilities to the provinces. In turn, the provincial governments are attempting to shift responsibility for making difficult decisions regarding resource allocation to communities and consumers. This trend has the potential to make providers more accountable to the communities they serve. What is the consumer's role in this process?

Charles and DeMaio (1993) note that roles and the context in which public participation exists must be defined for meaningful decision making to occur. Additionally, the level of participation of these representatives is important to note. Public or lay representatives may have a role as individual consumers of health services, or they may have a broader public or community perspective. Clarification of the roles that representatives have influences their levels of participation. Frequently, lay representatives are intimidated by the expertise of the various health professionals. Lay representatives do not always have the necessary knowledge to fully participate. Sometimes, the perspectives that they bring to the table are not valued. Consultation, participation, and opinions may be sought from public representatives for information gathering but may or may not be used when policy decisions are made. There is no guarantee that individual views will be taken into account. Representatives and professionals must understand the role of public representation. Public representatives may advocate for a specific group, but they need also to take responsibility for obtaining the knowledge necessary to be active participants in the decision-making process.

To be effective, public participants must be viewed as equal partners with the health policymakers. They need to be acknowledged and respected for the contributions they bring to the discussion. They need to be involved in the development, management, and operation of services as well as the assessment of need. "Control is no longer found in unilateral ownership or decision making. Instead, control is a function of the character and kind of risk sharing that service partners agree to bear together and therefore is negotiated between partners" (Krueger Wilson & Porter-O'Grady, 1999). In Canada, public participation on many district authorities is beginning to move toward a partnership with the professionals that will see greater public involvement in health care planning and decision-making responsibilities.

An example of the shift from consultant to active participant in decision making can be seen in the evolution of family advisory committees in children's hospitals. The primary mandate of these committees is to support and enhance the highest quality of family-centered care. An example of this mandate can be seen in the Winnipeg Children's Hospital's position statement on family-centered care (1999). Family advisory committees developed initially in the 1980s and early 1990s. Family input was explored through consultation, focus groups, and surveys. This information may or may not have been used in decision making with regard to hospital planning and policy. Over time, with clarification of roles and the sharing of knowledge and expertise to make decisions, strong professional and family partnerships have evolved.

■ IMPLICATIONS AND ISSUES FOR NURSES

As health care professionals and consumers of health, nurses play a pivotal role in health care delivery. They are influential by their sheer volume as well as the professional role they play. Public opinion polls continue to show that nurses are held in high regard. The public trusts nurses. Nurses are involved in all aspects of the health care continuum, and they are educated to act as patient advocates and to actively engage in health care education regardless of their practice sites. The consumer movement has placed greater demands on nurses to fulfill these roles.

Patient Advocacy

Advocacy is identified as a prominent role for nurses. Shellian (1997, p. 34), former president of the Alberta Nurses Association, describes advocacy as happening in the things nurses do to make a critical difference for people: "Advocacy in nursing is a quality we all recognize." The Canadian Nurses Association's *Code of Ethics for Registered Nurses* (1997, p. 17) states, "Nurses put forward, and advocate, the interests of all persons in their care. This includes helping individuals and groups gain access to appropriate health care that is of their choosing."

This advocacy role involves giving information to patients, speaking out for patients, and helping them speak out for themselves. Consumers need health information about particular conditions as well as information on how to navigate the health care system. They also need opportunities to discuss issues of concern. However, nurses may not feel comfortable or believe they have the knowledge and skills to address patient concerns. Additionally, many nurses do not believe they have the time to address the questions.

Informed consent exemplifies the role of the nurse as advocate. Nurses obtain consent for nursing care and give information about procedures. Although informed consent for surgery and many other procedures is generally viewed as the responsibility of the physician, the nurse is frequently in the position to ensure that the patient has been given all the necessary information to make appropriate decisions. The *Code of Ethics for Registered Nurses* (1997, p. 10) further states, "Nurses respect and promote the autonomy of patients and help them to express their health needs and values, and to obtain appropriate information and services."

Informed consent is a complex issue, and careful assessment of the patient's level of understanding is required. Different professionals may be involved. Nurses may view the responsibility of obtaining informed consent as solely that of the physicians. Lack of knowledge about a specific treatment or perceived lack of time may inhibit a nurse's involvement. However, nurses can assist patients in making informed choices by assessing their levels of understanding and helping them to question the benefits and risks of the proposed treatments.

What happens when the nurse believes that the patient does not have the needed information to make an informed decision? This leads to ethical and moral dilemmas for nurses as they are torn between their role of patient advocate and their loyalty to their employer and to the other professionals with whom they work. The events leading to the Winnipeg Pediatric Cardiac Inquest (Sinclair, 2001) exemplify this dilemma. Nurses questioned the information that had been given to parents, as well as the skill of the physician performing the procedures. They were torn between their role of advocacy for their patients and their loyalty to other professionals. At some point in their careers, most nurses face situations where they question the safety of practices they witness and this dilemma arises.

Nurses have a right and a responsibility to provide information to their patients even if the information is in conflict with physicians or other professionals. Ultimately, loyalty to other professionals must be limited by the good for the patient (Hinam, 1999). In addition to information regarding procedures, consumers are now demanding information about the competencies of health team members. Consumer groups such as the Coalition for Improved Access to Physician Profiles are demanding information about a surgeon's experience (*Winnipeg Free Press,* January 2001). In some jurisdictions, this demand has been acknowledged and access to information about a physician's professional experience and expertise is available.

Patient Education

Health education has always been a primary role for nurses. As consumers of health care become more informed, there is a greater demand for the education that nurses provide. As patient advocates, nurses have a responsibility to give their public the information needed to make intelligent decisions regarding their health care plans, including choices regarding treatments. Providing consumers relevant, current, and accurate information is an important role for nurses.

Consumers obtain their health information from many sources—family, friends, books, popular media, health information telephone centers, the Internet, and health professionals (Table 20.2). The accuracy and quality of this information will vary. It is difficult for nurses to assess the reliability of the multiple sources of information and make recommendations. The challenge for nurses is to help patients to sort the available information so they can make informed choices. It is important that consumers understand their role as primary providers of their own care, and health care professionals need to view themselves as partners providing professional expertise.

The many choices available influence consumers, and several strategies may be used to assist patients in obtaining health information. Nurses must use their assessment skills in deciding what information is needed, evaluating the patient's level of understanding, and identifying the supports needed to assist the patient in decision making. Information can be given to the patient, but, ultimately, it is up to the patient to use or not use this information. Nurses cannot be expected to be experts in all areas of health care, but, fortunately, specialization in nursing has created individuals with rich knowledge in their defined fields. For nurses, the challenge remains to teach consumers how to access information and resources appropriate to their individual needs and values so that they feel confident in making health care decisions and managing their own care.

TABLE 20.2 Statistical Breakdown: Consumer Use of the Health Line

Year	Total No. of Calls Received	Average No. of Calls Per Month
1992	10,584	882
1993	12,888	1,074
1994	27,876	2,323
1995	67,061	5,588
1996	90,707	7,559
1997	101,801	8,486
1998	102,551	8,546
1999	115,132	9,594

Source: www.thehealthline.com/consumer.htm

Complaints

As consumers learn more about their own health and the health care system, their expectations and demands increase. When the expectations and demands are not satisfied, complaints are inevitable—particularly when a system is faced with the financial, technologic, and human stressors that affect the current Canadian health care system. For the most part, institutions are rewarded more for fiscal responsibility than for improving the health of citizens. In Ontario, for example, an increase in complaints to the College of Nurses was reported (Beardwood et al., 1999). Originally, the primary source of complaints was employers, mainly hospitals; but the source shifted to the public. Beardwood and associates note that "ideological changes that have recognized the supremacy of individual rights and the importance of satisfying consumer expectations give much greater validity to patients' expectations" (p. 365). This report exemplifies the increase in numbers of complaints made to most health professional regulatory bodies across the country.

The effects of workplace stresses have changed working environments for nurses, often making it difficult for them to meet their professional standards. When nurses do meet their professional standards, it may be at personal cost. Media accounts abound of unsafe working conditions, delayed services, stress, and burnout for nurses. Nurses report workplace concerns to their employers and to their professional organizations. This has prompted some professional organizations to publish position papers and guidelines to deal with stress and workplace environments (Manitoba Association of Registered Nurses, 2000). Governments, regulatory organizations, and unions have undertaken numerous workplace studies. Changes in workplace environments will be slow given human and fiscal restraints within the current economic climate.

Nursing regulatory boards exist to protect the public, not the nursing profession. Public participation on regulatory boards serves to expand the regulatory bodies' awareness of changing health needs of the public and their preferred ways of meeting these needs to ensure that the regulatory body is responsive and accountable to the public that it serves. With the increased participation of the public on nursing regulatory boards, the general public's awareness of the role of these regulatory bodies has grown and these public representatives are aware of, and involved in, the complaint process. Criticisms of the complaints and discipline procedures of regulatory organizations have resulted in even greater public input into the discipline process.

Although complaints to regulatory bodies are increasing, they are still relatively few in comparison to the number of registered nurses. However, complaints regarding incompetent care may be underreported to regulatory bodies for a number of reasons. Although patient representatives in many institutions deal with complaints from the public, there remains a reluctance to register complaints with the regulatory bodies because this may necessitate a prolonged involvement in a complaint or disciplinary procedure or there may be fear of a wrongful dismissal.

Consumers may complain about deficient care to seek personal rectification or to advocate changes in the system. The complaint process is time consuming and dissatisfying to both the nurse and the complainant. "The process individualizes the problem and deflects attention from the problems of system change" (Beardwood et al., 1999, p. 370). It is likely that complaints and consumer involvement in the complaint process will continue to increase. The challenge is for nurse leaders within workplaces to examine systems to support nurses in their work environments. Those within regulatory bodies are also challenged to make the complaint and discipline process less cumbersome and dissatisfying to both nurses and the public.

■ SUMMARY

This chapter addresses the significance of the consumer movement on health care and particularly on the role of nurses. As consumers have influenced policy within the system and the accountability of governments and health care professionals, the consumer movement has led to many positive outcomes for individuals, groups, and the health care system as well.

Consumerism occurs at both the individual and the collective level. Consumers have voiced their rights and expect that health professionals will honor those rights. These expectations have been influenced by the shift from illness care to health promotion, the women's movement, and the aging population.

Consumers, however, must become partners in the process and not just recipients of service if they are to help themselves. Control of health and the health care system is not found in unilateral ownership or decision making. It will be found in a partnership between consumer and provider that will ultimately determine the direction for the health care system.

Nurses continue to play important roles as advocates and educators. Both roles are paramount in the informed consent process. It is not merely knowledge that is needed for consent but a partnership in which the patient bring values and preferences into an autonomy-enhancing model of informed consent.

Increased public participation in all levels of the health care system will challenge the concept of partnership. As consumers become more involved, they will take a more active role in the management of changes to the health care system. Leaders must critically work through the changes that are required to embrace the consumer-provided partnership.

Online Resources

Add to your knowledge of this issue:

Agency for Healthcare Research and Quality	**www.ahrq.gov/qual/kffhigh.htm**
Centres of Excellence for Women's Health	**www.cewh-cesf.ca**
Consumer Support Groups	**www.dmoz.org/Health/Support_Groups**
Consumers' Association of Canada	**www.consumer.ca**
The Hospital for Sick Children Family Advisory Committee	**www.sickkids.on.ca/fac**

REFLECTIONS on the Chapter . . .

1. Identify ways for the public to have more meaningful participation in health boards.

2. What does it mean to be a board member?

3. Identify and discuss some barriers to public participation.

4. What influence has the consumer movement had on the concept of informed consent?

5. Do you think the discipline process is the same across all professions? Should it be? Support your position.

References

Agency for Healthcare Research and Quality. (2001). Retrieved October 3, 2001, from www.ahrq.gov/qual/kffhigh.htm

Alberta Centre for Well-Being. (2002). Retrieved April 2002 from http://www.thehealthline.com/

Anderson, J. M. (1996). Empowering patients: Issues and strategies. *Social Science & Medicine, 43,* 697–705.

Beardwood, B., Walters, V., Eyles, J., et al. (1999). Complaints against nurses: A reflection of "the new managerialism" and consumerism in health care? *Social Science and Medicine, 48,* 363–374.

Blomqvist, A. (1979). *The health care business: International evidence on private versus public health care systems.* Vancouver: The Fraser Institute.

Calnan, M., & Gabe, J. (2001). From consumerism to partnership? Britain's national health service at the turn of the century. *International Journal of Health Services, 31*(1), 119–131.

Canadian Council on Health Service Accreditation Standards. (2005). Retrieved April 12, 2005, from http://www.cchsa.ca/pdf/ SurveyGuidelines2005.pdf

Canadian Nurses Association. (1997). *Code of ethics for registered nurses*. Ottawa: Author.

Charles, C., & DeMaio, S. (1993). Lay participation in health care decision making: A conceptual framework. *Journal of Health, Politics and the Law, 18*(4), 881–904.

Consumers' Association of Canada. (2001). Retrieved June 5, 2001, from http://www.consumer.ca/1480

Crichton, A. (1997). Community participation in health service policy making in Canada. *Bibliotheca Medica Canadiana, 19*(2), 66–69.

Foot, D. K. (with Stoffman, D.). (2000). *Boom bust & echo: Profiting from the demographic shift in the 21st century*. Toronto: Stoddart.

Gallant, S. J., Puryear, K., & Royal-Schaler, R. (1997). *Health care for women: Psychological, social and behavioural influences*. Washington, DC: American Psychological Association.

Griffiths, H. (1993, November/December). Supporting the advocacy role. *Nursing BC,* pp. 25–26.

Higgins, J. (1999). Closer to home: The case for experiential participation in health reform. *Canadian Journal of Public Health, 90*(1), 30–33.

Hiller, E., Landenburger, G., & Natowicz, M. (1997). Public participation in medical policy-making and the status of consumer autonomy: The example of newborn screening programs in the United States. *American Journal of Public Health, 87*(8), 1280–1287.

Hinam, I. (1999, December). Winnipeg's pediatric cardiac inquest: The ethical issues. *Canadian Operating Room Nursing Journal,* pp. 13–16.

Kerr, J., & MacPhail, J. (1991). *Canadian nursing: Issues and perspectives* (3rd ed). St. Louis, MO: Mosby Year Book.

Krueger Wilson, C., & Porter-O'Grady, T. (1999). *Leading the revolution in health care: Advancing systems, igniting performance* (2nd ed.). Gaitherburg, MD: Aspen.

Leigh, S. (1994). Cancer survivorship: A consumer movement. *Seminars in Oncology, 21*(6), 783–786.

Maharaj, R. (1999). The role of women's advocacy groups in shaping Canadian health care policy. *Women's Health Issues, 9*(5), 259–263.

Maloney, T., & Paul, B. (1991). The consumer movement takes hold in medical care. *Health Affairs, 10*(4), 268–279.

Manitoba Association of Registered Nurses. (2000). Supportive practice environments: A discussion paper. Winnipeg: Author.

Milburn, L., & Griffith, H. (1991). Economic issues in health care in nursing. In J. Creasea & B. Parker (Eds.), *Conceptual foundations of professional nursing practice* (pp. 107–128). St. Louis, MO: Mosby Year Book.

Minkler, M. (1994). Challenges for health promotion in the 1990s. *American Journal of Health Promotion, 8*(6), 403–412.

National Forum on Health. (1997). *Canada Health Action: Building on the legacy*. Ottawa: Author.

O'Connor, A. M. (1997). Consumer/patient decision support in the new millennium: Where should our research take us? *Canadian Journal of Nursing Research, 29*(3), 7–12.

Redden, C. (1999). Rationing care in the community: Engaging citizens in health care decision making. *Journal of Health, Politics, Policy and Law, 24*(6), 1363–1389.

Shellian, B. (1997). Registered nurses and advocacy: Helping others speak up. *AARN, 53*(3), 33–34.

Sinclair, M. (2000). *Report of the Manitoba pediatric cardiac surgery inquest*. [Online]. Winnipeg: Manitoba Provincial Court. Available: http://www.pediatriccardiacinquest.mb.ca

Singer, M. A. (1995). Community participation in health care decision making: Is it feasible? *Canadian Medical Association Journal, 153*(4), 421–423.

Storch, J. (1982). *Patients' rights: Ethical and legal issues in health care and nursing*. Toronto: McGraw-Hill, Ryerson.

Switankowsky, I. (1998). *A new paradigm for informed consent*. Lanham, MD: University Press of America.

Winnipeg Children's Hospital. (2001). *Position statement on family-centered care (1999)*. Winnipeg Free Press: Winnipeg.

Critical Questions

As a way of engaging with the ideas in this chapter, consider the following:

1. What do you imagine might be the prevalence of violence or abuse in your own community?

2. Imagine the range of situations that you might encounter where people have experienced violence or abuse.

3. Consider the actions of professionals that might silence the disclosure or reporting of experiences of violence or abuse.

4. Think of some reasons why professionals might be reluctant to address violence or abuse.

CHAPTER

21

Elizabeth Thomlinson

Violence and Abuse: Ending the Silence

This poem is reproduced with permission from Mabel Cook, a member of Mosakahiken Cree Nation, who has spent many years working to prevent abuse and violence within aboriginal communities. Her primary focus has been the youth of the communities. She has been a magistrate and currently is a community mediator in northern Manitoba.

Waiting to Be Seen and Heard

There are so many of us that cry out in agony
To no-one in particular because nobody cares to hear
People pass us by and never look beyond our exterior
Our bodies grow simply because it's the cycle of life.

When you look at us with contempt and mistrust
We feel that all you see is potential problems
Of young people not knowing how to be responsible
For you think we solve life's problems with violence.

Has it ever occurred to you to ask me how I feel?
We cry in vain in hopes that you will actually see
See the chaotic mess we strive to untangle
Trying to understand why you chose to hurt us.

Why don't you look deep within our very being
To find small defenseless children cowering in fear
Our growth was stunted because of a violent episode
One we did not ask for but received anyway.

You talk about us so negatively because we react in anger
Anger because we cannot tell anyone of our secret
Anyone who can take us on a journey of healing
Anyone who wishes to make us understand this cruelty.

You shattered what faith we had in humanity
For now we have built a wall around us where we cower
Cowering in fear wondering when you will come for us
To shatter our already battered and imprisoned spirit.

You have done much work on compiling information about us
Information that makes for good reading but does very little
We need you to take it to people who want to fight for us
Even the government sends men to war to kill others
    for freedom.

What about us? We are being killed Spiritually, Emotionally
Physically, Mentally, Sexually, and it is a slow death
We feel every fiber of our soul quivering in pain wanting
    freedom
Wondering who will see and hear to finally end this abuse.

— Mabel V. Cook

After completing this chapter, you should be able to:

1. Identify many forms of violence and abuse.

2. Analyze political, legal, and ethical factors related to violence and abuse.

3. Relate the effect of violence and abuse to the health of individuals.

4. Evaluate the impact of violence and abuse on the health care system.

5. Examine factors that contribute to the continued silencing of victims of violence and abuse.

6. Differentiate facilitators and barriers to resolution of various issues and generate strategies to address violence and abuse.

Since the late 1970s, there has been a growing recognition that violence and abuse in their many forms have a significant impact on the health of individuals specifically and on the Canadian health care system in general. According to the Canadian Nurses Association (CNA, 1996, p. 1), "violence is now recognized as a social act involving a serious abuse of power."

Violence consists of exerting power over another person to control, disempower, or injure the other. As a social act, violence crosses legal, ethical, and health care boundaries with serious moral, sociocultural, political, and personal ramifications for society (Hoff, 1994). Violence is perpetrated against people of all ages, in every socioeconomic sector of society, and in all societies around the globe. Young people, elderly people, and people with disabilities are among the most vulnerable. The long-term negative effects of violence have enormous implications for the victims as well as for all facets of society.

Discussion of violence is an everyday occurrence in the media. Although Canadian culture officially condemns violence, it is often glorified in film, television, books, and music. The long-held myth that the family is a safe haven for all of its members has been dispelled through frequent accounts highlighting the magnitude of the violence and abuse within that setting. In the workplace, there are ever-increasing numbers of stories of violent occurrences leading to injury and even death.

It is not possible in one chapter to present in-depth coverage of this complex topic. Rather, this chapter highlights some forms of violence, the association with the health of individuals, and the role nurses and the nursing profession can and should take to address issues of violence and abuse. There is a vast array of multidisciplinary sources of information, including print, film, and audio, on the topic of violence. This chapter is meant to stimulate a rudimentary recognition of the topic, and readers are encouraged to expand their knowledge and understanding through the numerous other sources that are available. To begin, definitions of the multiple forms of violence and abuse are presented in Box 21.1.

■ THE MANY FORMS OF VIOLENCE

Most people agree that violence is an act of physical force aimed at hurting, harming, or injuring another person, group, or object. The word *violence* is derived from the Latin infinitive *violare*, to violate, rape, or injure. Violation of another person not only may result in visible physical harm but also may result in emotional trauma that is as equally harmful as physical battering. Within this chapter, the terms *violence* and *abuse* are used interchangeably, although abuse may not entail physical trauma. The CNA (1996, p.1) focuses the discussion of violence on two major points:

- *Interpersonal violence* includes violence that occurs within relationships as well as that experienced from strangers and acquaintances. All types of violence are encompassed by this term, including violence against children, women, and elders; abuse of spouses or partners; violence within the context of

| BOX 21.1 | Forms of Violence and Abuse |

Physical

Slapping, kicking, hitting with a fist, beating, choking, shoving
Using a weapon against another
Forcibly restraining, confining, or kidnapping another

Sexual

Forcing another to perform sexual acts, e.g., fellatio
Forcing another to have sexual intercourse

Psychological

Name calling, humiliating another, verbally degrading another
Harming property or pets
Creating an atmosphere of fear and terror
Using threats and coercion
Witnessing assault or abuse of another (parent, grandparent, sibling, friend, etc.)
Infantilization

Financial

Taking or withholding money
Extorting funds or property
Taking control of all expenditures
Forcing another to stop working and become dependent
Selling the home or possessions of elderly people without their consent

Social

Imposing (forced) isolation from friends and other family
Monitoring all phone calls and connection with others

Physical Neglect

Failing to provide food, clothing, shelter, or medical care
Failing to supervise children or elders appropriately

dating; violence witnessed by children; and abuse and neglect of frail and vulnerable persons. Abuse may also be perpetrated by professionals.

■ *Violence in relationships* of kinship, intimacy, dependency, or trust can take the form of physical assault, emotional abuse, intimidation, sexual assault, neglect, deprivation, and financial exploitation. Although these forms of violence occur most often in families or within intimate relationships, they can also occur within the health care system.

The multiple definitions of violence and abuse influence how we view violence and where we place emphasis. Terms such as *family violence, domestic abuse, interpersonal violence*, and *violence in relationships* tend to downplay the gender relationships in violence and phrase the behavior in gender-neutral language. Although some authorities suggest that women are equally violent in their actions, the reality remains that most perpetrators of violence in families are heterosexual males, and the victims of the most violent crimes are women and children (Bunge & Locke, 2000; Canadian Public Health Association, 1994; Hoff, 1994). Terms such as *family violence* locate abuse within the family, diluting society's influence and effects. Nurses must be aware of how the terminology that is used affects the perceptions of professionals and society at large. The use of language that downplays gender relationships and societal influences is one of many issues that arise within the topic of violence and abuse.

■ HISTORICAL PERSPECTIVES ON VIOLENCE AND ABUSE

The abuse of children and of female partners has deep historical roots. Even today, abuse is condoned within many societies in the world. Throughout history, children have been sacrificed to appease the gods, killed if they suffer handicapping conditions, and beaten and tortured to rid them of demons or to educate them (Humphreys & Ramsey, 1993). It was only in 1962 that Dr. Henry Kempe coined the term *battered child syndrome* (Helfer & Kempe, 1968), which was the impetus for educational campaigns and increased efforts in America and Canada to protect children from violence and abuse.

Humphreys and Ramsey (1993) noted that it was the interaction of several factors that focused societal attention and helped raise public concern regarding child abuse. They suggested that the public was affected by the violence in Southeast Asia, namely the Vietnamese conflict, and the rising homicide rates in the United States. Other factors that heightened public awareness of violence were the women's movement and the interest demonstrated by social scientists studying the phenomenon. The combination of these variables led to multiple studies on violence and abuse, with resultant books and articles on the topic. Social agencies were formed, the Society for the Prevention of Child Abuse and Neglect was developed, and laws mandating the prevention of the abuse and neglect of children were updated. In Canada, child welfare falls within the mandate of individual provinces. Applicable legislation can be obtained from each provincial government's Web site.

Equally, the abuse of female partners has deep historical roots, with the Bible providing "the earliest prescription for physical punishment of wives" (Campbell & Fishwick, 1993, p. 73). According to these authors, documentation of wife beating can be found throughout European literature—women accused of adultery could be killed with impunity, and instructions for "correcting" wives by beating were available.

In other countries throughout the world, husbands may be punished only if their abusive behavior is "excessive" (Duffy & Momirov, 2000). Despite the efforts of the Indian government to suppress "dowry deaths," women continue to be murdered or harassed to commit suicide when husbands and families are not satisfied with the money and valuables brought to marriages. Media reports of the flogging of a Nigerian girl who had a child out of wedlock caused outrage around the world; however, the beating proceeded shortly after her infant's birth (Imam, 2001). Similarly, the violence by stoning and beating committed against women in Afghanistan for infractions such as having an ankle exposed highlight violence against women that is ongoing worldwide.

The prevalence of elder abuse only began to be recognized in the 1970s with initial efforts to "identify the kind and extent of abuse and neglect of seniors" (MacLean & Williams, 1995, p. xi). The Manitoba Association on Gerontology was the first provincial association to begin addressing this subject by developing guidelines to identify elder abuse and protocols for practice (Interdepartmental Working Group on Elder Abuse and Manitoba Seniors Directorate, 1993). In Canada, Elizabeth Podnieks, a nurse, is a leader in the study of elder abuse (Podnieks, 1985; Podnieks & Baillie, 1995; Podnieks et al., 1990). The national prevalence study that she undertook emphasized the scope of elder abuse in Canada and laid the groundwork for further research and intervention efforts.

There has been a tendency to treat violence from a generic perspective (Duffy & Momirov, 2000) without addressing the effects of class, race, sexual orientation, and ethnicity on the extent and impact of violence for aboriginal women, immigrant and refugee women, black women, people with disabilities, gay men, and lesbian women. The historical and cultural context adds a complex dimension to the analysis of violence and abuse.

■ STATISTICS IN THE CANADIAN CONTEXT

There is general acknowledgment that multiple factors are at play in the underreporting of violence and abuse. A personal need to keep any incidents of violence secret, shame on the part of the victim and the perpetrator, dependency of the victim on the perpetrator, ignorance of resources, fear of repercussions, and an inability to seek help because of forced restraint all contribute to a code of silence. For women living in rural and remote regions of the country, distance and a lack of resources hinder attempts to escape abusive relationships. This helps keep the true number of incidents of violence concealed. These factors compound the difficulties for young people, elderly people, people with disabilities, and immigrants and other women who do not know where to seek help and do not have the physical means to do so.

A leading study that attempted to ascertain the violence women experienced, especially by their intimate partners, was the 1993 Canadian Violence Against Women Survey (Bunge & Locke, 2000; Duffy & Momirov, 2000). Findings from this study indicated that 29% of women had experienced at least one episode of violence and that two thirds of these women reported that it had happened more than once. A second major survey undertaken to examine violence and abuse was the 1999 General Social Survey on Victimization (Bunge & Locke, 2000). About 26,000 people were selected through random-digit dialing and interviewed from February to December 1999. The findings from this survey, along with the findings from the Uniform Crime Reporting Survey (UCR2) and the Homicide Survey, form the basis for the report *Family Violence in Canada: A Statistical Profile 2000* (Bunge & Locke, 2000). The UCR2 collected information of criminal offenses reported to police. Victims only report these offenses after a lengthy process that includes multiple decisions concerning the implications of reporting. Equally lengthy and complex are the decisions made within the criminal justice system. Due to the complicated nature of this process, many cases are never reported.

Methodologic variations between surveys on violence and abuse result in differences in the data that have been compiled. Caution must be taken when comparing the results between studies because of these differences. There are often differences in time frames, definitions, and terminology between studies that may result in findings that require careful examination before any similarities and differences can be discussed.

Violence Against Women

Criticisms regarding the use of the terms *spousal abuse*, *conjugal violence*, *partner violence*, and *domestic abuse* center on the implication that the abuse that women direct against male partners is equal, in nature and degree, to that committed by men against female partners (Campbell & Fishwick, 1993). There remains a consensus in the statistics on violence and abuse that women continue to suffer the most severe, repetitive, protracted forms of abuse, often resulting in injury and requiring medical attention (Bunge & Locke, 2000; Dobash & Dobash, 1979). There is also concurrence in the research that female-to-male violence results from acts of self-defense (DeKerseredy & Kelly, 1993). This is consistent with the fact that men reported far greater incidents of hitting, kicking, biting, and having objects thrown at them than did women (Bunge & Locke, 2000). The concerns regarding the impact of terminology in focusing attention away from the reality of who constitutes the majority of abusers must be kept at the forefront while reading the following statistics.

Findings of the 1999 GSS suggest that, within the previous 5 years, 7% of people who were married or in common-law relationships experienced some form of violence from their intimate partners, with the rates for women and men being similar (Bunge & Locke, 2000). However, the report *Family Violence in Canada: A Statistical Profile 2000* emphasizes that the most severe and consistent forms of violence were reported by women. Women were three times as likely as men to report having been beaten (13% versus 4%). Women were also far more likely than men to be choked and sexually assaulted or to be threatened with a weapon. Men reported a higher incidence of being slapped, having something thrown at them, or being kicked, hit, and bit. During the same 5-year period, the police were involved in 37% of cases with female victims and 15% of cases with male victims.

A slightly greater proportion of women younger than 34 years of age reported being abused, as did more women in common-law relationships than those who were married (Bunge & Locke, 2000). Periodic bouts of heavy drinking, more than the frequency of the abuser's drinking, were related to episodes of violent behavior. A question that could be asked is whether the abuser became equally violent with people outside the home or confined the violent actions to those within the home.

Although this section focuses on violence and abuse within families, it must be noted that 23% of women are sexually assaulted by strangers (Matas, 2001). In 1997, there were 89 reported sexual assaults per 100,000 people in the population (Statistics Canada, 1997). The province of Saskatchewan reported the highest number of assaults, whereas Quebec reported the fewest. From the findings of anonymous surveys, it has been estimated that as many as 90% of sexual assaults, however, are never reported.

Comparisons with national studies in the United States and Great Britain produced findings that were similar to the Canadian statistics (Bunge & Locke, 2000, p. 26). Women reported being beaten or choked more often than men and were more likely to suffer injury when they were abused. Tham and colleagues (1995) noted that 40% of people presenting to psychiatric services reported a history of some abuse, whereas 24% reported being victims of domestic violence; the ratio of women to men in this group is 2.75:1.

Violence in Gay and Lesbian Relationships

Until recent decades, there have been relatively few studies of violence in gay and lesbian relationships. Ristock (2001) conducted a multisite qualitative study of violence experienced in lesbian relationships. Service providers (counselors, shelter workers, and social workers) who participated in focus groups noted that basing their efforts on heterosexual dynamics limited their practice. Ristock highlighted that some concerns were raised—chief among them that drawing attention to violence in lesbian relationships will detract from feminist efforts to raise awareness that violence perpetrated by men continues to be a significant social issue.

Although the focus on gender-based violence is challenged by the reporting of same-sex violence, these reports emphasize the need for the further examination of power and control as key factors in violence and abuse. Key questions that may be asked are Where is power held within a society? and What is the relationship between gender and power? Of importance in this discussion is the relationship to the social context in which this violence occurs. Victims of same-sex violence may fear being stigmatized as gay or lesbian and may expect their complaints will be trivialized (Duffy & Momirov, 2000). In a society that remains largely homophobic, the dynamics of violence within same-sex relationships are even more complex than those of opposite-sex relationships. This complexity will continue to contribute to the silencing of the issues in violent and abusive same-sex relationships.

Abuse and Neglect of Older Canadians

One of the leading studies on the abuse and neglect of older Canadians found that 4% of respondents reported financial, material, and verbal abuse by family members and other people (Podnieks et al., 1990). Ten years later, 7% of older adults in the GSS reported experiencing emotional abuse in the form of name calling, being put down, being isolated from friends and family, or being taken advantage of financially by a spouse, caregiver, or child (Bunge & Locke, 2000). One must keep in mind that older people may be reluctant or afraid to report abuse by family members for various reasons, among them dependency, feelings of shame, and fear of retaliation.

Little research has been undertaken on violence and abuse of elderly people living in institutions. Anecdotal and case study reports have been the source of information on abuse within residential care settings. Overt acts of physical abuse included extensive use of restraints as well as hitting, pinching, and shoving (Wiehe, 1998). Limiting freedom and choice, providing inadequate nutrition, and isolating people were among the more covert acts of abuse. In these cases, it was people who had responsibility for the care of the residents—the people who were in power—who often were the abusers.

In police-reported statistics of elder abuse, most offenders are strangers and people outside the family. According to statistics from the Incident-Based Uniform Crime Reporting Survey, older Canadians were 67% more likely to be abused by strangers than by family members (Bunge & Locke, 2000). Although the numbers are relatively small, people who deliberately target elderly people in home invasions and fraud are prominently figured in the media.

Violence Against Children and Youth

Child maltreatment is an all-encompassing term that includes physical, sexual, and emotional abuse and neglect of children. Although child maltreatment is recognized as a significant problem in Canada, no data set consolidates all of the provincial statistics to present a comprehensive national picture. Data on cases of child maltreatment are based on child welfare caseloads, police files on assault and homicide, and hospitalizations for violence-related injuries (Bunge & Locke, 2000). Child welfare is a provincial responsibility, and, although each province has legislation defining child abuse and neglect, a lack of common definitions across jurisdictions precludes the formation of a single national data set.

Although there are mandatory reporting laws for child abuse, it is accepted that official accounts of child maltreatment underestimate the prevalence because of the failure to report by perpetrators and victims, by community members who observe abuse, and by professionals who fail to recognize the maltreatment (MacMillan et al., 1997). According to the findings from the *Ontario Health Supplement* that focused on child physical and sexual abuse, males reported being physically abused more often than did females, whereas females reported more cases of sexual abuse. Girls also reported experiencing higher rates of physical and sexual abuse conjointly. A previous retrospective study of child sexual abuse in Canada (Badgley, Allard, & McCormick, 1984) provided similar statistics for child sexual abuse: 6% for males and 13% for females. It is thought that, despite the existence of mandatory child abuse reporting laws, as many as 90% of cases are not reported to child welfare authorities (MacMillan et al., 1997). At issue is why, with mandatory reporting laws for child abuse and neglect, underreporting persists. A question for professionals and for society is why and how this silence regarding a significant social and health problem continues.

Children and youth represented 60% of sexual assaults and 20% of physical assaults reported in Canada in 1999 (Bunge & Locke, 2000). Acquaintances were the primary abusers (52%), with the remaining perpetrators being family members (24%) and strangers (19%). Girls were victimized more often than boys in 80% of sexual assault cases and 53% of physical assault cases.

Violence in First Nations Communities

The Aboriginal Justice Inquiry in Manitoba noted that "violence and abuse in aboriginal communities has reached epidemic proportions" (Hamilton & Sinclair, 1991, p. 481). Among the health concerns of aboriginal community members were family violence and physical and sexual abuse, which they believed were prevalent in their communities (Smylie, 2001).

In one survey of community members, 63% of respondents reported they had experienced violence and abuse, whereas 76% were aware that family members had been abused (Thomlinson, Erickson, & Cook, 2000). However, only 37% disclosed their violence to people in authority. Fear of repercussions and a lack of trust that reporting would introduce a change contributed to this lack of reporting. According to the Report of the Royal Commission on Aboriginal Peoples, although it is impossible to ascertain the full extent of violence in aboriginal communities, the topic is distinctive from other communities in that "it [violence] has invaded whole communities and cannot be considered a problem of a particular couple or an individual household" (1996, p. 56). The interrelationship of poverty and social and economic marginalization of many aboriginal communities is believed to contribute to an increase in violence and abuse (Hamby, 2000).

Without efforts that will substantially change conditions in the community, attempts to address violence will continue to experience only minor success.

Dating Violence

As they do in other forms of violence, women suffer more severe, pervasive, and systematic victimization in dating relationships (Canadian Public Health Association, 1994) than do men. According to a survey of college and university students, 45% of women had been sexually assaulted while in a dating relationship, 79% had been psychologically abused, and 35% had been physically abused (DeKerseredy & Kelly, 1993). DeKerseredy and Kelly caution that although this survey pointed to high percentages of dating violence, these statistics should be regarded as underestimates for reasons similar to those of other forms of violence and abuse.

Violence in the Workplace

Studies on the violence nurses face in the workplace suggest that up to 70% of nurses have been abused or threatened on the job, including being hit, kicked, verbally abused, and sexually harassed (Canadian Public Health Association, 1994). According to Mireille Kingma, nurse consultant with the International Council of Nurses (ICN), "72% of nurses do not feel safe from assault in their workplace," and "97% of nurse respondents in a British survey knew a nurse who had been physically assaulted in the past year and up to 95% reported having been bullied at work" (ICN, 1999b). This topic has been extensively covered in Chapter 16 and is only mentioned here to remind readers that workplace violence and abuse represent an equally significant concern with their own specific issues.

One of the issues that is relevant to the safety of nurses and that ultimately affects the recruitment and retention of nurses in the workplace is the continued lack of reporting and tolerance of abuse against nurses. Of the 5,000 nurses who responded to a survey by the Manitoba Association of Registered Nurses (1989), between one fourth and one third noted that they chose to ignore abusive behavior directed toward them in the workplace. Factors affecting this decision are relevant to the analysis of this issue.

■ TRYING TO UNDERSTAND: THEORETICAL PERSPECTIVES

Since the 1970s, a number of theoretical approaches have been proposed in the attempt to understand factors related to the violence and abuse of people, mainly women and children (Campbell & Fishwick, 1993; Duffy & Momirov, 2000; Gelles, 1980). Gelles classified three different types of models: the psychiatric or intraindividual model, the social-psychological model, and the sociologic model. The focus of assessments and interventions varies depending on the type of model to which one subscribes: individuals, individuals in context, or society at large. Beliefs and myths regarding violence and abuse that arise from the underlying theoretical framework will affect how one chooses to interact with individuals who are experiencing abusive situations.

From Inside the Individual

Intraindividual explanations focus on abusive men as psychopaths and the women victims as masochists. Innes and associates (1991) noted that studies focusing on the mental health of men and women in abusive relationships demonstrated a bias against women by blaming the victims. Campbell and Fishwick (1993) contend that vestiges of the masochism myth remain today when authors suggest that a woman provoked a man to batter her. As early as 1979, Walker (1979) stated that by blaming the victims, men are ultimately excused of their abusive behaviors. Innes and associates (1991) further noted that men rarely demonstrate the same violent actions outside the home but confine their abuse to where they will avoid castigation.

Environment and Interaction

The social-psychological model focuses on the interaction of the environment and the individual and the family. In child abuse cases, Helfer and Kempe hypothesized that an interaction occurs between the child, the caretaker, and the circumstance that predisposes toward violence (Helfer, 1968). Social learning theory (Bandura, 1969) is the basis for the suggestion that growing up in violent homes predisposes children toward violent behavior (Duffy & Momirov, 2000). This model has been used to explain the intergenerational transmission of violence in which each generation of a family continues the violent and abusive behaviors that were perpetrated against them or that they observed against others in the family.

Tolerance of Violence

Sociologic models contend that violence and abuse occur in environments that tolerate, and even foster, violent actions. Garbarino's ecologic model of child abuse stresses the effect of the continued support of force in the care of children and multiple factors that affect the family (Garbarino, 1977; Garbarino, 1995; Garbarino & Kostelny, 1992; Garbarino & Sherman, 1980). A key component of this model is the incorporation of societal beliefs and values along with other factors that affect the family, such as housing, poverty, social supports, and reactions of others in the family and community.

Feminist Perspective

Feminist analysis emphasizes the role of patriarchal culture in legitimizing male violence against both women and children (Duffy & Momirov, 2000). The power and control that men hold in the corporate world, in government, in religious institutions, and in society as a whole facilitate male use of power and control in the home (Wiehe, 1998). Violence and abuse ensure continued control over women and children. Feminist analysis has contributed to the exploration of violence through examination of how race, culture, disability, social class, age, and sexual orientation affect the experiences that women of all ages have in society. Duffy and Momirov (2000) suggest that inclusion of violence in lesbian relationships in this dialogue has forced feminists to focus more attention on the issues of power and control rather than remaining concentrated on gender-based relationships.

Larger societal variables, including historical and cultural perspectives, are relevant to the analysis of violence within First Nations communities, among immigrant women, and among those living with disabilities. Prejudice, economic marginalization, and social powerlessness are key factors in the lives of both the abused and the abusers.

■ IMPACT ON HEALTH AND THE HEALTH CARE SYSTEM

Violence and abuse present formidable costs to society and to the health of individuals and families. These costs translate into expenditures to the Canadian health care system when victims seek medical care. Estimates have been made that more than 100,000 inpatient hospital days can be attributed to violence (Canadian Public Health Association, 1994). With hospital bed costs ranging from $400 to $800 a day in current dollars, this would result in expenditures between $40 and $80 million annually in Canada as a result of violence. There are no estimates of how many emergency room visits are related to violence, but at an estimated $150 per visit (hospital and physician costs), these visits would be a substantial drain on health care budgets. It is also not possible to estimate the amount of money spent on prescription drug use by battered women and other victims of violence and abuse.

Various sources estimate that abused women suffer losses of up to $7 million annually in wages and productivity (Duffy & Momirov, 2000). Financial costs to police, child welfare and victim counseling services, the court system, social services, shelters, and foster home care, as well as costs incurred for imprisoning offenders, for second-stage housing, and the incalculable costs in human suffering, contribute to the impact of violence and abuse on individuals and society.

Depression, feelings of powerlessness, alcoholism and drug use, ongoing difficulties to trust and develop relationships, and suicidal ideation and death are the individual costs to the victims of abuse and to children who witness violence and abuse (Sleutel, 1998; Wiehe, 1998). Battered women are at substantial risk for posttraumatic stress disorder (PTSD) (Wiehe, 1998), with rates ranging between 40% and 50% of serious depression and PTSD in samples of women who have been battered (Campbell, 1999).

The Canadian Public Health Association (1994) cites a significant relationship between attempted suicide and the experience of abuse and violence. One third of the respondents in one survey noted that they had attempted suicide as a result of their abuse (Thomlinson et al., 2000). Equally disturbing were the numbers of respondents in that study who continued to think about committing suicide.

One of the more frightening aspects of violence and abuse is the number of women who are murdered by intimate partners. One study of homicide revealed that 58% of female victims had been either married to or sexually intimate with their murderers (Dobash & Dobash, 1979). Other studies found that up to 71% of homicide victims were previously abused by their killers (Campbell & Fishwick, 1993; Wiehe, 1998). Battered women are extremely aware that the most dangerous time for them is when they decide to leave an abusive relationship (Langford, 1996). Over a 20-year period, from 1979 to 1998, three times as many wives as husbands were killed by their spouses (Bunge & Locke, 2000). For every 1 million couples, 10 wives and 3 husbands were murdered by their partners.

Physical and sexual abuse of children leads to severe, long-term emotional and academic problems. Abused children have difficulty concentrating, have little anger control, may suffer from eating disorders, and are at high risk for dropping out of school (Wiehe, 1998). Koniak-Griffin and Lesser (1996) found that child maltreatment was a significant predictor of self-injurious behavior and attempted suicide. In Canada from 1997 to 1998, childhood admissions for acknowledged cases of assault and other maltreatment such as battering, rape, fighting, strangulation, firearms, and stabbings were 2,359 per 100,000 population (Bunge & Locke, 2000). A total of 38 in every 100,000 children under the age of 1 year were admitted to a hospital as a result of child abuse. Considering that many more cases of abuse are never reported or go unrecognized, these are significant numbers. The cost to the health care system and in lost human potential and suffering because of the maltreatment of children and youth is incalculable.

There is a growing awareness that even if they themselves are not abused, children who live in a home where mothers are battered and where violence between parents occurs experience PTSD (Humphreys, 1993). Behavioral responses of these children include truancy, disturbed sleep patterns, decreased school performance, lack of positive peer relations, increased worry for their mothers, and fear. Children who are exposed to violence and abuse learn that violence is the way to settle problems and achieve their own ends (Beauchesne et al., 1997). Pynoos and Nader (1990) examined four main types of symptoms experienced by children who have observed violent and abusive incidents: PTSD, grief reactions, separation anxiety symptoms, and exacerbation or renewal of previous symptoms. They found that exposure to violence may have long-term detrimental effects on a child's cognitive development.

■ ISSUES FOR NURSES AND THE NURSING PROFESSION

Nursing associations at all levels, provincially, nationally, and internationally, advocate that nurses take an active role in addressing problems of violence by increasing their knowledge of issues associated with violence and abuse (Alberta Association of Registered Nurses et al., 1999; American Nurses Association, 1994; CNA, 1996). The associations advocate zero tolerance for interpersonal violence and violence in the workplace. What issues, then, should nurses be informed of and what information should they incorporate into their nursing practice?

Language

The use of gender-neutral language in discussing all types of interpersonal violence has diluted the issue so that there is a perception that violence and abuse are committed equally by men and women in society. A careful examination of the statistics on the types and circumstances surrounding any violence and abuse provides a more comprehensive picture of what actually is occurring. Nurses, as professionals and as members of society, have a role to play in recognizing that the use of a particular language can obscure and slant perceptions of what really is happening in violent and abusive relationships.

Lack of Understanding

A second issue arises from a lack of understanding about the pervasiveness of violent behaviors. Multiple myths about violence and abuse affect how health care professionals respond to, and treat, people involved in violent situations. One myth that continues to pervade society is that it is mainly people living in poverty who act violently toward others. Health care providers, then, do not consider that professionals and people from upper socioeconomic brackets could be victims or perpetrators of violence within their families. The effect of holding this perception is that poor people may be stereotyped as violent and the effects minimized as being part of the culture, whereas others receive little intervention because "it [violence] cannot possibly be happening in that home."

Other Issues

Other issues that require analysis include the following:

- The persistent underreporting of child abuse cases
- The question of whether there should be compulsory reporting of violence between adult partners who are treated within the health care system
- The need for a reporting mechanism for cases of abuse of elders who live in their own homes or the homes of family members, not in institutions
- The continuing belief that intervention in violence and abuse is not a health care issue but a social service issue
- The ongoing lack of reporting of violence against nurses in the workplace

■ BARRIERS TO RESOLUTION

The pervasiveness of abuse and violence through all ages, classes, cultures, and races and across genders and national and international political boundaries underlies and hampers efforts to address the issues surrounding the topic. This pervasiveness means that victims of violence, as well as the perpetrators, are in all sectors of society, including the health care professions. The strong need to deny abuse, to keep silent, pervades society. This social and political reality counters efforts for change. The silence that has permitted and even encouraged violence and abuse is complex, not easily understood, and universal.

A key factor that reinforces the silencing of abuse is a societal belief in the sanctity of the family: what occurs within the walls of the home is private. A belief that parents and spouses are permitted to control what goes on in the family and to discipline family members is another component. Gender-based power that underlies society, as was noted previously in the chapter, affects relationships at all levels. The perpetrators of abuse may be in positions of power in government, justice, and throughout the rest of society. Secrecy permits them to continue to abuse. Power in relationships such as nurse–patient interactions contributes to the opportunity for abuse to occur; there is sometimes little recognition given to the type and amount of power that health professionals hold over their patients.

Another element may be the helplessness that professionals feel regarding their inability to understand and to intervene in abuse between adults. It is easier not to ask questions about violence than to ask questions that might reveal an abusive relationship and not know how to interact and intervene. Professionals may subvert their assessments by the manner in which they ask questions regarding violence. Those who choose to speak out may be silenced by coworkers and others who wish to have the abuse and violence remain secret. The complex interactions that yield this ongoing silencing suggest there may be no easy solutions.

■ STRATEGIES FOR RESOLUTION

No one profession can successfully work toward ending the silence about abuse and violence in isolation from others. Developing partnerships with victims of violence will require a concerted effort by professionals to gain the confidence and trust that victims must achieve before alliances can be established. Although this is a time-consuming process, effective intervention programs can develop out of these alliances. To aid in developing understanding, interdisciplinary courses in the education setting are a beginning.

Interdisciplinary Education and Intervention

A key issue more than a decade after the federal government convened interdisciplinary consultations across the country to address violence and abuse is the persistent lack of interdisciplinary education programs and intervention protocols for health and social service professionals. This issue is particularly relevant to nurses because they are in key positions to advocate for patients, to educate others, to promote healthy relationships, to identify abuse and violence, and to intervene. To act, nurses must be knowledgeable about the topic, they must comprehend the education that the professionals with whom they work have, and they must understand the roles that each has in addressing violence and abuse.

A curriculum guide for nurses was developed by Hoff and Ross (1993) and then followed by an interdisciplinary curriculum guide for health care professionals (Hoff, 1994). Although some education on violence and abuse has been incorporated into curricula of health care professionals, the need for interdisciplinary courses to aid in developing a comprehensive prevention and intervention program remains.

Victims of violence continue to report that health care professionals focus on the injuries that have been sustained yet ignore any other aspects of the situation (Sleutel, 1998). Additionally, nurses and doctors acknowledged that they defer asking questions that may lead to disclosure of violence and abuse (Campbell et al., 1993). Moreover, victims have accused them of being judgmental, uncaring, and the least helpful category of professionals to whom they have gone for assistance (American Academy of Nurses Expert Panel on Violence, 1993, p. 87).

The CNA's *Code of Ethics* (1997), the practice standards and expectations for nurses across the country (Alberta Association of Registered Nurses et al., 1999), and the ICN (1999a) have set guidelines for zero tolerance of violence and abuse. This unanimity across all levels of nursing highlights the importance given to the problem presented by the diverse types of violence. Other associations and organizations have also recommended the need for the education of health care professionals (MacLean & Williams, 1995; MacLeod, 1991; McCullough, 1994). Despite this convergence of opinion and the consensus that everyone has the right to a life free of violence and abuse, the development of interdisciplinary curricula has been slow.

Political Action

The societal and cultural issues underlying the reticence to deal with issues involving violence and abuse are key factors affecting the procrastination in developing joint curricula.

In a circular fashion, the approach of health care professionals to focus on the short-term treatment of the signs and symptoms of violence places the onus on the individual to correct the problem and does not demand change within society. Compartmentalization and a focus on the physical effects of violence and abuse also, then, do not require that professionals accept responsibility to address the broader implications of abuse and violence.

Continued joint efforts of the professional associations at the national and provincial levels are needed for developing interdisciplinary curricula on abuse and violence. As with all other issues, there must be individuals within the various organizations who will advocate for these education programs. The efforts to lobby faculties of nursing, medicine, dentistry, physiotherapy, and occupational therapy must be undertaken by those who recognize and believe in the need to address this issue. An example of an organization that could be used in this lobby in Western Canada is RESOLVE (Research and Education for Solutions to Violence and Abuse), an interdisciplinary community and academic organization working toward ending abuse and violence (RESOLVE, 1999). Joint research and education organizations exist in other regions of the country (see Online Resources at the end of the chapter for several addresses and links), and the involvement of professionals from multiple disciplines, working with community members, strengthens the efforts and potentiates success. The commitment of time and energy to establish working relationships with members of other disciplines can facilitate efforts to address this issue.

■ SUMMARY

The enormity and pervasiveness of violence and abuse across society are emphasized and validated by the thousands of books and articles on the topic. The financial and human costs of violence are incalculable but extensive, affecting intimate relationships and all segments of society, particularly the vulnerable: elderly people, disabled people, First Nations members, immigrants and minorities, and children. Violence in the workplace affects nurses and other health professionals.

Nurses are in strategic positions to address issues of violence and abuse because they are among the most trusted professionals, are accessible to the public, and are often the first professionals met by those seeking health care.

Nurses, therefore, must become knowledgeable about violence and abuse, develop the skills to assess and intervene in cases of violence and abuse, and work in interdisciplinary teams to provide comprehensive care. To do any less is a disservice to patients and the profession.

Online Resources

Add to your knowledge of this issue:

British Columbia Institute Against Family Violence	www.bcifv.org
Family and Intimate Partner Violence Prevention Team	www.cdc.gov/ncipc/factsheets/ipvfacts.htm
Family Violence in Canada	www.statcan.ca/english/freepub/ 85-224-XIE/free.htm
Hot Peach Pages	www.hotpeachpages.net
Muriel McQueen Fergusson Centre for Family Violence Research	www.unbf.ca/arts/CFVR
National Clearinghouse on Family Violence	www.hc-sc.gc.ca/hppb/familyviolence
National Council Against Domestic Violence	www.ncadv.org
National Council on Child Abuse and Family Violence	www.nccafv.org
Research and Education for Solutions to Violence and Abuse	www.umanitoba.ca/resolve

REFLECTIONS on the Chapter . . .

1. What images do you have when you hear the terms *family violence, woman abuse,* and *abuse of the elderly*? Who are the main characters in your images and what are they doing?

2. Compile a list of accounts from newspapers, television, and radio from the past week that dealt with violence and abuse. What impact would these incidents have on the health of the population? Were health issues addressed in these accounts?

3. If you have had a patient divulge that she or he had been abused, what steps did you take to assist this person? What steps might you take having read this chapter? What resources could you draw on to guide your actions?

4. What attitudes have you heard expressed that would provide a caring atmosphere for any person (patient or nurse) who divulges abuse? What attitudes would hinder or suppress disclosing this type of information?

5. On which of the many facets of violence and abuse would you choose to focus your attention if you were asked to undertake a project of prevention? Where would you begin your efforts?

6. What resources are available in your work environment that would help you care for and deal with the emotional impact of working with victims of violence?

References

Alberta Association of Registered Nurses, College of Licensed Practical Nurses, & Registered Psychiatric Nurses of Alberta. (1999). *Joint statement on family violence* [Online]. Available: www.nurses.ab.ca/pdf/Joint_Statement_on_Family_Violence.pdf. Edmonton, AB: Author.

American Academy of Nurses Expert Panel on Violence. (1993). Violence as a nursing priority: Policy implications. *Nursing Outlook, 41*(2), 83–92.

American Nurses Association. (1994). *Workplace violence: Can you close the door on it?* (WP-5). Retrieved April 18, 2001, from http://www.nursingworld.org/dlwa/osh/wp5.htm

Badgley, R. F., Allard, H. A., & McCormick, N. (1984). *Sexual offences against children* (Catalogue No. J2-50/1984E). Ottawa: Department of Supply and Services.

Bandura, A. (1969). Social-learning theory of identificatory processes. In D. A. Goslin (Ed.), *Handbook of socialization theory and research* (pp. 213–262). Chicago: Rand McNally.

Beauchesne, M., Kelley, B. R., Lawrence, P. R., et al. (1997). Violence prevention: A community approach. *Journal of Pediatric Health Care, 11,* 179–188.

Bunge, V. P., & Locke, D. (2000). *Family violence in Canada: A statistical profile 2000* [Online]. Available: http://www.statcan.ca (Catalogue 85-224-XIE Canadian Centre for Justice Statistics). Ottawa: Minister of Industry.

Campbell, J., & Fishwick, N. (1993). Abuse of female partners. In J. Campbell & J. Humphreys (Eds.), *Nursing care of survivors of family violence* (pp. 68–106). St. Louis, MO: Mosby.

Campbell, J. C. (1999). *Safety planning based on lethality assessment for partners of batterers in treatment.* Paper presented at the Partnerships to Enhance Victim Safety Conference: Criminal Justice & Advocacy Responses to Domestic Violence, Troy, NY [Online]. Available: http://www.opdv.state.ny.us/

Canadian Nurses Association. (1996). *Interpersonal violence* [Online]. Available: http://www.cna-nurses.ca

Canadian Public Health Association. (1994). *Violence in society: A public health perspective* (Issue Paper). Ottawa: Author.

DeKerseredy, W. S., & Kelly, K. (1993). The incidence and prevalence of woman abuse in Canadian university and college dating relationships. *Canadian Journal of Sociology, 18*(2), 137–159.

Dobash, R. E., & Dobash, R. P. (1979). *Violence against wives.* New York: Free Press.

Duffy, A., & Momirov, J. (2000). Family violence: Issues and advances at the end of the twentieth century. In N. Mandell & A. Duffy (Eds.), *Canadian families: Diversity, conflict, and change* (pp. 290–322). Toronto: Harcourt Canada.

Garbarino, J. (1977). The human ecology of child maltreatment: A conceptual model for research. *Journal of Marriage and the Family, 39,* 721–735.

————. (1995). Growing up in a socially toxic environment: Life for children and families in the 1990s. In G. B. Melton (Ed.), *The individual, the family, and social good: Personal fulfillment in times of change* (Vol. 42, pp. 1–20). Lincoln: University of Nebraska Press.

Garbarino, J., & Kostelny, K. (1992). Child maltreatment as a community problem. *Child Abuse and Neglect, 16,* 455–464.

Garbarino, J., & Sherman, D. (1980). High-risk neighborhoods and high-risk families: The human ecology of child maltreatment. *Child Development, 51,* 188–198.

Gelles, R. J. (1980). Violence in the family: A review of research in the seventies. *Journal of Marriage and the Family, 42,* 873–885.

Hamby, S. L. (2000). The importance of community in a feminist analysis of domestic violence among American Indians. *American Journal of Community Psychology, 28*(5), 649–669.

Hamilton, A. C., & Sinclair, C. M. (1991). *The justice system and aboriginal people.* Winnipeg: Queen's Printer.

Helfer, R. (1973). The etiology of child abuse. *Pediatrics, 51,* 777–779.

Helfer, R., & Kempe, C. H. (1968). *The battered child.* Chicago: University of Chicago Press.

Hoff, L. A. (1994). *Violence issues: An interdisciplinary curriculum guide for health professionals* (H72-21/129-1995E). Ottawa: Mental Health Division Health Canada.

Hoff, L. A., & Ross, M. M. (1993). *Curriculum guide for nursing: Violence against women and children.* Ottawa: University of Ottawa.

Humphreys, J. (1993). Children of battered women. In J. Campbell & J. Humphreys (Eds.), *Nursing care of survivors of family violence* (pp. 107–131). St. Louis, MO: Mosby.

Humphreys, J., & Ramsey, A. M. (1993). Child abuse. In J. Campbell & J. Humphreys (Eds.), *Nursing care of survivors of family violence* (pp. 36–67). St. Louis, MO: Mosby.

Imam, A. (2001, April). Nigerian women's group condemns whipping [Online]. Available: http://www.web.net/~matchint/en/apr01/nlapr01_3.htm

Innes, J. E., Ratner, P. A., Finlayson, P. F., et al. (1991). *Models and strategies of delivering community health services related to woman abuse.* Edmonton: University of Alberta.

Interdepartmental Working Group on Elder Abuse and Manitoba Seniors Directorate. (1993). *Abuse of the elderly: A guide for the development of protocols.* Winnipeg: Government of Manitoba.

International Council of Nurses. (1999a). *Abuse and violence against nursing personnel* [Online]. Available: http://www.icn.ch/psviolence00.htm

————. (1999b, March 8). *Increasing violence in the workplace is a threat to nursing and the delivery of health care* [Online]. Available: http://www.icn.ch/prviolence_99.htm

Koniak-Griffin, D., & Lesser, J. (1996). The impact of childhood maltreatment on young mothers' violent behavior toward themselves and others. *Journal of Pediatric Nursing, 11*(5), 300–308.

Langford, D. R. (1996). Predicting unpredictability: A model of women's processes of predicting battering men's violence. *Scholarly Inquiry for Nursing Practice: An International Journal, 10*(4), 371–385.

MacLean, M. J., & Williams, R. M. (1995). Introduction. In M. J. MacLean (Ed.), *Abuse & neglect of older Canadians: Strategies for change* (pp. ix–xii). Toronto: Canadian Association on Gerontology and Thompson Educational Publishing.

MacLeod, L. (1991). *Freedom from fear: A woman's right, a community concern, a national priority* (C91-099010-7E). Ottawa: Secretary of State Canada; Multiculturalism and Citizenship Canada.

MacMillan, H. L., Fleming, J. E., Trocme, N., et al. (1997). Prevalence of child physical and sexual abuse in the community. *Journal of the American Medical Association, 278*(2), 131–135.

Manitoba Association of Registered Nurses. (1989). *Nurse abuse report.* Winnipeg: Author.

Matas, R. (2001, March 24). "He said if I ever told anyone, he will kill me when he gets out." *Globe and Mail,* pp. A9–10.

McCullough, I. (1994). *A challenge for health: Making connections within the family violence context* (Discussion papers on health/family violence issues H39-292/1-1994E). Ottawa: Health Canada.

Podnieks, E. (1985). Elder abuse: It's time we did something about it. *Canadian Nurse, 81*(11), 36–39.

Podnieks, E., & Baillie, E. (1995). Education as the key to the prevention of elder abuse and neglect. In M. J. MacLean (Ed.), *Abuse & neglect of older Canadians: Strategies for change* (pp. 81–93). Toronto: Canadian Association on Gerontology and Thompson Educational Publishing.

Podnieks, E., Pillemer, K., Nicholson, J. P., et al. (1990). *National survey on abuse of the elderly in Canada.* Toronto: Ryerson Polytechnic Institute.

Pynoos, R. S., & Nader, K. (1990). Children's exposure to violence and traumatic death. *Psychiatric Annals, 20*(6), 334–344.

Report of the Royal Commission on Aboriginal Peoples. (1996). *For seven generations* (Vol. 3). Ottawa: Libraxus.

RESOLVE. (1999). Winnipeg Foundation funds RESOLVE newsletter. In B. Comaskey (Ed.), (Vol. 1, p. 1). Winnipeg: Author.

Ristock, J. L. (2001). Decentering heterosexuality: Responses of feminist counselors to abuse in lesbian relationships. *Women & Therapy, 23*(3), 59–72.

Sleutel, M. R. (1998). Women's experiences of abuse: A review of qualitative research. *Issues in Mental Health Nursing, 19,* 525–539.

Smylie, J. (2001). A guide for health professionals working with aboriginal peoples: Health issues affecting aboriginal peoples. *Journal of the Society of Obstetricians and Gynecologists of Canada, 100,* 54–68.

Statistics Canada. (1997). *Graphical overview of crime and the administration of criminal justice in Canada, 1997* (Catalogue No. 85F0018XIE). Ottawa: Minister of Industry.

Thomlinson, E. B., Erickson, N., & Cook, M. (2000). Could this be your community? In J. Proulx & S. Perrault (Eds.), *No place for violence: Canadian aboriginal alternatives* (Vol. 1, pp. 22–38). Halifax: Fernwood Publishing and RESOLVE (Research and Education for Solutions to Violence and Abuse).

Walker, L. E. (1979). *The battered woman.* New York: Harper & Row.

Wiehe, V. R. (1998). *Understanding family violence: Treating and preventing partner, child, sibling, and elder abuse.* Thousand Oaks, CA: Sage.

As a way of engaging with the ideas in this chapter, consider the following:

1. What assumptions do you hold about the role of professional nurses in environmental health?

2. What knowledge would you need as a nurse to make a significant contribution to environmental health?

3. How might you account for the scarcity of knowledge in nursing curricula to support this area of nursing practice?

CHAPTER

22

Elizabeth Thomlinson

Environmental Health and Nursing

Across Canada, the relationship of the environment to the health of individuals and families is a serious concern. Emissions from gas plants and other environmental pollutants are just a few of the potential hazards to health. Individual nurses and the nursing profession can promote greater societal health through the traditional routes of nursing practice, education, and research.

After completing this chapter, you will be able to:

1. Identify some common environmental health hazards in your geographic region.

2. Examine the nursing profession's impact in addressing environmental issues.

3. Generate ideas about how individual nurses can affect issues of environmental health.

4. Evaluate how nursing curricula integrate health and the environment.

This we know . . . the earth does not belong to man, man belongs to the earth.
All things are connected, like blood which connects one family. Whatever befalls the earth befalls the children of the earth. Man did not weave the web of life; he is merely a strand in it.
Whatever he does to the web, he does to himself.

—*Chief Seattle, 1854 Suqwamish and Duwamish*

n a world that is increasingly affected by globalization; swift transportation; almost instant communication; global warming; the extinction of multiple species of plants, animals, and birds; and the rapid transfer of diseases around the globe, humans are as closely linked to the health of their environments as they were at the dawn of human history. Environmental hazards, the health of the earth, and the health of the earth's inhabitants are inseparable. The interdependence of all species on the earth and the physical environment cannot be overemphasized. The concepts of person, environment, health, and nursing, which form the metaparadigm of the nursing profession, underscore this interdependence, but a perusal of texts for nurses uncovered little discussion of environmental health.

Although this chapter does not focus on the conservation of natural resources, it does underscore how environmental hazards contribute to adverse health outcomes for humans. It is hoped that readers will examine the regions and communities where they live and work to gain awareness of the connection between their own environments and the health of the residents. The need to be aware of how environmental hazards impact human health is important for nurses regardless of their practice settings—community, long-term, or acute institutional care, or occupational health. All too often when concerns regarding environmental health issues surface, they are so far removed from the daily lives of most people that little attention is paid to the issues raised. Only when the media highlight major problems, such as the deaths from *Escherichia coli* (*E. coli*) bacteria resulting from contaminated water sources in Walkerton, Ontario (Ahluwalia, 2000), do citizens become concerned about the possibility of similar events in their own neighborhoods.

There is no doubt that human health is affected when the environment or ecosystem is damaged (McMullan, 1997). The term *environmental health,* as used in this chapter, refers to freedom from illness related to exposure to environmental contamination, hazards, or toxins that are detrimental to health. In the discussions that follow, the term *environment* includes the physical, social, political, legal, psychological, and cognitive environments of individuals, their families, and their communities. As scientific knowledge increases and social and political values change, the definition of, and factors related to, environmental health will also change.

Reference resources for this chapter include government agency Web sites, national and international nursing association Web sites, newspapers, and a variety of professional literature in addition to what is available in the Canadian nursing literature. A limited number of the many Canadian and American Web sites that are available for research and information are listed at the end of the chapter (see Online Resources). Readers are encouraged to examine the vast body of literature on the topic of environmental health, ranging from extensive research reports found in journals such as *Environmental Health Perspectives, Environmental Health*, and the *Ecologist* to general literature that alerts the public to issues of concern in the environment. The impact of Rachel Carson's books, including *The Silent Spring* and *The*

Sea Around Us, and the efforts of David Suzuki, among others, in raising awareness of the destruction of our physical world has been incalculable.

■ HISTORICAL LINKS BETWEEN ENVIRONMENT AND HEALTH

The effect that a healthy, or conversely an unhealthy, environment has on human health is not a recent discovery. Early civilizations were aware of the impact of the environment on health. The Minoans (3000 to 1430 BC), Mycenaeans (1430 to 1150 BC), and Romans (509 BC to 476 AD) all built extensive drainage and water systems as well as baths and toilets (McGuire & Eigsti-Gerber, 1999) in response to related environmental health hazards of pestilence and disease. Early Hebrew writings included a code on hygiene, and the ancient Egyptians (3100 BC to 600 AD) developed safe water and sewer systems. As civilizations rose and fell, this knowledge and the systems that had been developed were often forgotten or destroyed.

Plagues resulting from contamination of water sources and the spread of disease through animal vectors have been documented throughout history. Through the introduction of public health measures such as providing a clean source of drinking water and disposing safely of sewage and other wastes, great improvements were made in the health of populations; these key elements remain as important as ever (Clark, 1999; McDevitt & Wilbur, 2002). A major turning point in history, however, was the Industrial Revolution that began in Great Britain in the early 1700s and spread to Europe and North America. Industrialization resulted in a shift from what had been a rural, agricultural economy to one that was urban and factory-based with concomitant problems of pollution from large steel foundries and the burning of fossil fuels. The impact of the Industrial Revolution extended far beyond the production of goods and material to changes in governments, the use of resources in the world, material benefits for some of the world's population, and wars and exploitation of many populations. Modern transportation and communication, the globalization of markets, and the even more rapid destruction of habitats are evident today. Nurses have been integral participants in examining and changing some of the harmful environmental conditions to improve public health.

In *Notes on Nursing*, Florence Nightingale (1860, p. 5) observed that environmental factors had a key impact on health and disease:

In watching diseases, both in private homes and in public hospitals, the thing which strikes the experienced observer most forcibly is this, that the symptoms or the sufferings generally considered to be inevitable and incident to the disease are very often not symptoms of the disease at all, but of something quite different— of the want of fresh air, or of cleanliness, or of punctuality and care in the administration of diet, of each or of all of these.

Further, Nightingale noted that there were "five essential points in securing the health of houses" and, by extrapolation, the health of the population: "pure air, pure water, efficient drainage, cleanliness and light" (1860, p. 14).

Other nurses who actively advocated for safe water, sewage, and sanitation systems, which they incorporated into their health promotion and education practices, included Lillian Wald (1915) and Mary Breckenridge (1952; Eigsti-Gerber & McGuire, 1999). Wald was the founder of modern public health nursing, working in New York to improve the health of children in particular. Breckenridge incorporated principles of environmental health in her community health practice in rural Kentucky, which lowered infant mortality rates. Before the establishment of large hospitals and the focus on care in hospitals, most early nursing practice was carried out in the community. Nurses were cognizant of the environmental conditions in which their patients lived and worked. The shift to the majority of nursing practice being concentrated within institutions separated nurses from the environmental effects that had been more readily apparent.

Current environmental debates center on global warming as a result of the burning of fossil fuels (Foley, 2001; Last, Trouton, & Pengally, 1998), destruction of habitat around the world (Malcolm et al., 2002), and the potential for unrestrained population growth to outstrip the ability to produce enough food to feed the world's citizens (Brown et al., 2001). Multiple charters, agreements, summits, and conventions have been held to examine the health of the world's citizens, globalization and global issues related to the environment, access to safe water and food, global warming, the sociopolitical causes and impact of poverty, and the economic disparity that exists among nations within the context of a "sustainable global ecosystem" (Hilfinger Messias, 2001, p. 10). A proliferation of treaties and accords since the 1970s has resulted in more than 240 international agreements (Brown et al., 2001).

Brown and colleagues (2001) noted that the 1987 Montreal Protocol on Substances that Deplete the Ozone Layer led to the gradual phasing out of the use of chlorofluorocarbons that damage the stratosphere. The 1997 Kyoto Protocol to the 1992 United Nations (UN) Framework Convention on Climate Change has been much more contentious, with the United States refusing to ratify the treaty that requires industrialized nations to cut carbon dioxide emissions by 6% to 8% between 2008 and 2012. A major concern remains regarding the ability to police these agreements and end environmental crime that is fueled by greed and the self-interests of individuals, corporations, and governments.

While recognizing positive global effects linked to health, sanitation, and urban reclamation, Berlinguer (1999) raised concerns regarding pollution, depletion of natural resources, global warming, and the declining quality of life—particularly in urban centers and in developing nations. He noted that people in the lowest socioeconomic classes suffer the greatest damage because they lack the resources and facilities to preserve their health.

In all nations, the poorest residents tend to live in substandard housing in densely populated communities in close proximity to industrial areas where the potential for contamination and hazardous waste leakage is the highest (Chaudhuri, 1998). Within Canadian society, members of First Nations communities are especially at risk for health problems related to unsafe drinking water, lack of adequate sanitation, and substandard housing (Health Canada, 1999b). Environmental contaminants such as polychlorinated biphenyls (PCBs) used in electrical and hydraulic equipment, dioxins from bleaching wood pulp with chlorine, and mercury from old industrial practices and long-range transport have been found in fish and marine mammals throughout the country. This has resulted in a contaminated food supply, particularly for aboriginal people in the north and those who follow a traditional diet.

■ ENVIRONMENTAL HEALTH HAZARDS

Around the world, life expectancy has increased and morbidity and mortality have decreased as a result of significant improvement and availability of safe water and sewage systems and better nutrition and housing. Individuals, communities, and governments need to be conscious that these gains do not overshadow current and developing environmental problems. The World Health Organization (WHO) notes that about 2 million children younger than 5 years of age die annually because of unsafe drinking water and lack of sanitation. Air pollution is responsible for up to 20% of childhood mortality (WHO, 2001). A WHO task force has been established to promote the identification, assessment, mitigation, and prevention of environmental hazards specifically "to prevent disease and disability in children associated with chemical and physical threats" (WHO, 2001).

Various UN agencies participated in a global environmental assessment by providing data and information on environmental issues within their particular mandates (UN Environment Programme, 1999). This assessment was undertaken in response to the need to build a consensus on priorities regarding the environment. According to this report, increased industrialization around the world has contributed to environmental deterioration resulting from air and water pollution, waste dumping, and increasing ill health, especially among the poor. Environmental contaminants include biologic agents, inorganic and organic chemicals, radiation, and particulate matter (Box 22.1).

BOX 22.1	Selected Environmental Contaminants

Biologic Agents

Bacteria, such as *Escherichia coli*
Protozoa
Viruses
Fungi
Algae
House dust mites
Pollen grains
Moulds

Chemical Contaminants

Organic substances, such as fluorine, chlorine, bromine, iodine, nitrogen, sulfur, phosphorus, carbon, polychlorinated biphenyls (PCBs), DDT, dioxins, benzene, malathion, toluene, dioxane
Inorganic substances, such as ozone, nitrogen oxides, sulfur dioxide, lead, mercury, cadmium, arsenic, uranium, beryllium, chromium

Radiation

Microwaves
Ultraviolet light
Low-frequency electromagnetic fields
Sound

Particulate Matter

Fine dust
Smoke from forest fires and burning stubble
Asbestos
Cigarette smoke

Contaminants follow pathways from the time they are released into the environment until people, animals, or plants come in contact with them. These exposure pathways consist of five components that need to be examined when tracing sources of contamination (Health Canada, 1998). The components are:

- Source of contamination (e.g., emissions, waste water and disposal sites, volcanoes, fires, household products)
- Medium through which the contaminant travels (e.g., water, soil, air, food products)
- Point at which people come into contact with the contaminant
- Person, animal, or plant that is the receptor of the contaminant
- Route of exposure (e.g., inhalation [gases, vapors, or particulate matter], dermal contact [working in contaminated soil or swimming in contaminated water], or ingestion [contaminated food or water])

Many symptoms exhibited by people exposed to environmental contaminants can be attributed to other causes, making it difficult to establish an exact cause and effect. Therefore, it is important when assessing exposure to environmental contaminants to take as broad a perspective as possible to include all potential environmental factors.

Water Safety and Pollution

Water is fundamental to all life on the planet. Uneven distribution of this resource around the globe means that some regions, such as Canada, have an abundance of fresh water, whereas other regions, such as the Middle East and northern Africa, suffer from a shortage. It is estimated that 500 million people in the world live in countries that are short of water and that, by 2025, this number will dramatically rise to 3 billion (Mitchell, 2001). Water use worldwide has risen sixfold between 1900 and 1995, more than double the population increase.

In countries such as Canada, the abundance of water has led to waste and increased pollution of this resource. Although water is the ultimate renewable resource, major problems now exist in that water sources are polluted with chemicals, fertilizers, heavy metals, hydrocarbons, and raw sewage (Robson & Schneider, 2001; UN Environment Programme, 1999; Wanke & Saunders, 1996). Industrial waste, runoff from large-scale farming operations, and the dumping of garbage in uncontrolled waste sites lead to continued pollution. In the report *Health and the Environment,* Health Canada (1997) noted that, in a 1993 study, 40% of 1,300 rural wells in Ontario had undesirable levels of chemical or microbiologic contaminants. This report also stated that many Canadian residents have detectable traces of contaminants in their blood, hair, and body tissues.

Aquifers are being drained more quickly than they are being replenished. Global warming has led the atmosphere to retain more water in the form of vapor, which decreases the volume of water returned in the form of rain. An example of the overuse of subterranean water is the High Plains Aquifer that extends from South Dakota to Texas. The level of water has dropped by more than 40 m as the population uses the water for irrigating land that was once barren. Solutions to this water depletion suggested by American politicians and entrepreneurs are the bulk sale of water from Canada and the desalination of ocean water for human use. The short- and long-term effects on the environment of either of these proposals are not known.

The need to provide a safe drinking water supply has been highlighted by recent outbreaks of *E. coli* in the water supply at Walkerton, Ontario, and *Cryptosporidium* species found in the water in North Battleford, Saskatchewan. The *E. coli* outbreak led to multiple gastrointestinal illnesses and, ultimately, to the deaths of nine people (Ahluwalia, 2000). Contamination of the water sources from manure from cattle farms in the area and the inadequate treatment of the water are suspected causes of this outbreak. The impact of these outbreaks has heightened public awareness and increased the need to examine and question water safety in the communities.

Cryptosporidium, although not a new organism, is becoming more prevalent. Animals and humans shed this protozoan parasite in their feces. The consumption of contaminated water or food, ingestion of recreational water, or contact with infected people can lead to infection. There are potentially life-threatening consequences for immunosuppressed people who become infected (Physicians for Social Responsibility, 2001b). Proper filtration, distillation, or reverse osmosis processes must be used to ensure that the organism has been removed from the water supply. *Giardia lamblia (G. lamblia)* is another parasite endemic to the ecosystem. *G. lamblia* causes gastrointestinal infections and can also produce life-threatening effects in an immunocompromised person. Contamination of water supplies with various microbial contaminants leads to multiple "boil-water" alerts annually in all provinces.

In 2001, a government roundtable found that, although water quality is a serious problem throughout the country, there is particular concern regarding water supply to First Nations communities. A Health Canada report in 1995 signaled that 171 communities (one in five) had water systems that could negatively affect the health of the citizens (MacKinnon, 2001). Minimal improvements have occurred during the intervening years. As of 2001, there were no national regulations in Canada regarding water protection and safety, an indication that disasters can and will continue to occur.

Air Pollution

Many regions of the world suffer from air pollution that leads to illness and death. In South America, about 4,000 premature deaths are estimated to occur annually in Sao Paulo and Rio de Janeiro as a result of severe air pollution (UN Environment Programme, 1999). The very young and the very old suffer a greater burden from air pollution than do people in the interim age ranges. The risk from air pollution for children increases because they breathe more rapidly and inhale more pollutants per pound of body weight than do adults. A wide range of negative effects from air pollution include impaired pulmonary function; reduced physical performance; multiple visits to physicians, emergency rooms, and hospitals; and premature death (Health Canada, 1998).

Air pollutants are generated from burning fossil fuels, such as oil, coal, gasoline, and diesel fuel, in vehicles and power generators. Industries, such as pulp and paper mills, oil refineries, and ore smelters, contribute to air pollution. Oil, natural gas, and coal production has resulted in Alberta emitting 30% of the carbon dioxide, 26% of the nitrogen oxide, and 23% of the sulfur oxide emissions generated in Canada (Environment Canada, 2000). Asthma is a respiratory disease that can be triggered by airborne contaminants. Air pollutants, such as ground-level ozone, sulfur dioxide, and particulate matter, are believed to be key factors in increased asthma rates (Last et al., 1998). Pope and colleagues (2002) analyzed the mortality statistics of participants in the Cancer Prevention Study II who resided in American metropolitan areas where pollution data were available. They demonstrated that fine particulate air contamination is associated with cardiopulmonary and lung cancer mortality (Pope et al., 2002, p. 1137) and is a significant risk factor to population health.

An exponential increase in the incidence of asthma in children in Canada occurred in the 1990s. Rates of hospitalization for boys increased by 27% and for girls by 18% (Health Canada, 1997). This raised annual hospital admissions of children to more than 60,000. According to Last and associates (1998), hospital admissions in Ontario for acute bronchitis, bronchiolitis, and pneumonia in children younger than 1 year of age "can be attributed to the summer pollutants, ozone and sulphates" (p. 21). In the United States, asthma is the most prevalent childhood illness (Physicians for Social Responsibility, 1997). As well, since the 1970s, there has been a significant increase in the death rates from asthma of people 70 years of age and older in Canada and in the United States (Health Canada, 1997).

Some authorities suggest that it would cost $6 billion to implement a program to decrease air pollution by developing cleaner vehicles and fuels in Canada (Health Canada, 1998, p. 121). On the other hand, savings to the health care system are estimated to be $24 billion as a result of eliminating many of the negative health effects of air pollution. Improving ambient air quality in Canada alone could amount to $8 billion in health care savings over the next 20 years (Last et al., 1998). Last and associates (1998) suggest that the reduction of motor vehicle emissions would result in savings to the forest and agricultural sectors of the Canadian economy of between $11 and $30 billion.

Although chemically the same, ground-level ozone (found within 11 km of the earth's surface) and the "ozone layer" (found between 11 and 47 km above the earth in the stratosphere) need to be differentiated from each other. The ozone layer acts as a barrier against ultraviolet (UV) radiation (particularly UVB rays) from the sun (Health Canada, 1998). As this layer is damaged or destroyed by chlorofluorocarbons, more radiation penetrates to earth. The result is an increase in skin cancer, particularly melanomas. There is also evidence that UVB exposure increases the risk for cataracts (Institute of Medicine, 1995).

Ground-level ozone, or smog, forms when nitrogen oxides and volatile organic compounds react in the presence of sunlight (Health Canada, 1998). This occurs on hot, still, summer days, and the resultant air pollution can lead to adverse cardiac and respiratory effects. Again, those most affected are elderly and very young people. As the earth's average temperature rises, it is expected that more hot summer days with smog advisories or warnings will occur.

PCBs, dioxins, and other organic compounds can travel long distances through the air before being deposited on the land or in bodies of water. These toxins accumulate in the food chain, where they become a hazard to people who consume fish and wildlife as food, particularly when they are ingested faster than they can be excreted (Health Canada, 1998). There is grave concern that seals and other Arctic animals are contaminated and pose a risk to Inuit communities that rely on these animals as a source of food.

Chemical Pollution

Humans are slowly coming to realize the effects of the huge quantities of man-made chemicals that have been discharged into the environment since the 1940s (Physicians for Social Responsibility, 2005).

Excessive use of fertilizers, pesticides, and heavy metals such as arsenic, cadmium, lead, and mercury has polluted the land (UN Environment Programme, 1999). Local sources of contamination such as sewage and waste disposal and industrial discharge can be more readily identified. More diffuse contamination occurs through runoff from fields and lawns, motor vehicle emissions, and the long-distance contamination of acid rain (which develops from sulfur dioxide and nitrogen oxides from coal-fired power plants, smelters, and vehicular emissions). *The Health and Environment Handbook for Health Professionals,* prepared by Health Canada (1998, p. 38), notes that there are "300 industrial sites" in Ontario "that discharge directly into rivers and lakes" and "another 12,000 that dump their waste into municipal sewage systems that cannot adequately treat toxic chemicals."

Many of these chemical pollutants remain in the environment for long periods. They can be ingested and then accumulate in the tissues of humans if their excretion does not occur as quickly as their intake. Dioxins, furans, and PCBs build up in fatty tissue, whereas metals such as lead, mercury, and cadmium are stored in the liver, kidney, and bone. Mercury can be found in many lakes and rivers, where it converts to methyl mercury, a toxic substance that can affect the nervous systems of humans and animals (Environment Canada, 2000b). An additional concern is long-term arsenic ingestion (through drinking water), which increases the risk for skin, bladder, lung, kidney, and other cancers (Physicians for Social Responsibility, 2001a). The impact on human health of long-term low-level exposure to many chemical pollutants is unknown. Concerns focus on immune system suppression, neurologic and behavioral changes, and the role that chemical toxins play in initiating cancer.

The term *pesticide* refers to a variety of chemicals that control weeds (herbicides), bacteria (disinfectants), fungi (fungicides), insects (insecticides), and rodents (rodenticides). Pesticides are widely used in agriculture and forestry to protect crops and forests. Large amounts of fertilizer and herbicides are used annually in urban and suburban environments in the care of lawns and golf courses. In Canada, more than 500 active ingredients have been registered for use as pesticides (Health Canada, 1998). There is a growing movement within some towns and cities across Canada to ban the use of herbicides because of the risk to human health (Box 22.2).

Of grave concern are the implications for the health of residents who live in the immediate vicinity of toxic waste sites or who now live in what was once a contaminated industrial site (Carruth, Gilbert, & Lewis, 1997). There are no biologic markers by which the level of exposure can be determined for many of the chemicals that are discharged into the environment. Further, the long-term impact of long-term exposure to some contaminants, such as malathion, is not known. Key concerns related to long-term exposure include the following:

■ Those in lower socioeconomic conditions are often the people who live in areas closest to polluted sites.
■ As knowledge of chemical pollutants grows, standards may change (i.e., norms or levels that were once considered safe may be now considered a health risk).
■ Exposure to toxins may occur and may be undetected over extended periods of time.
■ Exposure to contaminants may occur through multiple pathways (air, water, soil) and enter the food chain in numerous ways, making detection more difficult.
■ Action to curb exposure to contaminants has not kept pace with society's abilities to detect contamination (Canadian Nurses Association, 2000).
■ Canada is without longitudinal research regarding the effects of individual contaminants as well as the combined effects from multiple sources of contamination (Canadian Nurses Association, 2000).

Inside Environments

The Ottawa Charter for Health Promotion (1986) credits adequate shelter as having a major effect on health. According to the report from the federal, provincial, and territorial governments, *Toward a Healthy Future: Second Report on the Health of Canadians,* one in five Canadians who rent accommodations is

BOX 22.2 Selected Environmental Health Concerns

Concerns Related to General Environmental Hazards

Cancer
Genetic mutation
Birth defects
Neurologic effects, such as cerebral ataxia, neuropathies, and encephalitis
Heat prostration, injuries, and death from weather and climate extremes
Joint and muscle pain or weakness
Organ damage
Reproductive damage
Developmental and behavioral abnormalities
Respiratory disorders such as asthma, bronchitis, and emphysema
Gastrointestinal diseases, such as cholera and other infections, caused by *Escherichia coli*,
   Giardia lamblia, or *Cryptosporidium species*
Death

Concerns Related to Nursing Workplace Hazards

Infectious diseases
   Hepatitis A, B, and C
   Tuberculosis, measles, rubella, influenza
   Human immunodeficiency virus (HIV)
Exposure to toxins
   Cytotoxic drugs
   Anaesthetic gas waste
   Ethylene oxide, gluteraldehyde, and formaldehyde
Radiation
Stress
Violence

living in substandard housing (Health Canada, 1999b). The people who most often live in these conditions are single-parent families, particularly ones in which parents are younger than 30 years old; people with mental health problems; and senior citizens living alone. Of grave concern are the inadequate housing and crowded living conditions in which aboriginal people live. This may be a major contributor to the fact that aboriginal children suffer from much higher rates of respiratory and other infectious diseases than do nonaboriginal children (Health Canada, 1999b).

Health Canada estimates that Canadians spend up to 90% of their time indoors in their homes, work sites, and other buildings. In addition to outdoor contaminants, which can also be found indoors, the inside air may contain tobacco smoke, formaldehyde, vapors from household products, carbon dioxide, and biologic agents such as bacteria, fungi, moulds, viruses, and mite byproducts (Health Canada, 1998). The health of the residents may be adversely affected if the concentrations of any of these contaminants rise too high. The growing trend toward weatherizing homes and buildings in the interest of conservation may result in a lack of adequate air exchange because the ventilation systems were not designed for these well-insulated and sealed buildings. Therefore, the potential for contaminant buildup increases.

A principal contaminant in indoor environments is tobacco smoke, including sidestream smoke emitted from cigarettes, pipes, and cigars between puffs and mainstream smoke exhaled by smokers. It is estimated that there are 300 deaths from lung cancer in nonsmokers annually in Canada as a result of environmental tobacco smoke (ETS; Health Canada, 1998, 1999b). In addition, ETS is considered a significant cause of cardiovascular disease and death in nonsmokers.

Canadian children are at an increased risk for health effects from ETS because they spend more time indoors than do children in many other countries. As mentioned previously, children have smaller airways and breathe more rapidly than do adults, thus inhaling more pollutants per kilogram of body weight. In the United States, authorities estimate that 11% of asthma cases, about 350,000 cases of bronchitis, and 152,000 cases of pneumonia are a consequence of ETS (Health Canada, 1998). More than one third of households with children younger than 15 years of age also have a smoker in the family. Authorities suspect that exposure to ETS during childhood may be associated with increased pulmonary disease and cancer (Health Canada, 1998).

There is a wide variation among provinces in the control and restriction of smoking in public areas. Restrictions against smoking range from being limited to designated smoking areas to a total ban on smoking on public premises. As the public becomes more aware and concerned with the health risks attributed to ETS, smoking bans may become more stringent.

Contaminated Social Environments

If consideration of environmental health risks is confined to the effects of pollution and hazards within the natural environment, a key component of the settings in which individuals and families live will be ignored. Impoverished neighborhoods with substandard housing, abject poverty, homelessness, visible signs of people who are substance abusing and drug dealing, and violence and crime within the community are examples of contaminated social environments. The impact on the physical, psychological, and emotional health of individuals living in such environments can be severe.

The national crime rate in Canada, including homicides, attempted murders, robberies, break-ins, motor vehicle thefts, and incidents of impaired driving, has doubled since the 1960s (Health Canada, 1999b). Of significant concern is the fact that the rate of young people charged with violent crimes is more than double the rate of a decade ago. The effects of violence in the schools and the impact of bullying, leading to teenage suicides, have been frequently in the news (Cox, 2002). There has, however, been a drop in the national crime rate since it peaked in 1991. An actual decrease of 19 homicides in which firearms were used (193 versus 212) occurred between the years 1996 and 1997. This is in contrast to the United States, where a proliferation of handguns contributes to an increased homicide rate. In that country, 17% of deaths in the workplace were homicides, with gunshots accounting for 82% of that total (Institute of Medicine, 1995). Almost 1,000 workers are murdered on the job annually in the United States, with homicide being the number one cause of women's deaths in the workplace (International Council of Nurses, 2001).

If the social environments in which people live are violent, degrading, and impoverished, there is a significant negative impact on the health of the residents. These negative effects are compounded by the toxic waste sites and heavy industry that are often near these communities. Health care professionals need to take into account the entire environmental context of the people and communities with which they are working.

■ NURSING AND ENVIRONMENTAL HEALTH

An ICN press release noted that "over 1 billion persons in developing countries live without adequate shelter or [un]acceptable housing, 1.4 billion lack access to safe water, and 2.9 billion people have no access to adequate sanitation" (International Council of Nurses, 2000). All of these environmental conditions continue a cycle of ill health that has negative consequences for the general welfare of individuals, families, communities, and nations.

The Canadian Nurses Association (CNA) position statement entitled *The Environment Is a Determinant of Health* states that "the CNA will work with others in the health and social sectors to influence decisions that impact the environment and thus human health" (CNA, 2000). Of particular concern are the long-term health effects of contaminants on children. In a joint statement, the CNA and the Canadian Medical Association (CMA) indicate that "a healthy environment is fundamental to life, and attention to the effect of the environment on human health is imperative if we are to attain the goal of health for all" (CNA/CMA, 1996).

Multiple sources note, however, that nurses consider themselves unprepared to address environmental health issues, nurses are not aware of regulations and policies that affect the environment and health, and nurses believe they are not competent to recognize the health effects of environmental contaminants (Bellack et al., 1996; Green, 2000; Institute of Medicine, 1995). It is important to question why, with the plethora of scientific and popular literature available on environmental health issues, nurses do not consider themselves to have the knowledge and skills required to address these issues.

First and foremost, nurses require knowledge about the particular environmental issues that affect their own health and practice of nursing. Nurses face particular health risks from infectious diseases, chemicals, radiation, air pollution (such as moulds) within their work sites, physical injuries, and even violence in the community and the workplace. To address these concerns, it is important to examine the roles nurses have involving environmental health, the competencies that are required, and the methods to achieve these competencies regardless of their work settings.

Practice Roles and Competencies

Nurses are frequently the only health care professionals who enter the homes, workplaces, and communities of the individuals and populations they serve (Institute of Medicine, 1995). Practicing nurses need the skills to identify environmental hazards that may be related to the health concerns faced by an individual or a population. According to Eigsti-Gerber and McGuire (1999), nurses require education to act as investigators, educators, and advocates in environmental health issues for individuals, families, and communities. To do this, they must be aware of the environmental hazards that cause or exacerbate particular diseases in the population. To assist in assessment, diagnosis, intervention, planning, and evaluation, nurses also need basic knowledge of the following:

- Potential hazards in a geographic region
- Routes by which people may become infected (exposure pathways)
- Prevention and control strategies
- Adult learning principles
- Referral agencies and resources (Institute of Medicine, 1995)

It is important to understand provincial and federal government legislation, policies, and regulations related to environment and health. As noted before, many Canadians are surprised to find that uniform standards for water safety do not exist in this country, a fact that was highlighted in the Walkerton *E. coli* illnesses and deaths. Knowledge of who should advocate for safety standards and regulations—as well as how to do so—is essential if change is to occur. (*Note:* The strategies of letter writing, presenting resolutions, and lobbying politicians and others in power, as outlined in Chapter 1, can be used to address issues that have been analyzed and clearly articulated.) Box 22.3 provides an example of a resolution presented to the International Council of Nurses by Canadian nurses.

It is also essential to recognize the ethical implications of actions undertaken by individuals, corporations, and governments that affect the environment and health. The enhancement of education on environmental health for nurses, who compose the largest group of health professionals, has the potential to affect significantly the health of individuals, families, and populations.

BOX 22.3	Example of a Canadian Nurses Association Resolution on Chemicals, Pesticides, and Contaminants

Whereas, People the world over are increasingly concerned about threats to the environment and are demanding that these be addressed by their government;

Whereas, There is increasing evidence that the extensive use of chemicals and pesticides has a negative effect on our environment and our health;

Whereas, There is evidence that certain substances such as polychlorinated biphenyls (PCBs) are concentrated in mothers' milk, and that some chemicals and pesticides are chronic carcinogens;

Whereas, One hundred (100) nations committed to ratify the World Declaration on the Survival, Protection and Development of Children and the Plan of Action following the United Nations World Summit for Children (September 1990);

Whereas, The Plan of Action addressed the need to preserve and create healthy environments for children;

Whereas, Findings of research into the effects of chemicals and pesticides on immune system competence would give guidance regarding necessary actions to protect children from the effects of these substances;

Therefore be it

Resolved, That the International Council of Nurses and its member associations call on all governments to support research on the role of chemical contaminants in altering immune system competence; and epidemiological studies on mothers and children to determine the effects of present contaminant loads on children.

Accepted by the International Council of Nurses Council of National Representatives: Madrid, Spain; June 1993 (CMA/CMA, 1996, #22).

Education and Professional Development

Requests from the public for information on health concerns related to the environment are growing (Health Canada, 1998). Many sources recommend that all nurses have a basic knowledge of environmental health hazards, risks, prevention strategies, and health promotion (Bellack et al., 1996; Green, 2000; Institute of Medicine, 1995; McGuire & Eigsti-Gerber, 1999). To suggest simply that environmental health be added into the already full curricula of nursing programs has the potential for failure before it is even considered. There must be an examination of how the content and skills required for practice could be integrated within various courses throughout undergraduate and graduate educational programs as well as continuing education programs for practicing nurses.

However, adding into every health history the question "Is there something in the environment that causes or exacerbates this condition?" would raise awareness of the impact of the environment both for nurses and patients. Continuing education programs could be developed on emerging concerns in environmental health, risk communication, and referral to resources and agencies. Some suggestions for incorporating environmental health information into a nursing curriculum are proposed in Table 22.1.

Research

Relatively little research with a nurse as the principal investigator or connected to a nursing organization has been conducted on environmental health (Institute of Medicine, 1995). Because of the complexity of health and environmental concerns, interdisciplinary research that included professionals from a wide range

TABLE 22.1	Integrating Environmental Health Issues Into Nursing Curricula	
Course	**Competency**	**Type of Content**
Health assessment	Assessment and critical reflection	History taking; educating regarding risk
Introduction to nursing	Basic knowledge	Concepts relating environment and health
Medicine, pediatrics, maternal/child, family	Assessment and critical reflection	Relationship of environmental factors, such as water safety and air pollution, to health
Research	Basic knowledge; issues related to implementation of studies on the environment	Current research on nursing, health, and the environment
Issues and trends	Assessment; advocacy; team relationships	Policies, issues, and trends
Leadership	Advocacy; ethics; ability to initiate projects	Policies, procedures, legislation, roles of professional associations
Community	Working in multidisciplinary teams; advocacy; basic knowledge regarding population health risks; community development; empowerment of patients	Hazards; exposure pathways; prevention; program planning

of disciplines could prove to be the most effective method to examine environmental health-related issues. Research on which to base best-practice standards and educational programming is desperately needed. The development of nurse researchers interested in conducting studies with nurses and other practicing professionals is of paramount importance. Primary to the conduct of research are the availability of and access to funding. Of equal value is the dissemination of the results of research to nurses, other professionals, government officials, and the public. Nurses are encouraged to publish and present in both professional and public arenas to achieve as broad a distribution as possible.

■ SUMMARY

Water safety, air purity or pollution, chemical spills and spread, the growing contamination of inside environments, and violent surroundings are serious environmental concerns across Canada, as is the relationship of the environment to the health of individuals, families, and populations whether in the home, community, or workplace. The information in this chapter represents a snippet of the volumes of literature available on the topic.

Individual nurses and the nursing profession can play a role in improving societal health through the traditional routes of nursing practice, education, and research. Examination of issues that arise within the topic of health and the environment is a complex process. Using a consistent process (such as the one presented in Box 22.4) is an effective method to examine critically the issues that arise. Questions that help clarify each stage of the analysis are included. See Chapter 1 for additional interpretation of the process.

BOX 22.4 Steps for Resolving Issues

Using a format that outlines the process in a stepwise fashion is a helpful strategy for resolving an issue. The example below addresses the effects of the environment on health.

Topic identification: Environment and health

Societal values: Greater concern if local? Less concern if more distant? Are there economic factors that will preclude resolution? What other points?

Nurses' assumptions: What perspectives are important here?

Conceptualization of the issue: What is the definition of the issue? An example of an issue related to the topic is that nurses continue to identify their lack of education and skills regarding the environment and health.

Significance of the issue: How important is the issue and to whom?

Analysis: What is the background? Who in society is affected? Who benefits by change in the issue? Who benefits by the situation staying the same? What are the politics that surround the issue? Who is involved? Are there ethical ramifications?

Strategies for resolution: What can be done? What will be most effective? Who will and should act on these strategies? What barriers will hamper resolution?

Online Resources

Add to your knowledge of this issue:

Canadian Nurses Association	www.cna-nurses.ca/cna
David Suzuki Foundation	www.davidsuzuki.org
Environment Canada	www.ec.gc.ca
U. S. Environmental Protection Agency	www.epa.gov
International Council of Nurses	www.icn.ch
International Development Research Centre	www.idrc.ca/ecohealth/indicators
National Academies Press	www.nap.edu
National Center for Environmental Health (U.S.)	www.cdc.gov/nceh
Physicians for Social Responsibility	www.psr.org
TOXNET (U.S.)	www.toxnet.nlm.nih.gov
World Health Organization	www.who.int/peh
Worldwatch Institute	worldwatch.org

REFLECTIONS on the Chapter . . .

1. Cite specific examples from courses in your nursing program that link health and environmental conditions.

2. Name three health issues related to environmental factors that have been in the news recently in your local region and in your province/territory. Were nurses evident in the discussions?

3. What evidence is there that global climate change will affect the health of individuals and communities across the globe?

4. What legislation has your provincial/territorial government or the federal government passed in the last year regarding pollution/contamination in the environment?

5. What types of medical waste might have an impact on the environment? What is the potential for contamination or pollution to occur from medical waste? Where and how might this contamination or pollution happen?

6. What impact will the spread of diseases such as the West Nile virus have on health and environmental issues for Canadians? What implications does the increasing call for the control of pesticides have for the spread of disease?

References

Ahluwalia, R. (2000, May). *Ontario's rural heartland in shock* [Television broadcast]. CBC TV News. Toronto.

Bellack, J. P., Musham, C., Hainer, A., et al. (1996). Environmental health competencies: A survey of U. S. nurse practitioner programs. *Journal of Nursing Education, 35*(2), 74–81.

Berlinguer, G. (1999). Globalization and global health. *International Journal of Health Services, 29*(3), 579–595.

Brown, L., Flavin, C., French, H., et al. (2001). *State of the world 2001.* New York: W.W. Norton.

Canadian Nurses Association. (2000). *The environment is a determinant of health: Position statement* [Online]. Available: http://www.cna-nurses.ca

Canadian Nurses Association/Canadian Medical Association. (1996). *Joint CNA/CMA position statement on environmentally responsible activity in the health sector* (pp. 1–6). Ottawa: Author.

Carruth, A. K., Gilbert, K., & Lewis, B. (1997). Environmental health hazards: The impact on a Southern community. *Public Health Nursing, 14*(5), 259–267.

Chaudhuri, N. (1998). Child health, poverty and the environment: The Canadian context. *Canadian Journal of Public Health, 89*(Suppl. 1), S26–S30.

Clark, M. J. (1999). *Nursing in the community: Dimensions of community health nursing* (3rd ed.). Stamford, CT: Appleton & Lange.

Cox, K. (2002, April 13). Teen gang demanded money, father says. *The Globe and Mail*, p. A9.

Eigsti-Gerber, D., & McGuire, S. L. (1999). Teaching students about nursing and the environment. Part 1: Nursing role and basic curricula. *Journal of Community Health Nursing, 16*(2), 69–79.

Environment Canada. (2000). *Clean air* [Online]. Retrieved April 14, 2005, from www.ec.gc.ca/air/introduction_c.html

Foley, D. (2001, May). *Fuelling the climate crisis: The continental energy plan.* Vancouver: David Suzuki Foundation.

Green, P. M. (2000). Taking environmental health education seriously. *Nursing and Health Care Perspectives, 21*(5), 234–239.

Health Canada. (1997). *Health and environment: Partners for life* (Cat. H49-112-1/1997E). Minister of Public Works and Government Services Ottawa Canada.

_____. (1998). *The health and environment handbook for health professionals* (Cat. No. H46-2/98-211-2E). Minister of Public Works and Government Services Ottawa Canada.

_____. (1999a). *A second diagnostic on the health of First Nations and Inuit people in Canada* [Online]. Available: http:www.hc-sc.gc.ca/fnihb/cp/publications/second-diagnostic_fni.htm

_____. (1999b). *Toward a healthy future: Second report on the health of Canadians* (Cat H39-468/1999E). Minister of Public Works and Government Services Ottawa Canada.

Hilfinger Messias, D. K. (2001). Globalization, nursing, and health for all. *Journal of Nursing Scholarship, 33*(1), 8–11.

Institute of Medicine Committee on Enhancing Environmental Health Content in Nursing Practice. (1995). *Nursing, health, & the environment.* Washington, DC: National Academy Press.

International Council of Nurses. (2000). *Poverty impacts on health: Nurses remind G8 leaders* (pp. 1–2) [Online]. Available: http://www.icn.ch/pr13a_00.htm

_____. (2001). *ICN on occupational stress and the threat to worker health* (pp. 1–6). Available: http://www.icn.ch/matters_stress.htm

Last, J., Trouton, K., & Pengally, D. (1998). Taking our breath away: The health effects of air pollution and climate change. Available: http://www.davidsuzuki.org

MacKinnon, M. (2001, July 18). Vital to improve water quality on reserves, group says. *The Globe and Mail*, p. A5.

Malcolm, J., Liu, C., Miller, L., et al. (2002). *Habitats at risk: Global warming and species loss in globally significant terrestrial ecosystems.* Gland, Switzerland: World Wide Fund for Nature.

McDevitt, J., & Wilbur, J. (2002). Locating sources of data. In N. Ervin (Ed.), *Advanced community health nursing practice* (pp. 109–148). Upper Saddle River, NJ: Prentice Hall.

McGuire, S. L., & Eigsti-Gerber, D. (1999). Teaching students about nursing and the environment. Part 2: Legislation and resources. *Journal of Community Health Nursing, 16*(2), 81–94.

McMullan, C. (1997). *Indicators of urban ecosystem health.* International Development Research Centre. [Online]. Available: http://www.idrc.ca/ecohealth/indicators_e.html

Mitchell, A. (2001, June 4). The world's "single biggest threat." *The Globe and Mail.*

Nightingale, F. (1860). *Notes on nursing: What it is and what it is not.* (Reprinted London: J.B. Lippincott Company. 1992: Philadelphia)

Ottawa Charter for Health Promotion. (1986). First International Conference on Health Promotion. Ottawa. Retrieved April 14, 2005, from http://www.ldb.org/inhpe/ottawa.htm

Physicians for Social Responsibility. (1994). *What you should know about* avoidable *risks of birth defects and other reproductive disorders.* Retrieved April 14, 2005, from http://www.envirohealthaction.org/upload_files/NEWBirthBro.pdf

_____. (1997). *Asthma and the role of air pollution: What the primary care physician should know* [Online]. Available: http://www.envirohealthaction.org/upload_files/asthmap01.pdf

_____. (2001a). *Arsenic: What health care providers should know* [Online]. Available: http://www.envirohealthaction.org/upload_files/arsenicfs.pdf

_____. (2001b). *Cryptosporidium: What health care providers should know* [Online]. Available: http://www.envirohealthaction.org/upload_ files/cryptofs.pdf

Pope, C. A., Burnett, R., Thun, M., et al. (2002). Lung cancer, cardiopulmonary mortality, and long-term exposure to fine particulate air pollution. *Journal of the American Medical Association, 287*(9), 1132–1141.

Robson, M., & Schneider, D. (2001). Environmental health issues in rural communities. *Environmental Health, 63*(10), 16–20.

United Nations Environment Programme. (1999). *Global environment outlook GEO-2000* [Online]. Available: http://www.unep.org/geo2000

Wanke, M. I., & Saunders, D. (1996). Survey of local environmental health programs in Alberta. *Canadian Journal of Public Health, 87*(5), 345–350.

World Health Organization. (2004). The precautionary principle: Protecting public health, the environment and the future of our children. Retrieved April 14, 2005, from http://www.euro.WHO.int/document/EEHC/ebakdoc09.pdf

Critical Questions

As a way of engaging with the ideas in this chapter, consider the following:

1. Consider the assumptions that you hold about people who are different from you in relation to age, race, gender, education, and sexual orientation.

2. Take a moment to consider how you might have come to hold such assumptions.

3. As you begin to read this chapter, consider how these assumptions position you in your nursing practice.

CHAPTER

23

Christine Ceci

When Difference Matters: The Politics of Privilege and Marginality

In what ways do differences matter and to whom? Although these boys appear to be friends of the same age, they may come from different cultures, economic levels, and belief systems. Photography by Larry Arbour. Used with permission from the Faculty of Nursing, University of Calgary.

Chapter Objectives

After completing this chapter, you will be able to:

1. Discuss multiple interpretations of difference.

2. Discuss social, political, and historical influences on our understanding of difference.

3. Explore the concept of difference as a relationship.

4. Critique the concept of difference as deviance.

5. Identify assumptions underlying ideas of normality.

This is a chapter about difference or, more specifically, about the challenges and resistances we encounter, both from others and from within ourselves, when we try to move beyond the superficial in our efforts to understand difference. The obvious approach calls on us to define differences, to list them, to create categories, to suppose that the significance of any particular difference is clear or uncontested. The obvious approach often assumes that the meaning of various "basic differences," reflected in categories such as sex, race, or class, is given to us—that trusting the evidence of our senses, we can read off the surface the difference of another. This is the kind of thinking we want to let go of in this chapter—the thinking that says to us that difference is simply a characteristic, a trait, or a description easily assigned to another whose difference is obvious to us.

This is not to say, however, that activities of defining or categorizing are not sometimes useful but rather to suggest they almost always stop too soon. Although we often may need to begin by organizing our observations, these definitions, categories, labels, and lists are inadequate in and of themselves for understanding difference. In fact, in this chapter, the tendency these activities have of locating difference outside ourselves and the processes of our own understanding is conceptualized as a problem. Further, this is posed as a particular problem for nurses in part because of the privileged access we have to other lives. As nurses, we encounter people in their most vulnerable moments and so have opportunity to cause harm by unthinking adherence to the false and damaging beliefs and assumptions often contained in categories and labels. A willingness to question our own thinking, then, seems an obviously necessary task for nurses.

■ A PHILOSOPHICAL APPROACH TO UNDERSTANDING DIFFERENCE

Raising questions about the meanings of difference requires that we examine the various ways difference has been constructed in historical and contemporary situations. By reflecting on the examples explored in this chapter, we can ask who has defined difference in various situations and for what purposes particular boundaries between groups have been inscribed. On what basis are claims to difference made? How have the meanings of particular differences been contested? In what ways do differences matter and to whom? The historical examples allow us the distance to reflect on how particular ideas of difference have played themselves out and also, when considered alongside contemporary situations, enable us to trace similarities and extend our analyses from one context to another. For the same reason (i.e., so we may observe the similarity in processes of differentiation), a variety of what are commonly viewed as differences are explored. In each case, however, the difference discussed (e.g., race or sex) is not understood as a thing in itself but rather as an outcome of social processes of differentiation. Difference, then, is understood in this chapter as a relational concept, whereby the meaning of any particular difference depends on relationship and context.

Admittedly, this is a more philosophical approach to difference than some readers may be expecting, but if we wish to understand the complexity of ideas of difference, we must be willing to raise questions of meaning, a project that requires from us a certain amount of thoughtfulness. As used here, *thoughtfulness* refers to a conscious and critical engagement with our current understandings of difference, an engagement that encourages us to question what we think we already know. This, then, is the purpose of this chapter: to "problematize" difference. We will proceed by exploring the discourses and ways of thinking that define difference and consider the social contexts and conditions through which differences come to matter.

Historical and Contemporary Considerations

Accounting for difference among people, in situation and status, in privilege and power, has long been a preoccupation of Western societies. From at least as early as Plato's argument for the naturalness of unequal social status for men, women, and slaves, the purpose of these narratives has been, with few exceptions, to explain and justify the prevailing social order. Throughout Western history, dominant belief systems suggested that people were positioned in particular ways in society because of inborn differences in capacities and worth. These differences were often understood as determined by what were considered unalterable laws of nature. The differences in situation between men and women, rich and poor, races and cultures were all informed by ways of thinking that assumed the properness and inevitability of existing social roles and hierarchies. These ways of thinking, which interpreted selected anatomic, biologic, and phenotypic differences as signs of inherent worth, were typically generated by people who occupied positions of privilege in the same social order they sought to justify. For example, even as late as 1919, the American psychologist H. H. Goddard could publicly argue that "the people who are doing the drudgery are, as a rule, in their proper places" (cited in Gould, 1996, p. 191).

The Significance of Marginalized Perspectives

Understanding and explaining difference, and arguing the grounds on which differences are seen to lie, continue to be major concerns in Western societies—but with one significant change. Many of those theorizing difference today have a stake in transforming rather than justifying existing social arrangements. For some, challenging what are considered inadequate interpretations of difference is related to awareness of the growing complexity of our societies, to increasing racial and ethnic diversity, and to the persistence of social inequities. In some respects, the presence of oppositional social movements (i.e., groups organized around a shared commitment to eradicate social, political, and economic inequities) has placed the need to rethink difference on the public agenda. Oppositional social movements question the validity of social norms and challenge ideas and practices viewed as contributing to the oppression, exclusion, and exploitation of marginalized groups. Marginalized groups—those that have been excluded from the social mainstream, including groups representing the interests of women, people of color, people living with poverty, gays and lesbians, and people with disabilities—pose alternative explanations for their experiences and positions in the social world. In doing so, they challenge the seeming naturalness of existing social roles and arrangements.

The challenges these movements offer are practical and material, having to do with access to resources and opportunities. They are also philosophical, having to do with how we perceive and interpret our worlds. Part of the challenge of oppositional social movements is the challenge they present to our commonsense understandings of society. For example, a challenge people living with poverty may pose to members of dominant groups is whether, in doing the "drudgery," they are, in fact, in their proper places or whether larger social and economic processes limit their opportunities. To understand this situation adequately, we need to ask who is doing what jobs in society. Are some groups disproportionately responsible for the dull, menial, and fatiguing work? How do we explain this? Similarly, some women have argued that it is not a law of nature that they be primarily responsible for the care of children and have instead raised questions about how the caring work of society is allocated and rewarded.

When given voice, members of marginalized groups point out the inaccurate and limited nature of many dominant social narratives—those common, familiar stories we draw on almost unthinkingly to understand our world. For example, there are dominant social narratives that explain the presence of poverty in our society. Chief among these are those that suggest that poor people are responsible for their poverty by virtue of their own inadequacies—this is the "flawed character" view of poverty (Banyard & Graham-Bermann, 1995). This explanation of poverty is partial and inadequate because it locates the "problem" of poverty inside the person and obscures the social, political, and economic arrangements that create and sustain poverty.

Marginalized groups also question the ability of those in positions of privilege to know or understand the experiences of less powerful groups. By contesting the adequacy of dominant perspectives and, hence, their reasonableness as the justification for existing social relations, and by offering alternative perspectives, marginalized groups challenge the authority of those in positions of privilege to speak for all of society. Developing more inclusive interpretations of society and more just practices involves taking these concerns of marginalized people seriously. It also involves recognizing that the experiences of many members of society are ignored or distorted by dominant social narratives. Although these narratives are commonly held to explain or describe all of reality, they more often depict only the experiences or situation of a particular social group.

The Insufficiency of Dominant Perspectives: False Universals

History holds many examples of these ostensibly universal discourses revealed instead to refer only to the experience of particular dominant groups. For example, understanding "man" as equivalent to "human" has, in many cases, been demonstrated to be a false universal. The falseness becomes apparent when excluded groups claim the benefits of these discourses or positions for themselves, but, because they are not members of dominant groups, their claims are disallowed or unacknowledged.

In 1929, to cite a well-known example from Canadian history, a particular group of Canadian women demanded to be considered persons under the law. They argued that, in practice, the apparently inclusive and gender-neutral legal concept "person" excluded women. Their argument demonstrated that their female bodies were, in this case, a difference from a male standard that mattered in terms of their rights and privileges in society. Yet many of those who successfully argued that this gender difference should not matter and who advocated for the legal personhood of Canadian white women did not similarly champion the legal rights of, for example, aboriginal women. In this case, "gender" for aboriginal women was inflected by race in a way that mattered for the status of First Nations women, whose right even to vote was not achieved until many decades after other Canadian women.

Similarly, in the late 19th century, when American white women organized to gain the right to vote, their failure to include women of color provoked ex-slave Sojourner Truth to ask, "Ain't I a woman?" Although she was, of course, biologically female, the dominant social ideology concerning women merged the term *woman* with particular and culturally specific ideals of femininity. "Real" women were gentle, passive, physically frail, in need of male protection, and white. "Real" women did not work the fields, never "plowed and planted, and gathered into barns" (Truth, 1851, cited in Trinh, 1989, p. 100). Truth's words challenged the then dominant conceptualization of "woman" because an affirmative answer to her challenge would have required a rethinking of what being a woman, in that time and place, meant. Her black body and her experiences as a black woman were differences that mattered in terms of her rights and privileges in society.

These two examples from "women's" history demonstrate how a supposedly neutral and inclusive category such as "woman" often disregards the experiences of entire groups of women who do not fit the tacit conceptualization on which it is based. These examples also suggest that practices of exclusion have adverse consequences for the status of those excluded.

Nursing and Exclusionary Practices

Organized nursing in Canada, particularly through the early 20th century, was not immune from this kind of exclusionary practice. In their efforts to elevate the status of nursing, the nursing profession and health care administrators promoted nursing as a bastion of feminine respectability. They defined nursing according to a particular paradigm of appropriate femininity that drew on racist and classist stereotypes to exclude certain women from education and employment. Canadian historian of nursing Kathryn McPherson (1996, p. 17) writes, "Because nursing relied on an image of feminine respectability to legitimate nurses' presence in the health care system and their knowledge of the body, respectability was constructed in a racial and national context." She also claims, based on the evidence of historical records, that "nurses' respectability and definition of gentility were European in origin. White, native-born Canadian women were expected to bring their superior sense of sexual and social behaviour to the bedside" (McPherson, 1996, p. 17). Although some women of color and immigrant women were able to obtain nursing training, they were expected to provide service only to their "own" communities. "In the eyes of hospital administrators and nursing leaders, Canadian women of non-European heritage could not be relied on to reflect the morality of health at the bedside" (McPherson, 1996, p. 17). In fact, until after World War II, "administrators remained convinced that the very presence of non-White attendants might exacerbate the health problems of White patients" (McPherson, 1996, p. 17). As McPherson (1996, p. 17) argues, these kinds of beliefs suggest that nursing's exclusivity was "not merely the innocent by-product of objective standards."

As a result, nursing in Canada was "the preserve of white and Canadian-born women" (McPherson, 1996, p. 17) for most of the 20th century. Although nursing shortages since World War II have necessitated an opening of occupational boundaries, issues of racism and workplace discrimination persist in nursing. In 1992, for example, a group of African-Canadian nurses successfully argued in front of the Ontario Human Rights Commission that they experienced racial discrimination and harassment in their workplace (McPherson, 1996). This suggests that, although the face of nursing has changed significantly in recent decades, nursing is also a product of a society in which whiteness is systematically privileged (Dyer, 1997). Having a body, a particular and specific body that is not only sexed but always simultaneously raced and classed, is almost always a difference that matters. The meanings and implications of these differences and others are considered in this chapter.

■ THE CHALLENGE OF DIFFERENCE

Part of the challenge that difference offers us is that our knowledge of the world is always limited by our positioning within it. This means that where and how we are located in the social world influences our experiences, our ways of thinking, and the discourses available to us to shape and express our understanding. Discourses consist of beliefs, assumptions, and statements that, although rarely conscious, form our possibilities for knowledge. A discourse of nursing, for example, includes the ways we speak of nursing as well as the ideas, rituals, practices, and social power relations that make nursing a recognizable entity. However, at any point in time, nursing is intersected and influenced by many, sometimes competing, discourses. For example, there are discourses that define nursing as caring, as vocation, or as skilled women's work, and there are others that emphasize the instrumentality or technical nature of nursing work.

To add to this complexity, our positioning in the world is often ambiguous, characterized by multiplicity rather than singularity. For example, a particular woman's understanding of what it means to be a woman is determined not only by her gendered difference from men but also by the many facets of her difference from other women. The meaning of being a woman will always be colored by the things a woman is and does, whether she is poor; whether she is a mother, a refugee, or a lesbian; whether she works as a nurse, an engineer, or a prostitute or receives social assistance. All of the features of her life texture what being a woman means, just as being a woman changes the meaning of all else that she is and does. What is significant here are the ways in which our circumstances and situations affect the nature of our experiences, what we take as fact, what we consider to be normal or natural, and the ways this changes over time and across society (Ceci, 2000).

The Canadian population is stratified by many relations of difference, and encountering difference is part of everyday life. But not all differences matter in the same way. Rather, it is our interpretations of difference—not specific differences in themselves—that influence whether and how they will matter. That our perspectives are limited and partial is not a problem, particularly not one that we can overcome. Limitedness is accepted simply as the character of our situation. However, in light of the limitedness of our perspectives, how do we proceed in a world with other people in it? To respond to this question, we can explore various interpretations of difference and hope to develop new understandings of what difference means in our lives and in our practices. Although difference as an issue is not resolvable, we can explore what it means to name difference. We can consider what it means to practise nursing with respect for difference. Our concern here is with both the meanings attributed to difference and the implications of these meanings in people's lives.

■ THEORIZING DIFFERENCE

We begin with two related questions. First, what does the term *difference* mean? And, second, what does it mean to theorize difference? A difference, to our common sense at least, is that which distinguishes one thing from another. Although this seems a fairly straightforward definition, it does not tell us whether difference is a feature of the thing itself or if distinguishing difference is a function of our habits of perception. That is, do we assign difference because something is different or because we are accustomed to perceiving it as different? Is it even possible to discriminate between these two activities? This is where theorizing enters the picture. Theories shape our seeing and our possibilities for interpretation. They "provide us with a way of ordering, understanding and capturing aspects of reality" (Cheek & Purkis, 1997, p. 160). Although theories can guide us in picking out features of the world that we then treat as significant, they can also blind us to other, equally important aspects of reality.

Theories organize the way in which a phenomenon such as difference will be perceived and represented (Cheek & Purkis, 1997). Described in these terms, theory is not just something located in books or classrooms; rather, all of our seeing and understanding should be thought of as theoretical. Our interactions with reality should be understood as informed beforehand by our beliefs, assumptions, and expectations. Like scientists, researchers, and others who consciously use theory, we too are guided in our lives, in our practices, "by a certain conception of the way things are" (Caputo, 1987, p. 215), by theories. For example, the primacy of race in social classification systems can be understood not simply as a reflection of a reality that contains people who have skin of various hues but as a testament to theories that say this must be important. Or, as Ahmed (1998, p. 27) writes, "bodies are never simply bodies: they are always inscribed within a system of value differentiation," a system that asserts which features of the body, which of its diverse aspects are worth paying attention to.

The Influence of Theories on Perception: Race as a Category

A good example of how particular theories influence our perceptions of the world is found in theories that suggest that racial differences are important units of analysis. Those who hold these views, consciously or unconsciously, will assume that just knowing a person's race can tell us important things about them. Race becomes a category that is "internalized into ways we think about other people . . . and ourselves" (Allen, 1996, p. 99), and stressing its significance leads us to perceive people initially and sometimes chiefly in terms of skin color and phenotype. Race, understood as visible difference, becomes one of the first things we see and interpret as meaningful when we look at a person. But is race, aside from the meanings we attribute to it, an important difference? And how do we know this? And then, how do we incorporate into our analysis the contemporary scientific evidence that demonstrates that race, as a meaningful biologic category, is not real (Alcoff, 1999)?

In societies that continue to categorize, classify, and rank people according to a conception of race that suggests innate, immutable differences among groups, how do we account for the fact that the "overall genetic differences among human races is astonishingly small" (Gould, 1996, p. 353)? How do we account for the fact that there are no such things as "race genes," or genes that are present in certain races but lacking in all others? Does knowing of this "remarkable lack of genetic differentiation among human groups" (Gould, 1996, p. 352) alter our understanding of what we have become accustomed to perceive as intrinsically and biologically distinct groups?

These are important questions because they ask us to reconsider our commonsense belief that race constitutes an obvious and important biologic difference among people. One would expect that these questions would direct us to seek other explanations, other than the biologic, for the tenacity of racial categorization and ranking in our societies. Yet despite significant efforts in this direction, "scientific" research seeking to establish innate difference among groups continues unabated (Brah, 1996).

The Classification of Bodies in History

A useful location from which to begin to rethink race and racial classification systems is history. Here we can see that race has not always been understood as especially relevant, even though in Western societies skin color and phenotype are currently considered important signifiers of difference (Weedon, 1999). Rather than disclosing fixed and stable natural categories, the salience of race as a significant social difference has changed over time. And because it has a history, we can see how human beings have made it. Specifically, its history reflects the development of the natural sciences in the 18th and 19th centuries. Racial categories were constructed by biologists and anthropologists as part of a project to order and classify the entire natural world (Alcoff, 1999; Gould, 1996; Weedon, 1999).

In addition, early scientists did not simply describe the realities they observed but rather interpreted difference in light of their pre-existing values, beliefs, and judgments. They ranked perceived differences in body type and appearance according to preconceived notions of character and worth. "The meanings attributed to nineteenth-century racial categories included value judgements about beauty, intellect, morality, emotionality, sexuality and other physical capacities" (Weedon, 1999, p. 153). These judgments, which always assumed the inherent superiority of the white race, came in handy because they "justified colonialism, the slavery of Africans, and the appropriation of African, Asian, and American land and human resources by whites" (Essed, 1996, p. 7). These practices came to be seen as the natural outcome of inborn inequalities between the "races."

In addition to interpretations of the meaning of skin color, 18th-, 19th-, and 20th-century scientists theorized links between particular physical features and what were believed to be inborn characteristics, such as intelligence or criminality. High foreheads, low brows, small heads, large jaws, big arms, as well as skin color were all interpreted as direct and uncomplicated reflections of character and capacity. Yet there are literally thousands of ways to measure the human body, and any investigator convinced beforehand by a theory, such as the hierarchic ordering of races, could easily choose the measurements, inadvertently or not, that would subsequently prove his or her theory true (Gould, 1996). These theories of the meanings of racial difference, which can be grouped under the general heading of biologic determinism or sociobiology, take bodies as "their referent and guarantee" and view bodies as the definitive and transparent source of differences among groups (Weedon, 1999, p. 13). Classifying people according to visible difference is a process that "seeks to systematize differences and to relate them to differences of character and worth" (Dyer, 1997, p. 20).

A Continuing Practice

Although one might expect this kind of thinking to have disappeared by now, in some ways, it has simply become more sophisticated. As outmoded and offensive as these views are, publications such as Herrnstein and Murray's (1994) *The Bell Curve: The Reshaping of American Life by Difference in Intelligence* and Rushton's (1995) *Race, Evolution, and Behavior* suggest that, no matter how often these concepts are exposed as vacuous by reputable thinkers, there will be someone—charlatan, fraud, or disingenuous scientist, politician, or social commentator—who is convinced that race and other physical features are important explanations and guarantees of social difference.

The Significance of Theorizing Difference

Recognizing that our understanding is theoretical and, therefore, that our interpretations of difference are informed beforehand by theory is important for at least three reasons.

First, this allows us to appreciate that certain features of the world, particularly those we tend to take for granted as naturally occurring, are, in reality, shaped by our pre-existing theoretical commitments and assumptions—commitments and assumptions we have simply by virtue of being born into a culture. For example, we may assume that race is an important biologically based difference among groups not only because of the "evidence" of our senses but also because our cultural and social experience supports this theory. It is, at some level, obvious to us.

Second, awareness of what we take for granted allows us to attempt to make the beliefs and assumptions that inform our theoretical views explicit rather than implicit. The theoretical perspective informing our assumption about the significance of racial categories is often called *biologic determinism*. This theory supports several propositions, including that of H. H. Goddard, which was mentioned earlier in this chapter: "The people who are doing the drudgery are, as a rule, in their proper places" (cited in Gould, 1996, p. 191). People are believed to be located where they are in the social world essentially for biologic reasons.

Third, consciousness of the specific ways of thinking that influence our understanding allows us to consider the reasons we might choose to hold one theoretical position rather than another. We might ask: What are the views of the people doing the drudgery concerning their proper place? Are their views even available to us? Why might people in positions of privilege hold the views they do? In what ways do social arrangements and the allocation of privileges and resources work to justify a particular social order and the ways of thinking that support it? If race is not an important biologically based category, what kind of category is it? Social? Political? What purpose does it serve?

■ DIFFERENCE AS DEVIANCE: A CASE OF BIOLOGIC DETERMINISM IN PRACTICE

Different theories—meaning different ways of ordering and interpreting the world—are more than just words. Theories have tangible effects in the world because of the ways in which they shape institutions and practices. The way something is understood, including the kind of problem it is seen to be, has implications for how we think it should be addressed. By focusing in some detail on a particular episode in Canadian history—the pre– and post–World War II preoccupation with the discourses and practices of social hygiene and eugenics—it is hoped that we can achieve some insight into how this happens. We can then take our understanding of this situation and use it to create new understandings of how issues of difference are theorized in our current contexts.

Part of the usefulness of knowing our own history lies in the ways it can help us to understand how others have attempted to respond to complicated issues, and perhaps even to locate the origins of our own ways of thinking. If we can do this, we can begin to recognize our beliefs as a particular way of thinking rather than the truth and reflect on how ideas we may hold have played themselves out in other times and places. Understanding how and why particular ideas may resonate for us or seem so obviously true offers us the opportunity either to take these ideas up more consciously and deliberately or to develop alternative points of view.

Eugenics and Social Hygiene in Canadian History

Eugenic discourses advocating the necessity of intervening in the course of human reproduction flourished openly in many Western countries for the first half of the 20th century fueled by the fears and uncertainties of a rapidly changing world and "consuming concern about the health and welfare of the race" (Dowbiggin,

1997, p. 165). In Canada, the social problems and public health challenges associated with increased immigration and urbanization led many prominent political figures and public health advocates, respected physicians, and psychiatrists to preach a gospel of social hygiene and racial purity rooted in the widespread fear that "traditional Canadian ideals, values and attitudes . . . were disappearing" (Dowbiggin, 1997, p. 134). Erroneously claiming that science could correct the hereditary "deficiencies" believed to cause poverty, crime, and vice, many influential public figures across the country advocated sterilization, segregation, and eugenic immigration restrictions as essential strategies for both public health and social reform (Dowbiggin, 1997). Swept up in the limitless possibilities for advancement that science seemed to offer, and by the expanding authority of medical and scientific discourses to pronounce on all areas of human life, claims that these measures would improve public health were claims that almost no one doubted (Paul, 1998). Faith in science, in its neutrality and objectivity, convinced many proponents that their positions were purely objective, inevitable, and rational responses to the "facts" of scientific knowledge. Such certainty did more than merely mask the cultural values latent in eugenic discourses; it made dissent seem both irrational and irresponsible.

As a pseudoscientific theorizing of difference, eugenic thinking was and is an argument for the biologic innateness of particular defining traits, most notably a belief in the hereditary determination of intelligence and character. Thriving particularly during the economically troubled 1930s, eugenic discourses explained social problems in terms of individual inadequacies, inadequacies defined in terms of, and relying for meaning on, pre-existing social structural relations of class, gender, and race (Valverde, 1991). The physically and mentally subnormal, the different, the deviant, the feebleminded, the unfit, and the defective were categories encompassing those with actual physical and mental illness as well as children who merely performed poorly on standardized tests, unmarried mothers, labor activists, aboriginal people, immigrants of color, and other nonwhites. These groups were assigned the blame for many social problems and were viewed as posing a threat to the smooth functioning of society through their supposedly inborn propensity for violence, crime, and aberrant sexual behavior. So widespread was this way of thinking that even labor unrest was understood by some not as the product of problematic social arrangements but as the result of defective brains (Dowbiggin, 1997).

During these years, it was clear to many influential Canadians that if a particular class of human life was to be preserved and enhanced, then preventive measures to control and contain those who threatened the existing social order, both through their dangerous behaviors and the economic burden their care represented, must be undertaken. This, a social argument, attained greater legitimacy and authority when it was rendered in scientific terms—terms that transformed complex social problems into mere matters of health and disease inviting medical intervention.

Although eugenic thinking could be found everywhere in Canada, only 2 of 10 Canadian provinces enacted sterilization acts—Alberta in 1928 and British Columbia in 1933. Other provinces debated these issues but chose not to create legislation, which is not to say that involuntary sterilization procedures were not performed across Canada without benefit of a law (McLaren, 1990). Eugenic policies, often framed in the language of social hygiene or cleanliness, were directed toward creating stronger, healthier societies through weeding out those deemed unfit in the dominant discourses of the day (Pernick, 1997). Across Canada, there was a general consensus, among dominant groups at least, that controlling the reproduction of some groups, segregating those deemed defective, and restricting immigration on eugenic grounds were warranted public health measures.

It is clear that the problems that eugenic policies were meant to address were very much problems of difference. As Canadian society was becoming more and more obviously heterogeneous, the fear that Canadian values and ideals were being lost was prevalent among more established groups. Eugenic policies were articulated from this center (i.e., by members of dominant groups) and had their greatest effects on society's weakest or most marginalized members. Differences that mattered were clearly framed by categories of class, race, and gender.

For example, in the case of eugenic sterilizations, the supposedly scientific and rational decisions made by eugenic boards clearly revealed the decided influence of social criteria of normality and value

(Dowbiggin, 1997; McLaren, 1990; Paul, 1998; Pernick, 1997). Those sterilized tended to be female, young and inexperienced, poor, rural, a member of a racial or ethnic minority group, and unmarried. In other words, those referred for sterilization procedures were rarely members of the dominant group; rather, as Pernick (1997, p. 1770) observed, "race, class, ethnic, religious and sexual prejudices determined who was defined as unfit."

Difference as Deviance: Assumptions of Normality

As noted previously, eugenic discourses explained social problems in terms of individual inadequacies, inadequacies that were thought to be reflected in and confirm one's proper position in society. These arguments typically focused on individual deviance from a supposed norm and gained legitimacy when they were communicated in scientific and medical terms that diagnosed those outside the dominant social order as diseased. Thus, complex social problems were transformed into matters of health and illness.

Although it is common to treat concepts of health and illness as matters of fact (Caplan, Engelhardt, & McCartney, 1981), ideas of both health and illness are only meaningful in relation to some prior conception about what is normal (Susser, 1981). And *normal* is not a neutral term with clear and self-evident meaning; rather, ideas of normality are constructed within particular sociohistorical contexts and always contain an evaluative element concerning what is understood to be usual, acceptable, and valued.

Concepts of normality require value judgments to be made, and their use implies the presence of a regulative structure that produces both the "normal" and the "not normal." Because ideas of normality are most often produced and employed by those in positions of social dominance, the experience and values of dominant groups tend to represent that which is then thought to be normal for everyone. For example, many school-aged children were labeled feebleminded or subnormal in the early decades of the 20th century after failing to pass standardized intelligence tests. These tests contained what we now recognize as "arbitrary norms of intellectual achievement" (McLaren, 1990, p. 38). Rather than providing objective, scientific measures of intelligence as it was then believed, these tests reflected the experiences and values of the dominant group who produced them. Children who were not members of this group were less likely to perform well. In some instances, then, what is conceived of as deviance from normality might be more usefully and accurately understood as a distant or marginal relation to a powerful center. This was certainly the experience of many Canadians labeled different or deviant during the years when eugenic policies and practices were prevalent.

Eugenic Practices and Public Health: Nursing Roles

In considering the role of nursing in the implementation of eugenic practices and policies, it is important to recognize that there were links between eugenic discourses and public health goals, beliefs, and values, what has been called "the convergence between genes and germs" (Pernick, 1997, p. 1769). With very little tolerance for difference, the supposedly defective, unfit, and subnormal were constructed in dominant discourses as deviant and diseased. And because public health nurses were concerned with protecting the health of society in general from any number of sources of disease, their goals were apparently congruent with those of the eugenicists whose interpretations of health and illness dominated public discussions.

Segregation, institutionalization, and restrictive immigration were all conceptualized as necessary social and mental hygiene measures intended to stop the spread of an unseen contagion, and to sterilize meant, in eugenics as in bacteriology, "to eliminate agents that cause disease" (Pernick, 1997, p. 1769). In some ways, nurses' actions in implementing these policies and practices, actions that included assessing children in homes and schools, identifying candidates for sterilization, making referrals to eugenics boards, providing operating room assistance, and assisting in the "Canadianizing" of new immigrants (Mansell & Hibberd, 1998), were simply extensions of the nursing role to care for the health and welfare of the population, at least as that task was then defined.

Nursing Practice and Dominant Thinking

This last point, however, is where difficulties for nurses may arise. Nursing and nurses are constituted within the dominant society and within the possibilities and constraints of particular sociohistorical contexts. The conduct of nurses, in this time and place, should be understood in relation to the lesser status of women in society, the subordination of nurses in the health care hierarchy, the rewards nurses received for compliance, as well as the absence of an alternative discourse or way of thinking about difference. Nurses consented to what was dominant in medical and societal thinking, to a particular understanding of difference influenced by the tenets of biologic determinism, a theory that we now clearly understand as informed by false beliefs and assumptions and as having caused significant harm to vulnerable people. This consent was not particular to nurses but rather a reflection of prevailing attitudes and beliefs or, as Mansell and Hibberd (1998, p. 9) have written, "nurses handled, managed, and controlled individuals in order to maintain a society that adhered to the wishes of the dominant group, of which they were part."

Significance for Contemporary Nursing

The purpose here, however, is not to suggest that nurses were right or wrong in terms of their participation but rather to consider the implications for ourselves, as nurses, of the possibility that we also may become the means through which social and moral harms are perpetrated. Nurses must consider these issues simply because they are often in the position of implementing policies not necessarily of their own making, of supporting and sustaining particular social and political arrangements of health care. It is a dilemma for nursing that, although much of our work, particularly in the area of public health, involves the care of socially, economically, and politically marginalized or disadvantaged people, the dominant voices in defining health and health care policies rarely come from these groups. In their roles as "conduits into the lives and social spaces of groups otherwise beyond the reach of social agents of authority" (Rafferty, Robinson, & Elkan, 1997, p. 3), nurses may have a special responsibility to be attuned to the differences of marginalized perspectives.

■ DIFFERENCE AS RELATIONSHIP

The meanings given to difference, whether that difference is named in terms of gender, race, class, intellectual ability, or sexual orientation, assume immediate significance for people because these meanings are used to circumscribe and explain experience, to influence both the lived meanings and material realities of a life. The meanings given to femaleness, for example, have been important to women "because they were used to determine and limit the social and economic spheres to which women had access" (Weedon, 1999, p. 10). Consider these words of the late 19th-century founder of social psychology, Gustave Le Bon: "All psychologists who have studied the intelligence of women, as well as poets and novelists, recognise that they represent the most inferior form of human evolution and that they are closer to children and savages than an adult, civilized man" (Le Bon, 1879, cited in Gould, 1996, p. 137). Le Bon goes on to describe women, who, with the rare exception, may be ignored as being "as exceptional as the birth of any monstrosity," as typically and naturally illogical, irrational, childish, capricious, and unreliable. Given that this is, in Le Bon's view, the nature or essence of woman's being, education for women, as well as any role for women outside the home, was seen not only as a wasteful indulgence but also as against nature and, therefore, dangerously aberrant.

As ludicrous as this now sounds, the importance for women lies not only in the aspersions cast on their characters and capacities, although these are not insignificant, but also in the ways in which these types of views have limited and constrained women's access to resources and opportunities for so many years. Women, in all their various social locations, have learned "who [they] are and how to think and behave through discursive practices" (Weedon, 1999, p. 104). As these social and political practices of thinking and theorizing have become entrenched through institutions such as psychology (medicine, religion, philosophy, and law), the difference of being a woman has come to matter in ways that have had and still have real material consequences for women. The meanings attributed to sex differences have justified the social, political, and economic inequality of women. These kinds of practice have had similar consequences in the lives of others who are marginalized and diminished on the grounds of their difference from a dominant group.

The difference of women, which is clearly meant to be understood as the difference between men and women, and most probably the difference between men and women of a particular race and class, is articulated by Le Bon as naturally occurring inferiority and lack. This is clearly not a neutral difference (e.g., one that would mean simply not the same). Rather, difference is organized in terms of a relationship in which one side is understood as being or setting the standard the other fails to achieve, a process still quite common in Western thinking.

Dualism and Difference

Western societies have tended to arrange many important features of the world into oppositional and exclusive dualities, necessary hierarchies whose meaning both reflects and sustains clear and pervasive differences in social power and status. Male/female, white/black, rich/poor, and straight/gay are examples of dualisms that organize difference in crude, yet highly effective, structures in which one side of the duality is clearly meant to be understood as superior to the other. The other in each case is named and defined in relation to the dominant group, whose power in some respects resides in the very capacity to create the kind of relationship that establishes "us here and them over there" (Trinh, 1990, p. 371), to name and to define those not themselves as "other." In the case of Le Bon, the claim is made that *us here men* are plainly the natural social masters of *them there women*—a crude but unquestionably effective process of differentiation and social categorization.

Limitations of Dualist Thinking

In dualistic thinking, difference is organized into simplistic, oppositional, and exclusive categories. This occurs despite the limited explanatory power such frameworks for understanding hold. As well as reducing our understanding of men and women, for example, to terms of difference and suggesting that women and men should only be understood in opposition to one another, dualistic thinking tends to erase differences among women and suggests that women should be understood only in terms of sameness—both clearly inadequate proposals. Strictly dualistic conceptualizations of difference limit our understanding of the multiple and shifting ways we are positioned in relation to others. A white middle-class or affluent woman may find herself and her opportunities limited in relation to the men in her life, but she may exercise power in her relation to other, less advantageously positioned men and women. Sometimes, the difference of gender may be in the foreground; at other times, race, class, and sexual orientation may be the differences that matter—sometimes singly, sometimes all at once.

Difference as a Relation Between Margin and Center

It is important to recognize that when we are perceiving difference, a relationship of some sort is being inferred, although the fact of relationship is often assumed rather than plainly stipulated. That is to say, there is a norm or a standard to which we refer, consciously or unconsciously, implicitly or explicitly, when we identify someone or something as different. The identification and production of difference, then, are bound up with assumptions concerning the socially, culturally, and politically relevant features of persons, which, in Western societies, have generally corresponded to the ways in which we are categorized according to gender, race, sexual orientation, and class. These differences mark people as different in relation to a dominant and presumably unmarked group, a group that in Western societies has tended to be composed of white, propertied, able-bodied, heterosexual males.

In this way, our identification of difference can be understood as the recognition of a particular relation between margin and center, between dominant and subordinate groups, with the differences that matter most arising in the context of relations of power. Relations of power are intrinsic to all social relations, but of particular concern are those that establish access to such things as resources, opportunities, and knowledge: "Power takes many forms, affecting access to material resources as well as questions of language, culture and the right to define who one is" (Weedon, 1999, p. 5).

Thus, besides trying to understand the processes through which difference is produced, understanding who defines whom as different is also always of significance. These relations of difference attain their significance for us when they result in structures of inequality or patterns of disadvantage: "Differences between individuals and groups—between sexes, classes, races, ethnic groups, religions and nations—become important political issues when they involve relations of power" (Weedon, 1999, p. 5).

Processes of Differentiation

Difference is produced through social processes of categorization. Some feature of a person is selected as significant and defined against a backdrop of dominant assumptions, beliefs, and values and in relation to that which is believed to be usual, or traditional, normal, or natural. These activities of selection and interpretation, however, cannot be thought of as politically neutral: "Both the construction of commonality among subjects and the assertion of difference between subjects are rhetorical and political acts, gestures of affiliation and disaffiliation that emphasizes [sic] some properties and obscures others" (Felski, 1997, p. 17). For example, designating income level as a person's most significant characteristic brings to the fore a single aspect of a person's identity while rendering invisible much else that the person is and does. Income level stands in for a more particularized explanation of life and circumstances and allows people living with poverty, for example, to appear as an undifferentiated mass. Conceptualizing difference as a relation rather than a thing in itself, and instead of a feature of people that exists independently of our theorizing about it, encourages us to inquire into the social relations through which differences that matter are produced.

For nurses, coming to understand the ways in which marginalized populations are related to the dominant social center means theorizing how apparently neutral differences are the result of structures of inequality or patterns of disadvantage affecting particular groups in particular ways. The prevalence of poverty among women provides a good example because women's poverty is both disproportionate and relatively intransigent. Women as a group are more likely than men as a group to live in poverty, and, although women have made gains in many areas of life, this situation has remained relatively unchanged. In 1997 in Canada, for example, 2.8 million women, or 19% of the total female population, were living in low-income situations (Statistics Canada, 2000). Although improved access to education, increased participation in the labor force, smaller family sizes, and changes in the structure of family living have improved the lives of many women, women in all age categories and family types are still much more likely to be poor than are men.

Single mothers and elderly women continue to be those with the greatest likelihood of living in poverty, and there is an especially high incidence of poverty among women of color, immigrant women, First Nations women, and women with disabilities. Each of these groups, in addition to being female, departs in some way from a dominant societal norm circumscribed by a white, middle-class, male, heterosexual, youth-oriented, able-bodied perspective. Not only is the other defined and named in relation to this dominant group but also relations of power and privilege are structured or shaped by this relationship.

For both women as a group and women with particular differences, distance from this center can be seen as having the power to shape both social relations and individual experience. Poverty, given this situation, could be theorized as being neither inherent nor accidental but rather as centrally about power, and society's economic organization could be one way in which relations of power are enacted in many women's lives, determining their success in obtaining both material and social resources. This type of thinking would stand in opposition to views that suggest women are disproportionately poor because they are flawed in some way. Being female in our society is clearly a difference that matters, a difference from a male norm, a difference whose consequence may be read in the likelihood of living in poverty.

Differences and Relations of Power

The social relations that work to construct the lived meanings, as well as the material realities, of differences such as gender, race, sexual orientation, and class can also be understood as relations of power. In fact, to raise the question of difference in the context of social relationships requires that we recognize that our interpretations of difference are always and in every case the "effects of many types of power relations" (Weedon, 1999, p. vii).

Attending to power means understanding that activities of labeling, defining, and categorizing are power moves and often result in some members of society being subjected to and by the power of others: "Those who claim a dominant position can presume the right to determine which aspects of identities are core, and by which aspect others will be known" (Kaplan, 1997, p. 34). The power exercised by dominant groups to name the differences that matter includes the capacity to determine the kind of difference something is understood to be. That is, is a particular named difference cultural, political, natural, or biologic? Is it normal or pathologic? Acceptable or perverse? Power is what makes differences matter—the power to impose definitions, to determine meanings, to shape reality.

For example, in a context in which heterosexuality is assumed dominant and is believed to be "normal," sexuality for gay men and lesbians, whether they wish it to or not, may become their significant defining feature, the aspect by which they will be known. To say of someone that "she is lesbian" has a different meaning and effect than to say "she is heterosexual" because, in our society at least, heterosexuality is assumed; it is not to be different at all. In naming a woman lesbian (which must be understood as different than naming oneself), a particular difference is called into being, a difference that matters in part because of its relation to a dominant center and to ideas of normality. In addition, a different kind of knowledge of the person is assumed, a knowledge that seems to be saying that the most important thing about this woman is her sexuality, and it is important not because of the meanings it holds for her but because it differs from a supposed norm. For those who are marginalized in relation to a dominant center, the consequences of being categorized in this way can be quite serious and range from having reduced access to resources and opportunities to the failure to have one's understanding or interpretation of one's own experience matter. A peculiar silencing occurs when what becomes most important about a person is how they are defined by others, by their perceived relation to the dominant group, to a supposed norm or center.

■ THE DISTINCT REALITIES OF OTHERS

It has become a cliché to suggest that, as a society, we must learn to live with difference. This can mean anything from halfheartedly agreeing to merely tolerating difference to the desire to embrace and celebrate diversity among people. Where we locate ourselves in this situation will depend, to some extent at least, on how we have chosen to interpret difference.

In the case of racial differences, for example, we have seen that, although many continue to believe that the meaning of race is located in biology, actual genetic differences between races are insignificant—the meaning of racial difference is not self-evident in the sense of being directly attributable to nature. Yet although race is a constructed rather than natural category, race, whether we are privileged or marginalized because of it, remains a compelling force in all of our lives, shaping our understandings of ourselves, our relationships with others, our possibilities and constraints.

Race in our social worlds is important because we attribute particular meanings to it. We should probably be willing to ask ourselves what it is, exactly, that we think race means. As we notice a person's skin color, his or her appearance, what do we think we already know about that person? Is reading off the surface in this way anything more than a reflection, not of the person but of ourselves, of our own and our society's beliefs, assumptions, and biases?

Similarly, the meanings of gender, sexuality, and economic status, to name only a few of the differences that constitute our social worlds, can also be understood in this way, as constructed within social relationships and as deserving of the same kind of questioning. These are categories that, like race, have the effect of seeming natural but that, to be realized, virtually always require value judgments backed up by the authorizing practices of various institutionalized discourses, such as those of medicine or law or religion. And these are only some of the most obvious differences, those that are enforced and reinforced by relations of power.

As nurses, in our privileged and intimate relationships with others, we must not only resist racist, sexist, classist, and heterosexist definitions of people, we must also be willing to reconcile the innumerable significant and insignificant ways we may differ from one another. Naming difference is not simply a descriptive act but one that creates a relationship that is often, although not always, a relation between margin and center, dominant and subordinate groups. In part because of the power we hold to influence events and experiences, we must take the distinct realities of others seriously. Nursing and nurses are embedded in a larger social world, and, because of this, we are not free of the constraints and prejudices that shape all of society. Yet "consequences are enacted by nurses, not as individuals, but because they are part of a larger system" (Liaschenko, 1998, p. 76). We have, perhaps, a greater responsibility than others for a critical consciousness of the beliefs, values, and assumptions that shape our thinking and inform our actions.

But what does this mean, this challenge that nurses practise with respect for the distinct realities of others? In the first place, it means that nurses must understand that there exist many competing discourses that make truth claims about people, that these truth claims do not exist equally, and that some versions of the world and some voices are privileged over others (Weedon, 1999). If, as Sherwin (1992, p. 222) has suggested, people's health needs "vary inversely with their power and privilege in society," then nurses need to recognize that quite often the people who are the focus of their attentions are also the ones whose voices are silent or silenced in determining the practices and processes of health care. Respect for difference, for the distinct realities of others, requires, at the very least, a willingness to re-evaluate what will count for us as important sources of knowledge and meaning. We must develop a capacity to hear the voices of the least powerful.

Second, nurses need to understand that they themselves are socially, culturally, economically, and politically situated. We are "located at particular positions, each of which enables and constrains the possibilities of experience" (Grossberg, 1996, p. 99). Our "situatedness" means we are not necessarily going to be able to understand the experience of others, and this knowledge of our limitations is simply the unavoidable character of our situations. But knowing of the partiality and limitedness of our own perspective can compel us to seek other views, to acknowledge that our own understanding is rarely adequate or sufficient (Strickland, 1994). Practising with respect for the distinct realities of others means recognizing that the singular significant characteristic of nursing practice is that someone else is there, someone who must be allowed to speak to us, to really tell us something.

Difference for nurses can mean diversity, a recognition of plurality and multiple points of view. This is important, but there is another meaning of difference that may be even more meaningful for nursing, a meaning of difference that has its roots in the essential alterity of others—the inescapable otherness of others. This is what Caputo (1993) calls the "difference that makes a difference" (p. 56) wherein "everything turns on a respect for difference, for the other one" (p. 60). This is difference that is singular, focused on this person, this particular other who is before me, here and now. The ethic of a nursing relationship is such that the presence of this particular other is fundamental rather than incidental to how we will proceed, an ethic that is compromised whenever we assume we already know the meaning of another person's life.

■ SUMMARY

In this chapter, difference has not been presented as an issue to be resolved but rather as a feature of the world that we must consciously consider. Difference is conceptualized as a relationship, the meaning of which is determined in part by how we choose to interpret our worlds. Familiar frames of reference, such as definitions or categories, have been presented as inadequate for truly understanding difference. These have been critiqued for the ways they mask complex and changing social relationships and conceal social processes of differentiation.

What has been raised for consideration in this chapter is how particular differences are constructed and how the meanings attributed to them come to matter in economic, social, and political domains. We are asked to think about how various categories of difference become invested with particular meanings rather than take the meanings of what are named as important differences to be self-evident.

Online Resources

Add to your knowledge of this issue:

Canadian Nurses Association	www.cna-nurses.ca
differences: A Journal of Feminist Cultural Studies (although not exclusively about gender)	muse.jhu.edu/journals/differences
University of Michigan Diversity Initiatives	www.rackham.umich.edu/StudentInfo/Diversity
Workplace Diversity Network	www.ilr.cornell.edu/depts/WDN
World Trust Foundation	www.worldtrust.org

REFLECTIONS on the Chapter . . .

1. From your practice experience, identify differences that seem to matter. Who has named and identified these differences as significant? In what ways do they matter and to whom?

2. Explore how difference is a concern or feature of your practice. What difference does it make to conceptualize difference as a relationship rather than a characteristic or trait?

3. Because difference is not an issue to be resolved, how would you proceed in your practice, given that the world is full of difference? Identify the assumptions and beliefs that influence your understanding and interpretation of difference.

References

Ahmed, S. (1998). *Differences that matter: Feminist theory and postmodernism.* Cambridge: University Press.

Alcoff, L. (1999). The phenomenology of racial embodiment. *Radical Philosophy, 95,* 15–26.

Allen, D. (1996). Knowledge, politics, culture, and gender: A discourse perspective. *Canadian Journal of Nursing Research, 28*(1), 95–102.

Banyard, V., & Graham-Bermann, S. (1995). Building an empowerment policy paradigm: Self-reported strengths of homeless mothers. *American Journal of Orthopsychiatry, 65*(4), 479–491.

Brah, A. (1996). *Cartographies of Diaspora: Contesting identities.* London: Routledge.

Caplan, A., Engelhardt Jr., H., & McCartney, J. (Eds.). (1981). *Concepts of health and disease: Interdisciplinary perspectives.* Reading, MA: Addison-Wesley.

Caputo, J. (1987). *Radical hermeneutics: Repetition, deconstruction, and the hermeneutic project.* Bloomington: Indiana University Press.

_____. (1993). *Against ethics: Contributions to a poetics of obligation with constant reference to deconstruction.* Bloomington: Indiana University Press.

Ceci, C. (2000). Not innocent: Relationships between knowers and knowledge. *Canadian Journal of Nursing Research, 32*(2), 57–73.

Cheek, J., & Purkis, M. (1997). "Capturing" nursing? Theories concealed in writings about nursing practice. *Social Science in Health, 3*(3), 157–163.

Dowbiggin, I. (1997). *Keeping America sane: Psychiatry and eugenics in the United States and Canada, 1880–1940*. Ithaca, NY: Cornell University Press.

Dyer, R. (1997). *White*. London: Routledge.

Essed, P. (1996). *Diversity: Gender, color, and culture*. (R. Gircour, Trans.). Amherst: University of Massachusetts Press.

Felski, R. (1997). The doxa of difference. *Signs, 23*(1), 1–21.

Gould, S. (1996). *The mismeasure of man* (Rev. ed.). New York: W. W. Norton.

Grossberg, L. (1996). Identity and cultural studies: Is that all there is? In S. Hall & P. Du Gay (Eds.), *Questions of cultural identity* (pp. 87–107). London: Sage.

Herrnstein, R., & Murray, C. (1994). *The bell curve: The reshaping of American life by differences in intelligence*. New York: Free Press.

Kaplan, A. (1997). How can a group of white, heterosexual, privileged women claim to speak of "women's" experience? In J. Jordon (Ed.), *Women's growth in diversity: More writings from the Stone Centre* (pp. 32–37). New York: Guilford Press.

Liaschenko, J. (1998). Moral evaluation and concepts of health and health promotion. *Advanced Practice Nursing Quarterly, 4*(2), 71–77.

Mansell, D., & Hibberd, J. (1998). "We picked the wrong one to sterilize": The role of nursing in the eugenics movement in Alberta, 1920–1940. *International History of Nursing Journal, 3*(4), 4–11.

McLaren, A. (1990). *Our own master race: Eugenics in Canada, 1885–1945*. Don Mills, ON: Oxford University Press.

McPherson, K. (1996). *Bedside matters: The transformation of Canadian nursing, 1900–1990*. Toronto: Oxford University Press.

Paul, D. (1998). *The politics of heredity: Essays on eugenics, biomedicine, and the nature–nurture debate*. Albany: University of New York Press.

Pernick, M. (1997). Eugenics and public health in American history. *American Journal of Public Health, 87*(11), 1767–1772.

Rafferty, A., Robinson, J., & Elkan, R. (Eds.). (1997). *Nursing history and the politics of welfare*. London: Routledge.

Rushton, P. (1995). *Race, evolution, and behavior*. New Brunswick, NJ: Transaction.

Sherwin, S. (1992). *No longer patient: Feminist ethics and health care*. Philadelphia, PA: Temple University Press.

Statistics Canada. (2000). *Women in Canada, 2000: A gender-based statistical report*. Ottawa: Author.

Strickland, S. (1994). Feminism, postmodernism and difference. In K. Lennon & M. Whitford (Eds.), *Knowing the difference: Feminist perspectives in epistemology* (pp. 265–274). New York: Routledge.

Susser, M. (1981). Ethical components in the definition of health. In A. Caplan, T. Engelhardt, & J. McCartney (Eds.), *Concepts of health and disease: Interdisciplinary perspectives* (pp. 93–106). Reading, MA: Addison-Wesley.

Trinh Minh-ha, T. (1989). *Woman, native, other: Writing postcoloniality and feminism*. Bloomington: Indiana University Press.

_____. (1990). Not you/like you: Post-colonial women and the interlocking questions of identity and difference. In G. Anzaldua (Ed.), *Making face, making soul: Creative and critical perspectives by feminists of color* (pp. 371–375). San Francisco: Aunt Lute Books.

Valverde, M. (1991). *The age of light, soap, and water: Moral reform in English Canada, 1885–1925*. Toronto: McClelland & Stewart.

Weedon, C. (1999). *Feminism, theory and the politics of difference*. Oxford: Blackwell.

As a way of engaging with the ideas in this chapter, consider the following:

1. Begin to think about the assumptions that you hold about nursing in First Nations communities.

2. How have you come to hold these assumptions?

3. What might be the influence of these assumptions and beliefs on the provision of health care to First Nations people?

CHAPTER

24

Fjola Hart Wasekeesikaw

Challenges for the New Millennium: Nursing in First Nations

Nursing students from the University of Manitoba Baccalaureate Nursing Program, Norway House, are dedicated to advancing health care among the First Nations. Front row (l-r): Cheryl McKay, Georgina Henry, Tena Flett, Harriet Hart, and Barb Queskekapow; back row (l-r): Tracy Fosseneuve, Allison Saunders, Kim Cooper, Glenda Muskego, and Stacy Dixon. Photograph by Lorraine Robertson. Used with permission from the University of Manitoba.

After completing this chapter, you will be able to:

1. Describe the relationship between the colonization of First Nations people and health-related issues.

2. Analyze the significance of concepts of population health in addressing issues of inequity.

3. Examine the different views of health held by the First Peoples in Canada, the First Nations.

4. Interpret the significance of cultural resurgence, community development, and the expressed need to widen the scope of health and transfer of health care services to First Nations communities.

5. Evaluate the role of nurses and nursing in the delivery of health care services to First Nations communities in Canada.

6. Examine the following issues confronting nurses in the provision of health care services to First Nations people:
   - Population demographics and the relationship to the health care needs
   - Transfer of health care services in relation to nursing issues
   - Need for cultural competence
   - Educational needs for nurses working in First Nations communities

This chapter introduces the reader to issues related to health, health care, and nursing for First Nations people in Canada and presents basic information to facilitate greater understanding of First Nations people. Key to understanding is recognition of the great diversity among First Nations communities and the views of health held by First Nations members. Also discussed are the relationship between the historical attempts for enfranchisement of First Nations people and health-related issues and the significance of cultural resurgence among First Nations in community development. How these factors influence the practice of nursing in Canada and how, in turn, nurses can potentially influence the health care of First Nations people will be explored. Additionally, current issues related to the nursing and delivery of health care to First Nations people will be identified.

■ DIVERSITY OF THE FIRST PEOPLES

The 560 First Nations in Canada constitute a diverse population of descendants of the First Peoples of North America. Many of these nations are further grouped into tribal councils, which provide unity and greater political power as well as combined resources among nations. Each First Nation has its own reserve land base, traditional territories, culture, and language.

First Nations are part of a larger group of aboriginal people. As defined in the Canadian Constitution Act, the term *aboriginal* refers to First Nations, Inuit, and Metis. All aboriginal people originate from 11 different language families (Smylie, 2000, p. 1072): Algonkian, Athapaskan, Haidan, Iroquoian, Kutenaian, Salishan, Siouan, Tlingit, Tsimshaian, Wakashan, and Inuit.

According to the Indian Act, an act of the Canadian Parliament, First Nations members are legally defined as "Indians." The Indian Act, first passed in 1876, was designed to administer programs to Indians for the purpose of assimilating them into Canadian society; the act also determined who was legally defined as an Indian. There have been many revisions to the Indian Act since its inception, but the purpose remains the same. Each person who is deemed to be legally Indian has a registration number to reflect her or his population number within her or his band or First Nations community.

Some First Nations members are also referred to as having "treaty" status. This term applies to those First Nations that signed treaties with the British or Canadian governments. Between 1817 and 1929, the First Nations conducted negotiations with the British government or with Canada in the right of the Crown, resulting in the signing of more than 20 international treaties. Through this treaty process, the Treaty Nations agreed to cede certain lands for use and settlement in return for specific guarantees. These guarantees are the treaty rights of First Nations. The treaties reserved lands and resources for continued use and existence as First Nations. The treaties also guaranteed specific social and economic rights to ensure continued strong First Nations governments. For example, the Natural Resources Transfer Agreements of 1930 guarantee that First Nations people residing in Manitoba, Saskatchewan, and Alberta have the right to hunt, trap, and fish—except for commercial purposes (Indian and Northern Affairs Canada, www.ainc-inac.gc.ca/index_e.html). Ultimately, the First Nations leadership guaranteed the right to be born and live as a First Nations person.

The term *Indian* originates from early explorers to North America who thought they had discovered India. First Nations members assert that the roots of this term are inappropriate and serve to reflect a history of colonialism. To reflect more appropriately that they are descendants of the First Peoples on this continent, the First Nations have determined that they would be identified accordingly.

■ EUROPEAN RELATIONSHIP WITH FIRST NATIONS

What is the significance of the impact of colonization on the lives and ways of living of First Nations families and communities in Canada? *Colonialism* (a result of colonization) is considered to be control by one power over a dependent area or people. It also refers to policy based on such control. Before contact with European colonizers, the First Peoples had their own systems of government, trade, and health care. After confederation, Canada began to displace the First Nations from their traditional territories to make room for the ever-increasing influx of European settlers. Government policies were developed to protect, civilize, and assimilate the First Peoples into Canadian society. The final outcome of these measures was cultural genocide. The process undertaken to achieve this end would greatly affect the mental, physical, and spiritual health of First Nations. The inherent oppressive and suppressive nature of these policies has had, and continues to have, far-reaching negative effects on First Nation governance and cultural identity.

Because of its extensiveness and the length of the time during which colonization took place, this chapter presents no more than a brief overview. The risk in attempting to discuss the historical highlights is the potential to oversimplify the European relationship with the First Nations and the long-lasting negative effects on the population. With this in mind, the history will briefly cover the following key phases:

- Cooperation, nation to nation
- Colonization and its effects on the health of First Nations members and their communities
- First Nations' cultural resurgence

Cooperation Among Nations

Colonization did not begin at the point of original contact between the Europeans and First Nations. Unlike the history between the First Peoples and European settlers in the United States, where wars established the dominance of European culture, the initial relationship between the First Peoples and first the French and then the British in Canada was one of mutual tolerance and respect. The social, cultural, and political differences between these societies were maintained. This reflected how First Nations related to each other. The newcomers came to a continent that was already inhabited by diverse nations of indigenous people who formed alliances and good relations with one another to access and distribute their tribal resources (Dickason, 1994, p. 76).

The First Peoples had their own economic, health, political, and social systems that were developed within their communities according to their traditions and the need imposed by their environments. When the first Europeans came into contact with the First Nations, each thought of the other as distinct and autonomous. Each nation continued to govern its internal affairs. Nations cooperated in areas of mutual interest and were connected in various trading relationships and other forms of nation-to-nation alliances.

The Royal Proclamation of 1763 demonstrates that the partnership between First Nations and the British Crown was one of cooperation and protection. In exchange for cooperation in the partnership that characterized the relationship between them at that time, the king of England extended royal protection to the First Peoples' lands and political autonomy. When Canada was formed in 1867, a legislative basis for dealing with the Indian people as nations had already been established.

Colonization and the Effect on First Nations

The written word reflects an author's attitudes and beliefs, and so it was that the plans of action or policies to carry out the government laws reflected the attitudes of the people who wrote these policies. The Indian Act was the legislative vehicle for implementing policies to civilize, protect, and assimilate the Indian people (Tobias, 1991). No single event marked the beginning of these colonial practices. Rather, they began with the attitudes of the time and laid the foundation for a series of actions that deemed the Indian people as inferior beings. Government laws still reflect these attitudes today; in doing so, these laws perpetuate a colonialistic attitude.

A series of actions led to the proclaiming of the Indian Act. This was one act of many that laid the foundation for the civilization program that was developed in 1828 and gave rise to the reserve system that became a social laboratory designed to enable Indian communities to adopt European values (Tobias, 1991). This program established Indians in isolated, fixed locations where they could be educated, converted to Christianity, and transformed into farmers. The goal was to eradicate the First Peoples' values through education, religion, new economic and political systems, and a new concept of property. Not only was the distinct cultural group to disappear but so, too, was the laboratory where these changes were brought about. It was assumed that each Indian person who became enfranchised would also take his share of the land from the reserve.

The Assembly of the United Canadas of the Gradual Civilization Act of 1857 provided the criteria for determining whether an Indian person qualified to become enfranchised. A special board of examiners determined each applicant's merit based on whether the person was educated, free from debt, and of good moral character. If so, the person was awarded 20 hectares of land within the colony and "the accompanying rights" as a citizen of the Dominion (Milloy, 1991, p. 147). One of the accompanying rights was the opportunity to vote in the country's elections. It was assumed that Indian people would sever ties with their communities and embrace colonial living and values.

The British North America Act of 1867, establishing the Canadian nation, also contained the forerunner of the Indian Act and placed First Nations, and lands reserved for them, under the legislative authority of the Canadian federal government. The Indian Act was amended almost every year to address unanticipated problems in carrying out the government policies. The need for policy revision also reflected resistance by First Nations people to change their values and cultural ways (Milloy, 1991). The amendments persisted on a course to erode the land base of First Nations, wipe out traditional political governance, and smother traditional ways of expression and living. Some effects of the amended Indian Act include the following:

■ *The erosion of the protected status of reserve lands.* In 1894, the government leased reserve land held by physically disabled Indian people, widows, orphans, or others who could not cultivate it (Royal Commission on Aboriginal Peoples, 1996a). These tracts of land were not surrendered, nor was approval required by the First Nations communities for the government simply to take over the land and lease it to European settlers. Later, in 1918, the leasing of reserve lands that had not been surrendered was broadened to include any uncultivated lands if the purpose of the lease was cultivation or grazing. Only Indian people who were able to cultivate their land were allowed to keep tracts of reserve land. This was in violation of treaty obligations connecting Canada to the Royal Proclamation of 1763, wherein Indian title to land and the need to obtain proper surrender of Indian lands were identified.

■ *The undermining of traditional political processes used by First Nations communities.* The federal government determined how First Nations community leadership was to be elected and interfered with the decision-making processes of the communities' affairs. The superintendent of Indian affairs determined the time, place, and manner in which the elections took place (Milloy, 1991). In addition, the governor could remove a chief or councilor from office if he thought the leader was dishonest, intemperate, or immoral. The interpretation of these terms and how they were applied to each case was left to the governor's advisors and departmental agents. The extent to which community members participated in the elections was limited to all males over the age of 21 years who could vote for their officials. The chief and council were forced to function within a foreign-designed and foreign-controlled system.

Federal authority also set a bureaucratic system of controlling the communities' affairs. The nature of the concerns in which the chief and council could make decisions was preset; in addition, each decision was subject to confirmation by the governor (Cassidy & Bish, 1989). The chief and council functioned within a narrow, federally controlled context, for example, making bylaws for a variety of purposes. Some of these bylaws include the control of band membership; provision of public health; regulation of commerce, traffic, construction, and buildings; assurance of the observance of law and order; prevention of disorderly conduct and nuisances; construction and maintenance of water supplies, roads, bridges, and other public works; regulation of animal populations; and removal of trespassers from reserve land. By interfering with the governing processes of First Nations communities, the federal government undercut the authority of the First Nations communities' leadership.

■ *The suppression of the traditions and values of First Nations.* In a concerted effort to extinguish any traditional beliefs and practices in the First Nations community, laws were enacted to ban all traditional ceremonies and to control Indian movement from one reserve to another (Milloy, 1991). It was thought that intertribal gatherings, celebrations, and ceremonies were the primary obstacles to Indian people becoming Christians. In 1884, the potlatch and the Tamanawas dance were prohibited, with a jail term of 2 to 6 months for any Indian who was convicted of engaging in or assisting with these dances. In later years, further amendments banned the practice of other traditional dances such as the Blackfoot Sun Dance. In part, the system was an attempt to control discussion between political and spiritual leaders living on various reserves. In 1885, Indian people were prohibited from traveling off their reserves without written authorization of the Indian agent on the reserve. These laws were designed to suppress historical, social, and political organization of First Nations societies and governments.

Government laws and policies have systematically assaulted First Nations in their spiritual practices and in their social organization, governance, and economic activities. For many First Nations, the residential school system in which the state and church attempted to capture and socialize First Nations children was the sharpest cut of all (Royal Commission of Aboriginal Peoples, 1996b). The residential school experience left in its wake dislocation and a strong sense of loss for individual students and their families, with rippling, cumulative, intergenerational effects on First Nations communities. Dislocation from one's community effected many losses, including culture, language, spirituality, identity, pride, self-respect, and ability to parent. This left many communities trapped between what remained of traditional ways of doing things and the fear of importing too much more of mainstream Canadian cultural values into reserve life. The residential school system insult to the spirit of the First Nations people has had, and continues to have, destructive effects on families and communities. It is important to recognize however, that colonization processes have not been successful in eliminating First Nations. Rather, they have propelled First Nations to embark on reviving traditions and proclaiming their identities.

Attitudes and policies reflecting the colonial system continue today because the present health care and government systems exist on a foundation of protection, civilization, and assimilation (Smylie, 2000). This has repercussions for the relationships between the First Nations people and their health care providers.

■ CULTURAL RESURGENCE OF FIRST NATIONS AND COMMUNITY DEVELOPMENT

The First Nations cultural resurgence and community development share similar roots and are closely intertwined. In the 1960s, First Nations people demanded the right to set their own cultural course. They spoke out about indigenous perspectives on development. Their voices were significant in creating a pathway on which community development could be used to bring about economic and social changes in First Nations communities.

Until 1951, when the Indian Act was revised, laws banned First Nations members from attempting to organize themselves. With the revisions to the Indian Act, First Nations members began the enormous task of developing political organizations to strengthen and improve the situations of First Nations people (McFarlane, 2000). Members began traveling from community to community, discussing issues and potential actions to change the conditions within the communities. Over the ensuing decade, tension between First Nations and the government of Canada developed. The early 1960s was a time when government control was so deeply entrenched that policy controlled almost every aspect of First Nations people's lives, interests, and concerns. For example, the Indian Act affected the family unit in that it provided for arbitrary enfranchisement of an Indian woman who married a person who was not registered as an Indian. Within a family unit, women's status as band members could cease depending on whom the female siblings married. Concomitant with this example, the Wildlife Act prohibits any Indian person from giving meat to a non-Indian. The non-Indian person in this case could be a sister who is enfranchised.

First Nations people set out to challenge policies reflecting a belief that Canadian institutions alone could prescribe solutions to the problems faced by First Nations people. They had different ideas about dealing with their own issues. Provincial organizations were developed to deal with concerns facing the status of Indian people. Nationally, the first status Indian organization, the National Indian Brotherhood, was started in December 1968. (*Note:* The term *status Indian* is applied to an Indian person who is registered under the Indian Act.) The National Indian Brotherhood gave a single voice to all status Indian people in Canada (McFarlane, 2000). Of particular significance was the First Nations response to the White Paper, a Canadian government policy statement in 1969 that aimed to abolish all First Nations rights, including rights to reserve lands. The First Nations response shifted the nature of the relationship the First Nations would have with the government of Canada; the response would be key in moving away from a relationship whereby Indian people were the wards of the state. First Nations governing their own affairs would provide a basis for developing community-specific health and healing systems.

■ MIYUPIMAATISSIIUM: BEING ALIVE WELL

Miyupimaatissiium, or "being alive well," is seen as an interdependent relationship people have with the natural world and with keeping one's spirit strong (Adelson, 1991; Hamilton & Sinclair, 1991; Malloch, 1989). Culture, language, and traditions used to express concepts similar to that of *being alive well* vary from one First Nations community to another. For example, to the members of a First Nations Eastern Ininiwuk—or "human beings"—community, also known as the Cree people, in the province of Quebec, Ininiwuk food is essential to miyupimaatissiium. Game and fish are requirements for miyupimaatissiium and symbolize essential aspects of Ininiwuk life.

To the people in this community, "eating well" means that one has been eating bush food, or food from the land, and from this, it can be assumed that there has been a good hunting season. In turn, a good hunting season signifies that one has the physical strength required to work in the bush. Miyupimaatissiium is evidence of an experienced hunter and of a woman who has the skills and ability required for preparing the meat and hides. The spiritual aspect of eating well is at the moment when the animal chooses to give itself to the hunter. The relationship between an Ininiwuk hunter and the animals hunted for food is based on mutual respect. A cyclical affinity between the Ininiwuk (human being), hunting, the land, and food incorporates all aspects of life and so too, being alive well. Miyupimaatissiium is a holistic concept encompassing people in relation to their environment and all that is within the universe. The Royal Commission of Aboriginal Peoples (1996c) identified that holism is an integral part of aboriginal health and healing systems.

Health Status of First Nations People in Canada

The First Peoples enjoyed good health in the Americas; then, as result of European contact, the decimation and extinction of many First Peoples followed. The effects of infectious diseases, such as smallpox, were devastating to the health and cultures of the First Peoples. They suffered many losses, ranging from decreased community sizes to a strong sense of personal and collective loss. The epidemics resulted in declining fertility rates because infected women were unable to conceive or carry their pregnancies to term and also in decreased chances of conceiving as a result of population loss and subsequent lack of partners. Loss of relatives and large numbers of community members resulted in loneliness, grief, and depression. Loss of leaders, warriors, and hunters, and the reduced size of communities, made it difficult to protect territorial boundaries (Ray, 1974). This resulted in migratory shifts in the tribal territories and the modification of economic roles from trappers to middleman traders. Canadian historian Olive Dickason presented to the members of the Royal Commission of Aboriginal Peoples reasons for the impressive state of good health of the First Peoples and then related the impact of infectious diseases on their health and well-being:

Some analysts argue that disease agents themselves were rare in pre-contact America until the tall ships began to arrive with their invisible cargo of bacteria and viruses. What is more likely is that Aboriginal people had adapted well to their environment; they had developed effective resistance to the microorganisms living along side them and had knowledge of herbs and other therapies for treating injury and disease . . . some . . . died prematurely. But more stayed well. Or recovered from illness, and thus lived to raise their children and continue the clans and the nations. Aboriginal populations fluctuated largely in relation to food supply.

Hundreds of thousands . . . died as a result of their encounters with the Europeans . . . infectious diseases were the greatest killer. Influenza, measles, polio, diphtheria, smallpox, and other diseases were transported from the slums of Europe to the unprotected villages of the Americas. . . . Aboriginal people were well aware of the link between the newcomers and the epidemics that raced though their camps and villages. During the eighteenth and nineteenth centuries, their leaders sought agreements or treaties with representatives of the British crown aimed at ensuring their survival in the face of spreading disease and impoverishment. In the expectation of fair compensation for the use of their lands and resources and in mounting fear of the social and health effects of Euro-Canadian settlement, many Aboriginal nations, clans and families agreed to relocate to camps, farms, villages or reserves distant from sites of colonial settlement. Many did so in the belief that the Crown would guarantee their wellbeing for all time. Given the gulf that separated Aboriginal and non-Aboriginal cultures, it is not surprising that the meaning of those oral and written agreements has been a matter of conflicting interpretation ever since (Royal Commission of Aboriginal Peoples, 1996c, p. 112).

Use of a Population Health Approach to Address Inequity

Population health includes a study of the determinants of health and disease, health status, and the degree to which health care affects the health of the community (Shah, 1998). An examination of the determinants of health helps to identify and then address inequities within the health care system (Evans, Barer, & Marmor, 1994). Many First Nations have identified the significance of clean drinking water; safe, uncontaminated food; reliable sanitation; comfortable housing and workplaces; and adequate employment as essential to the health of the population (Royal Commission on Aboriginal Peoples, 1996c). The health of

Transfer of Health Care Services to First Nations

As of March 2002, 284 First Nations communities—out of 599 communities eligible for transfer—have taken on the administrative responsibility for health care services—either individually or collectively— through multicommunity agencies or tribal associations (Health Canada, 2002). In addition, 41 First Nations communities are involved in the pretransfer process. Communities that have completed the transfer process are employers for nurses and other health care personnel in their communities.

Every community is unique in the manner in which it establishes its own health and healing system. The extent and manner in which traditional views about health are used in developing the system or in influencing existing health care services will lie with each community. The Royal Commission on Aboriginal Peoples (1996c) proposed that new aboriginal health and healing systems embody the following four essential characteristics:

1. Pursuit of equity in access to health and healing services and in health status outcomes
2. Holism in approaches to problems and their treatment and prevention
3. Aboriginal authority over health systems and, where feasible, community control over services
4. Diversity in the design of systems and services to accommodate differences in culture and community realities

The key to restoring well-being among aboriginal people originates from within aboriginal cultures (Royal Commission on Aboriginal Peoples, 1996c). There will likely be as many variations of health care delivery systems as there are First Nations communities in Canada. Self-determination in the development of community health care systems is essential.

■ CLIMATE FOR CHANGE: NURSING IN FIRST NATIONS COMMUNITIES

Nurses have played a vital role in the delivery of health services in First Nations communities over the past century. Nursing is at a critical crossroads in addressing the health care needs of people living in First Nations communities. Improving the overall health status of First Nations people is the impetus for creating more effective ways of delivering nursing care services that reflect the health and healing systems determined by each community or tribal council. Aboriginal nursing services are an integral part of a First Nations community's health and healing system. A community's processes for economic development and participation in transfer of health care services can serve as vehicles for making these changes. This would require nurses to learn how the First Nations community or tribal council in which they work views health and healing, whether community development is being used, what is being planned, and what changes have been made. Having this information will provide nurses with context and an understanding of the health care priorities selected by the community. These are important elements of a population health approach and the use of community development principles in providing nursing care in First Nations communities.

First Nations communities face many challenges, and some of these are barriers to the delivery of effective health care services (O'Neil et al., 1999, p. 147). Some of the barriers include the following:

1. *Scarce resources.* Beginning in 1995, the federal government capped increases in spending directed to First Nations and Inuit health services.
2. *No real autonomy for First Nations communities who have assumed administrative responsibility for health services.* Along with limited resources, a lack of planning for the increasing need for trained personnel to fill positions in a community's health and healing system, and a lack of resources to train personnel, communities have inadequate resources to develop new models of health programming. Unless nurses collaborate with community members and communities at large to overcome this major barrier, health programs to address the need will not be realized.

3. *Emphasis on curative services.* The Canadian health system's focus on curative services and the poor health of many First Nations communities mean that the limited health resources are focused on treatment services.

4. *Emphasis on physical health.* The Canadian health system ignores holistic health and culturally based health programming.

5. *Lack of attention to health promotion and disease prevention.* With the emphasis on curative programming, there are few resources for innovative health promotion and prevention.

6. *Lack of health service integration.* There is no single, concerted approach to improve health through addressing the determinants of health, including economic development, employment, housing, and education. This void is mainly because of the lack of integrated health services between the federal, provincial, and community jurisdictions.

7. *Diminished traditional role of women.* Reflective of Western models of governance that have replaced the traditional hereditary system, the role of indigenous women as central in sustaining the health of communities has been weakened.

8. *The legacy of enforced dependency.* Communities have had to rely on Canadian government-directed approaches to health services; thus, members have not had opportunities to develop integrated, effective First Nations health strategies.

Many First Nations face obstacles in delivering health care services to their community members. Subsequently, each of these barriers produces challenges for nurses and nursing. Current issues in the provision of nursing care to First Nations in Canada include the following:

- Significance of population demographics in relation to the health care needs of First Nations
- Effect of transfer of health care services and community development as a climate for change in providing nursing care to First Nations, including issues faced by nurses
- The need to develop cultural competence in providing meaningful nursing care to First Nations through education, research, and practice
- Barriers to accessing services in the health care system
- Scarcity of First Nations people in the health professions

Population Demographics

First Nations people are demographically distinctive from the Canadian population. They are similar, however, to the aboriginal population in that they are younger and experience higher fertility and mortality than the general population (Norris, 2000). Fertility and mortality affect the current and projected First Nations age-sex structure. The contrast between First Nations and the general population within the scope of current and projected age and sex configurations provides a basis for developing an understanding about the health care needs of First Nations people (Figure 24.1). Knowledge of the migration patterns of young First Nations women to and from reserves can also affect the nature of health care services provided both on and off the reserves. Demographic profiling serves as a valuable frame of reference within which to determine appropriate health care programming now and in the future.

In 1996, the median age of First Nations people was 25 years. The median age of the general population fell in the 35 to 44 year range. Also, 35% of children under the age of 15 years are First Nations, but this age group makes up only 21% of the general population. In contrast, only 7% of First Nations adults are 55 years of age or older, compared with 20% of the general population. However, analysis of census data and influencing factors suggests a shift to an aging First Nations population in the future. Although both the First Nations and general Canadian populations will be aging because of declining mortality and fertility levels, they will age differently. Norris (2000, p. 209) projects that between 1996 and 2021, the proportion of young people 18 years of age and younger in the First Nations population will decline from about 40% to 28%. The labor force and the elderly will significantly change, going from

FIGURE 24.1 (*Above*) Percentage distribution by age group and sex of aboriginal population; (*below*) percentage distribution by age group and sex of total Canadian population, aboriginal and nonaboriginal people. (*Source*: 1996 census data, *Statistics Canada*.)

between 4% and 9% to between 55% and 63% of the First Nations population during the same time period. The First Nations population will be shifting from youth into the older labor force age groups while the general population will be aging from the labor force age group into the retirement age group. The age configurations between First Nations and the general community will continue to differ in future decades. For example, the median age for First Nations people in 2021 is projected to be 32 years whereas in the general population it is expected to be 40 years. Infant, child, and teenage health programs are essential to prevent chronic diseases such as type II diabetes and heart disease from developing during the middle years in First Nations adults.

Fertility and mortality affect the age and sex configuration among First Nations people. Although higher than in the general population, First Nations fertility has been declining since the 1960s. This is attributed to the use of contraceptives. Consequently, the size of aboriginal families is decreasing numerically, and Native women are having children later and spacing them farther apart (Romaniuc cited in Norris, 2002, p. 175).

Mortality rates for First Nations have declined since the turn of the 20th century. However, the life expectancy of First Nations members continues to be shorter than that of the general population. In 1995, the life expectancy in the general Canadian population was 75.4 years for men and 81.2 years for women. That same year, the life expectancy in First Nations communities was 69.1 years for men and 76.2 years for women, with the leading causes of death accidents, poisonings, and violence.

The increase of First Nations people's life expectancy is due to the decrease in infant (a child who is less than 1 year of age) mortality and the influx of Bill C-31 registrants, who tended to be relatively young. In the early 1900s, about 25% of First Nations infants died within 1 year of their births. The infant mortality rate continues to be high among First Nations: two times higher than the national rate. Particularly alarming is the fact that First Nations babies between the ages of 28 days and 1 year died at a rate that was up to three times greater than the national average in 1995 (Norris, 2000).

Bill C-31 is the prelegislation name of the 1985 Act to Amend the Indian Act. This amended act eliminated certain discriminatory provisions of the Indian Act, including the section that resulted in Indian women losing their Indian status when they married non-Indian men. Bill C-31 enabled people affected by the discriminatory provisions of the old Indian Act to apply to have their status restored. Since 1985, about 105,000 people have successfully regained their Indian status (Department of Indian Affairs and Northern Development, 1997).

Most First Nations members who migrate do so between cities and reserves (Norris, 2000). Specifically, of those who migrated between 1991 and 1996, about 60% moved from reserves to urban areas and about 70% moved from the cities to the reserves. More First Nations people are moving to the reserves, and, as a result, reserves are serving more people. However, this gain is relatively small in relation to the reserve population. Norris (2000) surmises after the examination of the Department of Indian Affairs and Northern Development's 1996 Indian Register and adjusted census data that about 60% of registered First Nations people live on reserves. The initial percentage was adjusted for undercoverage and incomplete enumeration of reserves. The extent to which First Nations people migrate to and from reserves affects the health needs of First Nations, both on and off reserves.

Young First Nations women are similar to the general population and other aboriginal groups in that they tend to be the most mobile in a population (Norris, 2000, p. 184). In 1996, First Nations women, especially those between the ages of 15 and 24 years, migrated from reserves to urban areas significantly more so than men of the same age range. Women who attend postsecondary education influence this pattern. It is also noted that undercoverage in census among young adult males may attribute to these findings. Within the urban setting, First Nations people and, in particular, young First Nations women change their principal place of residence more than any other aboriginal group (nonstatus, Inuit, and Metis). This is with the understanding that aboriginal people tend to move at a higher rate than the general Canadian population (Norris, 2000). Between 1991 and 1996, among registered First Nations adults 20 to 24 years of age, 840 in every 1,000 registered First Nations women living off a reserve had moved, compared with 560 per 1,000 of young women living on reserve and 620 per 1,000 of young Canadian women in general (Norris, 2000).

Nursing Issues Related to Transfer of Health Care Services

Many nurses who are employed by First Nations communities that are administering their own health care services state the professional administrative structure and standards could no longer be guaranteed in their practice (ANAC, 1995, 2001a, 2001b). When the administration of health care services is transferred from Health Canada to a First Nations community, nursing service delivery also becomes the responsibility of that community. However, many communities were inadequately prepared through the transfer process to organize an effective system of nursing services (ANAC, 2000). Subsequently, nursing service structure and processes for supporting nurses at the community level were developed on an individual community or tribal council basis (ANAC, 2001b). The ANAC held nursing roundtables across Canada from 1986 to 1995 in which band-employed nurses clearly identified key issues surrounding health transfer, the delivery of nursing services, and the health of First Nations people in communities. Over the years, as communities completed the transfer process, these concerns became reality to the nurses.

In *Issues Verification: Current Nursing Workplace Issues and Best Practices in Aboriginal Communities: A Literature Review and Analysis,* ANAC (2002a) compiled the main workplace issues in the contemporary context by examining literature, surveys, reports, and other information ranging from the time of band nurse workshops to the present. One conclusion, in particular, was clear: Issues that were articulated more than 10 years ago at the ANAC Band Nurse Workshops continue to be pertinent. Indeed, they have now been identified as requiring strategic planning and research in the area of best practices. Issues related to transfer are identified in the following reports of the ANAC:

■ *Developing Best Practice Environments. Best Practice Model Development in Aboriginal Communities. Final Report. 2002b.*
■ *Supervision of Nurses in First Nation Communities: What Are the Gaps? A Literature Review and Analysis. January 2002c. Final Report.*
■ *Community Orientation for Newly Employed Nurses. Components of a First Nations Community Orientation Template. March 2002d. Final Report.*

Since the Indian Health Transfer policy was initiated in 1986, more than 40% of communities that were eligible have signed agreements for the health transfer initiatives. Although Health Canada has the structure and organization for delivering nursing services, First Nations communities did not have the experience and expertise to develop them, nor the financial resources to implement them.

Some key components for nursing services are nursing management and supervision, orientation, ongoing education, professional development, and a system of performance appraisal and evaluation. Substantive liability coverage and standards to practise nursing in the advanced role are also required to be available to nursing personnel. Standards of practice are established and regulated by professional nursing organizations. Only a few provincial professional nursing organizations have developed guidelines for use by employers and nurses to address advanced nursing practice.

A lack of understanding regarding the infrastructure required for nursing services may have been partly due to a shift in understanding about jurisdiction, self-government, and the role of the Medical Services Branch (MSB) of Health Canada. It was apparent that the nursing services department that was in place before transfer initiatives did not meet the nursing service needs of a transferred community. Communities gained through trial and error; others may have had the resources to redesign nursing services for their communities. Many communities engaged in the transfer process in isolation and so struggled to create effective community-based nursing services.

In the *Survey of Nurses in Isolated First Nations Communities: Recruitment and Retention Issues* (ANAC, 2000), several leaders from First Nations, who were considering transfer or were in pretransfer stages, and First Nations authorities, who had taken over management of nursing services, provided their suggestions and recommendations to address conditions successfully. One of these was to create mechanisms for First Nations authorities to exchange information and facilitate mutual learning and collaboration as they go through the transfer process. For example, the development of best practice models is one way of sharing solutions between communities and nurses. ANAC has identified a number of key issues directly related to the transfer of health care to First Nations communities:

1. Nurses, their employers, and professional nursing associations lack understanding about liability coverage as it pertains to scope of practice. Nursing legislation differs from province to province on the degree of protection provided to nurses who are functioning in advanced nursing practice. What are the implications of this legislation for nurses and employers?

2. Nurses are uncertain about how to support the community in which they are employed in the design of new program initiatives. Many transferred communities choose to take on this type of initiative by real-locating community funds. However, many First Nations communities consider the incorporation of cultural and traditional knowledge into these new health and healing systems as being desirable but unattainable. This is largely because of the cost of such initiatives and lack of personnel who have the skills to help the community create these kinds of systems.

3. Nurses who are newly employed in a First Nations community are unclear about the manner in which they can become involved with the community. This can be a challenge for the nurse because community members may view nurses as being part of the Western health care system. Or they may see that nurses "parachute" into a community to work only for a short time, and then they are gone. The legacy of colonization and illness prevail in some communities, and in others, only remnants are evident.

4. Nurses are not clear about the jurisdictions within which First Nations authorities are operating when considering the delivery of various community programs. In some cases, the jurisdiction rests with the First Nations government, whereas in other cases it may be the federal government. How does a nurse determine where the accountability for a program lies?

5. In some First Nations communities, the nurse reports to a non-nursing supervisor, such as the director of health. The nurse, supervisor, and community leadership may not be aware of the ramifications of this. There is potential that the supervisor may lack understanding about the role and function of nurses and may overrule nursing decisions, potentially eroding quality care.

6. Nurses may not be aware that nurse managers are key to creating effective community-based nursing services. Their role is pivotal in working with community leadership, health service directors, community members, and nursing staff to create mechanisms for effective quality nursing care.

Other issues that have been identified include the following:

1. Some band-employed nurses do not believe they have the respect of the community in which they are employed. This is evident when there is interference with the nurses' decisions.

2. The retention of nurses in First Nations communities depends on the quality of the practice environment. What are the key elements that need to be in place to ensure this quality is retained in the community workplace?

3. The employers of nurses may not be aware of the need for professional performance appraisal and evaluation.

Cultural Competence and Effective Health Care Programming

For many nurses, working with First Nations presents an opportunity to provide nursing care in a culture different from one's own. This also creates opportunities to positively affect nurse–patient relationships. Community development principles can affect the development of relationships with a community's leadership and its members (Shuster et al., 2001). Nurses who see themselves as partners with a community recognize that the strengths of the community will form a basis for organizing and improving the health of that community. The development of this kind of relationship could be profound for nurses as well as empowering and liberating for community members. This opportunity for deeper understanding and patience will help to convey an attitude that will foster the kind of relationship that First Nations patients would find helpful as they manage their health care needs.

Cultural competence includes an understanding of the perspectives and behaviors patients have about health and illness, family health care decisions, treatment expectations, and compliance with health care treatment plans (Lester, 1998). Cultural competence moves away from viewing how patients can fit into the nurses' world and way of doing things to examining how nurses may understand and fit into the patient's world (St. Clair & McKenry, 1999). Nursing research reinforces these elements of culturally competent approaches in the prevention and treatment of chronic disease among aboriginal people. For example, programming and services must take into account the historical, social, and cultural factors surrounding chronic disease (Gregory et al., 1999). Having this understanding influences how one will approach each patient within a community.

Nurse–patient relationships are affected by the perceptions that community members have about nurses and the nursing profession. First Nations people consider nurses and other health care providers to be a part of a health care system rooted in colonization. Indeed, elements of colonization continue today and affect nurse–patient relationships, in turn positively or negatively affecting access to health care services by First Nations members.

Access to Services

First Nations people experience a sense of isolation and marginalization when using general Canadian health care services (Dion Stout, Kipling, & Stout, 2001; Saunders, 1999). These experiences prompt many First Nations people to use health care services unwillingly or to avoid using them at all. A sense of isolation begins with having to leave one's home and community and, in many cases, travel great distances to access health services for specialized treatment. These distances tend to be geographic, but there are other kinds of distances, too: A key issue identified in the literature on aboriginal health is that aboriginal people face racism, prejudice, or insensitivity from the health care professionals from whom they are seeking services (ANAC, 2000; Royal Commission on Health of Aboriginal Peoples, 1996c).

One method to ensure that comprehensive care is available to First Nations people is to assess their experiences with mainstream health care services. After the barriers and supports for patients have been identified, health policies and practices can be instituted to provide equitable services to all patients. The effectiveness of nurse–patient communication can impose or remove barriers for persons seeking care. Dion Stout and colleagues (2001) compiled findings from the National Workshop on Aboriginal Women's Health Research held in Ottawa, in March 2001, and from results of research affiliated with the Centres of Excellence of Women's Health and Women's Health Bureau of Canada. Some of the most important findings include the following:

1. In an exploration of barriers and supports encountered by pregnant and parenting women entering addiction programs in Vancouver and Prince George, British Columbia, Poole and Isaac (2001) made a series of recommendations to redress the stigma, shame, and prejudice experienced by substance-abusing mothers and pregnant women. A number of supports were identified, ranging from those provided by families to those provided by health care professionals.

2. An assessment of the positive and negative aspects of aboriginal women's experiences with mainstream health care services was completed in the Carrier First Nation reserve community (Browne, Fiske, & Thomas, 2000). Health professionals were respectful of this community's cultural heritage and shared knowledge and decision making with patients about their health care. However, health professionals also learned that they dismissed or trivialized the women's concerns, judged in stereotypical negative ways, or demonstrated no regard for the patients' personal circumstances. The adoption of health policies and practices that incorporated the concept of cultural safety was among the recommendations made to address these concerns. Evaluation of other health service programs identified the following items as areas to address:

   ■ The importance of asking the aboriginal clientele themselves about their needs and priorities in accessing health care services
   ■ The need to provide support in tandem with services
   ■ The need for culturally appropriate services
   ■ The use of patient health outcomes as indicators for effective services
   ■ The need to be familiar with the socioeconomic issues relevant to patients
   ■ The development of awareness of the daily living contexts of patients
   ■ A knowledge of the history of community social supports

3. An assessment of the degree to which the service needs of aboriginal women were met by the Vancouver Native Health Society located in Downtown Eastside of Vancouver, British Columbia, was carried out by Benoit and Carroll (2001). Interviews with service providers and a series of focus groups with aboriginal women helped researchers to identify a number of access barriers, including the following:
   - A lack of sufficient security and anonymity while accessing clinic services
   - The use of Western approaches to counseling and the exclusion of more traditional aboriginal forms of healing
   - A general lack of female health care providers on staff

Guidelines and policy statements originating with health professional organizations can provide insight and significant information about developing culturally appropriate relationships with aboriginal people. Statements (Smylie, 2001) that have been developed in collaboration with aboriginal people and endorsed by the national aboriginal organizations add credibility to the content of the documents. Ethically, nurses are bound to respect culturally diverse clients (Canadian Nurses Association, 2002).

According to the College of Nurses of Ontario, patient-centered care requires that nurses recognize the patient's culture, the nurse's culture, and how both impact the nurse–patient relationship. Consequently, culturally sensitive care is the recognition of the similarities and differences between the patient's culture and that of the nurse. Nurses enhance their ability to provide patient-centered care by reflecting on how their own values and beliefs impact the relationship (College of Nurses of Ontario, 1999).

■ SUMMARY

Nursing in First Nations communities presents many challenges. At the forefront is the need to understand indigenous history, starting from the time when only First Peoples inhabited North America. The relationship of First Nations with the Crown of England and later the government of Canada beginning with the treaties and then the Indian Act, the goal of colonization to obliterate First Nations peoples' cultures and assimilate them into mainstream society, and First Nations' cultural resurgence and determination to obtain self-government are important parts of this history.

Both community development and transfer of health care services are integral to the development of culturally specific community health and healing systems. Population health is a way of identifying determinants of health to address inequities in health care. Nurses are also challenged to understand the relationship between population demographics and the development of relevant health programs. Nursing issues related to the transfer of health care services to First Nations communities will require critical analysis and collaborative efforts to effect optimal resolutions.

Online Resources

Add to your knowledge of this issue:

Aboriginal Nurses Association of Canada	anac.on.ca
Assembly of First Nations	www.afn.ca
Indian and Northern Affairs Canada	www.ainc-inac.gc.ca/pr/pub/ywtk/index_e.html
National Aboriginal Health Organization	naho.ca
Report of the Royal Commission on Aboriginal Peoples	www.parl.gc.ca/information/library/PRBpubs/ prb9924-e.htm

REFLECTIONS on the Chapter . . .

1. How have teachings regarding First Nations health care been included in your nursing program? Where are you able to obtain further information?

2. Using the determinants of health, examine the impact on the health of First Nations members and their communities.

3. Name four health care needs in First Nations communities. What are some strategies for dealing with them?

4. Using First Nations demographic data, determine two health issues that could become priorities by the year 2020.

5. Identify four approaches that will enhance nurse–patient communication with a First Nations person.

References

Aboriginal Nurses Association of Canada (ANAC). (1995). *Band nurse workshops, Halifax, Montreal, Saskatoon, Vancouver: Summary report, March 1995.* Ottawa: Author.

_____. (2000). *Survey of nurses in isolated First Nations communities: Recruitment and retention issues. Final report, September 8, 2000.* Ottawa: Author.

_____. (2001a). *The Aboriginal Nurses Association of Canada Submission to the Canadian Advisory Committee, November 19, 2001.* Ottawa: Author.

_____. (2001b). *Recruitment and retention workshop. Final Report, May 2001.* Ottawa: Author.

_____. (2001c). *Submission to the commission on the future of health care in Canada. Commissioner: Roy J. Romanow, Q. C. (November 1, 2001).* Ottawa: Author.

_____. (2002a). *Issues verification: Current nursing workplace issues and best practices in aboriginal communities: A literature review and analysis.* Ottawa: Author.

_____. (2002b). *Developing best practice environments* [Online]. Available: http://www.anac.on.ca/publications.html

_____. (2002c). *Supervision of nurses in First Nations communities: What are the gaps?* [Online]. Available: http://www.anac.on.ca/publications.html

_____. (2002d). *Community orientation for newly employed nurses* [Online]. Available: http://www.anac.on.ca/publications.html

Adelson, N. (1991). "Being alive well": The praxis of Cree health. *Arctic Medical Research, 50* (Suppl.), 230–232.

Benoit, C., & Carroll, D. (2001). *Marginalized voices from the downtown eastside: Aboriginal women speak about their health experiences.* Toronto: National Network on Environments and Health.

Berger, T. R. (1980). *Report of the Advisory Commission on Indian and Inuit Health Consultation.* Indian and Northern Affairs. Ottawa: Government of Canada.

Browne, A., Fiske, J., & Thomas, G. (2000). *First Nations women's encounters with mainstream health care services and systems.* Vancouver: British Columbia Centre of Excellence for Women's Health.

Canadian Nurses Association. (2002). *Code of ethics for registered nurses.* Ottawa: Author.

Cassidy, F., & Bish, R. (1989). *Indian government: Its meaning and practice.* Oolichan Books: Institute for Research on Public Policy: Lantzville.

College of Nurses of Ontario. (1999). *A guide to nurses for providing culturally sensitive care for registered nurses and registered practical nurses in Ontario.* Toronto: Author.

Department of Indian Affairs and Northern Development. (1997). Definitions [Online]. Available: http://www.ainc-inac.gc.ca/pr/pub/cana/def_e.html

Dickason, O. P. (1994). *Canada's First Nations: A history of founding peoples from earliest times.* Toronto: McClelland & Stewart.

Dion Stout, M., Kipling, G. D., & Stout, R. (2001). *Aboriginal women's health research, synthesis project.* Final report. Centres of Excellence for Women's Health Program, Women's Health Bureau, Health Canada. Ottawa: Government of Canada.

Evans, R. G., Barer, M. L., & Marmor, R. (Eds.). (1994). *Why are some people healthy and others not? The determinants of health of populations.* New York: Aldine de Gruyter.

Gregory, D., Whalley, W., Olson, J., et al. (1999). Exploring the experience of type 2 diabetes in urban aboriginal people. *Canadian Journal of Nursing Research, 31*(1), 101–115.

Hamilton, A. C., & Sinclair, C. M. (1991). *Report of the aboriginal justice inquiry of Manitoba: Vol. 1. The justice system and aboriginal people.* Winnipeg: Queen's Printer.

Health Canada. (1999a). *A second diagnostic on the health of First Nations and Inuit People in Canada* [Online]. Indian and Northern Affairs Canada. Available: www.ainc-inac.gc.ca/pr/pub/ywtk/index_e.html

_____. (1999b). *Ten years of health transfer. First Nation and Inuit control. April 1989–March 1999.* Ottawa: Minister of Public Works and Government Services Canada.

_____. (2002). *First Nations and Inuit control.* Annual Report 2001–2002. Retrieved April 24, 2005, from http://www.hc-sc.gc.ca/fnib/bpm/hfa/fnic_annual_report_2001_2002.htm

Indian and Northern Affairs Canada. Retrieved April 24, 2005, from http://www.ainc-inac.gc.ca/index_e.html

Lemphers, C. (1998). Perspective. Northern nursing: A type of advanced nursing practice. *AARN Newsletter, 54*(1), 11, 23.

Lester, N. (1998). *Cultural competence: A nursing dialogue.* Part one of a two-part article based on a roundtable discussion. *American Journal of Nursing, 98*(8), 26–34.

Malloch, L. (1989). Indian medicine, Indian health. Study between red and white medicine. *Canadian Woman Studies, 10*(2 & 3), 105–112.

McFarlane, P. (2000). Aboriginal leadership. In D. Long & O. P. Dickason (Eds.), *Visions of the heart, Canadian aboriginal issues* (2nd ed.). Toronto: Harcourt Canada.

Milloy, J. S. (1991). The early Indian Acts. In J. R. Miller (Ed.), *Sweet promises: A reader on Indian–white relations in Canada* (pp. 145–154). Toronto: University of Toronto Press.

Norris, M. J. (2000). Aboriginal peoples in Canada: Demographic and linguistic perspectives. In D. Long & O. P. Dickason (Eds.), *Visions of the heart, Canadian aboriginal issues* (2nd ed., pp. 167–236). Toronto: Harcourt Canada.

O'Neil, J., Lemchuk-Favel, L., Allard, Y., et al. (1999). Community healing and aboriginal self-government. In J. H. Hylton (Ed.), *Aboriginal self-government in Canada* (pp. 130–156). Saskatoon, Saskatchewan: Purich.

Poole, N., & Issac, B. (2001). *Apprehensions: Barriers to treatment for substance-using mothers.* Vancouver: British Columbia Centre of Excellence for Women's Health.

Ray, A. J. (1974). *Indians in the fur trade: Their role as trappers, hunters, and middlemen in the lands southwest of Hudson Bay 1660–1870.* Toronto: University of Toronto Press.

Royal Commission on Aboriginal Peoples. (1996a). *Report on the Royal Commission on Aboriginal Peoples. Vol. 1, Chap. 9.1: Protection of the reserve land base* [Online]. Ottawa: Government of Canada. Retrieved April 23, 2005, from http://www.ainc-inac.gc.ca/ch/rcap/index_e.html

_____. (1996b). *Report on the Royal Commission on Aboriginal Peoples. Vol. 2: Restructuring the relationship* [Online]. Ottawa: Government of Canada. Available: http://www.ainc-inac.gc.ca/ch/rcap/index_e.html

_____. (1996c). *Report on the Royal Commission on Aboriginal Peoples. Vol. 3: Gathering strength.* Ottawa: Government of Canada. Available: http://www.ainc-inac.gc.ca/ch/rcap/index_e.html

Saunders, W. (1999). Cultural sensitivity, a matter of respect. *Canadian Nurse, 95*(9), 43–44.

Shah, C. (1998). *Public health and preventive medicine* (4th ed.). Toronto: University of Toronto.

Shuster, S., Ross, S., Bhagat, R., et al. (2001). Using community development approaches. *Canadian Nurse, 97*(6), 18–22.

Smylie, J. (2000). Society of Obstetricians and Gynaecologists policy statement. A guide for health professional working with Aboriginal Peoples: The sociocultural context of aboriginal peoples in Canada. *Journal for Society of Obstetricians and Gynaecologists, 100,* 1070–1081.

_____. (2001). Society of Obstetricians and Gynaecologists policy statement. A guide for health professionals working with aboriginal peoples: Cross cultural understanding. *Journal for Society of Obstetricians and Gynaecologists, 100,* 157–167.

St. Clair, A., & McKenry, L. (1999). Preparing culturally competent practitioners. *Journal of Nursing Education, 38*(5), 228–234.

Tobias, J. L. (1991). Protection, civilization, assimilation: An outline history of Canada's Indian policy. In J. R. Miller (Ed.), *Sweet promises: A reader on Indian-white relations in Canada* (pp. 127–144). Toronto: University of Toronto Press.

Venne, S. (1997). Understanding Treaty 6: An indigenous perspective. In M. Asch (Ed.), *Aboriginal and treaty rights in Canada. Essays on law, equality, and respect for difference* (pp. 172–207). Vancouver: UBC Press.

Waldram, J., Herring, D. A., & Young, T. K. (1995). *Aboriginal health in Canada: Historical, cultural, and epidemiological perspectives.* Toronto: University of Toronto Press.

Young, K. (1984). Indian health services in Canada: A sociohistorical perspective. *Social Science and Medicine 18*(3), 257–264.

CHAPTER

25

Anne Bruce
Carol McDonald
Marjorie McIntyre

Opening the Conversation: Dilemmas and Possibilities of Spirituality and Spiritual Care

Used with permission from the photographer, Anne Bruce. ▶

Chapter Objectives

After completing this chapter, you will be able to:

1. Understand the relevance of spirituality for nursing practice.
2. Identify the different perspectives on spirituality and spiritual practices in nursing and related literature.
3. Consider how these perspectives are formed from underlying assumptions about the nature of spirituality.
4. Reflect on your own assumptions about the meaning of spirituality and the effects of these assumptions in your practice of spiritual care.
5. Articulate the barriers to providing spiritual care.
6. Generate possibilities for meeting the mandate of providing spiritual care to patients and families.

■ INTRODUCTION TO THE TOPIC: OPENING THE CONVERSATION ABOUT SPIRITUALITY

…Spiritual is that part of human beings that is responsive to beauty, searches after truth, appreciates kindness and compassion, accepts the obligations to care for fellow beings, motivates our efforts, energizes our lives, and opens the gates to laughter and tears. Spirit has little to do with religion, or as much, as he or she who has it, wishes.

Bevis & Watson, 1989

Spirituality is difficult to contain within language. Some authors see spirituality as a personal journey of discovering meaning and purpose in life (Fryback & Reinert, 1999). Others feel spirituality as a force like the wind that cannot be seen but is always felt (Cavendish et al., 2004). And yet others hear spirituality in the whispers of forest ponds or in music and in the silences before words. We, the authors of this chapter, acknowledge a view that no single understanding of spirituality can adequately embrace all human experience (Box 25.1), and yet we also recognize that the practice of nurses includes accompanying people during birth, old age, sickness, and death. As nurses, we engage with people during times of extreme vulnerability—when opportunities for spiritual awareness present themselves, and we are called to cultivate our capacities and willingness to engage openly with people at a spiritual level; this we see as integral to nursing practice.

   This chapter introduces spirituality and spiritual care in nursing as both a topic of interest and a conundrum with multiple dimensions, dilemmas, and possibilities. As an issue, spirituality is of widespread concern to the general public and poses challenges for nursing practice as we grapple with nurses' roles and

BOX 25.1	How Else Do People Refer to What We Have Called Spirituality?

Philosophy of life	Connection
	Love
Search for meaning	Peace
	Contentment
Inner resources	Personal strength
Personal beliefs	Religious beliefs/practices
Faith	Opening to the universe
Relationship with a higher power/god/goddess/nature	

BOX 25.2   Personal Assumptions

The lens through which I view the world is multihued. In part, my world view is shaped by my role and educational preparation in nursing and, in part, by my interest and practice in Buddhist interpretations of life and suffering.

capacities in providing spiritual care. However, unlike nursing problems that can often be resolved with adequate analysis and consultation, spirituality as a nursing issue is not seen as something to be solved but rather as a multifaceted topic that requires personal awareness, critical analyses, and the powers of curiosity and un/knowing to open possibilities for understanding and engaging spiritual connectedness.

Our intention in writing this chapter is to open a conversation about what we identify as some of the relevant questions that emerge with the topic of spirituality and spiritual care in nursing practice. The purpose is not to convince you, the reader, of anything at all about spirituality but rather to open spaces for you to wonder about and to explore the meaning that the topic of spirituality holds in your nursing practice. Our belief is that we bring ourselves to each encounter with clients. Although this may seem an obvious and taken-for-granted idea, the notion that we accompany ourselves to practice holds within it important assumptions that are central to the writing/reading of this chapter.

■ SITUATING THE TOPIC: PERSONAL/ PROFESSIONAL ASSUMPTIONS

Each of us comes to the conversation about spirituality with a history and a particular "situatedness" in the world. Our history is constructed of past experiences, beliefs, and values that have brought us to our current understandings of spirituality. From this position, we hold assumptions about the place and purpose of spirituality in our own lives and in the lives of others (Boxes 25.2 and 25.3). These assumptions are present to us in our nursing practice. Although some people may believe that we can extricate ourselves as nurses from ourselves as people, it is not always clear that we can or would even want to do this. And so, our assumptions about spirituality and spiritual care are with us in our conversations and in the practice of spirituality/nursing. At this juncture, it may be useful to contemplate the assumptions that are present for you as you engage with this chapter, assumptions derived from your personal and professional histories and your current "situatedness" in the world.

■ SITUATING THE TOPIC: UNDERSTANDING SPIRITUAL PRACTICES HISTORICALLY

As well as the individual assumptions that accompany us to this conversation, our understandings of spirituality and, in particular, our understandings of the dilemmas that arise when considering spirituality in nursing

BOX 25.3   Personal Assumptions

My spiritual life/practices are inseparable from the daily life that I live, and, while this life is situated by the tradition of a faith community, it is also deeply influenced by connection to the earth world: the sacred being of nature and animals.

practice are influenced by the ways in which spirituality and nursing have intermingled historically. You might wonder what this history has to do with your current nursing practice. We would suggest that our history is, in a sense, inescapable and that, although historical practice may not be clearly visible to us, it remains present and influences the ways in which nursing is understood by nurses and others.

The history of nursing in the western world has a close alliance with spirituality and spiritual practices. Long before the era of Florence Nightingale, credited with the founding of modern nursing, individuals who were organized around religious or spiritual ideals practised care of the sick. According to Nelson (1995), a nurse scholar and historian, nursing's inception can be traced backward through the 19th-century Sisters of Mercy and Sisters of Charity and the 17th-century origins of the Daughters of Charity to early Christian doctrine of St. Benedict, who elevated the care of the sick as service imbued with spiritual value. Nightingale is said to have studied with the Daughters of Charity in Paris, France, and to have "learned from them, how to become, and how to form a nurse" (Nelson, 1995, p. 37). Nightingale's so-called secular schools of nursing ascribed to ideals originating with Christian ideology. The influence of particular spiritual ideals is readily recognizable in our Canadian nursing history, where the earliest organized nursing practice arrived in the form of Augustine nuns from France in August 1639, decades before a Nightingale-model nursing school was established in Canada in June 1874. "For the Augustine nuns, caring and healing work was central to their Christian beliefs" (Carr, 2003, p. 472). The "training regimen" of Nightingale's schools and of nursing schools well into the 20th century sought to build capacity in nursing students for service and duty, building on a thinly veiled Christian morality.

Nelson (1995) asserts that Christian doctrine remains embedded in particular nursing discourse, now reinscribed as ideologies of humanism. "Humanism in nursing has resurrected the religious discourse and the spiritual dimension of nursing…Salvation has been redrafted to self-actualization" (Nelson, 1995, p. 37). Entire nursing curricula embrace humanism's ideals as foundational to nursing practice: valuing individual uniqueness, empowerment, freedom, and the caring relationship. Perhaps the most visible reinterpretation of spirituality in nursing from the 20th century onward is the widely held and seldom critiqued ideal of nursing practice as a "holistic" endeavor.

This cursory look at the history of the alliance of nursing and spirituality is important for a number of reasons, not the least of which is the recognition of the position from which this history has been written. Much of what we take to be an unbiased account of our past can also be understood as an interpretation of historical proceedings, recorded through the lens of people who are situated within particular social, cultural, political, and spiritual realities. Our nursing history has been written and interpreted from a position of Eurocentrism, in this case meaning that history has been interpreted through a Western world perspective that privileges Judeo-Christian ideology. Embedded in this position is the notion that kindness, compassion, charity, faith, hope, and service are primarily Christian attributes. And yet would we actually believe this when faced with the unspoken but implicit assumptions that kindness and compassion originated with Christianity or that these attributes are not esteemed in spiritual, philosophical, or social knowledge systems quite unrelated to Judeo-Christian ideology? How might nursing's history be understood differently through the lens of other positions in the world, positions that have been less privileged in the recorded history of the Western world?

■ SIGNIFICANCE OF THE TOPIC FOR NURSING: EMBRACING THE TENSIONS

Several considerations underlie the relevance of spiritual practice for nurses, including our position of access to patients' lives during times of spiritual crisis or suffering, the subscription of nursing discourse to "holistic care," and a growing mandate to categorize and account for spiritual care.

As we highlighted in the introduction to this chapter, nurses often have opportunities to be with people during birth, old age, sickness, and death, and, as nurses, we have privileged access to people during

BOX 25.4	What Might People Identify as Spiritual Practice?

Yoga		Conversation
Meditation		Reminiscing
Prayer		Being in nature
Practising kindness		Chanting
Listening		Singing
Ceremonies	Rituals	Traditional dance
Silence	Solitude	Sacred space
Making offerings		Sharing meals
Reading sacred text		Sacred art
Celebrations		Listening to/making music
Being close to important others		Mantra repetition

times of extreme vulnerability—when opportunities for spiritual awareness present themselves. These opportunities do not necessarily announce themselves as spiritual crises or awakenings, prompting us to plan for or execute "spiritual care," but they unfold in the ordinariness of days and evenings and nights, when we as nurses are already present and engaged with patients as they live out their lives. It is with the knowledge that these occurrences are surely and repeatedly lived by patients and families and nurses that we are invited to cultivate our capacities and willingness to engage openly with people at a spiritual level.

A "holistic" approach to nursing practice is a central tenet in innumerable nursing school curricula and is embedded in the philosophies of practice of countless individual nurses. One interpretation of the beliefs underlying holistic practice is "the mind, body and spirit are interdependent; the human spirit is the core of the person; a person's attitude and beliefs toward life are major etiological factors in health and disease" (Freeman, 2004, p. 165). In spite of the predominant understanding of holistic practice as inclusive of spiritual practices, many nurses feel poorly prepared to provide spiritual care to patients—and spiritual aspects of care are poorly represented in Canadian nursing school curricula (Olson et al., 2003).

Last, the relevance of spiritual practice in nursing is underscored when we recognize the provision of spiritual care as mandated both ethically and through overt and pragmatic means. The Canadian Nurses Association (CNA) *Code of Ethics* asserts that nurses "take into account the biological, psychological, social, cultural and spiritual needs of persons in health care" (CNA, 2002, p. 13). The impetus to attend to spiritual care grows as practicing nurses face increasing pressure to categorize and document all nursing practice, including practice that is spiritual in nature. For example, the Joint Commission on Accreditation of Healthcare Organizations (JCAHO) in the United States now requires that every patient receive spiritual assessment on admission along with appropriate care for those who request it (Taylor, 2003; Box 25.4).

■ ARTICULATING THE TOPIC AS AN ISSUE: PRACTICE DILEMMAS

This chapter invites us into a conversation on the topic of spirituality and nursing practice. We have selected one particular dilemma around which to focus our analysis and conversation. The issue, reflected in the nursing literature on spirituality, is the gap between positive attitudes toward spiritual care among nurses and the lack of spiritual care that is actually being provided by nurses. It seems that, although assessing and attending to the spiritual needs of patients and families is valued by nurses, many of us do not feel comfortable doing so.

Analyzing the Issue: Multiple Understandings

There are multiple ways of understanding the tension that arises between the ideal and the reality of spiritual care in nursing practice. Drawing on the research of Olson and coworkers (2003), we will analyze the issue by exploring different ways of understanding what contributes to the existing discrepancy between the valuing of spirituality in nursing discourse and the inadequacy of nurses' preparation and/or ability to address spiritual care in practice. We will engage with three understandings, or positions, that inform this issue. Embedded in each of these analyses are barriers to, as well as strategies that will promote, resolution. We will analyze the following understandings:

1. The nonscientific nature of spirituality does not easily fit within a science-based approach to nursing care (Price, Stevens, & LaBarre, 1995).
2. There is ambiguity about what is included in spiritual care in nursing (Price, Stevens, & LaBarre, 1995).
3. Nurses do not believe they have the knowledge necessary to adequately approach spiritual care (Chadwick and Piles, cited in Olson et al., 2003).

Engaging in a critical conversation about spirituality and spiritual care requires questioning the assumptions embedded within each of these ways of understanding the issue. We situate our discussion in a constructivist view; that is, we perceive knowledge not as unbiased or detached but as always generated, formed, and constructed within particular social, cultural, political, and material realities. This means that knowledge is never impartial but is always developed from and situated within a particular view of the world. One approach to making the "situatedness" of knowledge visible is to identify the taken-for-granted assumptions on which the knowledge is shaped or constructed. Our intention then, is not to resolve the challenges of how to provide spiritual care but to analyze and critique the issue with the view of opening spaces for you to develop your own interpretations.

Ways of Understanding: Scientific and Nonscientific

The non-scientific nature of spirituality does not easily fit within a science-based approach to nursing.

Price, Stevens, & LaBarre, 1995

Historical Influences of Science: Privileging a Dispirited Body

Although a spiritual heritage has been claimed in nursing, Wojnar and Malinski (2003) suggest that this spiritual legacy has been challenged by the separation of body from spirit in science. Interestingly, according to Burkhardt and Nagai-Jacobson (2002), this was not always the case, as when, around the 8th century, the body/spirit was established as connected yet separate in the Christian tradition. Later, in the 17th century, philosopher René Descartes proposed that the body and spirit are mutually exclusive. This belief became accepted in Western thought and paved the way for biologic and medical knowledge to become the dominant scientific view that persists today in North America. The body became the exclusive domain of science whereas the spirit and soul were relegated to philosophers, theologians, and priests. The modern era is marked by an unprecedented growth of scientific knowledge and power of the natural sciences. Indeed, natural sciences have been regarded as the zenith of human achievement (Couvalis, 1997).

This view of the world also reinforced oppositional thinking, a view where binaries are set up, known as *dualism*. In dualism, emphasis is given to separateness rather than to interconnectedness of phenomena. For example, dualistic thinking sees opposite positions of this versus that: science versus nonscience, body versus spirit, good versus bad. Although oppositional thinking is useful in distinguishing differences and categories, it is often inadequate when addressing complex human experiences. The complexity of human suffering or spirituality, for example, cannot be contained in simple categories. Instead, the messy, ambiguous nature of living and dying, of feeling health-within-illness, also needs to be acknowledged and valued. However, ambiguity, uncertainty, and un/knowing have not often been valued in nursing.

In the name of science, oppositional thinking has become almost uncritically accepted. Scientism, as distinguished from science, is a matter of putting too high a value on science as a branch of learning in comparison with other ways of knowing (Dzurec & Abraham, 1993). With scientism, the belief is that science is the most beneficial form of learning and, as such, it is good for all domains, including spirituality and philosophy, to be placed on a scientific footing. Consequently, we see scholars claim to have made history, politics, ethics, or aesthetics into a science and assume that these claims of scientific status are desirable (Sorell, 1991). In nursing, Kikuchi and Simmons (1994) provide examples in which nurse researchers attempt to answer philosophical questions such as What is the nature of health? and What is the purpose of caring? using exclusively scientific means, thereby demonstrating nursing's vulnerability to scientism. In recent years, however, many of the long-held tenets of science and ways of obtaining knowledge have been questioned. Previously held assumptions about reality and the nature of truth have been challenged both within traditional scientific communities and by feminists, critical theorists, and postmodern thinkers. Even so, science and perhaps scientism remain the dominant view within health care professions. The dominance of scientific knowledge has led to almost unquestioned acceptance of technology and secularism in social, political, and educational institutions.

Until recently, spirituality as a human phenomenon that is separate from the body and material world has been neglected by scientific inquiry. Increasingly, however, spirituality is receiving scientific attention as the body/mind/spirit split is challenged and shown to be too limited in understanding human health and well-being. Consequently, spirituality is being conceptualized in ways that promote clear distinctions and measurements that are congruent with the assumptions of scientific world views. Without minimizing the importance of scientific knowledge, the risk of scientism must also be attended to as we see the call in nursing for standardized language and interventions for spiritual care. Clearly, we must avoid the pitfalls of according science a privileged view at the expense of other ways of knowing spirituality while at the same time valuing the contributions of scientific knowledge.

In analyzing science, it is not our intention to throw out science or situate spirituality in opposition to science. Nevertheless, different ways of generating knowledge will shape our nursing practice differently. Through critical analysis, we can distinguish what kinds of knowledge and practices are left out, which are ignored or perhaps not legitimized, and where particular beliefs and power become dominant.

Natural Science and Human Science: Differing Approaches to Knowledge

In the academic milieu of the early 1980s, nursing attempted to legitimize its position as a discipline of science by privileging the natural sciences of medicine over what became known as human sciences (Kim, 1999). The natural sciences support a view where people are made up of different components continuously interacting with one another and the environment. This concept of person as an assemblage of traits and variables is inconsistent with a human science view. A decade later, the mood had changed; nursing science's position on "the person" (as a bio-psycho-social-spiritual being made up of components) was challenged by nurses valuing a human science perspective. Rather than seeing persons with components, the view from a human science perspective sees the person as a complex, evolving being, interconnected with the universe. The personal meanings of people's realities are considered of central importance in the investigations and practices of human science disciplines.

This is not to suggest that there is a single perspective of nursing theory/practice that draws on the human science view. Numerous nursing theories within human science value spirituality in nursing practice, among them the diverse approaches of Jean Watson, Betty Neumann, Martha Rogers, and Rosemarie Parse. When we consider the effect that differences in underlying assumptions have on how spirituality is understood and practised, we can suggest that to view spirituality as a component of a person would lead to different ways of practising than would to view spirituality as integral to our nature.

Ways of Understanding: Clarity and Ambiguity

There is ambiguity about what constitutes spiritual care in nursing.

Price, Stevens, & LaBarre, 1995

Embedded in this position is an assumption that clarity is required to overcome current ambiguity about what constitutes spirituality in nursing practice. As with the underlying assumption of the first position, a binary of "clarity versus ambiguity" is inferred in the language of this position. That is, it is assumed that clarity concerning spirituality is preferred over the existent situation of multiple and diverse understandings. Is it possible, or even desirable, to construct a single, clear, concise definition of spiritual practice that will adequately encompass all perspectives from ecologic, aboriginal, religious, and humanistic views, as well as from those views that cannot be easily identified? This assumption and its oppositional thinking are challenged as we explore other ways of approaching this dualism. In particular, we will consider both the differences between and the interdependence of spirituality and religion as well as the spiritual experience with conceptual understandings of spirituality.

Religion and Spirituality: Vehicle and Destination

It could be said that religion and spirituality are interconnected for some people some of the time, for some people all of time, and for some people none of the time. Given this, it seems important to understand them as separate and sometimes related concepts. A great deal of the research before 2000 has examined *religion* and *spirituality* as if they were synonymous (George et al., 2000) and has used the two terms interchangeably. Increasingly, however, nurses and others understand the importance of teasing apart the differences between religious traditions and our many interpretations of spirituality. Although religion and spirituality are seen as related concepts, religion is often linked to formal religious institutions whereas spirituality is seen as a broader idea that does not depend on institutional contexts. Religion is like a train journeying through and toward spirituality where we are cautioned not to mistake the vehicle for the destination (Borysenko, 1999). While for some, spiritual experience is not separate from their religious beliefs and practices, this is not the case for many who consider themselves spiritual yet not at all religious.

Spirituality as a Concept and as Lived Experience

Just as religion and spirituality are closely linked yet also very different, the interdependence of experience and concept can also be made. The nature of spirituality is complex as an experience and as a concept (Wojnar & Malinski, 2003). This distinction between experience and the conceptual representation of experience—how we understand spirituality through language—is rarely distinguished in current discussions of spirituality. Nevertheless, this distinction is important and may assist us in sifting through the many ways of understanding (conceptualizing) spiritual phenomena.

As with experiences of pain, many authors suggest that the experience of spirituality is unique to each person and can only be known by that person. From this perspective, the understanding of a particular person's spirituality is whatever the person says it is. Although our experiences are unique, at the same time there are also common themes and patterns of spiritual understanding that extend across groups of people. Through systematically examining how people describe their experiences, researchers generate categories and theories to better understand this human experience. The caution, however, is to avoid confusing individual experience (of each distinct patient and family) with a generalized understanding generated in concepts about spirituality. In nursing, we require embodied knowledge from the unique experiences of patients and families along with diverse sources of generalized conceptual knowledge, including nursing knowledge and empirical research.

If we accept the assumption that no single expression of spirituality can embrace all human experience, then it cannot reasonably be anticipated that nurses will know how to recognize or interpret the multiple possible expressions of spirituality or spiritual need. However, what nurses can do (and often do very well) is enter into and engage with the unique experiences of patients. From this standpoint, the central questions may not be What is spirituality? but rather How is spirituality lived between this patient/family and the illness, and how can we engage there with families? Nurses do not necessarily need to possess broad understandings of religious practices, theology, or cultural studies to provide spiritual care. Instead, nurses can be willing and able to engage patients with spiritual awareness about values, beliefs, and their experiences of illness.

Paterson and Zderad (1976) also emphasize the relationality of nursing in their focus on where nursing happens rather than what it is. "Nursing is an experience lived between human beings" (p. 3) "and is concerned with 'the between' of nurses and their others" (p. 44). Here, "the between" refers to a merging of nurse–patient boundaries into a space of authentic presence while maintaining one's capacity to question.

When I reflect on an act of mine (no matter how simple or complex) that I can unhesitatingly label "nursing," I become aware of it as goal-directed (nurturing) being with and doing for another. The intersubjective or interhuman element, "the between," runs through nursing interactions like an underground stream conveying the nutrients of healing and growth. In everyday practice, we are usually so involved with the immediate demands of our "being with and doing with" the patient that we do not focus on the overshadowed plane of "the between." However, occasionally, in beautiful moments, the interhuman currents are so strong that they flood our conscious awareness. Such rare and rewarding moments of mutual presence remind us of the elusive ever-present "between" (Paterson & Zderad, 1976, pp. 21–22).

This perspective resonates closely with definitions of spirituality and notions of spiritual care. According to Paterson and Zderad, it is important to explore and describe the nature of in-between experiences. This is significant, according to Paterson and Zderad, if we are to better understand how our interactions with others can have both humanizing and dehumanizing effects.

How we conceptualize spirituality within nursing discourse also shapes our clinical practice. The way we talk and write about spirituality shapes knowledge about the phenomenon—through writing/reading, we are making real, so to speak, and establish what spirituality is (Boxes 25.5 and 25.6). However, generating knowledge is not done in isolation, and we see health care institutions also mandating nurses to provide spiritual care. What conceptualization of spirituality do you want to support and foster? How might we proceed in a health care system and society that privileges "interventions" that can be measured and documented? An all-encompassing definition would be congruent with a science-based approach to nursing while the ambiguity of diverse and multiple definitions would more closely reflect differences encountered in people's experiences.

Is it possible to hold a space open in our thinking, where spirituality and spirituality in nursing practice are understood in multiple ways, as experience and concept, rather than narrowing our thinking to reach a clear and concise definition? We would suggest that in our wish to find simple definitions to these complex experiences, we risk generalizing and relying too heavily on the power of already privileged religious ideologies in our society. Rather than creating space for a range of spiritual practice, the search for "clarity" can lead us to marginalize, ignore, or trivialize spiritual practices that fall outside of the dominant norm. Perhaps then, developing comfort with the inevitable ambiguity of complex human experiences is also important.

Ways of Understanding: Knowing and Unknowing

Nurses do not believe they have the knowledge necessary to adequately approach spiritual care.

Chadwick and Piles, cited in Olson et al., 2003

Without minimizing the question of what nurses need to know to provide spiritual care, we would like to question the underlying assumptions embedded in this third position that infer an emphasis on knowing

BOX 25.5

Momentarily awake, pale gray-blue eyes washed out by morphine.
  Pin-point pupils, beady eyes peering into space.
You didn't want this, but are at the mercy of night guardians.
  Well meaning, yet inattentive . . . or unable to see?

"Good morning Martin".
. . . . You startle,
eyes flitting, seeking recognition,
hands grasping invisible objects in space.

"Hi, how are you" you whisper through dentureless jaws.
About to respond, but you're gone
drifting rudderless
    eyes rolling upward
        and away.

Are you able to be present
for the journey?
    You moaned and groaned too loudly,
so they took away
the/ir pain
    and hushed you into slumber
where we cannot go or witness,
you journey there alone . . . .

Source: Bruce, A. (2002). *Abiding in liminal spaces: Inscribing mindful living/dying with(in) end-of-life care.* Unpublished doctoral dissertation, University of British Columbia. Used with permission.

versus not knowing. Attending to knowledge, as this question implies, renders a valuing of "doing" and knowing in opposition to "being" and not knowing. The following discussion of these tensions may provide alternative ways of looking at spirituality.

The quest to know and define phenomena can be seen as part of a larger ideology or belief system. As mentioned, the model for generating nursing knowledge and practice has been embedded within a discourse

BOX 25.6

I am aware of the dance between definitive and non-definitive language. Although the question remains, how is this relevant for nursing practice, I hope to elude the pitfall of prescriptive discourse as my intention has always been otherwise. Death is not a problem to be remedied. Accompanying those in this journeying is also seeing the interplay of y/our dying and the limits of pre-scribed 'doing' . . . . . and yet . . . .

Source: Bruce, A. (2002). *Abiding in liminal spaces: Inscribing mindful living/dying with(in) end-of-life care.* Unpublished doctoral dissertation, University of British Columbia. Used with permission.

of science. Although this is changing, the push toward standardization of spiritual care and measurements of spirituality illustrates both the usefulness and continued dominance of this view. Once again, the issue is not that different ways of knowing are beneficial but rather that we need to be aware of and question the privileging of particular views at the expense of others. One such privileging arises in valuing knowing over un/knowing and is explored here for other possible interpretations.

Un/knowing as a Way of Knowing

Recognizing different modes of reality (such as spirit as supernatural) is difficult within the limited scope of language and ways of knowing in science (Wilber, 1998; Wolfer, 1993). For example, conventional scientific knowledge focuses on what is said, thereby excluding what is unsaid, or unsayable. By concentrating on what is certain and knowable, we often exclude the ambiguous, unknowable, and paradoxical. Conventional models of scientific knowledge depend on exclusion and function to privilege one voice or perspective over another. Through valuing what we can know of spiritual experience within a fixed idea of what is acceptable, we may ignore that which is "unknowable" or indescribable within spiritual experience. When exploring spirituality in nursing practice, careful attention to language and discourses can guide us to help people to live within the reality of their own spiritual experiences.

The question of what nurses need to know to provide spiritual care has practical implications when we consider that many nurses do not feel comfortable attending to the spiritual needs of their patients (McSherry & Ross, 2002), and nursing students seek guidance for developing spiritual awareness and engaging in spiritual discussions with patients and families (Pesut, 2002). Addressing spirituality from a scientific or a modernist view emphasizes knowing through establishing clear definitions that may lead to assessment tools and concept clarification. This could help to differentiate spirituality from other phenomena such as sense of coherence, caring, or connectedness. Although these ways of knowing contribute to nursing knowledge and practice, they also raise many other questions, including How are definitions determined? Who decides what definitions we will rely on? What world view or belief system is embedded within this knowledge? What happens when patients and families do not fit into particular views of spirituality? Even though themes related to spiritual experience may be identified across groups and aggregates, if spirituality, as some authors suggest, is whatever people say it is for them (Malinski, 2002), what pitfalls and potential harms do we face in privileging the views that are dominant or most commonly held?

Alternative ways of knowing may complement and yet put into question modernist approaches to spirituality. Where the modernist approach is based in a historical era when there was increased growth in the valuing of freedom, individuality, and scientism, views from a postmodern perspective challenge the nature of modern assumptions. Modernism, although largely located in the 19th and early 20th century, continues to inform some schools of thought, particularly those of the natural sciences whereas postmodernism critiques of modern thought are increasingly prevalent in nursing scholarship.

Munhall (1993) challenges modernist assumptions about knowledge in exploring unknowing as a way of knowing. Munhall introduces "unknowing" as a state of mind and a way of knowing that brings another dimension to understanding complex human experience. Unknowing is viewed not simply as a gap in knowledge that must be filled but as an ability and way of knowing that is interconnected with conventional knowing. After all, knowing that we do not know opens us to learning and new possibilities. Munhall calls for unknowing to be included as another pattern of knowing (Box 25.7).

Cultivating Abilities to Engage With Spiritual Openness: A Way of Being

We support the view of nurse scholars who suggest that spiritual care is multifaceted and wide-ranging, much of which does not demand or require specialized knowledge (Ross, 1997; Wright, 2002). If we are practising nursing in an interdisciplinary setting, what aspects of care are within the purview of nursing and

BOX 25.7

Let us not talk *about* death,
Let us talk . . . with/in
. . . . open-enededness
forming and dissolution.
trans/forming, per/forming,
constantly dissolving
becoming anew
abiding in spaces between thoughts.

Let us talk
nursing
as witnessing
mindful of empty spaces and places
   of self/no self
   of birth, old age, sickness and death.
Mindful of basic impermanence
of living and dying,
abiding in spaces
of ceaseless transitioning . . . . .

Source: Bruce, A. (2002). *Abiding in liminal spaces: Inscribing mindful living/dying with(in) end-of-life care.* Unpublished doctoral dissertation, University of British Columbia. Used with permission.

what areas can best be referred to other health care/spiritual care practitioners, such as aboriginal healers, pastors, shamans, and priests? And what aspects of spiritual care can be attended to within direct nursing care?

Recent research reports that patients and families appreciate and see spiritual care from nurses more as a way of being rather than as specific interventions (Sellers, 2001). The most frequently identified descriptors of spiritual care included being treated with kindness and respect ("it's the little things"); talking and listening; praying; connecting (being genuine, showing interest); providing quality temporal care (keeping the room tidy, not letting the patient suffer); and mobilizing religious and spiritual resources (referrals to clergy, providing spiritual music or readings; Taylor, 2003, p. 587, 588).

Some patients have reported that they do not want nurses to be spiritual care providers based on the perception that nurses are not qualified and an assumption that differing beliefs between patients and nurses would be a barrier to spiritual care (Taylor, 2003). Other participants in the same study saw nurses as appropriate spiritual care providers because nurses were perceived as those who are there during vulnerable experiences and recognize experiences that would prompt a desire for spiritual care. Patients without family or particular spiritual or religious support were seen to particularly benefit from nurses with spiritual awareness. Taylor identifies several prerequisites to the provision of spiritual care from the perspective of patients in her research (Box 25.8). Most significantly, patients stated "nurses need to establish some respect and relationship with patients prior to providing spiritual care" (Taylor, 2003, p. 589). This finding supports an understanding that spiritual practice may be most appreciably delivered through a "way of being" with patients rather than through the influences of scientific or modernist knowledge.

BOX 25.8

Prerequisites to Spiritual Care

<u>Personal</u>: Having a spiritual awareness; establishing trusting relationships

<u>Relational</u>: Possessing a caring attitude; developing rapport first; conveying warmth and interest; assessing patient receptivity

<u>Professional</u>: Meeting patients' expectations for what nurses might do; having appropriate training if needed

Source: Taylor, J. E. (2003). Nurses caring for the spirit: Patients with cancer and family caregiver expectations. *Oncology Nursing Forum, 30*(4), 585–590.

■ IDENTIFYING BARRIERS: FURTHERING OUR UNDERSTANDING

The following are some barriers to nurses providing spiritual care.

1. Our lack of knowledge of our nursing history and the influence of this history on our current understandings of spiritual care in nursing practice
2. An unexamined Eurocentric perspective of spirituality that privileges Judeo-Christian ideologies
3. The dilemma of defining *spirituality* and *spiritual care*. Definitions and clarity, regarding both concepts and interventions, lend themselves to accounting for evidence-based practice and meeting mandated requirements for care. However, this kind of clarity is located within a particular world view and understanding of knowledge that may not move us any closer to the actual provision of meaningful spiritual care for patients and families.
4. The idea that there is, or should be, a single understanding of spirituality and of approaches to spiritual care in the face of the lived realities of multiple understandings and meanings of spirituality

■ GENERATING STRATEGIES: FUTURE POSSIBILITIES

The following are some possibilities for nurses to remain open and provide spiritual care.

1. Make clear our personal and professional assumptions about spirituality and recognize the influence that these hold on our practice.
2. Always search for the taken-for-granted assumptions on which knowledge is shaped or constructed.
3. Pay careful attention to language and discourse because it is important in helping others live within their own spiritual realities.
4. Develop curricula and opportunities for nurses in practice to expand their comfort with the inevitable ambiguity of complex human experiences.

■ SUMMARY

Through this chapter's conversations, poems, and reflections on the literature, we have intended to open the possibilities for multiple understandings of spiritual practice for nurses. One might assume from the language used in the literature regarding spiritual care (*kindness, gentleness, caring*) that good nursing care is spiritual in nature. However, as we consider this evocative idea, we are left with the notion that it is something more—that spiritual practice involves accompanying patients and families on their journeys of suffering and hope and joy in ways that allow them to be present to the journeys themselves.

Online Resources

Add to your knowledge of this issue:

American Holistic Nurses Association	**www.ahna.org/home.html**
Canadian Holistic Nurses Association	**mypage.direct.ca/h/hutchings/chna.html**
Canadian Wellness Directory of Alternative Medicine Professionals	**www.canadianwellness.com/alternative/ alternative_associations.asp**
Care Nurse	**care-nurse.com**
International Association for Human Caring	**www.humancaring.org**

REFLECTIONS on the Chapter . . .

1. Does everyone have spiritual experience? What words do you use to refer to your spiritual life/practices?

2. In your practice, what have you observed about the spiritual nature of people and how does that fit with nurses' practice?

3. Identify the assumptions and beliefs you hold about spirituality and the provision of spiritual care to patients and their families.

4. How do your assumptions align or differ from those held by the authors of this chapter and/or the literature they include?

5. Is there a mandate for nurses to provide spiritual care in your province? If so, how does this compare with the CNA *Code of Ethics* mandate?

References

Borysenko, J. (1999). *A woman's journey to God: Finding the feminine path.* New York: Riverhead Books.

Bruce, A. (2002). *Abiding in liminal spaces: Inscribing mindful living/dying with(in) end-of-life care.* Unpublished doctoral dissertation, University of British Columbia.

Burkhardt, M., & Nagai-Jacobson, M. G. (2002). *Spirituality: Living our connectedness.* Albany: Delmar Thomson Learning.

Canadian Nurses Association. (2002). *Code of ethics for registered nurses.* Retrieved April 19, 2005, from www.cna-nurses.ca/ cna/documents/pdf/publications/codeofethics2002_e.pdf

Carr, T. (2003). The spirit of nursing: Ghost of our past or force for our future? In M. McIntyre & E. Thomlinson (Eds.), *Realities of Canadian nursing: Professional, practice, and power issues.* Philadelphia: Lippincott Williams & Wilkins.

Cavendish, R., Luise, B. K., Russo, D., et al. (2004). Spiritual perspectives on nurses in the United States relevant for education and practice. *Western Journal of Nursing Research, 26*(2), 196–212.

Couvalis, G. (1997). *The philosophy of science.* Thousand Oaks: Sage.

Dzurec, L. C., & Abraham, I. L. (1993). The nature of inquiry: Linking quantitative and qualitative research. *Advances in Nursing Science, 16*(1), 73–79.

Freeman, J. (2004). Holistic healing modalities. In B. Kozier, G. Erb, A. Berman, et al. (Eds.), *Fundamentals of nursing: The nature of nursing practice in Canada.* Toronto: Prentice Hall.

Fryback, P. B., & Reinert, B. R. (1999). Spirituality and people with potentially fatal diagnoses. *Nursing Forum, 34*(1), 13–22.

George, L., Larson, D., Koenig, H., et al. (2000). Spirituality and health: What we know, what we need to know. *Journal of Social and Clinical Psychology, 19*(1), 102–116.

Kikuchi, J., & Simmons, H. (1994). *Developing a philosophy of nursing*. Newbury Park: Sage.

Kim, S. (1999). Critical reflective inquiry for knowledge development in nursing practice. *Journal of Advanced Nursing, 29*, 1205–1212.

Malinski, V. (2002). Developing a nursing perspective on spirituality and healing. *Nursing Science Quarterly, 15*(4), 281–287.

McSherry, W., & Ross, L. (2002). Dilemmas of spiritual assessment: Considerations for nursing practice. *Journal of Advanced Nursing, 38*(5), 479–488.

Milligan, S. (2004). Perceptions of spiritual care among nurses undertaking post registration education. *International Journal of Palliative Nursing, 10*(4), 162–171.

Munhall, P. (1993). "Unknowing": Toward another pattern of knowing in nursing. *Nursing Outlook, May/June*, 125–128.

Nelson, S. (1995). Humanism in nursing: The emergence of the light. *Nursing Inquiry, 2*(1), 36–43.

Olson, J., Paul, P., Douglass, L., et al. (2003). Addressing the spiritual dimension in Canadian undergraduate nursing education. *Canadian Journal of Nursing Research, 35*(3), 94–107.

Paterson, J., & Zderad, L. (1976). *Humanistic nursing*. New York: National League for Nursing.

Pesut, B. (2002). The development of nursing students' spirituality and spiritual care-giving. *Nurse Education Today, 22*, 128–135.

Price, J. L., Stevens, H. O., & LaBarre, M. C. (1995). Spiritual caregiving in nursing practice. *Journal of Psychosocial Nursing, 33*(12), 5–9.

Ross, L. (1997). The nurse's role in assessing and responding to patients' spiritual needs. *International Journal of Palliative Nursing, 3*(1), 37–42.

Sellers, S. C. (2001). The spiritual care meanings of adults residing in the midwest. *Nursing Science Quarterly, 14*, 239–248.

Sorell, T. (1991). *Scientism: Philosophy and the infatuation with science*. London: Routledge.

Taylor, J. E. (2003). Nurses caring for the spirit: Patients with cancer and family caregiver expectations. *Oncology Nursing Forum, 30*(4), 585–590.

Wilber, K. (1998). *The marriage of sense and soul*. New York: Random House.

Wojnar, D., & Malinski, V. (2003). Developing a nursing perspective on spirituality and healing: Questions and answers following a letter to the editor. *Nursing Science Quarterly, 16*(4), 297–300.

Wolfer, J. (1993). Aspects of "reality" and ways of knowing in nursing: In search of an integrating paradigm. *Image: Journal of Nursing Scholarship, 25*(2), 141–146.

Wright, M. C. (2002).The essence of spiritual care: A phenomenological enquiry. *Palliative Medicine, 16,* 125–132.

Critical Questions

As a way of engaging with the ideas in this chapter, consider the following:

1. What occurs to you when you think about future or emerging issues for the profession of nursing?

2. How, in your own life, have recollections of your history influenced your actions or understandings of the future?

CHAPTER
26

Carol McDonald
Marjorie McIntyre
Elizabeth Thomlinson

Professional, Practice, and Power Issues: Thinking Back, Looking Ahead

Used with permission from the photographer, Yvonne Oliver.

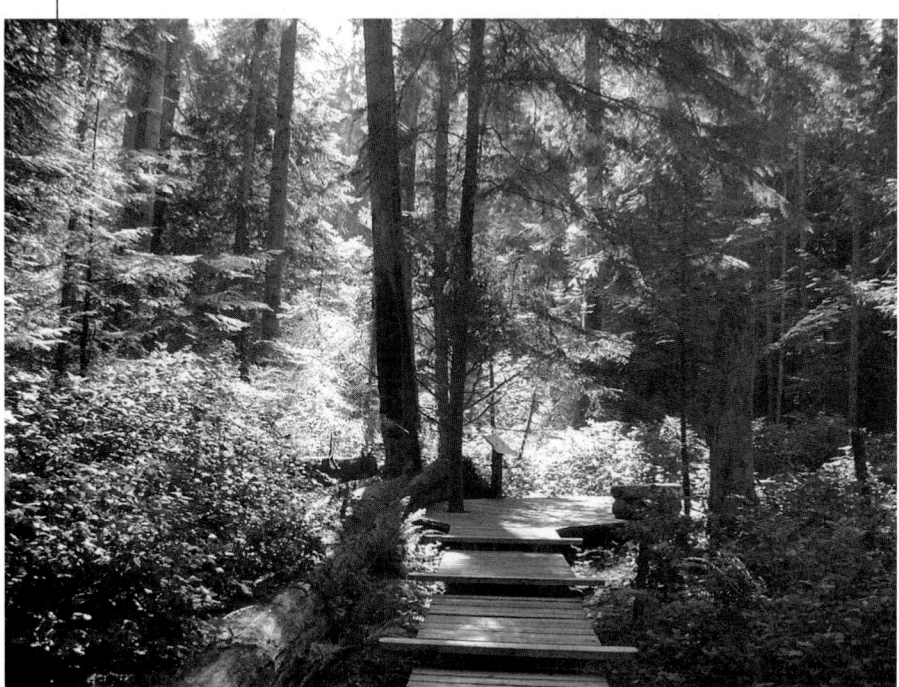

After completing this chapter, you will be able to:

1. Describe the way in which any account of history can be understood as a partial interpretation of historical realities.

2. Discuss trends that will have an impact on the future of nursing and health care.

3. Identify some of the issues on the horizon for the discipline of nursing.

ooking ahead to the issues that we anticipate, to the changes we await, to the trends we now observe coming to fruition, begins, perhaps surprisingly for us, with a look to the past. The very recent past includes the writing of the second edition of this text, and, in this chapter, we will revisit some of the emerging issues in nursing practice and health care. Beyond this, we will explore the idea of writing our nursing history anew as we face the future. With the knowledge and experience of our nursing history and our current circumstances in nursing education and professional practice, we would suggest that nurses are well positioned to engage with issues that will make a difference in our world.

■ RECLAIMING OUR PAST

The point is to write about and render historical what has hitherto been hidden from history.

Joan Scott, 1992

In Chapter 1, we launched this text with the notion of the influence of history on our current understandings: "An in-depth analysis of issues brings us the opportunity to reopen our nursing and health care history. This reopening is more than a return to the history that has been dominantly recorded; rather, it can be seen as an occasion to excavate the historical understandings that have been silenced, diminished, or erased" (p. 6). Although history has been variously addressed in the chapters of this text as well as in other nursing literature, what we are proposing is not only continued excavation but an excavation of depth and disruption, one that interrupts our assumptions and rethinks and reclaims our past. History, understood in this way, is more than what has been written in this and other texts; it includes what has not been written, what was overlooked or simply obscured in the dominant accounts of history. History understood differently opens us to the possibility that the past and the present could be otherwise—and necessarily changes our view of and our potentials for the future.

■ LOOKING TO THE FUTURE

Of the many frameworks to envisage the future, the framework introduced by Henchey, a Canadian futurist, highlights four imagined futures: a *possible future* that is unlikely to happen, a *plausible future* that could happen, a *probable future* that is likely to happen, and a *preferable future* that we prefer to happen (Roy, 2000; Ward-Murray, 2000).

▪ A *possible future* is one that might happen but for which the probability is very low. This is the kind of future that is difficult to imagine ever happening—even in one's wildest dreams. Such a future would have a real focus on health promotion and disease prevention and the funding support necessary to achieve change. In such a future, community members and politicians fully collaborate with educators and practitioners toward a common goal of health for all.

▪ A *plausible* future is one that could happen. It is one in which society and nursing evolve to include governments that work to protect the environment and thereby alter the health care needs of the world's residents. Development of a comprehensive home care system across Canada that permits citizens who wish to remain in their homes during periods of ill health and infirmity is a plausible future.

■ A *probable future* is one that is based on current trends and one that is likely to happen. If changes to modify or reverse current situations do not happen, today's realities are likely to be our future realities. Unless there are significant changes in the nutritional and exercise habits of Canadians, the increasing numbers of Canadians now developing diabetes will continue—and so will the concomitant effects on the health care system (Zinman, 1998).

■ A *preferable future* is one that is desirable, one that addresses the hopes and wishes of the profession and society. A preferable future is one in which nurses are autonomous, accountable decision makers with both the authority and resources needed to provide competent ethical care to patients and their families. Rogers (1997) suggests that an effective strategy to plan for the future is to develop future scenarios and work back from what has been envisioned. By stepping into the future, we are unencumbered by current and past "experiences, knowledge and the dominant values and beliefs in the sociocultural environment" (p. 32). Considering the possibilities for what each of these futures could hold provides a vision for the profession and a direction for future goals. By working through the scenarios one has envisioned, each with different consequences, one can make decisions and choices regarding the actions needed to bring about the preferred scenario. Nurses are well positioned to participate in cocreating a vision for health and health care for Canadians and members of the global community.

■ TRENDS AFFECTING THE FUTURE

According to Roy (2000), major trends will have an impact on health, health care delivery, and the nursing profession: These include the information explosion, changing demographics, changes in health care delivery systems, and the consumer movement. Throughout the previous chapters in this text, these trends have either been highlighted or interwoven into the various discussions. What follows are some issues that arise from, and must be analyzed and resolved within, each of these trends. It is important that readers consider a sixth trend that is having an effect on health and health care delivery: the global changes in trade, travel, disease patterns, and climate that are occurring at an ever-increasing pace.

The Information Age

The explosion of information technologies and systems has radically changed how interactions between and within governments and all other organizations, including the health care system, are conducted. Information that is now available regarding individuals and their health needs could be stored in microchips and electronic cards.

The issues of confidentiality, individual privacy, and the potential for abuse by employers and others who gain access to this information raise serious concern. The growth in telehealth and telemedicine—the transmission of imagery over the telephone that permits the treatment of illnesses within distant communities—will have an effect on northern and rural health care delivery (Lindeman, 2000). Lindeman suggests that this information expansion will result in the further growth of virtual universities and a need for ongoing education throughout one's working life. The availability of information through Internet technology has the potential either to provide misinformation or to educate the public regarding any subject possible. Are nurses prepared and actively developing credible information for responsible distribution? Are nurses analyzing what is currently available, or are nurses allowing others to decide what information will be available? In Chapter 14 of this book, Care and coauthors critically examine multiple issues related to the information age. Readers are encouraged to examine these issues and the implications for their own practice.

Changing Demographics

One of the many demographic changes influencing future directions is a population that is living longer. This phenomenon increases the chances that more health care services will be required to support this longevity. The health care professionals needed to provide such care are also aging faster than they can be replaced. Many concerns have been raised regarding whether there will be adequate numbers of health care providers in the future.

The aging of the populace has implications within Canada and other industrialized nations (Frean, 2002). Increasing numbers of people with chronic conditions could place great demand on the health care system, ultimately affecting how the system is structured. In nursing and other health and social science disciplines, there has been a deluge of research studies supporting the need for the health care system to shift its focus from illness care to health promotion and disease prevention. These studies and discussions have yet to influence changes in the health care system to the degree that is needed

Another demographic change is the ongoing shift in immigration to this country. Canada is continuing to receive more migrants from Asia and Africa than from European countries, as was common in the past. This results in diversity in the population that is not yet reflected in the student body, or in the faculty, of most nursing education settings. An issue that requires immediate attention is the preparation of nurses to work with people from many different cultures. In addition, adequately prepared interpreters are needed to assist health care professionals in the provision of culturally appropriate care.

A present and even greater future concern rests with the health of and health care delivery for aboriginal peoples. First, given the size of Canada's existing aboriginal population, the number of aboriginal students and graduate nurses reflects neither the number nor the nature of nurses needed to meet the complex needs of aboriginal people. Second, given the predicted increase in growth of First Nations communities, attention must be urgently given to attracting aboriginal students into nursing as they begin to graduate and enter the workforce (see Chapter 24). Coupled with the lack of aboriginal persons in nursing is the recognition that there are many health challenges faced by aboriginal peoples in Canada (Federal, Provincial and Territorial Advisory Committee on Population Health, 2000).

Another demographic change that will affect health care is a shift of population in much of rural Canada as more people move off farms to towns and large urban centers (Brethour, 2002; Rothwell et al., 2002). This migration means that alternative methods of health care delivery must be found for rural and remote regions of the country. Besides the changes brought on by geographic shifts of people requiring nursing care, there is also a widening gap between the wealthy and the poor throughout all of North America (Roy, 2000) as well as between the industrialized and agrarian-based nations around the globe. This disparity between the haves and the have-nots may ultimately lead to greater difficulties and disputes throughout the world. Nurses need to prepare to be active participants in this demographically changing world.

Changes to the Health Care Delivery System

Of the many changes to the health care delivery system since the 1990s, the alterations and closures of institutions, specifically hospitals, have affected access to health care by Canadians. Current terminology, such as *restructuring*, *rightsizing*, *downsizing*, and *regionalization*, emphasizes the ongoing structural and organizational changes in health care—both institutionally and nationwide. In Chapter 3, Storch discusses how important it is for nurses and other Canadians to understand the evolution and current state of Canada's health care delivery system as well as what drives it. Drawing on Coburn and Rappolt's analysis of the current state of the Canadian health care system, Storch helps us understand how the "logic of medicare," coupled with the "internationalization of capital," has led to the disempowerment of nursing and the enabling of globalized industry to manipulate health care. Storch encourages nurses to position themselves to be part of the change "by attending to the history, current status, and future projections for health care; by being listening and caring caregivers; and by taking action individually and collectively to influence greater attention to social determinants of health and better health care provision for their patients" (p. 51).

One outcome of the random restructuring of the Canadian health care system in the 1990s was that many nurses lost their jobs and new graduates could not find work. This resulted in decreased enrollments in nursing schools and a subsequent loss of nurses to the United States or from the profession altogether. Admissions to nursing schools and faculties in Canada had decreased from 12,170 in 1990 to 9,969 by 2002, while the Canadian population continued to grow (Advisory Committee on Health Human Resources, 2000; CASN, 2005). Governments have not acknowledged the drastic impact their restructuring exercises had on the exit of nurses and on the decreased numbers entering the profession. Time is now required to educate the numbers of nurses needed for the system. The actions of the Manitoba government and the attempt by the Saskatchewan government to decrease the educational requirements of nurses (see Chapter 11) are stopgap measures that will ultimately have a further negative impact on the profession.

The Consumer Movement

In Canada, an increasingly enlightened public is having an impact on health and health care delivery. Inspired by the vast amounts of information available on the Internet, in the press, and during public campaigns, the public is demanding changes in the delivery of, and access to, health care. Activists, such as those working with the Friends of Medicare, have mounted campaigns in Alberta against the privatization of the health care system and the dismantling of medicare (Friends of Medicare, 2002). These activists face formidable opposition from the insurance industry and some governments, which suggest that sweeping changes to the current system would enable public health care funding to be reduced and private for-profit health care to be introduced.

The need to inform patients fully regarding their health care options and the pros and cons of treatment has altered the manner in which many physicians provide information regarding risks, benefits, and options for treatment before the signing of treatment consent forms (see Chapter 20). In Chapter 18, Hardingham discusses issues related to informed consent, moral dilemmas, and legal concerns that are influencing both patients' and nurses' options and decisions about treatment.

Global Changes

Globalization and international trade agreements can affect the future of health care for Canadians. Large multinational companies are suing governments in Canada, Mexico, and the United States because of decisions that did not permit them to build industries that have the potential to pollute the countryside or to import and export potentially harmful chemicals. These companies claim these restrictions are illegal under the North American Free Trade Agreement (Knight, 2001). No one yet knows how these actions may affect the health and health care of ordinary citizens. Concerns have been raised that there is the opportunity through international trade agreements for private insurance and medical care companies from outside Canada to enter the Canadian health care arena.

Another global issue that will affect health, health care, and nursing is the displacement of populations that is occurring, particularly in Africa and Asia. The movement of vast numbers of immigrants and refugees, often propelled by natural disasters, such as the tsunami of December 26, 2004, and manmade disasters, such as famine and war, will create changes in every country in the world. In North Africa, the Sahara creeps ever farther south, spreading desert terrain and dislocating many other populations. Global warming has the potential to alter species' habitats to an extent that can only be imagined (Malcolm et al., 2002; see Chapter 22). The extent to which these habitats will shift, the spread of diseases and parasites to previously moderate and cold climates, and the changes in vegetation and weather patterns resulting from climate change are all unknown. How nurses can remain current in the midst of these ever-escalating changes will be another major issue.

■ POSSIBILITIES FOR RE-VISIONING THE FUTURE

In considering the issues on the horizon of nursing, we find ourselves asking the following questions: What is the potential for social justice in nursing? What would it mean to understand nursing practice as political activism? Is it realistic to locate the responsibility for political action with the individual nurse? How can we understand and address the tension between the expectations placed on nurses and the realities of discordant views and an absence of support from the institutions in which we are educated and practice? It is our suggestion that the answers to some of these complex questions lie in further understandings of our history, in our socialized practices as women and as nurses employed in hierarchical institutions such as hospitals, universities, and governments.

Some nursing analysts (Porter-O'Grady, 1998) have suggested that, as a group, nurses are reluctant to face issues head on and that we undermine the actions of others inside and outside the profession. An alternative viewpoint suggests that nurses as a group are neither passive nor inactive but that we have been socialized in particular ideologies of what it means to be a nurse and what it means to be a woman. Conservative ideologies have undermined the initiative of some women to act in direct, challenging, and powerful ways. The challenge is to disrupt discourses that promote and sustain powerlessness and to support one another in raising the profile and the esteem of the nursing profession.

Equally important is the inability to articulate fully the difference that nurses make to the health and health care of citizens. The study by Tourangeau and associates (2002) that found that having more registered nurses on a unit led to lower mortality (after 30 days) for acute care patients needs to be emphasized to both consumers and governments. The challenge will be to educate employers and society about what nursing practice includes and the value of attracting and keeping registered nurses in the system. In addition is the challenge of the attitudes demonstrated by governments and employers toward a profession that has remained largely female. In Chapter 19, McDonald claims, "Ideas about women and women's work and whether this work requires significant knowledge, responsibility, and skill contribute to the devaluing of nurses' work by society" (p. 335). She reminds us that to "challenge effectively what is taken for granted about the role of gender and its powerful influence on nurses' work, we must be willing to notice difference and to acknowledge the way that differences, such as gender, class, race, ethnicity, and sexual orientation, matter in the ways our identities are lived and viewed by the world" (p. 345).

One of the greatest challenges the profession faces is the current and projected nursing shortage. Not only are there shortages of nurses for specialty clinical areas and particular regions of the country as in the past but there are projected shortages that will affect all areas of health care. The Canadian Nurses Association (CNA) has highlighted an impending shortage of nurses who have the skills and knowledge to meet the health care needs of Canadians. According to Ryten's research study commissioned by the CNA, "Canada could face a shortage of up to 113,000 nurses by the year 2011 unless nursing, government and educators act now" (Sibbald, 1998, p. 22). This report further suggests that the "current pool is not renewing itself at a sufficient rate" (p. 23) and that, as currently practicing nurses retire and increasing numbers of nurses leave the country or leave the profession, the shortage in Canada could reach between 59,000 and 113,000 nurses within the next decade. An issue raised for Canada and other countries experiencing shortages is the "poaching" of nurses by the wealthier provinces and countries. A major issue created by a shortage of nurses is that we do not have enough nurses available to mentor, support, and be preceptors for nursing students and new graduates, including new faculty in nursing education programs.

Another challenge the profession faces is the need for leaders to speak out against future actions that can be detrimental to providing health care in this country. There is a dearth of nurse leaders who are prepared to pursue aggressively and generate changes required within the profession and society at large. In Chapter 16, McIntyre and McDonald note that "downsizing and restructuring have undermined existing leadership structures and the vision the CNA documents provide for nursing. Significantly, positions such as the chief nursing officer are being eroded. In some instances, they have disappeared altogether" (p. 294). This raises important questions about how we might look to our history and ask how we might reclaim our leaders for the profession. Increasingly, nurses in leadership positions have been co-opted through a business model in the heath care system to positions where, instead of being able to lead, mentor, and support nurses as they have in the past, nurse leaders find themselves in adversarial positions to practicing nurses as they carry out the employer and government expectations. It is not so much that we are suggesting that we return to a leadership style from the past but that we might reclaim from the past the mentorship, support, and leadership of nurses in their practice. It is important to point out that it is the nature of hierarchical, fiscally driven structures, whether in hospitals, public health units, home care agencies, universities, colleges, or government institutions, that contribute to the loss of nursing leadership that supports patient/client care. As important as the focus on fiscal responsibility is, what such a focus overlooks is the covert losses in patient care and the erosion of nursing leadership to the profession.

The acuity level and complexity of the conditions of patients in hospitals challenge the provision of care. The rapid turnover of patients, the availability of diagnostic and treatment modalities, and shortened hospital stays mean that the acuity level of patients in hospitals has risen significantly. Concomitantly, the level of illness of those being cared for in their homes, either by family members or home care nurses, is also much more acute. The impact this has on nursing practice has not been fully articulated.

The scope of practice for registered nurses will continue to evolve as an issue for the profession. Although the re-emerging nurse practitioner movement carries with it many unanswered questions and considerable tensions, the movement is undeniably an exciting and significant recognition of the contribution that nurses can make to Canadian health care. As we look to our past, the evolution of the nurse practitioner movement over the previous 4 decades has been far too often under the influence of government and medical authorities' needs and whims. The possibilities for the enormous contribution that nurse practitioners could make to the health of Canadians now rest in the hands of educators, regulators, and nurses. In this and other important issues for the profession, nurses have increasing opportunities to further both the discipline and relationships with other health care providers. In addition to the expanded scope of practice for nurse practitioners, the composition of nursing teams and scope of practice in care settings continue to evolve. In these practice teams, registered nurses with diplomas and baccalaureate and graduate degrees work collaboratively with licensed practical nurses, nurses' aides, and care attendants. Complex boundaries and negotiations for scope of practice and delegation of responsibilities are accompanied by the opportunity for leadership, mentorship, and professional collaboration.

These issues on the horizon, and those beyond our view, will shape the future of the nursing as a professional and a practice discipline. The ways in which we articulate, understand, and respond to these issues are open to the individual and collective interpretations of both the history and the future directions of the discipline. Our history, as it is known, has the capacity to tell us who we are. In another sense, our history as it is still emerging and becoming known, has great potential to inform our directions. A willingness to engage deeply with the salient issues of the discipline includes a critical interrogation of our historical and current realities—professional, practice, and power issues. It is, however, through political action in education, health care, and government arenas, and through the recognition of nursing practice as entwined with social justice, that we have the opportunity to make a difference.

References

Advisory Committee on Health Human Resources. (2000).The nursing strategy for Canada. Ottawa: Health Canada [Online]. Available: www.hc-sc.gc.ca/english/pdf/nursing.pdf

Brethour, P. (2002, May 16). Small farms fading away. *Globe and Mail*, p. A7.

Canadian Association of Schools of Nursing. (2005). The national student and faculty survey of Canadian schools of nursing. [Online]. Retrieved April 19, 2005, from http://www.causn.org/Databases/table_4_2002_2003.pdf

Coburn, D., & Rappolt, S. (1999). The "logic of medicare": Variants of capitalism and medical dominance. Contextualizing profession-state relationships. In D. Coburn, S. Rappolt, I. Bourgeault, et al. (Eds.), *Medicine, nursing and the state* (pp. 139–167). Aurora, Ontario: Garamond Press.

Federal, Provincial and Territorial Advisory Committee on Population Health. (2000). *Toward a healthy future: Second report on the health of Canadians*. Ottawa: Health Canada.

Frean, A. (2002, May 17). U.K. frets over plunging fertility rate. *Calgary Herald*, p. A27.

Friends of Medicare. (2002). Do you know what the Alberta government has in store for your health care system? [Online]. Available: www.keepmedicarepublic.ca

Knight, D. (2001). Lawsuits spark calls for changes in NAFTA. [Online]. *South-North Development Monitor*. Available: http://www.twnside.org.sg/title/spark-cn.htm

Lindeman, C. (2000). The future of nursing education. *Journal of Nursing Education, 39*(1), 5–12.

Malcolm, J. R., Liu, C., Miller, L. B., et al. (2002). *Habitats at risk: Global warming and species loss in globally significant terrestrial ecosystems.* Gland, Switzerland: World Wide Fund for Nature.

Porter-O' Grady, T. (1998). A glimpse over the horizon: Choosing our future. *Orthopaedic Nursing, 17*(2), S53–S61.

Rogers, M. (1997). *Canadian nursing in the year 2020: Five futures scenarios.* Ottawa: Canadian Nurses Association.

Rothwell, N., Bollman, R., Tremblay, J., et al. (2002). Migration to and from rural and small town Canada [Online]. *Rural and Small Town Canada Analysis Bulletin, 3*(6). (Catalogue no.21-006-XIE.) Ottawa: Statistics Canada. Available: http://www.statcan.ca

Roy, C. (2000). The visible and invisible fields that shape the future of the nursing care system. *Nursing Administration Quarterly, 25*(1), 119–131.

Sibbald, J. (1998). Special news report. The future supply of registered nurses in Canada: A new study commissioned by the Canadian Nurses Association urges immediate action to avert a shortage. *Canadian Nurse, 94*(1), 22–23.

Tourangeau, A., Giovannetti, P., Tu, J., et al. (2002). Nursing related determinants of 30-day mortality for hospitalized patients. *Canadian Journal of Nursing Research, 33*(4), 71–88.

Ward-Murray, E. M. (2000). Creating nursing's future: Issues, opportunities, and challenges. *Nursing and Health Care Perspectives, 21*(6), 305–306.

Zinman, B. (1998). Diabetes: The magnitude of the problem. *Proceedings from the National Forum on Diabetes* (pp. 5–16). Ottawa: Canadian Diabetes Association.

Taking Action: The Mighty Pen

T here are many ways of taking political action. One that has been used since time immemorial is writing letters; another is proposing resolutions. These pages feature sample letters to governmental officials, such as the minister of health, and sample resolutions, such as one submitted to the Canadian Nurses Association.

■ LETTERS TO PUBLIC OFFICIALS

Letter to the Minister of Health

_____

[Date]

The Honorable _____, P.C., M.P. Minister of Health
House of Commons Ottawa, Ontario K1A OA6

Dear Minister _____:

The registered nurses of [name your region] are concerned that if no action is taken today, many Canadians will soon be deprived of the quality health care to which they are entitled. This will happen because there will be too few qualified registered nurses to provide the care that is needed. Seventy-five percent of health care professionals are nurses. The stark reality is that Canada faces a severe shortage. [Add an example.] This is happening across Canada.

We are writing today to lend our support to the position advanced by the Canadian Nurses Association in its presentation to the House of Commons Standing Committee on Finance. Their brief "The Quiet Crisis in Health Care" outlines a proposal that could greatly alleviate the looming crisis.

My colleagues and I would like to meet with you at the earliest opportunity to discuss our proposal. I will contact your office to set up a meeting.

Sincerely,

_____

[Signature]

Alternative Letter to the Minister of Health

[Date]

The Honorable _____, P.C., M.P. Minister of Health
House of Commons Ottawa, Ontario K1A OA6

Dear Minister _____:

I would like to bring to your attention a problem that has been largely ignored by politicians, but one that Canadians will soon be facing if no measures are taken.

Seventy-five percent of health care professionals are nurses. The reality is that Canada faces a severe shortage of registered nurses with the knowledge and skills to meet the future needs of Canadians. Nurses across the country are using the term a *quiet crisis* to emphasize not only the gravity of this situation but also the fact that this problem has gone largely unrecognized.

The good news is that there is time to act, and the nurses of Canada have put together a proposal that we believe will largely alleviate the problem.

We believe the federal government should invest in the following three key areas:

- nursing recruitment and retention
- nursing research that improves patient care and quality of life
- the dissemination and uptake of evidence to provide the best patient care

Should you wish further information on the nursing proposal, please call me or contact the Canadian Nurses Association at 1-800-361-8404.

Sincerely,

[Signature]

Adapted from Canadian Nurses Association (1998). *The Quiet Crisis in Health Care*. Lobby Kit.

Letter to a Member of Parliament

_____

[Date]

[Name]
[Address]

Dear Member of Parliament _____:

Last September, the Canadian Nurses Association (CNA) presented startling evidence to the House of Commons. The CNA testified that the costs of restructuring have been high, both for nurses and for their patients. The Standing Committee on Finance heard that the nursing profession is seriously affected by the increased casualization of the workforce, whereby approximately 25% of nurses are now working for multiple employers.

I am one of those nurses.

[You might want to personalize this part by explaining how this is impacting patient care. Here is an example of what you could write:]

I hold jobs for as many as three agencies at one time. In any week, I see patients in one location one day and in another the next. As challenging as this is for me, the impact of continuity of care is enormous. I am not able to conduct comprehensive assessments and to adequately implement a plan of care that involves all of the patients' needs. This is not enough time to provide the care these people deserve. The focus of my activity each day is not on the patients whom I should be caring for but rather on constantly reorienting myself to the physical facility and how to work in this particular unit. How would you like to have a nurse care for you who does not know how to get emergency help when required?

As such, many experienced nurses are leaving the profession and many new graduates have left Canada, Those who remain, like me, are demoralized, which is why I would like to add my voice to the growing number of Canadian nurses asking that the next federal budget takes into account a nursing investment.

Sincerely,

_____

[Signature]

_____

Adapted from Canadian Nurses Association (1998). _The Quiet Crisis in Health Care_. Lobby Kit.

■ LETTERS TO THE EDITOR AND OTHER MEDIA AUTHORITIES

Write a letter to the editor of a newspaper or journal outlining an issue for the purpose of moving that particular issue toward resolution. If a meeting is planned with a local politician, include a news release to the local media to highlight the activities initiated for resolving an issue.

_____

[Date]

[Editor's Name]
[Name of Newspaper, Magazine, or Journal]
[Address]

Dear Editor:

I would like to draw your attention to a serious problem. Amid Canadians' increasing alarm over the quality of the health care system, the impending shortage of registered nurses has gone largely unnoticed by governments.

Seventy-five percent of health care professionals are registered nurses, and the stark reality is that Canada is facing a serious shortage. Already in our communities the shortage is negatively affecting patient care. Canadians will soon be deprived of the care they require because there will be too few qualified nurses to provide it.

Federal politicians have been saying that the next federal budget will be a health budget. The nurses of Canada are saying the next budget needs to include an investment in quality nursing care.

Sincerely,

_____

[Signature]

_____

Adapted from Canadian Nurses Association (1998). *The Quiet Crisis in Health Care*. Lobby Kit.

■ RESOLUTIONS SUBMITTED TO AN ASSOCIATION

A resolution submitted to the Canadian Nurses Association at the June 1998 Annual Meeting follows:

Resolution 5   Prescription Drugs

WHEREAS, Pharmaceuticals have an important role to play in preventing illness, promoting and maintaining health, assisting with diagnosis, controlling pain and suffering and improving quality of life;

WHEREAS, The role of pharmaceuticals in the health care system is becoming increasingly important;

WHEREAS, Between 1975 and 1994, expenditures per person (adjusted for inflation) on drugs have more than doubled—increasing from $108 to $232;

WHEREAS, For the same time period, drug expenditures as a percentage of total health spending rose from 8.7% to 12.7%;

WHEREAS, Public spending on prescription drugs pays for less than half of their cost (45%);

WHEREAS, Most provinces provide prescription drug plans for seniors and welfare recipients;

WHEREAS, Four provinces provide some coverage to all residents. However none provide first dollar coverage. The drug plans of British Columbia, Saskatchewan, Manitoba and Quebec include co-payments and/or deductibles;

WHEREAS, Twelve percent of Canadians have no insurance coverage for drugs;

WHEREAS, The National Forum on Health has recommended that the Canadian federal/provincial health insurance system move toward integration of prescription drugs as a fully funded component of publicly funded health care;

WHEREAS, Health Canada and Saskatchewan Health sponsored an invitational conference on National Approaches to Pharmacare in Saskatoon (January 1998) that examined the related issues;

WHEREAS, One of CNA's corporate objectives is to act in the public interest for Canadian nursing and nurses, providing national and international leadership in nursing and health issues;

BE IT RESOLVED THAT Promoting and facilitating the realization of the recommendation of the National Forum on Health with respect to integration of prescription drugs as a fully-funded component of publicly funded health care be designated as a priority of CNA for the next three years.

Source: Directions for a Pharmaceutical Policy in Canada. *A report prepared for the National Forum on Health, 1997. Submitted by the Manitoba Association of Registered Nurses.*

Index

Note: Page numbers followed by f, t, and b indicate figures, tables and boxed text, respectively.